Sustainable Tea Plantation Management

G.D. Banerjee
BA (Hons), MA (Eco), LLB, Pragya (Hindi)
Deputy General Manager,
Production Credit Department,
National Bank for Agriculture and Rural Development,
Plot No. C-24, G- Block,
Bandra-Kurla Complex,
Post Box No.8121, Bandra (E), Mumbai-400051, Maharashtra

Sarda Banerjee
BA (Eco), MA (Eco), BEd
Freelance Columnist
A2/42, Nabard Nagar, Thakur Complex,
Kandivili(e), Mumbai-400101, Maharashtra

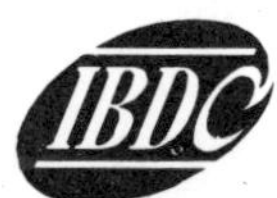

International Book Distributing Co.
(Publishing Division)

Published by

INTERNATIONAL BOOK DISTRIBUTING CO.
(Publishing Division)
Khushnuma Complex Basement
7, Meerabai Marg (Behind Jawahar Bhawan)
Lucknow 226 001 U.P. (INDIA)
Tel. : 91-522-2209542, 2209543, 2209544, 2209545
Fax : 0522-4045308
E-Mail : ibdco@airtelbroadband.in

First Edition 2008

ISBN 81-8189-148-1

© Smt Shikha Banerjee
All Rights Reserved

No part of this publication may be reproduced, stored in a retrieval system, or transmitted, in any form or by any means, electronic, mechanical, photocopying, recording or otherwise, without the prior written permission of the publisher.

Composed & Designed at :
Panacea Computers
3rd Floor, Agrawal Sabha Bhawan
Subhash Mohal, Sadar Cantt. Lucknow-226 002
Phone : 2483312, 9452295008, 9335927082
E-mail : prasgupt@rediffmail.com

Printed at:
Salasar Imaging Systems
C-7/5, Lawrence Road Industrial Area
Delhi - 110 035
Tel. : 011-27185653, 9810064311

Dedicated to Bhagaban Sri Rama Krishna,
Rama Krishna Mission and Math, Belur Math, Howrah,
India and The Holy Mother Sarada Devi,
Rama Krishna Mission & Sarada Pith,
Belur Math, Howrah, India

Basudev Banerjee
IAS
Chairman, Tea Board,India

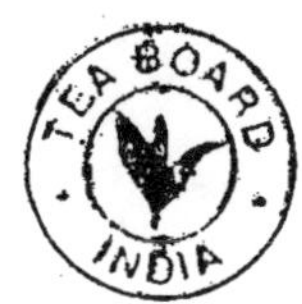

14, B.T.M. Sarani (Brabourne Road),
Kolkata - 700 001
E-mail: tboardcp@cal3.vsnl.net.in

Foreword

The Tea industry provides the largest formal employment in the country. Of the total work force approximately half are women. Women are mostly engaged in plucking tea leaves. They are also employed in other field operations like weeding, irrigation, pruning etc. The tea farming community consists of mostly tribal, scheduled caste and other backward classes. Tea is the common man's beverage. Tea plantations are placed both under agriculture and industry classification. It is an industry in the sense that tea is a processed and manufactured commodity. It is an agricultural crop and is grown on land.

This book on "Sustainable Tea Plantation Management" covers an over view of the tea industry. The Indian tea brief dwells on tea farming, manufacturing, geographical location, distribution of estates by size group and age, extent of new planting, modes of disposal of crop, exports of bulk teas and value added items.

I am sure, the present publication will be useful not only to the academicians and researchers but also to the students, tea companies, tea associations and those involved in tea trade etc. in various capacities.

Basudeb Banerjee
Chairman, Tea Board India

PREFACE

The treaty on "**Sustainable Tea Plantation Management**" consists of 16 Chapters. **Chapter I** outlines an overview of tea industry, which covers farming and manufacturing; geographical locations (tea regions of North and South India), area, production and yield according to revenue zones and size of estates. All estates were divided in to several size- classes in terms of area under tea and production to understand overtime changes in the nature of concentration. The Lorenz curve for six different years; 1957, 1971, 1982, 1995 and 2004 are indicative of the fact that there exists substantial inequality in distribution of area and production among tea estates in North and South India throughout the period. Age group of bushes, extension, replacement and replanting; disposal of tea through various auction centers and export under forward contact and ex-garden sale; export and product diversification and export market, major imposts (cess, excise duty and rebate) on type of tea and labour deployment in field and factory, as also productivity and labour per hectare have been analyzed. Besides, wage employment relationship (labour employed, money wages, real wages, wage cost, productivity of labour and profit after tax as per centage to net worth), implementation of various developmental schemes, important decisions taken up by the respective appropriate agencies to strengthen development of tea industry and action points for further accelerating the tempo of growth of the industry in Nagaland, Orissa , Purulia, Uttaranchal Hill have presented in this chapter. Further, the roles of development banks, issues of small growers with polity prescriptions have been reviewed, identified and documented.

Chapter 2 deals with sustainable tea cultivation that by definition is a method of growing green tea leaves and processing the same for greater human consumption through maximum utilization of all available resources without polluting environment. The wide vistas opened up the exim scripts and competitiveness, which presented opportunities and challenges. Indian tea industry pronounced policy shift from the hitherto conservative "residual approach" to one envisaging "production of exports". The pace of production growth needs to be sustained by consistent and adequate level of resource generation. This is currently difficult under the prevailing taxation structure. The main plank of progress would be perceived in terms of business, trade, and economy / society. There is no denying that investment would tend to flow more readily to areas that afford it a safe labour and attractive returns. Much against its gain and certainly at variance with the major task - that of tea production - the tea industry is being called upon to assure rates that are best left to government. Owing to its aging asset profile and predominance of its agro-based operations, asset valuations, capitalization and securities of tea companies have been typically based on historical and written down values distorting the under valuing the industry's resource raising potential. Updating asset values will greatly facilitate the process of modernization and expansion of tea industry. This chapter briefly asses yhe impact of new planting in attainment of sustainability. New plantings increase area, yield, exports, prices . Grabbing of sizable area by the migrants and local encroacher, techno-institutional subjects, utilization of improper man power, faulty planning of lay out, optimum exploitation of capital inputs, role of rejuvenation pruning/deep rooted grasses as rehabilitation crops/green crops in young and heavy pruned areas have bearing on low yield in tea in replanted area.

Chapter 3 entails management of natural resources for sustainable livelihood in tea plantation workers. To fulfill the above objective, attempt has been made to dovetail the role of soil conservation tillage together with tea bushes and mulching and shade trees, weed control, non conventional sources of energy like solar energy, briquettes of organic resides, tree plantation (firewood and other bio-mass) and human energy. Role of perfect plucking such as good plucking, several flushes, tipping (timely and regularly), frame forming and re-centering, tips of plucking, productivity of plucker and reduction in plucking cost, good culture practices, plucking management, suitable drainage etc., planting of tea leaf in water and soil environment, spacing of tea based on depth of drains, ground water table and surface runoff have been spelt out in this chapter. Application for sustainable tea plantation management necessarily confines foliar fertilizer, and point injector fertilizer and avoidance of sickness, amalgamation of sick units with healthier units, improvement in tea prices, reduction in costs and proper management are the answesr of sustainable livelihood of tea plantation.

Chapter 4 encompasses competitiveness economy and ever changing environment. The quality and performance of tea management determines both the survival and success of any enterprises. The Indian tea industry has built up a crop, which in number and quality far exceeds that of any other producing country. "Tea plant that has been brought to light will be found capable, under last century's was 20th. It is 19 th or 20th management of being cultivated with complete success for commercial purpose". In this chapter attention has been drawn to the reader on (i) stages of tea development, (ii) management as social process, (iii) middle class temperament of tea management, (iv) tea management's performance and productivity, (v) model building, (vi) production planning and (vii) productivity of labour and productivity of tea estates. All these are required for sound and detailed programming for each and every item of work. Plucking and labour deployment of plucking, correlation between plucking round and requirement of labour plucking and plucking productivity, role of management in plucking productivity (plucking strategy), cost effective strategies, have been explored. Cost and quality control through introduction of improved methods of management (maintenance of reasonable productivity and quality of tea and enhancement of higher productivity and quality of tea at lowest possible cost), ensuring better financial management (generation of own cash to meet financial obligation, working on the principle of sound finance, credit worthiness), assuring financial planning - short term and long term, and extending coordination have been examined.

Chapter 5 concentrates on various issues that have relevance in sustainable development of tea industry. These issues are covered mainly in national perspectives. These are collected from various journals, mainly, the Assam Review and Tea News, TAI News Letter, Chakibat, Tea Chronicle, National dailies, Kurukshetriya, Agriculture Today, Kishan World etc and put in place in this chapter with a view to keep the reader abreast the recent developments that have been taking place in the tea sector.

Chapter 6 includes some aspects of green tea. It covers the method of processing, and type of manufacturing. Under the type of manufacture, Japanese technology like Steaming, Cooling, Rolling/Drying, Rotary Drying, Twisting and Final drying has been discussed. Similarly, under Chinese Technology various procedures viz., Primary Planning, Rolling, Rotary Planning, Final Panning has been dwelt upon. Soviet Technology which is another area has also been forecast in this chapter along with Indian Practices. Production of green tea in India during 1961 to 2005 along with world production and exports of green tea have been analysized in order to assest the share of green tea to total exports. Moreover nutritional and medicinal values of green tea have been explore.

Chapter 7 defines sustainable tea plantation management, explores scope for intervention in such management, maintain natural resources and improve property on sustainable basis, identify natural factors and their contribution in tea production and suggest indicators of sustainable plantation management. In the process, field management with particular focus on land preparation, transplantation and cultural practices, pruning young infills, manuring, pest and diseases, soil-water-nutrient management, organic matter management, soil conservation, human resource management, crisis management, environmental hygiene and sanitation have been evaluated. This chapter depicts the most important areas of concern for tea industry. These are management of cost of production, productivity of land and labour management, employer-employee relation, training, safety of workers, monitoring and control of processing variables in tea manufacture.

Chapter 8 makes an attempt to assess the thrust areas/critical eyes of tea industry. These require special attention of the governments (Central & State), tea associations, tea board, research bodies etc. Some of these are innovation in tea bushes, organic cultivation of tea, violation of pesticide and residual limits, lack of planning premises while planning for business, action plan, stand on own instead of taking a crunch, close interaction between industry and research institutes, multiplicity of forms and returns, Tea and Control/ Coordination, now quality matter, reminding the commitments etc..

Chapter 9 incorporates the marketing channel of tea which covers marketing system of tea, modes of disposal, seven marketing modes (direct consignment to London auction, direct sale by forword contract to overseas buyers, consignment to London auctions, direct factory sale to Indian buyers, direct marketing of loose tea in wholesale market and self packeting and export to packet overseas) etc. Besides, primary marketing of tea, development of auction markets in the world, auction facilities, auction system, advantages of auction sale, ex-garden sale, min auction etc. have been placed in this chapter. To strengthen the auction system, Tea Board formed a committee headed by S S Ahuja, the then Deputy Chairman, Tea Board to "study the existing rules of all the public tea auction Centers in India and suggest changes where, necessary to bring improvement in the auction system". The committee on auction rules also known as Ahuja Committee submitted its final report. The committee identified eleven areas like (i) auction day (ii) catalogues, (iii) promt date, (iv) brokers commission, (v) size of lots, (vi) division of lots, (vii) withdrawal of lots, (viii) sale of outlets, (ix) warehouses rent and insurances, (x) closing catalogue and (xi) distribution of sample. The Ahuja committee submitted four interim reports and a final report, the recommendations of which were accepted by the Chairman of the Tea Board.

Chapter 10 throws light on thrust areas of tea industry. These are being debated by the scholars, planters, tea associations, policy makers, traders, research institutes and others involved in tea trade and industry. Some of the thrust areas include deployment of child labour, destruction of tea waste, simplification and rationalization of sale tax, pesticide residue in tea, land for extension, incentive under section 80 HHC, export incentive, land for extension, depreciation of tea bushes, infrastructure, revamping tea industry, variation of tax rates at the auction centres, incidence of tax, fiscal reforms etc.

Chapter 11 describes the role of research bodies in sustainable development of tea industry. Direction of R & D in Tea, technological innovations of Tea Research Association (TRA), fruits of R & D activities, research policies of TOCKLAI, TRA & CSIR Round Table Conference, formation of Indian Institute of Plantation Management (IIPM), Tea Research Institute of United Planters' Association of Southern India (UPASI), ICAR projects - UPASI Krishi Vigyan Kendra (KVK), Tea Board - Research Institute, and National Tea Research Foundation have been revisited.

Chapter 12 highlights issues relating to sustainable development of tea industry in international perspective. German tea importers were satisfied with the corrective measures adopted by India Tea growers to control application of pesticides and phasing out of child labour. The remarkable growth in demand for liquid tea in Japan, pitching for a common tea market among SAARC countries with arrangement for collective marketing in international markets, chalking out a two-prolonged strategy to retain the single largest market for plantation companies in the Commonwealth of Independent States (CIS), uninterrupted supply of wide range of tea (by India to Britain) with requirement of quality conscious market, growth of black tea market in Japan, new packaging regulation in Japan have been narrated. This chapter further illustrates Indo-CIS trade in tea, minimum residual level of checks, tea in European countries, trade protocol between Indian and Russian Federations of Coffee and Tea, Symposium in Vienna and Austria, tea in UK, privatization of Sri Lanka tea, first world tea festival in Russia, publicity of Indian Tea in Russia, tea exports to Egypt, tea becoming favorite beverage in China, tea in Italy gaining popularity, trade fair in Germany etc.

Chapter 13 documents the health aspects of tea. The first and second UK tea convention held in 1990 and 1993 respectively claimed that tea is the whole some healthy beverage which is rich in vitamins and minerals. The most important message of the UK Tea Convention was that tea should be promoted as healthy drink. The convention emerged research evidence on health benefits of tea consumption. The United States Tea Association scientifically documented the traditionally held belief that tea is good for health. It has the therapeutic value and aids digestion and body's fluid balance. It has some action on atheroscierosis. The research findings on health aspects of tea includes (i) anti inflammatory action, (ii) antimutagenic and carcinogenic effects of tea, (iii) reduction of lung neoplasia, (iv) antitumor activity, (v) blocking of endogenous nitrosamine, (vi) inhibition of heptocarcino genesis induced by a flatoxin, (vii) tea catechins and cardiovascular conditions. Further, Tea Trade Health Research Association (TTHRA) was created to manage and administer a joint research effort between the Tea Council of the USA, the Tea Council of Canada and the UK Tea Packer Association to further scientific knowledge about the human health benefits of tea. The focus is specially directed to the black tea and its role in preventing/inhibiting the formation cardiovascular diseases and certain forms of cancer. Dr Chung of the American Health Foundation studied the effect of tea on lung and tiver carcino genesis. Dr. C S Yang of Rutgers conducted a study entitled "Effect of Black Tea and Green tea on spontaneous Tumorigenesis in A/J Mice". Dr Young investigated spontaneous cancers. Besides tea has weight reducing and anti sunscreen properties. It is a time-honoured health giving beverage.

Chapter 14 makes a comparative study between India ad world with reference to some growth variables like area, production, and exports over a period of 46 years commencing from 1958 to 2004. Further world imports, world tea prices realized at different auction centers remedial measures to restrict fall in tea prices at the auctions, export promotion measures, international tea convention and FAO meet have been assessed with data base. In the process, Indian tea scene has been discussed with due weightage to production, export, direction of exports, marketing, product diversification, internal consumption, taxes and duties and import duty.

Chapter 15 envisages strategies for international tea marketing/tea trade and tea promotion. Marketing of any product along with other three essential P's namely product improvement, pricing and packaging is essential condition for promotion. Even for a primary commodity like of tea promotion is important in sustaining long-term demand. Efforts to promote Indian tea abroad were started in 1894 when Industry started promotional campaigns in US, Germany, Italy etc. Organized internal exercises to promote tea as beverage did not start until prolonged depression in tea prices brought the tea producing countries together and made them realize that a joint action was necessary for their survival. The formation of Indian Tea Marketing Expansion Board (ITMEB) in 1935 and establishment of Institutional arrangements called the Tea Council came into being in eight countries. The task of the generic promotion to protect the beverage tea from the onslaught of other competing beverage was organized. Subsequently, generic promotion programme was launched. The roles of FAO, GATT, UNCTD and ITPA (International Tea Promotion Association) were encouraging and they established a working group on long-term measure with the following terms of conditions -

- To make recommendations concerning the need and justification for long term action
- To consider long term internal cooperation to achieve prices that are equitable to the consume, remunerative to producers and capable of ensuring satisfactory level of export earnings for exporting countries vis-a-vis their government for consideration. The group submitted the report. The recommendations have been discussed and some of these have been implemented.

Chapter 16 illuminates the objectives of Indian International Millennium Tea Convention held in New Delhi in 2000. The convention concentrated on (i) review of tea industry scenario (ii) establishment of health credentials of tea and (iii) revisit of the emerging marketing concepts that could draw on health aspects of tea and help repositioning it as a beverage of the new millennium. The experts from various tea producing countries presented papers. The Chairman of Consultative Committee Plantation Association, Shri R S Jhawar welcomed the delegates and Shri Murasoli Maran, the then Minister of Commerce and Industry addressed the convention. The major recommendations have been presented in the chapter.

The authors are grateful to Prof Emeritus Amiya Kanti Gupta, Department of Economics and Politics, Visva Bharati Cenral University, Santiniketan for going through the manuscript and providing valuable suggestions to enrich the book. His continuous guidance, inspiration and help have enabled the authors possible to complete the journey of writing this book. The authors are indebted to their father/grand father Dr. Indranarayana Banerjee and mother/grand mother Chhayarani Banerjee for their moral support in this venture. The best tribute could have been paid to them if the publication was brought out during their life time. Let their blessing shower on the authors from the heavenly abode. Thanks are due to Srimati Shika Banerjee, wife/mother and Srijeet Banerji son/brother respectively for assisting in many ways in publication of the treaty. The authors are obliged to M/s. Interrnational Book Distributing company, lucknow, Uttar Pradesh. India and their staff members for taking trouble in printing the book. The authors are sure the present publication will be useful to the academicians, researchers, students, planners, policy makers, tea companies and those involving in tea manufacturing and trade. Last but not the least the authors are highly indebted to those who directly and indirectly helped in publication of the book.

G.D. Banerjee
Sarda Banerjee

CONTENTS

List of Tables

List of Tables As per Appendix

Tables As Per Annexure

Chapter 1

Tea Industry in India - An Overview

Tea occupies an important position in the national and world economy today. Indian tea occupifies one-fourth of total world area under tea and a little less than one-third of the total production and export. It earns foreign exchange and provides direct and indirect employment to a large number of population. In view of this, it is very worth-while to have an overview of the industry covering the structure of tea industry. This it helps in better understanding of the total setting or frame-work within which it functions. This total setting is provided by a whole complex of features which are characteristic to the industry. There are eight some-what broad heads which furnish the setting of the industry. These are (i) farming and manufacturing (ii) geographical location, area, production, yield, size etc. (iii) marketing (iv) export (v) internal consumption (vi) major imposts (vii) labour and (viii) finance.

1. Farming and Manufacturing

It starts from preparation of "seedbed" to packing of tea. Seedlings are grown in the nursery generally for one to two years and are transplanted in the field. The transplantation of the young tea plants require levelling and deep hoeing of the shade tree. Proper growth of tea plants demands planting of shade tree, application of manures and fertilisers in required doses, maintenance of good drainage, control of pest attacks and plant diseases. Besides, pruning and plucking are essential operations for inducing vegetative growth and ensuring continuous supply of "green flushes" as well as improving quality of manufactured tea.

Withering : The plucked green leaves are spread out in racks made of wire mesh or hession cloth arranged in withered sheds. They are kept for a period of 18 hours for a good 'wither'. During this period they lose a good deal of moisture and become placid for rolling which breaks down the leaf cells and releases the juice and enzymes contained in them. The withered leaves are fed into the rolling machine which twists the leaves and breaks the leaf cells. As a consequence the leaf juice oozes out and becomes subject to the action of atmosphere. A process of oxidation (called fermentation) begins to change colour and release its characteristic aroma. The degree of rolling required will depend on the condition of the wither and requirements of manufacture.

Rolling and Fermenting : The rolled leaf leaves the roller in the shape of twisted ball and is placed under roll-breakers. The rolled leaf finally obtained from roll-breaker is taken to the fermenting room of the floor which may be either tiled or cemented or platforms. The atmosphere of the fermenting room is kept cool and humid, sometimes with the help of wet screens or suitable water sprays. Fermentation is a process of oxidation during which the rolled leaf undergoes certain chemical changes. The time taken for fermentation, which depends on various factors, may vary from 20 minutes to 60 minutes.

Drying : Having received the desired degree of fermentation, the fermented leaves are removed to the driers. The drier consisting of large enclosed chamber has moving trays inside it where the fermented leaves are put. Hot air from the drier enters into the chamber and the moving trays travel in this hot air and get the necessary degree of descication. The nature of drying and intensity of heat will affect the quality of tea. The adjustment of temperature and the speed of machine requires expertise and experience.

Grading and Packing : The manufactured tea which comes out of the driers is then sorted and graded with the help of sooting machines which are mechanically vibrated sieves or tables. This helps in sifting tea and separating them into particulars of different sizes. The larger particulars are often cut into smaller bits with the help of cutting machines before grading. The grading of tea only refers to size of the processed leaf and not to its quality or flavour. The two main classifications in grading are leaf grade and broken grade. Broken grades include small particulars resulting from the sifting or sorting of tea and the leaf grade consists of larger particles left after broken grades are removed. The important leaf grade are orange pekoe, pekoe etc. and the important leaf grades are broken orange pekoe, pekoe, fanning, dust etc. After tea is sorted and graded, it is packed for despatch. The container almost in universal use for packing tea is plywood tea chest with an aluminium foil lining.

2. Geographical Locations, etc.

In India, tea growing regions are located in monsoon belt - Assam, West Bengal and the foothills of the Himalayas in the North and the moist slopes and the plateus of the Western Ghats in the South. The climate and the soil of these widely separated locations exhibit wide variations, the impact of which is naturally noticed in wide difference in productivity and cultural practices.

Tea Region in North- East India : The tea districts of North-East India take the shape of a triangle, the apex of which is Sadiya in Assam. They could be spelt into five districts/regions viz. (i) Assam Valley (ii) The Surma valley or Cachar (iii) Darjeeling (iv) Dooars and Terai and (v) Tripura. Although Assam Valley is covered by high mountains, almost the entire area is a level plain. Conditions are ideal for tea plantation especially towards the east of the valley. In the Surma valley, the tea areas of Cachar are covered with small hillocks or tillahs interspersed with low-lying bits of flat land which are often waterlogged. Tillahs and beels where they have been drained, carry the tea in Cachar. The climatic conditions here are less favourable compared to Assam Valley. Tripura, geographically, is more or less a continuation of the Surma valley but climatic conditions are probably more difficult due to droughts. The Darjeeling tea area is a hilly district. The Dooars and Terai form a long narrow strip adjacent Himalayas interspersted by a number of hill streams which during monsoons often inundate the area causing serious damages and interruptions to communications. Besides these main tea areas of North-East India, the other areas of tea cultivation in

Northern India are Ranchi, Dehradoon and Kangra valley the three widely separated regions. The Ranchi gardens are situated on Chhotanagpur plateau about 2000 ft above the sea level. The soils are regarded as poor. The Dehradoon tea plantations are situated in the valley between Himalayas and Sivalik hills. Here the soils resemble that of Assam tea areas. The Kangra valley tea gardens are very weak. The valley lies in the foothills of Himalayas in the Punjab. The climate is said to be too cold and the rainfall unevenly distributed for successful tea growth. Recently, non-traditional areas like Arunachal, Mizoram, Meghalaya, Manipur, Orissa and some parts of Kerala and Karnataka have been explored for tea cultivation.

Tea Regions in South India : The tea districts in South India are located in the hills and slopes of Western Ghats. The Nilgiri hills situated in the north of Palghat is an important tea area. The Nilgiri-Wynaad and Malabar-Wynaad tea districts which are situated on the strip between Nilgiris and the Malabar coast at an average elevation of 3000 ft south of the Palghat lie in Annamalai and cardamen hills. On the slopes of Annamalai hills lies the Annamalai tea district. The Kanandevan is situated in the hills of Travancore–Cochin at an elevation of about 5000 ft. In south Travancore, the tea districts are located at an altitude averaging 3000 ft. In the Nilgiri hills of Tamil Nadu and Western Ghats of Kerala the rainfall ranges between 2000 mm and 3000 mm with a similar dry spell. Warmth, the second essential pre-requisite, favours the Southern tea region and induces luxuriant growth of flushes resulting in high volume of yields. The hill slopes in South India have deep and rich forest loam well suited to tea. South Indian tea soils have lower humus content than North and thus require more fertiliser inputs. Two varieties of tea leaf are mainly grown in India - the China and the Assam. The former is a tall bush having soft leaf and is mostly grown in Darjeeling district. The latter is a shorter bush with coarse leaf. It does not have flavour and is liked mainly for liquor. The Assam tea is grown in the plains of Assam and in South Indian plantations. Number of tea estates, area owned and crop produced and yield per kg by district and states 1951 to 2005 have been in corpotrated in Tables 1 to 8.

Area, Production and Yield of Tea : Tea is mainly produced in Assam, West Bengal, Tamil Nadu and Kerala. It is also produced to a small extent in Tripura, Karnataka, Himachal Pradesh and Uttar Pradesh. At present tea is cultivated on an experimental basis in the states of Manipur, Sikkim, Orissa and Arunachal Pradesh. The state-wise distribution of tea under tea production and yield is given in Table 1.1.

Total area under tea stood at 331 thousand hectares, of which North India constituted 77.6 per cent and South India 22.4 per cent in 1961. Among tea growing states in North India, Assam accounted for 48.9 per cent followed by West Bengal 25.1 per cent and other states 3.6 per cent. Similarly, among tea regions of South India, Kerala formed 11.8 per cent followed by Tamil Nadu 10 per cent and Karnataka 0.60 per cent. As regards production, as much as 354 million kg was recorded in the year 1961 out of which North India produced 77.1 per cent and South India 22.9 per cent. State-wise data showed that Assam constituted the lions share to the extent of 51.4 per cent followed by West Bengal 24.3 per cent and "other states" 1.4 per cent. Tamil Nadu and Kerala produced 10.9 per cent each of total production followed by Karnataka 1.1 per cent. Yield per hectare worked out to 1070 kgs for India as a whole, while it was 1064 kgs for North India and 1091 kgs for South India. Among the various states of North India, yield rate of Assam–tea–estates was 1,123 kgs per hectare while it was 1215 kgs tea estates in Tamil Nadu.

The estimated Area under tea in the year 2005 increased to 528 thousand hectares exhibiting an average annual rate of growth of 1.1 per cent, while the average annual growth rate of production was 3 per cent. This clearly indicates that production has enhanced mainly due to improvement in yield rate.

Area, production and yield of tea per hectare during 1918 to 2005 is shown in Table 1 of the Appendix.

Zone-wise Area, Production and Yield : Tea growing regions are classified into revenue units or zones. The new classification came into effect from 9.9.1986. All earlier seven zones have been restructured

Table 1.1 State-wise area, production and yield of tea during 1961 to 2004

State	1961			1971			1981			1991			2005		
	A	P	Y	A	P	Y	A	P	Y	A	P	Y	A	P	Y
(1)	(2)	(3)	(4)	(5)	(6)	(7)	(8)	(9)	(10)	(11)	(12)	(13)	(14)	(15)	(16)
Assam	162	182	1123	182	224	1227	195	276	1413	229	380	1456	263	472	794
	(48.9)	(51.4)		(51.0)	(51.5)		(52.1)	(50.6)		(55.0)	(55.2)		(49.90)	(53.0)	
West Bengal	83	86	1043	88	104	1176	91	124	1362	101	143	1418	120	186	1550
	(25.1)	(24.3)		(24.6)	(23.9)		(24.3)	(22.7)		(24.3)	(20.8)		(22.7)	(20.9)	
Other*	12	5	417	13	4	307	13	4	307	11	7	636	15	6	666
	(3.6)	(1.4)		(3.7)	(0.9)		(3.5)	(0.8)		(2.6)	(1.0)		(2.8)	(0.6)	
North India	257	273	1064	283	332	1175	229	404	1353	341	538	1549	398	664	1670
	(77.6)	(77.1)		(79.3)	(76.3)		(79.9)	(74.1)		(81.9)	(77.0)		(75.4)	(74.5)	
Tamil Nadu	33	40	1215	35	57	1661	37	78	2109	38	101	2644	75	144	1920
	(10.0)	(10.9)		(8.8)	(12.9)		(9.9)	(14.3)		(9.1)	(14.7)		(14.2)	(16.2)	
Karnataka	2	1	992	2	3	1589	2	4	1878	2	3	2071	3	5	1666
	(0.6)	(1.1)		(1.5)	(0.9)		(0.6)	(0.9)		(0.5)	(0.5)		(0.6)	(0.8)	
Kerala	39	40	994	37	43	1164	36	58	1611	35	54	1557	52	76	1462
	(11.8)	(10.9)		(10.4)	(9.9)		(9.6)	(10.6)		(8.4)	(7.8)		(9.8)	(8.5)	
South India	74	81	1091	74	103	1398	75	140	1863	75	158	2125	130	225	1920
	(22.4)	(22.9)		(20.7)	(23.7)		(20.1)	(25.7)		(18.0)	(23.0)		(24.6)	(22.5)	2517
All India	331	354	1070	357	435	1221	374	544	1455	416	685	1652	528	889	
	(100.0)	(100.0)		(100.0)	(100.0)		(100.0)	(100.0)		(100.0)	(100.0)		(100.0)	(100)	1683

Note :- Figures in brackets indicate percentage of total others include Tripura, Himachal Pradesh, Uttaranchal, Bihar, Manipur. Sikkim, Arunachal Pradesh, Meghalaya, Nagaland and Orissa.

i) A = Area in thousand hectare, P = Production in million kg, and Y = Yield in kg per hectare

ii) Tea cultivation in non-traditional areas other than Tripura, Himachal Pradesh, Uttar Pradesh started from 1975 onwards.

Source : Tea Statistics, Tea Board, India, Kalkata

to only two zones. The details of area, production and yield rate of tea according to various zones are given in Table 1.2. Yield rate of Zone I was higher than that of Zone II during the last three ten years (1995-2005).

Size-wise Distribution of Tea Estates : Tea production is perennial in South India and seasonal in North India. In North India, the number of tea estates registered with the Tea Board was 2521 but a little more than three-fourths (77 per cent) of them are large in size with area above 100 hectares (371 hectares) each. There were 6978 registered tea estates in South India with preponderance of small estates having an area of less than 8.09 hectares each which accounted for 96 per cent of the total. It is estimated that there are also about 10,000 small tea estates in the south which are not registered with the Tea Board. Total area under tea and production of tea in the North is three times of the south.

There were 125220 tea estates registered with the Tea Board in India in 2005. About 9 percent of tea estates cover 80 per cent of the total area under tea in North India. In contrast, South India, with about 20 per cent of total area under tea had 91 per cent of total number of tea estates (Table 1.3)

Lorenz Ratios of Acerage and Production Distributions

The structural pattern of tea industry in India in these two regions may be illustrated with the help of Lorenz curve. A Lorenze curve which departs from the line of equal distribution shows the extent of departure from equal distribution. The more the actual curve departs from the line of equal distribution, the greater is the extent of divergence from equal distribution. All the estates were divided in several size classes and then the share of each of these classes in the total area under tea and production was worked out as shown in Tables 10-15 of Appendix for the years 1957, 1971, 1982, 1990 to understand overtimes changes in the nature of concentration. The Lorenz curves for the six different years are indicative of the fact that there exists substantial inequality in the distribution of area and production among estates in the North

Table 1.2 : Excise-zone-wise Area. Production and Yield of Tea During 1995-2005

Tea Revenue units	Area in hectare as on December			Production in thousand Kg.			Yield in Kg/hectare		
	1995	1997	2005	1995	1997	2005	1995	1997	2005
(1)	(2)	(3)	(4)	(5)	(6)	(7)	(8)	(9)	(10)
Zone-1 (North India)									
Dibrugarh	68998	70,022	87,583	143,931	146,435	162,214	2,086	2,091	1,852
Lakhimpur	4,494	4,361	6,555	8,678	8,494	9,506	1,931	1,949	1,450
Sibsagar (a)	62,810	62,751	78,168	98,186	110,278	122,083	1,659	1,575	1,561
Darang (Excluding Barsola Circle)	32,962	33,435	42,354	67,297	69,889	74,206	2,042	2,090	1,752
Total Zone-1 (North India)	169,264	170,570	213,660	318,092	335,096	368,009	1,879	1,965	1,722
Zone-II (North India) Barsola circle of Darrang	7322	8,140	9,056	13,241	13,351	15,291	1,808	1,640	1,752
All other North India districts	162,647	164,690	201,880	237,298	249,781	287,612	1,459	1,517	1,425
Total Zone (North India)	169,969	172,830	292,440	250,539	263,132	303,482	1,474	1,522	1,437
Total North India	339,133	343,400	242,904	568,631	598,228	671,419	1,676	1,742	2,164
Zone - II (South India) (All South Indian district)	87,832	87,845	108642	187,385	181,999	228029	2,133	2,072	2,090
Total South India	87,832	87,845	108642	187,385	181,999	228,029	2,133	2,072	2,072
Zone I Total	169,64	170,570	213660	318,092	335,096	368009	1,879	1,965	1,722
Zone II Total	257,801	260,675	314590	437,924	445,131	521551	1,699	1,708	1,690
All India Total	427,065	431,245	528250	756,016	780,227	889560	1,770	1,809	1,703

(a) excluding Mikir hills and NOrth Kolkata

Source : Tea STatics, Tea Board, India, Kolkata

Table 1.3 : Size wise area, Production and Yield during 2005

		Up to 10.12 hectare	Above 10.12 to 50 hectare	Above 50 to 100 hectare	Above 100 to 200 hectare	Above 200 to 400 hectare	Above 400 hectare	Total
		(1)	(2)	(3)	(4)	(5)	(6)	(7)
I.	**North India**							
1.	No. of estates	40,833	1,276	1,034	1,650	2,126	2,580	(49,500)
2.	Area in hectare	6,555	5,185	12,055	37,313	94,755	24,156	(397,450)
3.	Production in thousand	11,528	6,364	17,498	50,315	147,675	430,686	664066
4.	Yield (kg/hectare)	1,758	1,227	1,452	1,348	1,558	1,782	1,670
II.	**South India**							
1.	No. of estates	74,647	495	109	126	255	88	75,720
2.	Area in hectare	28,104	4,776	4,098	10,384	40,740	25,752	88,592
3.	Production in thousand kg	57;,217	4,988	3,958	16,317	88,295	54,720	225494
4.	Yield (kg/hectare)	2,035	1,044	967	1,571	2,167	2,125	1,980
III.	**All India**							
1.	No. of estates	115,480	1,771	1,143	1,771	2,381	2,674	125,220
2.	Area in hectare	34,659	9,961	16,153	47,697	135,494	284,286	528,250
3.	Production in thousand	68,744	11,352	21,456	66,630	235,970	485,408	889,560
4.	Yield (kg/hectare)	1,982	1,140	1,328	1,397	1,742	1,707	1,685

Source : Tea Statistics, Tea Board, India, Kolkata

and South throughout the period.

A Lorenz ratio - an index of inequality – measures the degree of concentration. The more equal the area and production distribution, the closer the ratio to zero and the greater the degree of inequality, the closer the ratio to one. The Lorenz Ratio is calculated with the help of the following formula :-

$$\frac{L = 1 - \sum_{j}^{n} = 1 \quad nj \left(\Sigma Y_j + \Sigma Y_{j-1} \right)}{NY}$$

where nj : Number of tea estates in jth class

Σ_{yj}: Summation of area or production of classes j

Σ_{yj-1}Summation of area and production of classes j-1

Table 1.4: Lorenz Ratio or Gini Coefficient of Area and Production.

	North India		South India	
Year	**Area**	**Production**	**Area**	**Production**
(1)	**(2)**	**(3)**	**(4)**	**(5)**
1957	0.39	0.46	0.90	0.85
1971	0.38	0.45	0.85	0.81
1982	0.39	0.48	0.85	0.83
1990	0.39	0.49	0.86	0.84
1999	0.39	0.50	0.87	0.85
2005	0.04	0.52	0.88	0.86

Source : Data Complied fromthe Various Issues of Tea Statitics, Kolkata

N : Total number of tea estates

Y ; Total acerage under area or production

It is clear from the above table that Lorenz ratios of area and production are higher in the South than those of the North and this concentration has not declined over time since 1957 at all. A large number of small estates, particularly in South, constitute a large percentage of total estates and control small percentage of total area and production. The extent of dominance of a few producing units over the total production activity is quite remarkable.

Area Under Different Age-groups : Bushes are the assets of tea estate owners as they provide green leaf which are basic raw materials for made/green tea. In view of this one must know the composition of assets which may indicate the phase-wise replacement or otherwise

Table 1.5 Area Under Different Age-group of Buses in 2005.

Age (in years)	Area under tea in hectare					
	North India	Per-centage	South India	Per-centage	All India	Percentage
(1)	(2)	(3)	(4)	(5)	(6)	(7)
Below 5	30458	5.8	3349	0.6	33807	6.4
5 to 10	36447	6.9	8982	1.7	45429	8.6
11 to 20	47432	9.0	9618	1.8	57050	10.8
21 to 30	58417	11.0	11343	2.2	69760	13.2
31 to 40	41940	8.0	10885	2.0	52825	10.0
41 to 50	30373	5.7	11359	2.2	41732	7.9
Above 50	152383	28.8	75264	14.3	227647	43.1
All India	397450	75.2	130800	24.3	528250	100.0

Source : Teat Statistics, Tea Board, India, Kolkata

so as to ensure constant flow of income by way of plucking green leaf from bushes. Here composition of assets means area owned by different age-group of bushes.

The bushes are classified into three age-groups namely tender (below 5 years), economic (5 to 50 years) and old (above 50 years). In the first group, the quantum of green leaf plucked per plant hardly commensurate and in the last group, green leaf plucked per plant reduces. Data presented in the above table brought out the fact that 50.5 per cent of total area under tea contains bushes which attain the economic age-group while it is 43.1 per cent for old age bushes and 6.4 per cent for tender bushes.

Rehabilitation Programme

Since more than two-fifths area is covered by over-aged bushes, it requires a rehabilitation programme in the form of new planting (extension, replacement and replanting) in a phased manner. It is pertinent to record here that about 5000 hectares are brought under new planting annually. Let us have a look at this aspect. (Table 1.6)

Table 1.6 : Extensions, Replacement and Replanting of Tea during 1952 to 2005

(Area in Hectare)

Year	Extensions	Replacement	Replantings	Total
1952-53	1,116.83	180.00	1,199.70	2,496.53
1962-63	2,224.86	401.13	1,571.16	4,197.15
1972-73	1,632.98	180.36	1,109.22	2,922.56
1982	1981.93	188.83	1,355.55	3526.51
1987	3070.50	476.73	1,195.33	4,742.13
1988	2780.05	374.31	1,303.88	4,458.24
1989	2553.29	381.65	1,402.56	4,337.50
1990	2,525.05	376.62	1,394.61	4,296.28
1991	2,423.05	343.90	1,495.68	4,262.63
1992	2,392.75	518.62	1,282.15	4,193.48
1993	2,462.53	450.47	1,338.65	4,251.65
1994	3,503.33	464.54	1,324.40	5,292.27
1995	1,642.26	235.46	1,280.47	3,158.19
1996	4,879.63	1,409.66	1,755.96	8,045.25
1997	2,639.45	1,006.57	1,421.17	5,067.19
1998	4019.37	1109.21	1495.89	6624.47
1999	2029.33	913.66	1320.21	5263.20
2000	2844.94	796.00	1197.35	4838.29
2001	2606.02	632.00	959.68	4197.70
2002	2750.15	749.25	1075.15	4574.55
2003	2850.75	805.25	1109.79	4765.79
2004	2995.50	945.38	1150.75	5091.63
2005	3025.45	1095.25	1257.45	5378.15

Source : Teat Statistics, Tea Board, India, Kolkata

3. Primary Marketing

Tea, being a perishable commodity, should be disposed of quickly as economic viability of tea industry depends crucially on profitable disposal of products. There are various modes of disposal of tea, namely, auction, ex-factory and forward contract. Among the different modes, the public auction centre plays the most important role since the major part of production is channalised through it. (Table 1.7 and 1.8)

4. Exports and Product Diversification

India's export of tea during the last four decade or so have shown an increasing trend. It increased from 195 million kgs in 1951-52 to 180 million kgs in 2005. On an average, India exports 200 million kgs annually. If one follows the export figures during the last 55 years, it reveals that India reached the highest level of exports to the tune of 242 milliong kgs in 1976-77 followed by 233 million kgs in 1956-57. From 1977-78 onwards onwards exports were between 177 to 214 million kgs except a few years. The details of exports are given in Table 16 of the Annexure.

India exports huge quantity of tea invative added forms like pocket tea, tea bags, instant tea, further at present organic tea, scented tea are also exported. Details of value added tea during the last four decades are given in Table 17 of the Annexure.

Export Markets

Indian tea is exported to 80 countries in the form of bulk tea. East Europe accounted for about 50 per cent of total exports of Indian tea followed by "West Asia and North Africa, West Europe, Asia other than West and America. Market-wise export of tea is given in Table 1.9. Further, country wise and region wise export of Indian tea through out the world are depicated in Table 4 of the Annexure.

5. Internal Consumption

Domestic demand of tea had grown enormously in so far as volume

Table 1.7 : Primary Marketing of Indian Tea

Name of the Region/Auction Centre	1999		2000		2002		2003		2004	
	Qty in .kg	Percentage to total sale	Qty in th.kg	Percentage to total sale	Qty in kg	Percentage to total sale	Qty in kg	Percentage to total sale	Qty in kg	Percentage to total sale
(1)	(2)	(3)	(4)	(5)	(6)	(7)	(8)	(9)	(10)	(11)
North India										
Kolkata Auction	95,926	15.55	87,801	14.09	105,730	16.74	133765	20.64	117956	17.81
Guwahati Auction	159,427	22.84	145,072	23.28	131,424	20.80	138664	21.39	127067	19.91
Siliguri Aucton	79,145	13.30	86789	13.93	73,293	11.60	87090	14.34	91989	13.89
Amritsar Action	968	0.10	556	0.09	507	0.80	190	0.03	146	0.02
Sub total of North India	344,966	51.39	320128	51.39	310954	49.22	359709	55.49	337158	50.91
London Auction	-	-	-	-	-	-	-	-	-	-
Total Auction	344,966	51.39	320128	.39	310,954	49.22	359709	55.49	337158	50.91
Export under forward ccntract	36,032	4.66	32,866	5.28	33,794	5.32	35609	5.49	38921	5.88
Ex garden sale	269,752	44.05	270,155	43.34	287,000	44.43	252959	39.02	286105	43.21
Total sale	640,750	100.00	623,259	100.00	631,748	100.00	648277	100.00	662184	100.00
South India										
Cochin Auction	66,132	0.88	59,632	29.42	58196	28.15	50633	22.03	54599	23.66
Coonoor Auction	70,967	28.82	79,285	39.12	60665	29.35	40586	17.66	44279	19.19
Coimbatoor Auction	33,274	9.47	20,262	10.00	26,658	12.90	22331	9.71	18400	7.97
Tea serve	-	-	-	-	-	-	4403	1.91	18527	8.03
Kolkata Auction	2,188	2.27	1,371	0.68	76	0.04	109	0.05	1363	0.59
Guwahati Auction	-	-	-	-	-	-	-	-	28	0.10
Sub total South India	172,561	71.44	160,550	79.22	145595	70.43	118062	51.36	137196	59.45
London	-	-	-	-	-	-	-	-	-	-
Total Auction	172,561	71.44	160,550	79.22	145595	70.43	118062	51.36	137196	59.45
Export under F/C	6,995	2.86	5,543	2.73	6240	3.02	8041	3.50	8727	3.78
Ex-garden sale	26,160	25.70	36538	18.05	54,891	26.55	103749	45.14	84858	36.77
Total Sale All India	206,166	100.00	202,676	100.00	206,726	100.00	229852	100.00	230781	100.00
Indian Auction	07,527	57.10	480,768	58.21	456,549	54.44	477771	54.41	474354	53.12
London Auction	-	-	-	-	-	-	-	-	-	-
Total Auction	507,527	57.10	480,768	58.21	456,549	54.45	477771	54.41	474354	53.12
Export under F/C	43,027	397	38,429	4.65	40,034	4.77	43650	4.94	47648	5.34
Ex-garden sale	296,368	38.93	306,738	37.14	341,891	40.78	356708	40.62	30763	41.54
Total sale	846,922	100.00	825,935	100.00	838,474	100.00	878129	100.00	892965	100.00

Source - Tea plantation Industry in India between 1850 and 1992 - Structural changes by Dr G.D. Banerjee

Table 1.8: Quantity and Price Realised at Various Auctions during Last 5 Years 1987 to 2005

AUCTION	1987		1992		2002		2003		2004		1997		2005	
	Q	AP	Q	AP	Q	AP	Q	AP	Q	AP	Q	AP	Q	AP
(1)	(2)	(3)	(4)	(5)	(6)	(7)	(8)	(9)	(10)	(11)	(12)	(13)	(14)	(15)
Kalkata	132,628	28.97	112,912	43.86	94,776	76.36	96,584	80.15	99412	81.52	88,870	79.80	96,452	87.33
Guwahati	147.651	24.83	149,695	40.02	137,794	68.68	139,412	70.15	142,429	69.98	148,670	67.67	145,226	75.15
Siliguri	80,583	23.61	82,395	37.25	71,791	63.48	75,607	67.75	80,066	70.15	67,001	86.95	86,145	74.66
Amritsar	429	14.26	406	28.82	507	24.47	610	25.85	681	29.54	744	41.89	717	45.43
Cochin	52,221	22.67	58907	52.21	58,907	52.21	59,214	43.47	62,252	44.42	63,523	61.57	65,815	73.31
Coonoor	27,439	19.27	34,196	30.63	74,555	41.47	78,415	42.56	79,812	43.15	73,298	57.13	82,145	45.12
Coimbatore	31,524	20.98	17,141	32.29	25,118	44.98	26512	45.75	15,057	41.30	16,473	50.05	17,245	49.15
London	10,132	122.0@	6,666	116.60@	Nil	Nil	Nil	Nil	2,475	126.70@	1,657	148.31@	Nil	Nil

* Combination of black and green tea, Q = Quantity; AP = Average Price (Weighted) @ Average Price in Pence per Kg.,

Source : Tea Market Reports.

intake is concerned. At the break of the independence, domestic consumption of tea was about 31 per cent of total production. In 2005 at 720 million kg, it had gone up to 81 per cent. Between 1971 and 2005, domestic consumption has grown at a compound rate of 4.5 per cent against the corresponding production growth rate of 2.6 per cent. The domestic demand, however, cannot be expected to grow at this rate in the coming years as has been evident from the decadal decelerating trend. Between 1960 and 1970, the growth rate was 5.2 per cent. It however, reduced to 4.36 per cen during the period from 1980 to 2000 It declined to 3.7 per cent during the period from 1980 to 2005. Again from 2000 to 2005 domestic demand declined 2.05 per cent.

Data presented in the table below showed that India's domestic demand is increasing at an estimated level of 10 to 15 million Kgs a year and with a considerable demand pull in the internal market, it is extremely different to find surplus for exports. The details of internal consumption is given in Table 1.10.

Factors Determining Internal Consumption

There are various demographic, economic, social and psychological factors that determine the demand for a commodity like tea in a developing economy like India. Income, prices of tea and its substitutes and complements, changes in consumer tastes, preferences, population and social satisfaction are some of the important factors in this regard. Another factor is urbanisation, the pace of which, in the developing countries, is very rapid.

It was empirically established that income elasticity and price elasticity of demand for tea are 1.18 and 0.256 respectively. Dr. Sibranjan Mishra in this Ph.D theses showed that an increase in income by 1 per cent will bring about, other things remaining constant, an increase in consumption by 1.81 per cent. That means income exerts a significant positive influence on consumption. But consumption of tea does not change with changes in the prices of tea. Other peculiarity is that present consumption is more in urban areas than in rural areas. Thus, it is expected that volume of consumption of tea will increase in view of the

Table 1.9 (a) : Market-wise exports of tea.

Name of Country		Quantity in thousand kg			Value in thousand Rs.			Unit-Price (Rs./kg)		
		1995-96	1996-97	1997-98	1995-96	1996-97	1997-98	1995-96	1996-97	1997-98
I. WEST EUROPE										
(a)	EEC	34,554	36.789	38.037	2782,190	3081620	377048	80.52	83.76	99.13
(b)	Other West Europe	564	433	251	73763	43596	31063	130.79	100.68	123.76
Sub-total of West Europe I		35118	37222	38228	2855953	3125216	3801545	81.32	83.96	99.29
II.	East Europe	90307	71912	110533	6284726	5084780	10290132	69.59	70.71	93.10
III.	America									
(a)	North America & West Indies	3282	4705	4520	205345	444255	401324	62.57	94.42	88.79
(b)	Latin America	01	64	23	111	4152	2167	111.00	64.88	94.22
Sub-total America III		3283	4769	4543	205456	448407	403491	62.58	94.03	88.82
IV.	West Asia & North Africa									
(a)	West Asia	22357	29926	32799	1855829	2406203	3059382	83.01	80.41	93.26
(b)	North Africa	7230	7510	8398	371838	303357	529186	51.43	40.39	63.01
Sub-total of West Asia & North Africa IV		29587	37436	41197	2227667	2709560	3588568	75.29	72.35	87.11
V.	Asia other than west	5150	11263	12118	443065	843553	1216431	86.20	74.90	100.38
VI.	Africa other than North	2031	3623	1375	119264	217595	105743	58.72	60.06	76.90
VII.	Australia and Ocenia	773	947	719	48167	59123	47297	62.31	62.43	65.78
Grand Total		166239	167172	208773	12184298	12568167	19453207	73.29	75.18	93.18

Note-(i) EEC includes United Kingdom, Irish Republic, Denmark, the Netherlands, Germany, Belgium, Italy, France, Greece, Spain, Portugal; (ii) Other West Europe covers Austria, Finland, Norway, Sweden, Switzerland, Cyprus, Iceland; (iii) East Europe includes Lithuania, Russian Federation, Latvia, Turkmenistan, Estonia, Georgia, Tajikistan, Ukrain, Kazakhstan, Azerbaijan, Slovenia, Uzbekistan, Moldova, Belarus, Bulgaria, Czechoslovakia, Hungary, Poland, Romania, Kyrgyzstan, Armenia; (iv) North America and West Indies incorporates USA, Canada, Trinidad and Tobag Canary Island, Bahamas; (v) Latin America covers chili, Medico, Uruguay, Argentina, Panama, Venezuela, Guatemala; (vi) West Asia covers Iran, UAE, Qatar, Kuwait, South Arabia, Bahrain, Jordan, Yemen, Syria AD Sep. (vi) North Africa covers ARE, Libya, Sudan, Tin Morocco. (vii) Asia other than west thichudes Afghanistan, Bangladesh, Burma, Hong Kong, Japan, Malaysia, Singapore, Nepal, Philippines, Pakistan, Thailand, Turkey, Cyprus, Korea, Sri Lanka, China, Taiwan, Bhutan, Indonesia, Maldives, Mongolia (viii) Africa other than North covers Ghana, Mauritius, Nigeria, Djibouti, South Africa, Liberia, Ethiopia, Zambia, Zimbabwe, Tanzania, Kenya, Sierra Leone, Guinea, Congo R, Republic, Guinea Bissau, Ivory Coast and (ix) Australia and Oceania covers Australia, Fizi and New Zealand.

Table 1.9 (b) Market wise Exports of tea during 2001-03 to 2003-004

Name of Country		Quantity in thousand kg			Value in thousand Rs.			Unit-Price (Rs./kg)		
		2001-02	2002-03	2003-04	2001-02	2002-03	2003-04	2001-02	2002-03	2003-04
I. WEST EUROPE										
(a)	EEC	1456	392	584	286150	110282	137684	196.53	188.33	267.86
(b)	Other West Europe	232	15	14	27838	2886	2893	119.99	192.66	206.64
Sub-total of West Europe I		1686	407	602	313988	113168	140541	186.23	189.24	233.45
II.	East Europe	21342	14277	12399	2193341	1394400	1228236	102.77	97.66	99.06
III.	**America143.35**									
(a)	North America & West Indies	1512	1502	1385	230366	215313	267931	152.36	143.35	193.45
(b)	Latin America	3	0	0	943	0	3	314.00	0	0
Sub-total America III		1515	1502	1835	231309	215313	267934	152.67	143.15	146.01
IV.	**West Asia & North Africa**									
(a)	West Asia	17498	16804	16946	2368018	2275445	2143748	135.33	135.41	126.50
(b)	North Africa	172	19	46	15158	2555	6040	88.13	134.47	131.30
Sub-total of West Asia & North Africa IV		17670	16823	17072	2383176	2278000	2149788	134.86	135.41	125.93
V.	Asia other than west	474	374	1151	86154	60759	117196	181.75	162.46	101.82
VI.	Africa other than North	4	0	29	631	63	0	157.75	0	108.21
VII.	Australia and Ocenia	29	229	1009	2773	22619	151140	106.65	98.99	149.79
Grand Total		42719	33606	34103	5211372	4084322	4057973	121.99	121.54	119.31

Source - Global Tea Trade - Dimensions and Dynamics by Dr GD Banerjee

Details of Country wise exports of tea are given in Table 4 of the Annexure

Table 1.10 : Estimates of Internal Consumption (Quantity in million Kg.)

Year	Quantity	Increase or decrease	Percentage increase or decrease
1971	221	—	—
1972	233	12	5.43
1973	244	11	4.72
1974	258	14	5.73
1975	272	14	5.45
1976	287	15	5.22
1977	302	15	5.22
1978	320	18	5.96
1979	322	12	3.75
1980	346	14	4.22
1981	360	14	4.05
1982	372	12	3.33
1983	386	14	3.76
1984	400	14	3.62
1985	415	15	3.75
1986	430	15	3.62
1987	446	16	3.72
1988	462	16	3.58
1989	480	18	3.90
1990	500	20	4.17
1991	511	11	2.20
1992	524	13	2.54
1993	537	13	2.48
1994	550	13	2.42
1995	562	12	2.18
1996	580	18	3.20
1997	597	17	293
1998	615	18	3.01
1999	633	18	2.92
2000	653	20	3.15
2001	670	17	2.6
2002	685	15	2.24
2003	695	10	1.45
2005	710	15	1.43

Source : Tea Statistics, Tea Board, Calcutta.

trend towards industrialisation. It should be noted that rural areas are also getting into the habit of drinking more and more tea. Cultural change which is taking place in rural India is likely to boost in volume the demand for tea.

6. Major Imposts

Tea is a major source of revenue to the national exchequer. The major imposts are excise duty and cess on tea production as well as various central and state taxes like sales taxes, entry tax, agricultural income tax etc. These are given below :-

I. Cess, Excise Duty and Rebate (w. e. f. 9.9.86)

1.	The rate of Cess on Teas Produced: (w.e.f. 15.8.86)	
(a)	In the Sadar Sub-Division and Kurseong Sub-Division excluding the areas under the jurisdiction list No. 31, 29, 33, 20, 21, 22, 23 and 24 comprising Siliguri Sub-Division of New Chumta Tea Estate, Simulbari and Marionbari Tea Estate of Kurseong Police Station in Kurseong Sub-Division of the District of Darjeeling in the State of West Bengal.	Rs. 08 per kg
(b)	In all other tea growing areas of India other than 'a' mentioned above.	Rs. 0.15 per kg
2. EXCISE DUTY:		
	(Excise zone has been restructured from the earlier number of seven zones to only two zones w.e.f. 9.9.86)	
LOOSE TEA :		Rate off Excise Duty
(a)	On loosse green tea (irrespective of the zone of production).	Rs. 0.11 per kg.
		Green tea is exempted from Excise Duty w.e.f. 1.4.1988
(b)	Loose Black Tea	
(i)	On tea produced in Zone-1 i.e. the teas produced In the district of Darrang, Dibrugarh, Lakhimpur, Sibsagar, Jorhat and Sonipur but excluding Barsola circle in the district of Sonitpur.	Rs. 1.50 per kg.
(ii)	In other areas in the territory of India other than the area included in the Zone-1	Rs. 0.50 per kg.

Concession in respect of levy of excise duty to certain sections of the industry

(A) Where the tea manufactured in a factory owned by a co-operative society registered under any law relating to co-operative societies is assessed according to the rate specified above the duty leviable on such tea shall-

(a) In respect of district of Darrang under the State of Assam be 0.66 per kg.

(b) In respect of other areas be reduced by 10% of such rate subject to the condition that-

(i) No member of such co-operative society owns a holding exceeding 10 hectares cultivation of tea plants, and

(ii) That the green leaves are not purchased by such co-operative society from any grower who has holding exceeding 10 hectares under cultivation of tea plants.

Explanation

The grower does not include the Tamil Nadu Govt. Tea project.

(B) Where the tea manufactured in a Bought-leaf factory is assessed according to the rates specified for all zones, the duty leviable on such tea shall-

(a) In respect of the district of Darrang in the State of Assam be Rs. 0.66 per kg.

(b) In respect of other areas be reduced by 10% of such rate.

(C) As per Central Excise Notification No. 241/87 dated 29.10.87' "Bought leaf factory" means a factory which-

(i) has worked for at least six months during the financial year immediately preceding the financial year in which the duty is levied; and

(ii) has purchased not less than two thirds of the green leaf processed by the factory in the preceding financial year from any grower who has a holding not exceeding 10 hectares of land under cultivation of tea plants.

Package Tea:

(a)	Tea packed in unit containers of content not exceeding 25 gms. ordinarily intended for sale to consumers in those pack.	Rate Rs. 0.44 per kg. plus the duty for the time being leviable for loose tea which has not already been paid (w.e.f. 11.3.86)
(b)	Tea packed in unit containers of content exceeding 25 gms. but not exceeding 20 kgs. whether or not ordinarily intended for sell to consumers in that pack.	Rate Rs. 1.10 per kg. plus the duty for the time being leviable for loose tea which has not already been paid (w.e.f. 11.3.86)
(c)	Tea packed in bags for consumption known as tea bags.	There is no Excise Duty on tea bags but duty leviable for loose tea should be paid if such loose tea is used for manufacture of tea bags. (w.e.f. 15.5.86)
Instant Tea:		Rate 11% plus duty for the time being leviable on loose tea (w.e.f. 11.3.86) per kg

3. Rebate Allowed on Export (w.e.f.3.9.86) Loose Tea:

A. Loose Tea

A rebate on Excise duty @ 50 paise per kg. on loose unblended/blended tea exported out of India is granted w.e.f. 9.9.86.

With effect from 4.2.86 the rebate is granted on export @ 50 paise per kg on loose un-blended/blended teas exported out of India provided the duty of excise so paid is not less than 50 paise per kg.

Full rebate of Excise Duty has been granted on loose tea exported out of India w.e.f. 27.4.1988.

B. Package Tea:

(i) A rebate of excise duty @ 50 paise per kg on loose unblended tea which is used in the manufacture of blended tea and packet tea exported out of India is granted w.e.f 9.9.86.

(ii) A rebate of additional excise duty on export of packet tea at the following rates are also granted w.e.f. 9.9.86.

(a)	Tea packed in any king of container containing not more than 25 gms. net of tea.	0.44 p. per kg.
(b)	Tea packed in any kind of containing more than 25 gms. but not more than 1 kg. net of tea.	Rs. 1.10 per kg.

c. Instants Tea:		The whole of the duty of excise leviable on instant tea provided that the duty of excise has already been paid on loose tea used in the manufacture of such instant tea w.e.f. 1.3.86.
d. Loose Tea		Rebate of Excise duty granted on exports of Bulk tea w.e.f. 23.7.83 has been withdrawl w.e.f. 1.2.1985.
4.	**Cash Compensatory Support w.e.f. 1.4.89**	w.e.f. 1.4.89 the C.C.S has been granted at the following rates on f.o.b. value of exports (valid up to 31.3. 1992

Description of the Product:

			Rates of CCS
(a)	Tea Bags	....	8%
(b)	Packet Tea, Tea Caddies and Tea Chestlets.	....	18%
(c)	Instant Tea.	....	8%
(d)	Quick Brewing Black Tea.	....	12%

5.	**Corporate Income Tax**	@ 40% on taxable income, plus 15% surcharge as per ordinance issued on 15.10.90. With effect from the Budget year 1992-93 the rate was 45% plus 15% surcharge, With effect from Budget year 1993-94, the rate was again 40% plus surcharge of 15%. The surcharge was reduced to 7.5% in 1996-97 Budget. In 1997-98 Budget, the surcharge was abolished and corporate tax was reduced to 35%. In 1999-2000 Budget surcharge @ 10% was re-imposed.

6.	**Central Sales Tax:**		
Is generally levied @ 4% on Inter-State Trade or Commerce. However,			
(i)	Central Sales Tax on teas sold at Calcutta auction	....	3%
(ii)	Central Sales Tax on teas sold at Siliguri auction	....	2%
(iii)	Central Sales Tax on teas sold at Guwahati auction	....	Nil

7. Agricultural Income Tax:

Tea is only agricultural and plantation crop which has been given a special status wherein 40% of the income tax is taxable under the Central Income Tax Act and balance 60% is chargeable under Agricultural Income Tax of the concerned State Governments.

8. The Excise Duty Leviable on Loose Packet & Instant Tea has been Removed

w.e.f. 27.2.1993. However, as a result of withdrawal of relevant exemption notification 925% excise duty on instant tea has become effective w.e.f. 1996-97 Budget period.

B. Duties and Taxes in Different States in India.

Assam:			
(a)	State Sales Tax :	(i)	w.e.f. 28.3.89, 2% Assam Sales Tax is levied on teas sold in the Guwahati Auction (Except orthodox tea)
		(ii)	Teas bought for export in Guwahati auction are exempted from this tax.
		(iii)	7% Assam Sales Tax is levied on private sales within Assam on·purchases outside auction.
(b)	Assam Taxation on (Specified land) (amendment Act, 1994)		@ Rs. 2.50 for Rs. 0.18 every killogram of green tea leaf. w.e.f. 15.5.94. The rate is 30 paise for every kg of green leaf produced on Assam valley. The rate is 27 paise in Cacher.
West Bengal :			
(A)	**West Bengal Sales Tax:**	(a)	On teas sold in auction held in Calcutta or Siliguri 4% (w.e.f. 1.4.90) except:
		(i)	Teas sold for exports Nil
		(ii)	Teas sold to registered dealers for resale in West Bengal.......1%.
		(iii)	Teas sold for blending in West Bengal....2%.
		(b)	On teas sold other than in auctions in Calcutta or Siliguri....4% (w.e.f. 1.4.90). except
		(i)	Sales for export against prior order only...Nil.
		(ii)	Sales to registered dealers for resale in West Bengal....1%.
		(iii)	Sales to registered dealers for blending in West Bengal....... 2% but resale after blending.
Note : Govt. of W.B. levies additional sale tax @ 10% of the total amount of sales tax payable w.e.f. 1.1.1995. This lexy is applicable to dealers selling teas in West Bengal.			

(B)	**West Bengal Entry Tax**	Withdrawn in 1995-96 Budget.					
(C)	**West Bengal Purchase Tax with effect. from 1st October, 1982.**	On teas purchased for blending in West Bengal and subsequent transfer to other States for sale 3%.					
(D)	**West Bengal Rural Employment and Production Cess applicable to tea produced in West Bengal only.**	8 paise per kg of green leaf produced.					
(E)	**West Bengal Primary Education Cess**	4 paise per kg of green leaf produced.					
(F)	**West Bengal Agricultural Income Tax:**			Till 31.3.91	w.e.f. 1.4.91	w.e.f. 1.4.93	w.e.f. 1.4.96
		(1)	Upto Rs. 1 lakh	65%	65%	65%	50%
		(2)	Above Rs. 1 to 2 lakh	75%	75%	70%	50%
		(3)	Above Rs. 2 to 3 lakh	75%	75%	70%	50%
		(4)	Above Rs. 3 to 5 lakh	75%	75%	70%	50%
		(5)	Above Rs. 5 to 10 lakh	75%	80%	70%	50%
		(6)	Above Rs. 10 lakh	75%	88%	70%	50%
	* Based on Budget of 91						

Tamil Nadu		
(A)	State Sales Tax :	5% (Effective from 12.3.93)
(i)	On sale of tea at Auction Centre at Coonoor and Coimbatore.........	Exempted
(ii)	On tea sold for exports	5%
(iii)	On tea sold to outside auction	Exempted (provided the tea sold has already suffered tax in the state)

Note: In regard to local sales surcharge @ 15% and additional surcharge @ 5% on tax due and additional sales tax as applicable is also leviable. On the sales affected in the Madras city, surcharge @ 15%. On tax due and additional tax as applicable are also leviable on the sales affected in the other areas.

B	Tamil Nadu Agricultural Income Tax:	
(a)	Where the total agricultural income does not exceed Rs. 25,000.	45% of total agricultural income.
(b)	Where the total agricultural income exceeds Rs. 25, 000 but does not exceed Rs.1,00,000	50% of total agricultural income.
(c)	Where the total agricultural income exceeds Rs.1,00,000 but does not exceed Rs.3,000.	55% of total agricultural income.
(d)	Where the total agricultural income exceeds Rs. 3,00,000 but does not exceed Rs.10,00,000	60% of total agricultural income.
(e)	Where the total agricultural income exceeds Rs. 10,00,000	65% of total agricultural income.
Kerala		
A.	Kerala State / Sales Tax :	
		Rate of Tax
(i)	For sale of Cochin auctions	7%
(ii)	For export sale through Auctions	Nil
(iii)	Tea sold other than (i) and (ii)	7%

Explanation:- Where a tax has been levied in respect of manufactured tea, the tax if any, levied and collected in respect of green tea leaves from which such manufactured tea is produced, shall be refunded.

Levy of Charges :		
(i)	For turn over not exceeding	Rs. 10 lakh 5% of basic ST
(ii)	For turn over exceeding	Rs. 10 lakh 10% of basic ST
B.	**Plantation Tax :**	
i)	On the first 3 hectares	Nil
ii)	Above 3 ha but below 4 ha	Rs.100 per ha in excess of 3 ha.
iii)	Above 4 ha but below 8 ha	Rs.150 per ha in excess of 3 ha.
iv)	Above 8 ha but below 15 ha	Rs.200 per ha in excess of 3 ha.
v)	Above 15 ha but below 25 ha	Rs.250 per ha in excess of 3 ha.
vi)	Above 25 ha	Rs.350 per ha in excess of 3 ha.

Cess, Excise Duty and Rebate (w.e.f. 1.4.1997)

The Rate of Cess on Teas Produced (w.e.f. 1.4.97)

(a)	All tea produced in Sadar sub-division and Kurseong sub-division excluding the areas of jurisdiction of tea estates numbering 31, 29, 33, 20, 21, 22, 23 and 24 comprising Siliguri sub-division of New Chumta Tea Estate, Simulbari and Marionbari tea estates of Kurseong police station in kurseong sub-division of the district of Darjeeling in the state of West Bengal	Rs.0.12 per kg
(b)	All teas except those produced in the areas specified above in (a)	Rs.0.30 per kg

Excise Duty:

With effect from 24.6.1998 central excise duty @ 8% advalorem was leviable or packet tea of size above 100 gms and below 200 gms falling under sub-heading No. 0902-10 of the excise tariff. However w.e.f 1999-2000 Budget, the excise duty @ 8% of packet tea was withdrawn and excise duty at specified rate of Rs.2.00 per kg became leviable on "Tea, including the waste" under sub-division 090-00.

Taxes Levied in Other Tea and Non-tea Producing States/ Union Territories.

Sl. No.	State	Central Sale Tax	State Sale Tax	Other taxes
1.	Andhra Pradesh	4%	10%	CST without form C, 10%
2.	Bihar	NA	10%	Additional Tax 1%, CST without form 'C' 10%
3.	Delhi	2%	5.5%	-
4.	Goa, Daman, Diu	NA	4% w.e.f. 30.5.95	
5.	Gujrat	4%	8%	12% for packet tea below 20 kgs 8% for packages above 20 kgs + Surcharge 10%, Octorai 1%.

6.	Haryana	4%	4%	C.S.T without form 'C' 10%
7.	Himachal Pradesh	4%	7%	-
8.	Madhya Pradesh	NA	8%	On loose tea and 10% on tea in packets
9.	Maharashtra	4%	8%	Surcharge 10%
10.	Meghalaya	4%	7%	Surcharge 1%
11.	Mizoram	-	-	-
12.	Nagaland	4%	6%	-
13.	Orissa	4%	12%	Entry tax 1%, CST without form 'C' 12%
14.	Pondichery	3%	3%	-
15.	Punjab	2%	4%	-
16.	Rajasthan	4%	4%	-
17.	Tripura	8%	8%	-
18.	Uttar Pradesh	4%	6%	-
19.	Sikkim	4%	8%	-

7. Labour

Tea plantation industry in this country has special feature. It provides employment opportunities to the rural people living in the remotest area. It is one of the highly labour intensive industries. The average daily number of labours employed in this sector was estimated at about 14 lakh in 2005. This is on the high side as compared to other industries. Tea plantation can also provide maximum employment per household. Besides, quite large number of workers are engaged in this industry.

Labourers are employed in tea industry both in field and factory operations. They are mainly resident and outside workers. Resident workers are the permanent labour of the estate where as outside are temporary or casual labour. Both resident and outside workers are again divided into male, female, children and adolescent depending upon the nature of work involved. The details of labour employment according to field and factory are depicted in Table 1.11. Rates of daily wages for tea plantation labour in North and South India are given in Annexure. Table below shows the details of Labour wage settlement in Kerala/Tamil Nadu and Karnataka along with guidelines of labour liaison committee are depicted in Tables 5 and 6 of the Annexure.

8. Labour Employment-Field and Fatory

It is observed from the data that about 13.01 lakh workers representing 90.8 per cent of the total workers are engaged in field operation and 1.30 lakh account for 9.20 per cent in factory operation. Majority of the workers, i.e. 9.25 lakh, are resident workers and a few, i.e. 3.76 lakh, are outside workers. In terms of percentage, 9.25 per cent are living within the estate and 28.8 per cent outside the estate. Out of a total of 9.20 lakh workers, male workers account for 47.8 per cent followed by female workers 47.8 per cent and adolescent & children 4.6 per cent.

Table 1.11: Average Daily Number of Labourers Employed in Field and Factory in 2005.

(in Number)

Operation/Category		Male	Female	Adolescent	Total
	(1)	(2)	(3)	(4)	(5)
A.	North India				
(i)	Field				
(a)	Resident	252941	311410	24791	629142
(b)	Outside	91220	157990	32660	281870
Sub total of field (a+b)		384161	469400	57451	911011
(ii)	Factory				
(a)	Resident	72195	6500	500	79195
(b)	Outside	31450	4015	900	36365
Sub total of factory (a+b)		103656	105151	1400	115560
Total North India (i+ii)		487806	479915	58851	1026572

B.	South India				
(i)	**Field**				
(a)	Resident	999333	101273	550	201156
(b)	Outside	84457	103655	100	188212
Sub total of field (a+b)		183790	204928	650	389268
(ii)	**Factory**				
(a)	Resident	10854	1159	12	12025
(b)	Outside	2270	456	-	2726
Sub total of field (a+b)		13124	1615	12	14751
Total South India (i+ii)		196914	206543	662	404019
C.	**All India**				
i)	**Field**				
(a)	Resident	3992274	412683	25341	830298
(b)	Outside	175677	261645	32760	470082
Sub total of field (a+b)		767951	674328	58101	1300380
ii)	**Factory**				
(a)	Resident	83049	7659	512	91220
(b)	Outside	33720	4471	900	39091
Sub total of factory (a+b)		116769	12130	1412	130311
Total (i+ii)		**684720**	**686458**	**59503**	**1430691**

Further estimated average number of labour employed according to districts during 1992-2004 is depicted in Table 20 of Appendix.

Productivity of Land and Labour

On an average, labour employed per hectare is estimated at 2.41 which is lower than South India average of 3.13 and higher than North India average of 2.21. (Table1.13) Output produced per labour is calculated at 710 kgs in India, while it was 639 kgs for South India and 738 kgs for North India. Productivity and labour per hectare during 2005 is given below:-

Table 1.12 : Labour/production per hectare and production per labour during 2005.

State	Labour per hectare (No.)	Production per hectare (in kg.)	Production per labour (in Kg.)
(1)	(2)	(3)	(4)
Assam	2.72	1603	7055
West Bengal	2.30	1882	817
Others @	0.81	587	726
North India	2.21	1630	738
Tamil Nadu	3.50	2146	613
Karnataka	2.12	2641	1247
Kerala	2.44	1675	688
South India	3.13	2003	639
All India	2.41	1713	710

*Others include Tripura, Bihar, Uttaranchal, Himachal Pradesh, Sikkim, Arunachal Pradesh and Manipur.

Source : Tea Statistics, Tea Board, Kalkata.

9. Wage Employment Relationship

Tea industry plays a crucial role in employment generation of our country. In this context, possible relationship between wage and employment has been examined during the period 1961-2005 based on data available from Tea Statistics for West Bengal. Labour employment includes aggregation of various categories of labour without taking into consideration quality difference of labour and specialisation of female labour in particular operation. Money wages are defined as wages at current prices, real wages are expressed by deflating money wages by all India consumer price index and wage cost is obtained by deflating money wages by product prices. Wage cost also reflects the real burden of wages on the producers. Absorption of labour is inversely related to changes in real wage cost. The following table describes changes in growth of employment, real wages, wage cost, productivity of labour and profit after tax as percentage of net worth. (Table 1.13)

Table 1.13 : Index number of Wages, Productivity and Profit

(Base 1961 = 100)

Year	Labour employed	Money wages	Real wages	Wage cost	Productivity of labour	Profit after tax as percentage to net worth
(1)	(2)	(3)	(4)	(5)	(6)	(7)
1961	100	100	100	100	100	100
1962	101	140	104	110	105	101
1963	104	148	108	120	108	103
1964	102	180	110	138	115	101
1965	103	180	118	140	125	102
1966	105	185	112	135	110	104
1967	106	210	115	140	115	120
1968	105	210	110	160	131	160
1969	106	258	122	165	138	80
1970	104	258	120	150	129	82
1971	105	275	120	155	128	190
1972	108	275	126	160	110	155
1973	107	300	131	168	125	124
1974	109	320	135	170	127	180
1975	108	340	127	175	130	305
1976	108	340	128	185	126	260
1977	109	355	132	175	125	385
1978	109	355	131	178	125	385
1979	109	360	130	180	131	260
1980	108	378	133	185	135	135
1981	109	390	135	190	139	270
1984	110	398	137	193	141	275
1985	111	400	135	194	143	270
1987	112	405	136	195	143	271
1989	114	408	136	196	144	272
1990	115	408	136	198	144	272
1991	115	408	136	199	144	273
1992	115	500	136	202	144	275

(1)	(2)	(3)	(4)	(5)	(6)	(7)
1993	116	502	136	205	145	276
1994	116	503	136	207	145	279
1995	116	505	137	209	145	281
1996	116	510	137	215	146	255
1997	117	515	137	220	146	257
1998	117	520	138	235	146	259
1999	117	520	138	245	147	290
2000	118	510	139	240	145	276
2001	117	515	139	245	145	276
2002	117	520	140	250	147	275
2003	118	525	140	250	147	275
2004	117	525	140	250	148	276
2005	118	525	140	240	148	275

Note: *Columns 2 and 5 obtained from Tea Statistics, Tea Board, column 3 is computed by dividing money wages by consumer index number obtained from the Annual Report on Currency and Finance, Reserve Bank of India. Column 4 is computed by dividing money wages by product prices obtained from Tea statistics. Column 6 is obtained from currency and finance.*

Employment recorded a very mild growth of 18 per cent over a period of 44. Although money wages increased by 5.25 times, real wages showed a persistent marginal increase (40 percent). This may be due to sharp increase in consumer prices of industrial workers. Similar trends are observed in the movement of wages at constant product price i.e. wage cost. While real wages increased by 40 per cent, wage cost increased by 140 per cent. It should, however, be noted that prices during this period increased by more than four times.

When there is a slow growth of real wage cost, we may expect a rise in employment. Unfortunately, it did not happen. The decline in rate of growth of wage cost is not a sufficient factor to increase employment. Other factors like productivity of labour and profit may be treated as relevant explanatory variables.

The increase in average physical productivity may reduce the burden of rising cost of production. But productivity of labour has not shown any significant move to mitigate the burden of wage increase. Again, the movement in the profit after tax as percentage to net worth is slow and eratic during the period. The inadequate generation of internal resources due to slow flow of paidup capital and declining rate of retained earnings that can be ploughed back may explain to some extent the generation of employment of a slow pace. Thus, it is empirically analyzed that employment growth in tea industry does not exclusively depend on wage-cost. Average physical productivity of labour and profitability of estates are also relevant in this regard.

10. Term Finance

The growing internal off take calls for substantial increase in tea production in the coming years so that domestic requirements can be met and India's share to world export (28 per cent) is maintained. The basic strategy is to increase the production of tea and improve its quality. To achieve this it is necessary to adopt various short term and medium term measures as explained earlier. Further, tea cultivation has to be extended on a wider scale to non-traditional areas, keeping in view the suitability of climate etc. The process had already been started since 1980 onwards. This would take some time to field result. Along with the increase in production, the existing manufacturing capacity has to be augmented for scientific processing of larger crop. Provision has to be made for renovation and modernisation of tea factories and for construction of new labour houses and ancillary buildings.

Though the major part of the increased output of tea would, no doubt, come from the large estates, socio-economic considerations necessitate special efforts to improve productivity and income of the existing large number of small units which are commonly called family gardens. As regards the small planter, it is necessary to provide technical and financial support to them by adopting a cluster approach. Besides construction of modern tea factories in the cooperative sector, establishment of colonal multiplication centres for supply of improved planting materials and setting up demonstration plots are other activities which are required to be taken up in the interest of small tea planters.

11. Development and Finance - Tea Board

To meet the above resources, the industry would call for substantial support from the existing institutional set up comprising the Tea Board, the National Bank for Agricultural and Rural Development (known as National Bank), the Industrial Development Bank of India (IDBI) and others.

The Tea Board implements various development schemes for increasing production, productivity and quality of tea in India. The particulars of the development schemes implemented during the year 1999-2000 under report are noted below. Briefly, the position with regard to financial outlay sanctioned by the Government *vis-a-vis* the disbursement made during the year was as under:

Table 1.14: Financial Outlay & Disbursement.

(Rs. in lakhs)

	Fund Component	Outlay Sanctioned	Funds Disbursed
1.	Loan Schemes	1000*	1034.11
2.	Subsidy Schemes	1000	1025.09
3.	Grant-in-Aid for R & D Scheme	700	749.08
	Total	2700	2808.28

**Internal accrual Source-Tea Board Kolkata, Annual Report*

The period under report marks the completion of Third year of the 9th Five-Year Plan period. The summary particulars of actual funds disbursed during the first three years of the plan period are shown in the Table below:

Table 1.15: Utilisation of Plan Funds during first 3 (three) years of 9th plan period.

(Rs. in crores)

1999-00	10.34	10.25	7.49	28.08
1998-99	11.59	10.08	7.56	29.23
1997-98	12.38	8.88	4.26	25.52
Total	34.31	29.21	19.31	82.83
Approved outlay for 9th Plan period	50.00	47.00	33.00	130.00
Utilisation during the first years of 9th Plan period	68.62%	62.14%	58.51%	63.71%

Scheme-wise disbursement during first years of 9th Plan period is given in Annexure-IV.

Sanctions accorded by the Development Committee/ Board during the year 1999-2000.

Loan Schemes

During the year, sanction was accorded for a sum of Rs. 11.11 crores as loan for the following three major activities :

Rs. in lakhs

1.	Extensions and replantation under Plantation Development Scheme	227.00
2.	Irrigation under Plantation Development Scheme	382.60
3.	Tea processing and packaging machinery under Tea Processing and Packaging Development Scheme	501.70
	Total	1111.30

Other Sanctions/Approvals & Important Decisions taken by the Board during 1999-2000

i. Inclusion of southern districts of Tripura for financial assistance under the Board's Tea Development Scheme for North Eastern States for control of Jhum cultivation.

ii. The Board approved organising productivity seminars in Assam in collaboration with Indian Institute of Plantation Management, Bangalore, Assam Tea Planters' Association (ATPA) and Tea Board on a cost sharing basis between ATPA and Tea Board.

iii. Setting up of a Task Force to look into production, manufacture, export and R&D needs of Green tea.

iv. Opening up of an office of the Board in Itanagar, Arunachal Pradesh with an estimated outlay of Rs. 3.00 lakhs.

v. Based on the recommendation of a Technical Committee set up by the Board to review the usefulness of Tea Area Rejuvenation Pruning and Infilling with or without Interplanting, the Board approved continuation of the scheme during the 9th Plan period and affected minor modifications in maximum pruning height from ground level as under :

For Infilling - 20" for Assam/Assam hybrid and 14" for China/ China hybrid.

For Interplanting - 18" for Assam/Assam hybrid and 12" for China/China hybrid.

vi. Sanctioned Rs. 7.00 lakhs for purchase of a mini bus by Assam Agricultural University, Jorhat for small growers' advisory service.

vii. Admitted the request of the tea companies for waiving the additional interest and for accepting defaulted outstanding dues with normal interest. During the period under report, nine companies (eleven of cases) settled their outstanding dues in full and an amount of Rs. 16.92 lakhs was waived on account of additional interest.

viii. As per the directives of the Board, the default position of various tea companies was brought to the notice of tea Producers' Associations for settlement of dues.

ix. Approved constitution of a sub-committee for finalising the winners of Tea Board Awards for the year 1998.

x. Approved proposal for new plantation in Kotagiri/Gudalure tribal area under the banner of the Nilgiri Adivasi Welfare Association (NAWA) for financial assistance under the Board's Small Growers' Development Scheme.

xi. Admitted withdrawing the aspect of verification of Tea Marketing Control Order, 1984 in compliance with respect to all applications under the Development Schemes of the Board.

xii. Accorded ex-post facto sanction for a sum of Rs. 6.58 lakhs towards setting up of 14 demonstration plots covering an area of 5.6 hectares by M/s. Tripura Tea Development Corporation.

xiii. Accorded ex-post facto sanction of Rs. 14.10 lakhs for the Trade Information Centre in Mumbai.

xiv. Sanctioned Rs. 20.00 lakhs for 10 lakh strength nursery to be raised during the year under report by the Department of Industries, Government of Mizoram, for the small growers. Ex-post facto approval for Rs. 10.00 lakhs was also accorded towards reimbursement on account of five lakh plants raised and distributed during 1998-99.

xv. Sanctioned Rs. 11.35 lakhs to Assam Agricultural University for continuation of Small Tea Growers' Advisory programme during 1999-2002.

xvi. Based on the proposal received from the Department of Agriculture, Government of Himachal Pradesh, the Board considered acceptance of applications for rejuvenation pruning and infilling activity from small growers of Himachal Pradesh for grant of subsidy for the same area where rejuvenation has been carried out 20 years back by availing subsidy from Tea Board.

xvii. Accorded approval of fund support to the tune of Rs. 6.00 lakhs to M/s. Indian Institute of Plantation Management, Bangalore for conducting a study on Benchmarking for Indian Tea Industry.

xviii. Approved fund support to the tune of Rs. 32.10 lakhs to UPASI, Coonoor for continuation of Small Tea Growers' Development Scheme involving training, demonstration and nursery activities for the years 2000-01 and 2001-02.

xix. Sanctioned Rs.20.00 lakhs for setting up of a nursery in Keonjhar district of Orissa for distribution of sapling among small growers to be set up by Integrated Tribal Development Agency, Keonjhar as advance against subsidy payable under New Area Development Scheme on completion of planting.

xx. Sanctioned a sum of Rs. 2.40 lakhs for study tour of small growers of South India to Assam tea growing areas, including TRA, Jorhat and Assam Agricultural University.

xxi. The Board approved Rs. 2.43 lakhs to IIPM, Bangalore for conducting an in-depth evaluation study on INCOSERVE, Coonoor.

xxii. Admitted fund support to the tune of Rs. 3.00 lakhs for creating a corpus fund for organizing productivity seminars on regular basis by the Plantation Productivity & Management Council, Assam.

xxiii. Sanctioned Rs.7.00 lakhs for system analysis and preparation of Oracle package of the Finance Branch in Head Office, by M/s SQL Star Limited, Hyderabad.

xxiv. Approved in principle the cost sharing of two-thirds of expenditure of Rs.19.15 lakhs (Rs. 6.38 lakhs being one-third to be borne by UPASI towards capital cost) for setting up of a tea nursery and creation of infrastructure for UPASI Advisory Centre for Karnataka.

xxv. Approved Rs. 10.00 lakhs each during the financial year 2000-01 for setting up of a Small Growers' Development Council and a Specialty Tea Register.

xxvi. Admitted grant of Rs. 6.50 lakhs for meeting one-fourth of budgetary deficit of M/s IIPM, Bangalore.

xxvii. Earmarked Rs. 10.00 lakhs for the financial year 2000-01 towards the scheme of extending incentive for acquiring Quality Assurance Certification in Tea - ISO 9000 and Hazard Analysis on Critical Control Point (HACCP).

1. Nagaland

An action plan for development of tea in Nagaland has been drawn up. The important action points include the following :

a) Setting up of farmers' co-operative societies with the State Government's participation.

b) Arranging training on nursery techniques and new planting.

c) Extension of technical support by TRA.

d) Preparation of a comprehensive project plan for systematic development of tea with appropriate financial backing from various agencies - NABARD, commercial banks, Tea Board, etc.

e) Organisation of a seminar to create awareness amongst the local farmers.

f) Study tour was organized by Tea Board for the farmers of Nagaland to visit Nilgiris.

2. Orissa

A task force has been set up to assist the State Government of Orissa in formulating a scheme for setting up a tea plantation for the benefit of tribal farm families in and around Banspal block of Keonjhar district. Subsequently, the task force met twice in Keonjhar to firm up the proposal and identification of the suitable areas for planting tea.

Accordingly nursery was set up so as to raise the plants locally and to take up planting during June/July, 2001.

3. Purulia (West Bengal)

The project site was visited by a technical team comprising Senior Advisory Officer of TRA and Director of Tea Development from Tea Board. The land is under rehabilitation crops. It is proposed to take up planting during the ensuing monsoon months. Since the nursery set up at Purulia got damaged due to the recent storms it is proposed to set up a nursery at TRA's premises at Nagrakata and transport the plants for planting at Purulia. This would also facilitate the small growers in North Bengal in getting good planting material from TRA.

4. Award Scheme

As the claims received from the gardens for the year 1998 were inadequate, the last date for submitting the claims was extended upto 29th February, 2000. The gardens have been advised to submit their claims for the year 1999 as well, so that the Awards for 1998 and 1999 may be given out at one go. The processing of the application is underway.

5. Visit to Uttaranchal Hills

The Senior Assistant Director of Tea Development from Head Office was deputed to accompany Mr. Arun Kumar Srivastava, Board Member, to visit the tea areas in Kumaon Hills. They visited the various plantation sites from 25th to 29th February 2001. It has been reported that the young tea is faring well and the locally processed (hand made) tea has been found to be of good quality.

6. Management Training Programmes

The following two modules have been finalized in consultation with the Producers' Associations and IIPM, Bangalore and guest faculties from other institutions:

Module-1 : One day seminars on Total Product and Productivity Management held in April 2000 at the following places :

a) Dibrugarh on 24th April 2000;

b) Tinsukia on 25th April 2000;

c) Jorhat on 27th April 2000;

d) Tezpur on 28th April 2000;

Following topics were covered during the seminars :

a. Improved Processing Technology

b. On-line process controls on :

   i) Energy usage

   ii) Quality of tea

c. Garden level improvement strategies

A course fee of Rs. 500/- per participant was levied.

Module-II : Two-day programmes on Human Resource Management held at the following places :

a) Binnaguri on 4-5 April, 2000

b) Terai on 7-8 April, 2000

c) Dibrugarh on 4-5 May, 2000

d) Jorhat on 9-10 May, 2000

e) Tezpur on 11-12 May, 2000

f) Darjeeling

g) Cachar

7) Conferences

i) The Millennium International Conference on Renewable Energy Technologies was held in Chennai on February 9-11, 2000. Considering the importance of renewable energy technologies in the coming years, a sum of Rs. 1 lakh was contributed from the Board. Three officers of the Board were deputed to attend the conference.

ii) India International Millennium Tea Convention was held in New Delhi from March 22-24, 2000. Senior officers of the Board were deputed to attend the convention.

iii) North Bengal University organized a seminar on tea on 12th April, 2000. A sum of Rs. 30,000 was granted towards the seminar expenses to the University.

Development Schemes

During the period under review, the below noted eight new schemes and three old schemes were implemented :

New Schemes of 9th Plan Period

i) Plantation Development Scheme
ii) Tea Processing and Packaging Development Scheme
iii) Tea Development Scheme for North Eastern States for control of Jhumcultivation
iv) New Area Development Scheme
v) Small Grower's Development Scheme
vi) Marketing Development and Export Promotion
vii) Human Resource Development Scheme
viii) Research and Development Scheme

Old Schemes

i) Plantation Finance
ii) Tea Machinery and Irrigation Equipment Loan Scheme
iii) New Tea Unit Finance Scheme
iv) Replantation Subsidy Scheme

Old Schemes which have been Amalgamated with the New Schemes

i) Plantation Finance Scheme, Replantation Subsidy Scheme, Tea Area Rejuvenation Subsidy Scheme and the irrigation component of the Tea Machinery and Loan Scheme have been amalgamated and merged with the new scheme - Plantation Development Scheme. All the applications received under the old schemes are now dealt with under the new scheme if the field activity is found to have been commenced on or after the new scheme came in for implementation.

ii. Tea Machinery Loan Scheme and scheme for setting up of co-operative factories have been merged under the new Processing and Packaing Development Scheme.

iii. New Tea Unit Finance Scheme has been merged under the New Scheme - Tea Development Scheme for North Eastern States for the Control of Jhum Cultivation. Non-traditional areas in other parts of the country are dealt with under the New Area Development Scheme. The loan component of the scheme has been discontinued w.e.f 1st April 1998.

iv. Special Input and Interest Subsidy Scheme for Nilgiris and other schemes operated under the erstwhile development grant schemes have been merged with the new scheme - Small Growers' Development Scheme.

v. Special Area Development Scheme has been merged with the new scheme - New Area Development Scheme.

Old Schemes which have been Discontinued with effect from 1st April 1998

i) Darjeeling Interest Subsidy Scheme.

ii) Interest Subsidy Scheme for Extension Planting.

iii) Interest Subsidy Scheme for Irrigation and Drainage.

The salient features of the above schemes and the particulars of financial support extended through them to the tea industry during the year under report are as under:

1. Plantation Development Scheme

This scheme was introduced in the year 1997-98 by amalgamating erstwhile Plantation Finance Scheme, Replantation Subsidy Scheme and Irrigation component of the Tea Machinery and Irrigation Equipment Loan Scheme. It provides for financial assistance by way of long term loan and subsidy for motivating the tea garden owners in undertaking production oriented field developmental activities covering extension planting, replacement planting, replanting, rejuvenation pruning, infilling and irrigation.

The Activities Supported and the Nature of Assistance Rendered Through this Scheme Include:

	Activity	Nature of Assistance
1.	Extension Planting	Long-term loan @ 80% of unit cost
2.	Replanting/Replacement Planting	Loan plus subsidy@ 25% of unit cost subject to the condition that loan plus subsidy put together would not exceed 80% of the unit cost
3.	Rejuvenation Pruning & Infilling with or without Interplanting	Subsidy only 25% of unit cost
4.	Irrigation	Long-term loan @ 80% of unit cost subject to a ceiling limit of Rs. 50 lakh per garden

The rates of loan are Rs. 1,00,000 and Rs. 1,28,000 per hectare for tea estates in the plains and hills, respectively. In case of an applicant availing subsidy for replanting and replacement planting under the Replantation Subsidy Scheme, the amount of loan shall be reduced to Rs. 69,000 per hectare and Rs.88,000 per hectare for gardens in plains and hills, respectively.

The duration of loan for Extension Planting/Replanting/Replacement Planting would be 15 years and for Irrigation it would be 10 years.

The loan will bear a simple interest as applicable from time to time. A rebate of 3% would be allowed for timely repayment. The security for the loan would be equitable mortgage of the fixed assets of the applicant tea garden. In the case of irrigation equipment, the security is the hypothecation of the irrigation equipment purchased with the loan provided by the Board.

For plantation activities, 50 per cent of the sanctioned loan would be released immediately after sanction for commencement of the planting. The balance 50 per cent would be released only after completion of the planting in the approved area in three to four annual instalments for proper upkeep and maintenance of the planted area. For irrigation equipment, 80 per cent of the unit cost will be released in one instalment.

The main source for funding the loan component of the scheme is the recoveries under the erstwhile Plantation Finance Scheme. As per the directive of the Government, the Board is allowed to utilise the amount recovered from its borrowers and off-set the same against the Board's dues to the Government.

The source of fund, which are used for the purpose of lending, include the following :

i) **The plantation loan instalment repaid by the loanees.** The loan is repayable in eight annual instalments commencing from the 7th anniversary of disbursement of 1st instalment of loan. In the case of irrigation, the loan is repayable in ten annual instalments.

ii) **Interest on the loan paid by the loanees.** The interest is payable at the prescribed rate annually. On the normal interest for plantation loan, 1 per cent deferment is allowed for the first five years. The interest so deferred is covered during the 6th and 7th year along with the normal interest. For irrigation equipment no deferment in interest is allowed. The interest is required to be paid annually along with loan instalment.

iii) **Penal interest and commitment charges.** The loanees are liable to pay additional interest @ 1 per cent per month on the

i) The subsidy per hectare is as under

Subsidy for uprooting and replanting or replacement of old and uneconomic tea sections	Rate per ha. from 08.10.97 to 31.03.98 (Rs. per ha)	Rate per ha. from 01.04.98 (Rs per ha)
Plains	30,200	31,000
Hills other than Darjeeling	37,900	40,000
Darjeeling	45,500	45,000

ii) Tea Area Rejuvenation and Consolidation Activity

	From 08.10.97 to 31.03.98	From 01.04.98
Purpose	**(Rs. per ha.)**	**(Rs. per ha.)**
Rejuvenation pruning and infilling only	12,000	13,000
Rejuvenation, infilling and inter-row planting	16,400	17,000

Rates of subsidy per ha. and the mode of disbursement under Plantation Development Subsidy Scheme since its inception i.e. from 08.10.97.

i) For Uprooting and Replanting : Rs./ha.

	From 01.04.98			From 01.04.98		
	For Replanting			For Replacement Planting		
Instalment	**Plains**	**Hills**	**Darjeeling**	**Hills**	**Plains**	**Darjeeling**
1st	15600	19900	25500	24400	20000	30500
2nd	7300	9000	10000	4500	4500	5000
3rd	7300	9000	10000	4500	5700	5000
4th	—	—	—	4500	—	5000
Total	30200	37900	45500	37900	30200	45500

	From 08.10.97 to 01.04.98			From 08.10.97 to 01.04.98		
	For Replanting			For Replacement Planting		
Instalment	**Plains**	**Hills**	**Darjeeling**	**Hills**	**Plains**	**Darjeeling**
1st	16000	21000	25000	25000	20500	30000
2nd	8000	10000	10000	5000	4500	5000
3rd	7000	9000	10000	5000	6000	5000
4th	—	—	—	5000	—	5000
Total	31000	40000	45000	40000	31000	45000

ii) Tea Area Rejuvenation Pruning & Consolidation Activity.

From 08.10.97 to 01.04.98				
	Big growers		Small growers	
Instalment	**With Infilling**	**With Interplanting**	**With Infilling**	**With Interplanting**
1st	7200	9840	8000	11000
2nd	2400	3280	4000	5400
3rd	2400	3280	—	—
Total	12000	16400	12000	16400

From 01.04.98				
	Big growers		Small growers	
Instalment	With Infilling	With Interplanting	With Infilling	With Interplanting
1st	7800	10200	8500	11500
2nd	2600	3400	4500	5500
3rd	2600	3400	—	—
Total	13000	17000	13000	17000

defaulted dues. The commitment charge is levied, if the loanee fails to draw the second subsequent instalment as per the prescribed schedule of release. The Subsidy for Replanting/ Replacement Planting and Rejuvenation Pruning and Infilling is given only after ensuring completion of the field operation in the area approved by the Board. The subsidy is disbursed in three instalments. The release of each instalment of the loan and subsidy is to be preceded by field inspections either by the Board's field officers and/or by the panel of inspectors drawn from the nominations received from the major Producer Associations.

2. Tea Processing & Packaging Development Scheme

This scheme was introduced in the year 1997-98. It provides for necessary financial assistance to the needy tea gardens/factories for renovating as well as augmenting the processing capabilities, including setting up of new tea factories under co-operative sector, replacement of worn out tea processing machinery in the existing factories, creating facilities for packaging, generation of power required for processing and transport vehicles such as tractors, trailers and light commercial vehicles.

The amount of loan and subsidy disbursed during the first three years of 9th Plan Period under the Scheme is as under

(Rs. in lakhs)

Year	Loan	Subsidy
1997-98	72.89	149.77
1998-99	413.45	300.35
1999-2000	591.73	334. 06
Total	1078. 07	784.18

The Board would extend financial support by way of term loan to procure approved items of tea machinery/equipment, LCV and packaging machinery through the suppliers approved for the purpose by the Board. Eight per cent of the value of the machinery item would be given as loan which is repayable in ten equated annual instalments along with interest.

The rate of interest would be 18 per cent p.a. A rebate of 3 per cent would be allowed for timely repayment.

The maximum loan that can be sanctioned to any tea estate would be limited to Rs. 50 lakh for machinery items and 80 per cent of c.i.f. value plus 80 per cent of import duty subject to the maximum ceiling limit of Rs. 50 lakh for tea packaging/machinery.

In the case of State Corporations or other public sector organizations and co-operatives, the Board's loan for setting up a tea factory for processing green leaves shall be limited to 50 per cent of the cost involved towards plant and machinery. Application for such loan shall be entertained following successful planting of tea in a minimum approved area of 50 hectares. Priority would be given for setting up of co-operative tea factories in the North Eastern non-traditional States during the 9th Plan Period.

The main source of funding the loan component of the scheme is the recoveries under the erstwhile Tea Machinery and Irrigation Equipment Hire Purchase Scheme and Tea Machinery and Irrigation Equipment Loan Schemes. As per the directive of the Government, the Board is allowed to utilise the amount recovered from its borrowers and offset the same against the Board's dues to Government.

The sources of fund which are used for the purpose of lending include the following:

1) **The loan instalments repaid by the loanees.**

   The loan is repayable in ten annual instalments for machinery item and five annual instalments for transport items, like tractor/LCV.

2) **Interest on the loan paid by the loanees.**

   The interest is payable at the prescribed rate annually along with loan instalment.

The amount of loan disbursed during the first three years of 9th Plan Period under the scheme was as under.

(Rs. in lakhs)

Year	Loan
1997-98	46.62
1998-99	435.01
1999-2000	385.47
Total	867.10

3. Tea Development Scheme for North Eastern States for the control of Jhum Cultivation

This Scheme primarily seeks to serve as a vehicle for social transformation in the non-traditional tribal North Eastern States. It aims at weaning away the farmers from the traditional practice of jhuming/shifting cultivation and enthusing them to take up tea cultivation. This not only provides an opportunity for the jhumias to settle permanently in one place and provide them with regular income but also helps in arresting of denudation and degradation of forest wealth in the North Eastern Region.

i) The scheme, which has been introduced from the 9th Five-year Plan i.e. from 8.10.97 in place of erstwhile New Tea Unit Finance Scheme, provides for grant of Subsidy for new planting. The rates of subsidy are given below. The subsidy is paid in two equal instalments. The first instalment of subsidy is payable on completion of planting from own source and 2nd instalment, after 12 months from the date of completion of planting provided the planted area is maintained satisfactorily.

ii) The scheme is applicable to all who, in the opinion of Tea Board, would be in a position to undertake individually or as a group viable project having a minimum area of 200 hectares under tea in a compact block as far as possible so as to sustain a viable tea factory. Individual tea growers are also eligible provided there is reasonable prospect of having sufficient numbers of such units in close proximity so as to sustain a central tea factory which may be set up eventually in the area for processing green leaves from the small holdings. Individual growers, irrespective of the size of the land holding and extent of area, can claim subsidy for the planted area provided there is a tie-up arrangement with a nearby tea factory for sale of green leaves to be harvested from the field.

Rates of Subsidy

	From 8.10.97 to 31. 03.98	From 1. 4.98	For growers holding less than 5 ha.
Instalment	**Rs./ha.**	**Rs./ha.**	
1st	18950	20000	40000
2nd	18950	20000	40000
Total	37900	40000	80000

The total amount of subsidy disbursed during the three years was as under

Year	Subsidy
1997-98	38.52
1998-99	59.58
1999-2000	92.57
Total	190.77

iii) Financial assistance for planting tea is 25 per cent of the unit cost as capital subsidy. Small growers holding less than 5.00 hectares are eligible to receive subsidy at the rate of 50 per cent of the unit cost.

4. New Area Development Scheme

i) This scheme would aim at encouraging setting up of new plantation in the area found to be suitable but remained hitherto unexplored for tea cultivation in the non-traditional tea growing areas other than North Eastern States, viz. Sikkim, Uttar Pradesh, Himachal Pradesh, Orissa and five blocks in Kishanganj district of Bihar, certain isolated pockets hitherto not brought under tea cultivation in the traditional tea growing states such as Kerala, Karnataka and Tamil Nadu.

ii) The scheme, which has been introduced from the 9th year Plan Period i.e. from 8.10.97 in place of erstwhile New Tea Unit Finance Scheme, provides for grant of subsidy for new planting.

The subsidy is payable in two equal instalments. 1st instalment of subsidy is paid on completion of planting and 2nd instalment, after 12 months from the date of completion of planting provided the planted area is maintained satisfactorily.

iii) The Scheme is applicable to all who in the opinion of Tea Board would be in a position to undertake individually or as a group viable project having a minimum area of 200 hectares under tea in a compact block as far as possible so as to sustain a viable tea factory. Individual tea growers are also eligible provided there is reasonable prospect of having sufficient numbers of such units in close proximity so as to sustain a central tea factory which may be set up eventually in the area for processing green leaves from the small holdings. Individual growers, irrespective of the size of the land holding and extent of area, can claim subsidy for the planted area provided there is a tie-up arrangement with a nearby tea factory for sale of green leaves to be harvested from the field.

iv) Financial assistance for planting tea is 25 per cent of the unit cost as capital subsidy.

Rates of Subsidy for New Planting and Mode of Disbursement

Instalment	Rs./ha. (Plains)	Rs./ha. (Hills)
1st	13800	16800
2nd	9200	11200
Total	23000	28000

The total amount of subsidy disbursed during the first three years of the 9th Plant was as under

Year	Subsidy
1997-98	18.10
1998-99	21.50
1999-2000	29.84
Total	69.44

5. Small Growers Development Scheme

This scheme provides for a comprehensive developmental package for the overall development of the small growers sector which would include subsidy for new planting, imparting training on modern aspects of tea cultivation and manufacture, supply of planting materials and other inputs at subsidised cost, orgainsing study tours, field advisory visits, etc.

- Through the scheme, during the 9th Plan, it is proposed to provide capital subsidy at the rate of 25 per cent of the unit cost for taking up new planting by the growers in their holdings, the size of which shall be less than 10.12 hectares.
- In order to ensure the availability of good quality planting material in the areas of small growers' concentration, tie-up arrangement would be made for setting up of tea nurseries through nodal agencies like State Government departments, agricultural universities, voluntary organisations and private entrepreneurs.
- One of the major reasons attributed for the lower productivity in small tea gardens is the adoption of outmoded cultural practices. In order to make the small growers aware of the benefits of adopting improved cultural practices, demonstration plots would be laid out in the important areas of small growers' concentration in collaboration with UPASI TRI in South India and CSIR in Himachal Pradesh (Palampur), Assam Agricultural University in Assam.
- For imparting training to small growers on modern aspects of tea growing and manufacture, it is proposed to strengthen the training centre and a mini tea factory, already functioning at Coonoor, for the South Indian farmers and set up a new centre in Assam in collaboration with Assam Agricultural University for the farmers

Rates of Subsidy & Mocs of Disbursement

Instalment	Year	Subsidy Disbursed
1st	13800	16800
2nd	9200	11200
Total	23000	28000

of North Eastern India. The training centres will have facilities to organize several on-campus as well as off-campus training programmes for the various sections of the small growers' community.

- Keeping with the adage that seeing is believing, it is proposed to organize several study tours for the small farmers to visit various tea growing regions of the country

6. Marketing Development and Export Promotion Scheme

This scheme would cover market research survey, uninational campaign for Indian tea in selected markets, brand promotion support to Indian companies for launching the brands in the international markets, generic campaign for tea in new markets and setting up of an umbrella unit in India to meet the requirements of product and packaging standards in international market.

Based on the aforesaid objectives, the activities to be undertaken during the 9th Plan Period have been grouped broadly into two categories :

i. Activities which will be conducted entirely by Tea Board and

ii. Where the Boards' support would be provided to Indian exporting companies/organisations in their Export Promotion and Market Research work.

a) The activities to be conducted by the Board are as under:

i. Commissioning market research surveys to buildup market information and data bank, brand position, competitiors, strategy, growth of new/innovation on tea based products, etc.

ii. Uninational campaign for restoring the position of Indian tea in select markets where our Indian teas are/have been taken over by other suppliers (like UK, Ireland, Egypt, Russia, Poland) five target markets.

iii. Uninational campaign for improving the position of Indian tea in major markets where positive trends are noticed while India's share is not high (like USA, Canada, Germany, Saudi Arabia, Morocco, Japan, Pakistan)-seven target markets.

iv. Exchange visits of delegations to and from India and holding buyer-Seller meets.

v. To set up India Tea Pavilion in major/specialised international fairs where selected major exporters would also be invited to participate.

vi. Production of publicity materials for trade and consumer education in various international languages, including films, audio visual aids, gift items, publicity literature, posters, etc.

b) Assistance to Indian Exporters

i. Lending support to association/consortium of exporters for conducting specific market research in new and potential markets limiting the Board's support to 50 per cent of projected cost with a ceiling of Rs. 10.00 lakh in each project.

ii. To provide brand promotion support to Indian exporting companies towards promotion/marketing cost based on a 3-year programme of the company, with the Board's share of cost restricted to 50 per cent of the company's projected cost, limited to Rs. 2.00 crore for each programme.

iii. To support exporting companies in their independent participation in fairs/exhibitions. Financial support limited to Rs. 1 lakh to each beneficiary.

iv. Assisting the companies in preparation of publicity materials, product literature, etc. (50 per cent of cost limited to Rs. 5 lakh to each beneficiary).

v. Providing assistance to Indian Institute of Packaging for research and field test of tea packaging material both for bulk and consumer packaging, in compliance with international parameters on such packaging, bar coding, etc.

vi. To support organizations/consortium of companies to set up umbrella packaging unit with the Board's assistance one unit each for North India and South India.

The total amount of subsidy disbursed during the first three years of the 9th Plan was as under

(Rs. in lakhs)

Year	Subsidy Disbursed
1997-98	65.00
1998-99	347.04
1999-2000	365.06
Total	777.10

vii. Assisting Indian exporting companies for import/installation of modern machineries on packet tea, tea bag, ready-to-drink manufacture, etc. (limited to 33 per cent of machine cost).

7. Human Resource Development Scheme

This scheme aims at development of human resources for efficient working of the tea producing units. It would, during the 9th Plan Period, seek to:

Strengthen

- Indian Institute of Plantation Management, Bangalore
- Training Centre for Small Growers and Manufacturers
- Comprehensive Labour Welfare Schemes implemented by ITA & UPASI and imparting technical training by TRA and UPASI TRI

The total amount of subsidy disbursed under HRD Scheme during the first three years of the 9th Plan was as under

(Rs. in lakhs)

Year	Subsidy Disbursed
1997-98	7.52
1998-99	17.95
1999-2000	18.03
Total	43.50

The Scheme will be executed through the following agencies:

a. Indian Institute of Plantation Management
b. Indian Tea Association
c. Tea Research Association (TRA)
d. UPASI Tea Research Institute
e. Tea Board

8. Research and Development Scheme

Research would cover :

i. Agricultural and agronomical aspects, including biotechnology.
ii. Integrated pest management and plant protection measures.
iii. Manufacture and quality improvement
iv. Upgradation in nutrition management and use of micronutrients
v. Exploration of use of bio-control and bio-fertilisers for enhancing productivity and soil health.

The total amount of subsidy disbursed during the first three years of the 9th Plan was as under

(Rs. in lakhs)

Year	Subsidy Disbursed
1997-98	426.00
1998-99	756.49
1999-2000	749.08
Total	1931.57

Would also cover :

i. Strengthening of extension services and technology transfer to tea growers and manufacturers
ii. Setting up of Trade Information Centre
iii. Computerization of activities of Tea Board

Old Schemes

1. Tea Plantation Finance Scheme

This scheme was introduced in the year 1962-63 for advancing term loan to tea estates for undertaking replanting, replacement planting and/or extension planting. Since inception of the scheme, the Board has drawn a total amount of Rs. 18.63 crore as loan from Government as on 31. 3.98.

In addition to the loan drawn from Government, the other sources of fund which were used for the purpose of lending included the following:

i) *The plantation loan instalment repaid by the loanees.* The loan is repayable in eight annual instalments commencing from the seventh anniversary of disbursement of first instalment of loan.

ii) *Interest on the loan paid by the loanees.* The interest is payable at the prescribed rate annually. On the normal interest for plantation loan, 1 per cent deferment in allowed for the first five years. The interest so deferred is covered during the sixth and seventh years along with the normal interest. The interest is required to be paid annually along with loan instalment.

iii) *Penal interest and commitment charges.* The loanees are liable to pay additional interest @ 1 per cent per month on the defaulted dues. The commitment charge is levied, if the loanee fails to draw the second subsequent instalment as per the prescribed schedule of release.

During the year 1999-2000 no repayment has been made to the Government against the outstanding loan. In lieu of it, in line with the directive of the Government, a sum of Rs. 1.42 crores towards

The amount of loan disbursed during the first three years of the 9th Plan Period is as under

(Rs. in lakhs)

Year	Subsidy Disbursed
1997-98	279.97
1998-99	137.85
1999-2000	56.91
Total	474.73

interest and Rs.0.45 crores towards principal were transferred to the Tea Board Tea Fund Loan Account, for implementation of Plantation Development Scheme. With this book adjustment the total remittance made to the Government so far adds upto Rs. 7.16 crore towards principal and Rs. 11.89 crore towards interest.

During the year 1999-2000, a sum of Rs.0.57 crores was disbursed. This brings the total loan disbursed since inception of the scheme to Rs.27.44 crores. The total extent of area planted out with financial support under the scheme since its inception is 14863.89 hectares.

This scheme has since been merged with the Plantation Development Scheme which came into operation w.e.f the first year of the 9th Plan Period i.e. 1997-98. However, in order to honour the past commitments, it has become necessary to continue with the scheme for some more time till the entire past commitment is discharged.

2. Tea Machinery and Irrigation Equipment Scheme

This scheme was introduced in the year 1960. It provided for advancement of loan to tea estates/tea factories to acquire tea machineries, irrigation equipment and tractors on deferred payment basis (hire purchases) for replacing old and worn out tea machineries and creating transport and irrigation facilities. In May 1980, the scheme was enlarged to include, imported tea packeting/bagging machineries for facilitating value addition. With effect from 1st April 1995, this scheme, was converted into loan scheme. From 1997-98, this Scheme was merged with the New Scheme - Tea Processing

The amount of loan disbursed during the first three years of the 9th Plan Period was as under

(Rs. in lakhs)

Year	Subsidy Disbursed
1997-98	772.08
1998-99	172.50
1999-2000	-
Total	944.85

and Packaging Development Scheme. The amount recovered from the hirers/loanees under the scheme on account of the loans advanced upto the period ending 31st March, 2000 would be transferred to the Tea Processing and Packaging Development Scheme. During 1999-2000 the recovery (Principal & Interest) was Rs. 2.32 crore. During the period under report no payment has been made to the Government against the outstanding loan. In lieu of it's in the line of the directive of the Government, a sum of Rs. 2.48 crores was transferred to 'Tea Board Tea Fund Loan Account' for implementation of Tea Packaging & Processing Development Scheme.

3. New Tea Unit Finance Scheme for non-traditional areas

This scheme was introduced in the year 1982-83. It provided for financial assistance by way of long term loan and capital subsidy for setting up new tea plantations in the non-traditional areas. The areas declared as non-traditional for the purpose of the scheme include Arunachal Pradesh, Manipur, Meghalaya, Mizoram, Nagaland, Orissa, Sikkim, Garhwal and Kumaon Hills in Uttaranchal, non-tea growing areas in the districts of Idukki and Wynaad in Kerala, Kodagu district in Karnataka, Kodaikanal and Annamalais in Tamil Nadu, N.C. Hills and Karbi Anglong district of Assam, southern districts in Tripura and Mandi and Chamba districts of Himachal Pradesh.

During the year 1995-96, the rates of loan and subsidy were revised and were made applicable to all cases where planting had been undertaken on or after 1.10.94. During the year under report the rate of loan was Rs. 63,200 per hectare and subsidy Rs. 37,900 per hectare. The entrepreneurs were required to invest @ Rs. 25,000 per hectare. While the scheme envisaged grant of loan and subsidy for a comprehensive tea project of at least 200.00 hectares with a provision for setting up of a tea manufacturing unit, the scheme also provided for subsidy to small farmers taking up planting with their own resources upto 50 hectare provided they were registered with Tea Board and entered into a tie-up arrangement with a nearby tea manufacturing unit for sale of green leaves.

Particulars of area brought under tea and the fund disbursed since inception of the scheme are given below

A. Big Growers

(Rs. in lakhs)

States	Proposed area in Hect.	Sanctioned area in Hect.	Planted area in Hect.	Amount disbursed	
				Loan	Subsidy
Arunachal Pradesh	2421.00	1567.92	968.57	418.47	218.92
Manipur	425.00	357. 00	233. 03	99.80	42.51
Nagaland	621.51	97.42	13.42	12.18	1.14
Kerala	170. 00	170. 00	151.36	56. 00	32.14
Orissa	775. 00	210. 00	210. 00	52.50	31.50
Tamil Nadu	3000. 00	1500. 00	988. 00	395.20	244.62
N.C. Hills (Assam)	800. 00	200. 00	200. 00	80. 00	50. 00
Total	8212.51	4102.34	2764.38	1114.15	620.83

B. Small Growers

(Rs. in lakhs)

States	Proposed area in Hect.	Sanctioned area in Hect.	Planted area in Hect.	Amount disbursed	
				Loan	Subsidy
N.E.India and S.India	1818.10	1297.46	1297.46	—	171.68
Grant Total (A + B)	10050.10	5399.80	4061.84	1114.15	792.51

In the 9th Five Year Plan starting from 1997-98, the loan component of the scheme had been dispensed with. Therefore, any application received after 1.4.97 was eligible for subsidy component only. The applications received prior to 1.4.97, however, continued to receive both loan and subsidy under the scheme.

The loan is recovered in eight annual instalments commencing from

i) Replantation Subsidy Scheme

(Rs. per hect)

Subsidy for uprooting and replanting or replacement of old and uneconomic tea sections	Rates of Subsidy
Plains	30,200 (10,400)
Hills other than Darjeeling	37,900 (12,400)
Darjeeling	45,500 (15,000)

i) Tea Area Rejuvenation and Consolidation Subsidy Scheme

(Rs. per hect)

Rejuvenation Pruning and Infilling only	12,400 (3000)
Rejuvenation, Infilling and Inter-planting	16,600 (4000)

Figures in brackets are pre-revised rates.

the seventh year after disbursement of the first instalment of loan. Thus, a moratorium of six years is allowed towards principal. The interest on the outstanding loan is waived for the first three years. The interest is payable from the fourth year onwards.

This scheme has been merged with the new schemes - Tea Development Scheme for North Eastern States for control of jhum Cultivation and New Area Development Scheme for covering the non-traditional areas other than the North East. In order to honour the sanctions accorded earlier, it has become necessary to continue with the scheme for some more time.

4. Tea Replantation and Rejuvenation and Consolidation Subsidy Schemes

These schemes were introduced in the year 1968 and 1975 respectively. The rates of subsidy were revised during the year 1995-96. The rates of subsidy during the year under report were as follows:

During the year 1987-88, the Replantation Subsidy Scheme was enlarged to include no or minimum tillage replantation and progressive replantation with no or minimum tillage for tea estates in South India.

The total amount of subsidy disbursed during the first three years of 9th Plan Period was as under

(Rs. in lakhs)

Year	Subsidy Disbursed
1997-98	382.09
1998-99	133.16
1999-2000	84.77
Total	600.02

Rates of subsidy per hectare and the mode of disbursement under Replantating Subsidy Scheme since its inception in 1968

From 1968 to 1971-72			From 1972 to 1978-79		From April 1979 to August 1980	
Instalment	**Plains**	**Hills**	**Plains**	**Hills**	**Plains**	**Hills**
1st	1500	1800	1800	2100	3000	3400
2nd	1100	1200	1200	1300	500	800
3rd	400	500	500	600	500	800
4th	400	500	400	500	—	—
5th	100	400	100	400	—	—
6th	—	100	—	100	—	—
Total	3500	4500	4000	5000	4000	5000

1. **For uprooting and Replanting (Rs. per hect.)**

From Sept. 1980 to Sept. 1994 for replanting				From Sept. 1980 to Sept. 1994 for replacement planting		
Instalment	**Plains**	**Hills**	**Darjeeling**	**Plains**	**Hills**	**Darjeeling**
1st	5400	6400	8000	6400	8800	10800
2nd	2500	3000	3500	1000	1200	1400
3rd	2500	3000	3500	1000	1200	1400
4th	—	—	—	2000	1200	1400
Total	10400	12400	15000	10400	12400	15000

2. Tea Area Rejuvenation Pruning & Consolidation Subsidy Scheme from 1975 to Sept 1994

	Big Growers		Small Growers	
Instalment	**With infilling**	**With interplanting**	**With infilling**	**With interplanting**
1st	1200	1600	2400	3200
2nd	1200	1600	600	800
3rd	600	800	—	—
Total	3000	4000	3000	4000

From October 1994

	Big Growers		Small Growers	
Instalment	**With infilling**	**With interplanting**	**With infilling**	**With interplanting**
1st	4800	6560	8000	11000
2nd	4800	6560	4000	5400
3rd	2400	3280	—	—
Total	12000	16400	12000	16400

The Rejuvenation Pruning and Consolidation Subsidy Scheme, which was applicable only to the tea gardens of South India, Darjreeling Hills, Himachal Pradesh, Tripura, Hills of Uttar Pradesh and Tillah areas of Cachar has since been extended to the plain gardens of North Bengal and Assam vide Government Order No. T-17015/1/92 Plant A dated 6.12.95 enlarging the scope of the scheme to a great extent.

The activities of replantation and rejuvenation have been merged with Plantation Development Scheme introduced from the 9th Five Year Plan, Keeping in view the past commitments, the scheme was continued during the year under report.

Other Development Activities

During the period under report, several developmental activities have been undertaken for the benefit of small tea growers. Besides direct assistance by way of subsidy for replantation and rejuvenation, grant-in-aid was provided to various nodal agencies for implementing the development schemes on behalf of the Board. These agencies included.

- UPASI Tea Advisory Service, Coonoor - for the small tea growers in South India
- Assam Agricultural University - for the small tea growers in North East India

The North Eastern States account for 55 per cent of all India tea area and 53 per cent of total production as shown below

Table-1.16 : Area and Production

Name of the State		Area under tea (ha)	Production (m. kg)
1.	Assam	230978	462.78
2.	Tripura	6100	7.17
3.	Manipur	400	0.08
4.	Arunachal Pradesh	2000	0.95
5.	Nagaland	456	0. 03
6.	Meghalaya	267	-
7.	Mizoram	400	-
8.	Sikkim	172	0.12
Total for N.E.		240773	471.13
All India		436057	870.40
% Share of N.E.		55.22	54.12

- Himachal Pradesh Krishi Vishvavidyalaya
- CSIR, Palampur - for the small tea growers in Himachal Pradesh and
- Various State Government Agencies- for the small tea growers in non-traditional States such as Arunachal Pradesh, Mizoram, Manipur, Meghalaya, Nagaland, Sikkim and Tripura.

Financial Assistance extended to North Eastern Region

A brief note on the activities undertaken & financial assistance extended to North Eastern Region are given below :

The Boards' activities for which the financial support is being extended through the Plan Schemes include :

- Extension of tea area in all the non-traditional North Eastern States.
- Replanting of old and uneconomical sections.
- Rejuvenation & consolidation of existing tea areas.

The funds disbursed and the activities supported during the last three financial years are shown below

Table 1.17 : Activities supported and financial assistance extended during last three financial years 1997-98 to 1999-2000.

(Rs. in lakhs)

	Purpose	Amount disbursed	Amount disbursed	Amount disbursed
		1997-98	1998-99	1999-2000
1.	Extension of tea area	101.89	131.68	176.66
2.	Replanting/rejuvenation & infilling	260.21	295.11	193.46
3.	Small growers development	89.14	99.43	138.01
4.	Irrigation facilities	178.60	76.56	164.10
5.	Machinery items	246.50	293.93	189.55
6.	Grant-in-aid to TRA/AAU/Others	221.27	576.69	611.32
Total for North East		1097.61	1473.40	1473.10
Total for All India		2551.68	2923.79	2828.10
% for the N.E. out of the total disbursement		43%	50%	52%

- Improvement of the quality through replacement of old and worn out tea machinery.
- Creating irrigation facilities in the tea gardens.
- Extending advisory services to the small growers through the Assam Agricultural University.
- R&D support to the big gardens through TRA.
- Organising management training programmes for the plantation managers through Indian Institute of Plantation Management.

- Organising study tours for the small farmers from North East to visit small tea gardens in Nilgiris.
- Organising training programmes on modern aspects of tea growing for the small growers through TRA.
- Setting up of tea nurseries for the supply of planting materials to the small tea growers.

Finance

The primary source of revenue of the Board is the proceeds of a cess levied and collected by Central Excise Department on all teas made in the country in terms of provision contained in Section 26 of the Tea Act. The rate of cess has been enhanced with effect from 1st April, 1997. At present, the rate of cess charged on Darjeeling and other than Darjeeling varieties of made teas are @ Re. 0.12 per kg and Re. 0.30 per kg, respectively, in terms of the provision contained in Section 25 of the Tea Act. The other major sources of sustenance of the Board are grants, subsidy and loan released to it by the Government of India under Section 26A of the said Act. The Board has also some other minor sources of revenue such as fees on licenses, interest on loans and advances and miscellaneous receipts such as sale of liquid tea, sale of green leaves, gain in foreign exchange, sale of application forms and other publications, etc. All the proceeds of cess, grants, subsidy and loans are accounted for as receipts into the Consolidated Fund of India by the Government and subsequently appropriated with the approval of Parliament and then apportioned to the Board by its administrative ministry, viz. Ministry of Commerce. In other words, all funds available to the Board under Section 26 and 26A of the Tea Act are routed through the medium of the Annual Union Budget. Such funds are then applied to the functions of the Board enshrined in Section 10 of the Tea Act subject to the delegation of financial powers of the Government and/or under the provisions of the Act and subordinate legislation thereto. The Budget of the Board comprises of two constituent elements, viz., Cess and Plan.

3.1 Cess Proceeds

The estimated collection of cess during the year under review was Rs. 2698 lakh. The total amount released by the Government during the year 1999-2000 was Rs. 1350 lakh under Section 26 of the Tea Act.

Plan Proceeds

The same constitutes the following :

Receipts during the year 1999-2000 under different heads were as under

A. Receipts - Cess

Rs. in lakhs

1.	Money received under Section 26 of the Tea Act	1350.00
2.	Fees realised on account of licences/permits, etc. issued by the Board	1.03
3.	Miscellaneous receipts (including sale of green leaves, sale of liquid tea, gain in foreign exchange, etc.)	46.78
4.	Interest on advances and loans	1.80
	Total	1399.61

Expenditure during the year 1999-2000 were as under

B. Expenditure - Cess

1.	Administration, including Library	751.46
2.	Tea Promotion in India	101.55
3.	Tea Promotion outside India	234.04
4.	Labour Welfare	10.17
5.	Pension	275.03
6.	Works	1.49
7.	Housing Scheme for officers and staff	9.28
8.	Advance to employees (Net)	23.81
9.	Other payment	8.72
10.	Transferred to Market Development & Export Promotion Scheme	267.47
	Total	1683.02

C. Expenditure - Research & Development Grants - Plan

Rs. in lakhs

	Rs. in lakhs
Research and Development	773.58

D. Expenditure - Plan Loan

Rs. in lakhs

1.	Tea Plantation Finance Scheme	56.91
2.	Hire Purchase/TM & IE Loan Scheme	–
3.	Tea Board Tea Development (Loan) Scheme	591.72
4.	Tea Processing & Packaging Development (Loan) Scheme	385.47
Total		1034.10

E. Expenditure - Plan Subsidy

Rs. in lakhs

1.	Replantation Subsidy Scheme	84.65
2.	New Tea Unit Finance Scheme	–
3.	Darjeeling Interest Subsidy Scheme	–
4.	Small Growers' Development Scheme	100.32
5.	New Area Development Scheme	29.80
6.	Tea Development Scheme for the North Eastern States for Control of Jhum Cultivation	92.52
7.	Human Resource Development Scheme	18.01
8.	Market Development & Export Promotion Scheme	316.39
9.	Plantation Development Scheme	333.68
10.	Special Area Development Scheme	1.16
Total		976.53
Total of C + D + E		2784.21

Source : 46th Annual Report 1999-2000, Tea Board

3.3 R & D Grants

During the year 1999-2000, a sum of Rs.747.83 lakh was received from Government towards Research and Development Grants for old and ongoing schemes and new schemes under Section 26A of the Tea Act.

3.4 Subsidy

A sum of Rs. 1000 lakh was received by way of adjustment of opening balance of Rs. 20.39 lakh during the year under Section 26A of the Tea Act.

3.5 Loans

During the year under review, no amount was released by the Government under Section 26A of the Tea Act towards loans since the Computerisation

Computerisation

During the year under review, the Board has taken a positive step for computerisation of its activities of the Finance Branch. The work is now in progress and it is expected that full computerization of the activities of Finance Branch will be implemented from the next financial year, i.e. 2000-2001.

Role of Development Banks in Promotion of Tea Industry

Every morning almost all Indians take a hot cup of tea but how many would pause over a sip and think of crores of rupees rolling around the big tea business. Recently, one might have read about one kg of Assam Orthodox tea fetching Rs. 1500 in the German market. Tea not only has vast domestic demand but also have very ambitious potentials for expansion in foreign market. Even the industrialists like Tata has not forgotten to reap rich profits from tea. Tea is a highly expensive investment due to long gestation period for commercial exploitation as well as heavy overheads required for processing and marketing. This expensiveness entails need for large credit inputs and that is where the financial institutes come into play in a big way to extend credit to tea industry. There are a number of on-going schemes in Assam and North-East India with refinance support of national banks.

Introduction of Tea Plantation in Non-tradation Area-A Fresh momentum

Introducing tea plantations in non-traditional areas which include Arunachal Pradesh, Manipur, Meghalaya, Mizoram, Nagaland, Orissa, Sikkim, Garhwal and Kumaon hills in Uttaranchal, non-tea growing areas in the districts of Idukki and Wyanad in Kerala and Kodagu in Karnataka has given fresh momentum. India is the largest producer and exporter of tea. She accounts for one-third of world's tea production and an equal share in world's exports. There are 1,25,220 registered tea estates in the country covering an area of 528250 thousand hectares with an annual production of over 889 million kgs in 2005 North India, which includes Assam, West Bengal, Tripura, Bihar, Uttar Pradesh, Himachal Pradesh, Manipur, Sikkim, Arunachal Pradesh and Nagaland, as per Tea Board, alone produces 660 million kgs representing 75 per cent of total production of tea in the economy and owns 49,500 tea estates with an area of 3,97,450 hectares constituting 80 per cent of total area under tea. Among the various states in North India, Assam and West Bengal produce 455 million kgs and 200 million kgs respectively while other states together contribute nine million kgs. Yield of tea has been worked out to 1670 kgs per hectare which is slightly lower than all India average of 1685 kgs per hectare. It may, however, be mentioned here that production of tea during 2005 has been estimated at 889 million kg, of which North India produces 644 million kgs (76 per cent). Assam, West Bengal and "other states" produce 380 million kgs, 157 million kg and 7 million kgs respectively.

Analysis of data during the last five years showed the fact that area and production of tea increased by equal proportion (5 per cent). Area under tea increased mainly because of establishment of new estates and party operation of New-planting in the form of extension, replacement and re-planting, while production enhanced on account of improvement in yields Tea is one of the highly labour intensive industries. It employes daily 14 lakh workers which account for 11 per cent of total workers employed in private sectors. Majority of workers i.e. 91 per cent are engaged in various operations in field, while a few i.e. 9 per cent are in factory operations. Women workers are generally employed in field operations and male workers, barring a few, are in factory operations. More interesting feature of this industry is that number of bonafide dependents of the resident "workers on roll" has been estimated at 10 lakhs.

All India figure reveal that on and average 1679 kgs of tea per hectare is produced by employing 2.40 number of workers per hectare when production per labour has been worked out to be 700 kgs. In North India, lesser quantum of output per hectare (1722 kg) was realised by developing more number of workers (2.23) per hectare when production per labour is less (734 kgs.). This clearly shows that there is a scope for improving production per hectare and per labour in North India.

North India, on an average, exports 162 million kgs of tea to different countries of the world. This constitutes 30 per cent of the total production. Taking into account the total exports India, North India claims, major share accounting for 80 per cent of total exports. In value terms, North India earns on an average Rs. 581 crore rupees which form 83.35 per cent of total export earnings (Rs 697 crore). The main purchasers of North Indian teas are USSR, UK, UAE, ARE, Afghanistan, Iraq, Iran, West Germany, Yugoslavia, Saudi Arabia, Sudan, Tunisia, Ireland, the Netherlands etc.

Role of National banks for Agriculture and Rural Development (National Bank)

National Bank is actively involved in supporting the promotion of tea industry in general. Besides providing refinance support to financial institutions, National Bank is engaged in project formulation, technical guidance and support for research and development activities for healthy growth of the country.

National Bank provides medium term and long term credit to tea industry for the following purposes:

a) New planting, re-planting, replacement planting, including maintenance expenses upto bearing stages and initial expenses to be incurred for clearing and preparing of land for setting up the plantations and for construction of roads.

b) Vacancy infilling, including maintenance expenses upto bearing stage.

c) Intensive cultivation for mature plantation with less than optimum yield to enhance productivity.

d) Construction of tea factory, purchase and installation of processing machinery, electrification etc.

e) Construction of labours houses and supervisions quarters.

f) Land development and soil conservation measures for new and existing planting.

g) Purchase of neglected estates or virgin lands. It forms part of integrated schemes covering both acquisition if land or estates and its development.

To fulfil the above purpose, the National Bank prepared various models in consultation with the representatives of various tea associations. Tea Research Associations, Tea Board, Tea Producers' and Manufacturers' Association and State Governments. One of the unique models is "financing small tea growers."z

Release on Surplus Land for Cultivation of Tea in Small Holding

Based on release of surplus land from the tea estate for cultivation of tea in small holding by the State Government model scheme for financing small growers has been formulated by the National Bank, This idea was already in vogue in South India and Kenya.

Small Tea Growers-Some Facilities

The scheme pre-supposes that the land allotted would be virgin one in the vicinity of existing tea estates with factories. These estates will purchase the green leaf from the small growers and also provide them with necessary technical guidance in their own interest. The small growers will receive technical guidance in the matter of field management which include (i) selection of planting material, (ii) land preparation, (iii) plant population and planting, (iv) pit-digging, (v) mulching, (vi) pruning, (vii) tipping and plucking, (viii) manuring (young tea and mature tea), (ix) weed control, (x) pest and disease control, (xi) shade tree, (xii) drainage, (xiii) irrigation and (xiv) fencing. All these will help the small growers to keep abreast of the latest development in cultivation and cultural practices in tea. National Bank has prepared a scheme indicating the total cost to be incurred for cultivation of one hectare of tea.

Issues of Small Tea Grower

At the instance of the Governor of Assam, the representatives of the National Bank held discussion with him to explore the possibility of evolving a suitable scheme for accommodating the unemployed youth by ensuring adequate finance and thereby reducing unemployment problem to some extent. It revealed that the problem of unemployment could be tackled to a large extent by encouraging them to take up tea plantation scheme. In the light of the scheme, the National Bank discussed some of the issues like (i) subsidy or margin money, (ii) allotment of land to youths for establishment of tea estates on a long term basis, (iii) credit support etc. National Bank also offered some suggestion on these points. it was suggested that Government Tea Board should provide the subsidy/margin money to youths. It was also suggested that the responsibility of identifying entrepreneurs, guiding them, supervising the implementation of the project, helping in marketing etc., be entrusted to a nodal officer either in industry department of agriculture department of district level. For processing of green leaf a tie-up arrangement with the big estates may be attempted. The existing facilitate available with Assam Tea Corporation will remain. To facilitates the credit flow, National Bank will prepare the banking plan district-wise or state-wise for smooth implementation of the scheme. In the light of the above, National Bank desires state Government's initiatives in formulating suitable action plan and strategy for harvesting the natural resources and channelising the energy/enthusiasm of vast youth resource.

Following the implementation of Tea Board's scheme for providing financial assistance in the form of log term soft loans and capital subsidy for the prospective entrepreneurs to set up new plantation in the non-traditional areas, National Bank has been receiving composite projects for plantation and processing facilities for such areas and tea units have been insisting on sanctioning of loans for the said purpose. Since the two channels of financing the same project are not desirable, the matter was taken up with the Tea Board and Ministry of Commerce, Government of India, to rationalise the system of providing Tea Board loans and subsidy.

The revised system relating to new tea projects in non-traditional areas where bank financing is involved is given below:

a) Tea Board's liability in respect of concerned projects would by quantified and the amount involved, both loan and subsidy, would be placed at the disposal of concerned financing bank. The bank shall work out the financial package as per the schedule jointly agreed to by the Tea Board, financing bank and National Bank.

b) Technical and financial appraisal of such projects would be conducted jointly by them.

c) Necessary arrangements for joint inspection of the works in progress would be made.

d) Documents and operational procedure would be decided jointly by Tea Board and financing bank.

Future strategy of National Bank depends on successful Implementation of these schemes. To do justice, National Bank may ensure timely evaluation of these schemes and narrow down the gap between the anticipated and realised results. This would help in bringing out new light in the system.

The productivity of the tea industry can be increased by bringing more area under extension, replacement, and re-planting (which is about one per cent of total tea area); uprooting of uneconomic bushes; infilling of plants in between the rows; application of fertilisers, pesticides and weedicides in required doses and in time; undertaking scientific methods of pruning; adopting better plucking standard; providing adequate finance through various development schemes; engaging skilled labour; arranging timely internal and external marketing studies and research at micro level may be undertaken by the planters and manufacturers to boost up the productivity of tea industry.

Small Tea Growers

The problems identified by small tea growers are many. Unless the issues are properly addressed, tea cultivation in small batches will not be remuneration. The Techno Economic cell Tea Board concluded a survey of small tea growers in Assam sometimes in first quarter of 2003. The report has been published. The major findings and policies are presented below:

1. Registration of Tea Gardens

Issues:

There are around 5600 small tea growers in 12 districts of Assam, of which only 293 are registered with Tea Board. The main reason for non-registration gardens were absence of patta or ownership title for the land.

Registration of small growers is essentially for identification of units, compilation of area, production and planning programmes to benefit them.

Policy Presciprtions:

The Government of Assam should quicken the process of allotting the vested land to the deserving growers. This may help in getting Tea Board's registration and obtaining financial assistance from Bank and the Tea Board.

Wit the emergence of sizeable number of small tea growers in Assam, the Tea Board's extension service may have to be strengthened by opening a Sub-Regional Office in Dibrugarh.

2. Size of the garden

Issues:

Although the surveyed gardens has ownership titles for the land, but they have not registered with the Tea Board either being unware of the benefits of such registration or due to expenditure involved in preparing survey maps, etc.

The number of growers in Assam would be substantially more than that indicated by the Small Tea Grower's Association.

Small growers in Assam were deprived of the necessary scientific and technical and advice from the Tea Research Association.

Most of the small tea growers did not receive the benefit the training in tea cultivation from recognized institutions like Assam Agricultural University, Tea Research Association and such others did depend on their commonly acquired knowledge on land preparation, cultural practices, selection of planting materials, timely application of inputs like fertilizers, chemicals etc.

Of the total area (341.38 ha), only 40 per cent (138.13 ha.) was utilized for tea and the rest was either under cover of other crops (11 per cent) or lying vacant (49 per cent).

Survey revealed that about 166.13 ha. of additional area was available for tea cultivation among the small gardens. Such land was available as degraded forest and wasteland lying unused or marginal land along the state boundary areas.

Policy Prescriptions:

Besides simplifying the procedure for registration, the small growers have to be enlightened about the desirability of registering their gardens.

The felt need, therefore, is to prepare a small tea growers directory of

Assam indicating the location and name of the owners of small tea gardens.

The Advisory Service of the Tea Research Association to small tea growers may be extended at subsidized rate. Further, All-Assam Small Tea Growers Association may augment in resources to improve and supplement is services.

The Assam Agricultural University may establish a few training centres at suitable locations and organise 'or-campus' and 'off-campus' training programmes for the various sections of these small growers. The Tea Board may consider providing grant-in-aid to Assam Agricultural University for the purpose.

Necessary steps may be initiated for extension of the tea area within the periphery of the garden. The small growers in the districts of Cachar may be motivated to bring more area under tea.

It will be worthwhile for the state to allow such land to small growers for growing tea.

3. Field Practices and Cultural Operations

Issues

The major problems in procuring planting material were distance from source, non-availability of the desired variety, high mortality rates of planting materials, high costs, etc.

None of the sample gardens had artificial irrigation. Almost all the gardens reported non-availability of perennial source of water.

The sample gardens adopted closer spacing and average number of bushes per ha. ranged from 12,000 to 16,000 with renegotiable vacancy level.

The average yields of green leaf per ha. is 3,925 kg. which is estimated at 872 kgs. of made-tea per ha. Such a low average yield rate was on account of sizeable area under tea containing bushes of four years of age group at a non-pluck-able stage.

Small tea growers are facing the problem of procuring essential inputs such fertilizers, weedicides/pesticides, etc. High price inputs, compulsion to purchase in bulk, transport, and irregular availability of material in the retial market were some of the other factors.

Majority of the sample garden, except in Sonipur, adopted seven to ten days plucking rounds while some gardens in Dibrugarh adopted more than ten-day plucking round. Sometimes, young bushes were also plucked for ready hurting the future health of the bushes.

Policy Presciprtions:

Tea Board may set up nurseries and demonstration plots for trail plantations at centralised spaces to supply suitable planting material to small growers and provide knowledge on improved cultural practices. Tea Board may also consider extending the benefit of special input and interest-subsidy scheme in Nilgiri to the non-registered small growers as well.

There is a need to constantly monitor development schemes of the Tea Board as applicable to the small growes vis-a-vis the level of utilization and constraints and operational bottlenecks encountered by them.

A suitable irrigation scheme may be formulated in consultation with State Government. As a short-term measure, the state may consider sinking sufficient number of deep tube wells to meet the immediate irrigation needs of the small growers.

Considering the young age of the bushes coupled with high density, the future of plantation under small growes segment of Assam seems to be promising. necessary assistance may be available from financial institutions. Tea Board, research bodies and state agricultural bodies to compensate for the poor infrastructure and inadequate technical know-how and procedural formalities in obtaining such financial assistance may be simplified as mush as necessary.

Considering the low productivity of poor shape of the economy of the small growers segment, they may be allowed suitable concession in respect of agricultural income tax and tax under Assam Taxation (On Specified Lands) Acts, 1994.

Co-operative efforts may have a positive role in ensuring regular availability of essential inputs at a reasonable prices.

Small growers have to be provided training to build up awareness among them on sound cultural practices and upkeep of bushes.

4. Crop Disposals and Price Reaslisation

Issues

Almost the entire quantity of green leaf plucked by the small growers is sold to the factory owned by the large growes directly or through middlemen. Transport of such green leaf to the factory, which are located more than ten kms, away, reduces the quality of the leaf and thereby the price.

Some growers sold green leaf to the factory based on bilateral agreement. Some used the services of the selling agents, negotiated the price in absence of any agreement. More small growers sold green leaf on the basis of annual agreements, which fetched higher average price than any other made.

Policy Prescriptions

To mitigate the problem of marketing of green leaf, the Tea Board may set up a cooperative tea-processing unit at a suitable place, to ensure a ready market for small tea growers.

Bank loans are generally not available in the absence of standing sale agreement between the buying factory and small growers. Such prior sale contracts were not always possible due to uncertainty of crops and fluctuations in prices. A possible solution could be establishment of a co-operative tea factory.

Conclusion

A planned increase in the countries' tea production and improvement in its quality would need extensive support in the shape of scientific research on tea culture and manufacture and wide application of results of such research. The research efforts have necessarily to be supported by well organised extension services for dissemination of the results of research. All these would necessitate the tempo of current research like tissue culture etc., and advisory work for tea industry. For effective application of the findings of research, it would be necessary to organise suitable technical training course of for persons employed in tea industry as well as for those who opt for a career in tea particularly in the non-traditional area. These proposals got momentum in the eight and ninth Five Year Plans and accordingly National Tea Research Foundation was constituted to look into various aspects of current research on tea.

To fulfill the above development strategy it is needless to say that the tea industry requires huge finance. P.R. SenGupta, ex-secretary, in his article "Tea Board, India on Finance for Development" - A new dynamic approach to (TAI News Letter, Vol 21, No. 5, May 1985) indicated that the industry was required to invest over Rs. 5000 crores up to 2000 AD (1985 onwards) on both capital and revenue account. Based on per year investment of Rs. 333 crores (5,000 ÷ 15) and an escalation of 20 per cent in investment cost for a period of eight years commencing from 1992, the total investment has been estimated at Rs. 3,200 crores (333 x 8 x 1.20) which is required for development finance of the industry.

The economic viability of the tea industry, however, depends on profitability and productivity of tea industry. Profitability depends on realisation on more remunerative prices and reduction in cost of production. Realisation of per kg of tea depends on market forces of demand and supply, Government control over prices and quality of tea. Reduction in (a) cost of inputs - fertilisers, manures, weedicides, fuel and electricity, factory sundaries, repair and renovation of tea machinery and building, packing-material etc. (b) labour cost, (c) head office cost, executive and staff salary, (d) depreciation,

(e) marketing and transport, (f) interest and (g) duties and taxes. Thus, to reduce the cost of production technological improvement both in field and factory operations as well as institutional measures are called for. Technological improvements in field and factory and subsequent redaction in cost are the sole responsibility of the tea estates. The institutional measures viz. taxation, finance and labour, which are of prime importance, can be undertaken by the Government agencies. Both sets of measures are important. The institutional measures create the climate conducive to nursing the industry back to health and technological and operational measures take advantage of improved climate.

Chapter 2
Sustainable Tea Cultivation

This chapter deals with sustainable tea cultivation, which by definition is a method of growing green tea leaves and processing the same for *greater human consumption through maximum utilization of all available resources without polluting environment*. The most important consideration of this type of tea production is to keep all kinds of losses to a minimum. The ultimate aim is to reduce cost of production. All available resources are to be utilised judiciously to meet increasing demand for tea of good liquor and flavour. The quality and quantity both have to be considered while fulfilling the need of increasing population. Presently many developing countries, including India, face problem of inadequate supply of this beverage. Hence, the only alternative is to exploit production. The solution to this problem exists in *modern technology, which should be utilised along with traditional technology in a harmonious way so that tea production may remain sustainable*. This is today's demand. The intensive utilisation of land without conserving soil fertility and soil structure lead to springing up of deserts and, therefore, productivity of land has to be maintained. Tea is a commercial crop in this India. Farmers of the country, especially in North-Eastern India, are willing to switch over to tea from other crops, as soil is suitable for growing tea. Keeping this in view, attempt has been made to include rates of new planting (extension, replacement and replanting), rejuvenation pruning, deep rooting grasses as rehabilitation crop, green crops in young and heavy pruned tea in attainment of sustainable tea production in India.

Opening of wide vistas with the introduction of Exim Scripts

The wide vistas opened up consequent to the introduction of Exim-scripts and the competitiveness that the scheme imparted to tea exports, presented *opportunities as well as challenges*. On the one hand, Indian trade exporter with very little import requirement stood on the threshold of great opportunities but, on the other hand, tea exports had to face necessarily *the pangs of short term dislocation*. Government's growing disenchantment with the gains of bilateral trade mechanism did not wholly satisfy India's requirement of certain vital goods. The tremendous support extended by the government towards lending a sharper edge was exports. In tune with government eagerness to impart greater "automaticity" and "user-friendliness" within the institutional framework of government departments, the Tea Board simplified export-licensing operations. Revolutionary *changes in the political and economic structure of the erstwhile Eastern Bloc countries, which formed the mainstay of Indian exports, rapid dismantling of trade barriers and emergence of an economically integrated Europe in 1992 threw up the imperatives of a reformulated export strategy for Indian tea.* As one learns to do business under the "open" rules being increasingly evident world-wide, competitiveness through quality and price assumes new urgency. With the persistent efforts jointly of industry and government, a high-powered Indian tea delegation visited Europe. This visit was a reflection of government's clear thinking on the need for aggressive promotion. The industry resolves to promote and establish the clear superiority teas. The mission was wholly in tune with the Government of India's conviction in regard to trade policy reform, which is one of the important instruments for restructuring the Indian economy. The delegation impressed upon importing countries that Indian tea export now stand poised for growth consequent to the pronounced policy shift from the hitherto conservative *"residual approach" to one envisaging "production for exports"*.

Pace of Production Growth to be Sustainable

Even if there is slow–down in internal consumption growth the thrust to tea exports that both the government and industry covet will be rendered a non-starter if the industry fails to push ahead with it's job of augmenting production. The *pace of production growth needs to be sustained by consistent and adequate level of resource generation. This is currently impossible under the prevailing taxation structure.*

Notwithstanding the rationalisation of corporate income tax rates, whatever concessions were envisaged by the Centre have been completely negated by the penal taxation rates of the State governments. If tea production growth is really perceived to be in the national interest, the Centre and State governments must address themselves to this problem and affect well conceived tax reforms. *For too long has tea served as the proverbial milch cow for the state exchequers, which have raised their tax rates to unconscionable levels. Besides high rates of agriculture income tax, tea continues to be slapped with plethora of state cesses and duties*. Betraying a pronounced lack of political will to broaden the tax base, State governments have eagerly preyed on the tea industry, lulled perhaps by the transitory improvements in its fortunes. Planning and policy-making at the state level have rarely displayed any concern towards a stable regime and short-sighted fiscal measures on the grounds of revenue expediency continue to undermine competitiveness and growth prospects of this export-oriented sector. It is, therefore, quite in the fitness of things that the tea associations have strongly pursued their taxation proposal in regard to reframing Section 33AB of the Income Tax Act to allow for advance spending on development oriented activities. It is in consonance with the desired export thrust that a change in Section 80HHC of the Income Tax Act which conferred benefits to the producer tea exporter at par with those enjoyed by exporters in the sectors. Given are the Government's clear appreciation of the imperatives and the active support of the Commerce Ministry on these matters.

The Plank of Progress in terms of Business, Trade, Economy or Society etc.

The main plank of progress would be perceived in terms of business, trade, the economy or society and the political milieu in which various activities are conducted. There is no denying that investment will tend to flow more readily to areas which afford it a safe labour and attractive returns. Located as they are in remote areas, tea estates remain particularly vulnerable to socio-political tensions that continue to prevail in the North East. Much against its gain and certainly at variance with its major task – that of tea production – *the tea industry is being called upon to assume roles that are best left to government.* While an enhancement of industrial potential through a more rational tax structure may be identified as the need of the hour, attention must also be focussed on the industry's ability to raise adequate finance to sustain its growth plans. Owing to its ageing asset profile and the predominance of its agro-based operations, asset-valuations, capitalisations and securities for *tea companies have been typically based on historical and written-down values distorting and under-valueing the industry's resource raising potential. The Government and more importantly lending institutions must adopt a more supportive stand to admit revaluation of assets at current* values in so far as loans and their securities are concerned. *Updating of asset values will greatly facilitate the process of modernisation and expansion of the tea industry.* This assumes even greater importance in the North-East States. The tea industry's direct commitment to its own employees continues to receive the highest priority. In keeping with the best of traditions, pay scales of clerical, medical and technical staff and those of the other monthly-rated employees have been amicably negotiated. Negotiations for revision of pay scales for sub-staff grades in gardens reached their ultimate stage and an agreement is now imminent. Notwithstanding the sense of achievement that underlines the amicable working relationship between employer and employee, one *must eventually address the problem of productivity in tea units.* The lingering question remains as to whether managements can retain a strong motive for achieving productivity gains if every gain is appropriated either by the state through taxation or is diverted to higher levels of wages. Tea plantations, in common with the rest of agriculture, are labour intensive and every measure of productivity is concerned with the *volume and kind of labour utilised in the production process.* If rigid conditions are imposed on the kind and level of employment for given types of operations and for size of establishment and flexible use of labour is resisted at every turn, the opportunity for change would be severely limited if not non-existent. While on the subject, one cannot but touch on the vital area of *Employer-Employee relations* is no far as they impinge on the labour laws of our country. It should be appreciated that the relationship is dynamic in character and labour laws themselves must reflect the changing socio-economic scenario in which they operate. There is a growing perception, in the context of the need for improved productivity, that our labour laws suffer from rigidities and offer undue protection to employees irrespective of their performance or conduct during wars. Rationalisation and simplification of labour laws assume importance towards restoring some equity and imparting a degree of discipline necessary to make the "*Made in the India*" label work.

Sustainable Tea Production – Areas of Concern Role of new Planting

The tea industry in India is one of the oldest and well-organized industries and plays an important role in our economy. It has now reached a most significant stage of its development and holds a pride a place in the industrial and trade structure of the country. It accounts for about 10 per cent of country's foreign exchange earnings and contributes about rupees one thousand crore to national economy. Besides, it provides direct and indirect employment to a large section of population and helps in accelerating the growth of ancillary industry. A review of the growth rates of area, yield and production over the past few years indicated the sluggish pace of development of area under tea in India, i.e. at average linear rate of 0.74 per cent per annum during the same period; while yield has increased at a significant average linear rate of 2.24 per cent per annum, and since independence, the consumption of tea in India, the leading tea drinking country in the world, has gained a momentum for its accession in the spectrum of daily beverage for some refreshment and stimulation. Gradually, *the consumption of tea has reached such a level that it has set the industry thinking about a future probably contingency of disharmony and dis-equilibrium in the process of production, export and internal consumption of India tea.* It is difficult to starve our domestic market when our people have got the habit of this drink. Because of the importance of tea in our economy, it will be necessary to know the factors that stand on the way of increase in production.

Effects of Different Componants on the Increase in Tea

In the first place, it should be noted that by adopting a *suitable scheme of decomposition*, the effects of different components like area and yield on the increase in tea over the period were computed. It was observed that the yield effect was the most important force in this regard. *Seventy-two per cent of the total increase in output was accounted for by yield effect.* A look at the relevant statistics reveals that the area under tea in India has increased only from 3,16,000 hectares in 1950 to about 528,250 hectares in 2005. Among the main impediments to the expansion of area under tea is that the required *areas of planted land are just not available* in the traditional tea growing states. Land is no longer *an acquirable asset for a plantation as any reserve of land available in or near a plantation is subject to the land ceiling laws.* Also, lands close to the estates are either *substandard or belong to the near by people or the government.* A considerable portion of the remaining land, which is partially rich, is under government forest. In view of increased demand for forest product, it is very difficult to increase land further to the disadvantage of the tea estates. Another important point is that in the last fifty five years, *the migrants as well as the local encroachers have also grabbed a sizeable area close to the tea estates.* As a result, there is very little space left for expansion. So, future scope for *increasing production through extension of area is limited. Crop intensity is the answer.*

Techno-Institutional Subjects

There are some techno-institutional subjective factors that play a dominant role in not expanding yield rate. Tea is a crop of *high location specificities.* It requires a particular type of agro-climatic condition. Expansion of tea cultivation is inhibited to some extent because of the absence of a specific type of climatic condition. It is true, till now, that the plantation is neither planned nor carried on systematically. As a result, the pace of plantation is not only slow and sluggish, but also freakish. It is true that an expansion of production through replacement, re-plantation and new extension requires heavy investment for deforestation, leveling of land, proper drainage, management for cultivation and other activities. *Because of the ever-increasing cost of production, the rate of profit which the industry is been earning is very low and fast declining.* An analysis of the sources and *uses of funds of tea plantations reveals the inadequate generation of internal resources that can be ploughed back and the industry's excessive dependence on long-term assistance from financial institutions and government grants and subsidies. The industry depended 90 per cent on internal resources and 10 per cent on the external resources in 1950-51* whereas, share of internal resources in financing its economic activities in *2000-05 declined to 4 per cent.* This peculiar situation can be explained in terms of slow flow of *paid up capital and in the declining rate of retained profits – because of rising costs, tax liabilities, increasing amount of money being paid as interest, higher percentage of dividends in profits.* With the low unattractive level of profit, it would be difficult to sustain any sizeable programme of rehabilitation worth the name for a significant period.

Utilisation of Inproper Man Power, Fautly Planning of Layout, Optimum Exploitation of Capital Inputs, Uneconomic Tea Bushes etc.

It should be mentioned that due to *inefficient utilisation of manpowers, faulty planning and layout*, there is under-employment in some gardens. Some redundant *labour is carried on the rolls due to poor management, tradition or any other circumstances*. These planters cannot readily vary such basic inputs as labour, which are more or less fixed. Again, some capital inputs are not used *to the optimum available capacity*. There remains some *excess capacity for some specific and indivisible inputs* maintained on the plantations. Another significant reason for low productivity could be the existence of higher *proportion of old economic bushes of tea*. The main thrust of tea production rests on mature tea bushes. The general view is that tea bushes take five years to start yielding at reasonable economic level but after 50 years, the yield is not economic. In 2005, about 38 per cent of total area in Terai, 79.6 per cent of total area in Darjeeling and 49 per cent of total area under tea in Dooars was occupied by bushes that had outlived their optimum economic life. *They were over-aged, debilitated and obsolete uneconomic bushes*. Again, of late, many of the planters have resorted to only *light pruning*, as this gives quick yield. They also try to increase production by *spraying fertilizers on bushes as this increases yield immediately*. But all these methods have deleterious impact on the life span of the bushes.

These quick profit-yielding strategies should be examined carefully. All in all, there is much of ad hocism in matters of this industry. *A well-knit rehabilitation programme is essential.* Rehabilitation of the used land includes thorough deep ploughing, harrowing, levelling, sub-soiling, rest under a cover crop for at least two years and proper manuring. There is a need for undertaking infilling, replantation and replacement planting. If the unit is retrievable, cost of rehabilitation is smaller than that required for setting up a new unit. A flourishing tea industry would ultimately be a better source of revenue than a languishing one.

Economic Viabaility Depends on Profitability and Productivity etc.

The economic viability of the tea industry depends on it's profitability and productivity. Profitability depends on realisation of more *remunerative prices and reduction in cost of production*. The price realisation per kg of tea depends on market forces of demand and supply, government control over prices and quality of tea. Reduction in cost per kg of tea depends on several components like (a) cost of inputs - fertilizers, manures, wedicides, fuel for vehicle, electricity, factory, repair and renovation of tea machinery, buildings, packing materials, etc; (b) labour cost; (c) head office expenses, executive staff salaries; (d) depreciation; (e) marketing and transport; (f) interest; and (g) duties and taxes. Thus, to reduce the cost of production, technological improvements both in field and factory operations as well as institutional measures are called for. The technological improvements in the field and factory and subsequent reduction of costs are the sole responsibility of tea estates. The institutional measures viz. taxation, finance and labour which are of prime importance, can be undertaken by the government agencies. Both sets of measures are important. *The institutional measures create a climate conducive to nursing the industry back to health and technological and operational measures take advantage of the improved climate.* The productivity of the tea industry can be increased by bringing more area under extension, replacement and replanting, up rooting of un-economic bushes, infilling of plants in between the rows, application of fertilizers, pesticides and weedicides in required doses and in time, undertaking scientific methods of pruning, adopting better plucking, providing adequate finance through various development schemes, engaging skilled labour, arranging timely internal and external marketing, etc. Studies and research at micro level were undertaken to boost up the productivity of the tea industry.

Role of Rejuvenation Pruning - New Thoughts

Rejuvenation pruning is generally not prescribed in June, July or August. During these months, the sun scorch on bare frames is bound to fall. At the time of pruning care must be taken that each bush is left with minimum two lungs. Little purpose is served when these lungs are left on weak branches. A good supervision is required to ensure that the branches on which these lungs are left are healthy. After the growths of about three new leaves, which may start showing in March, these lungs should be pruned with a sharp knife at the level of pruning. Following aspects may be considered while rejuvenation pruning is undertaken :-

- The branches found to be diseased after rejuvenation pruning should be cut back to the point where healthy wood is found in the month of January followed by immediate bitumen painting on the surface of the cut. The frame of the bushes left un-pruned must be cleaned up to remove diseased parts and pests.
- Pruning height of 16 inches, on an average, is considered to be good. However, this may not be strictly followed because removal of knots and disease affected branches are the main job in rejuvenation pruning. The height of pruning must be decided considering this aspect. It is very common to find a few bushes the collars of which are rotted badly. Such bushes should be uprooted.
- A minimum of 80 kgs nitrogen fertiliser per ha with the same quantity of potash should be applied in the year of rejuvenation during spring. The quantity of potash should actually be based on soil' available potash content.
- In the month of January in the second year, the plucking table should be leveled off followed by the judicious pruning after the first half of December. The type of pruning depends entirely on

the condition of bushes and at times instead of pruning, a skiffing may be found useful.

- Shade nursery should be opened two years before undertaking requirement at a spot to meet the requirement of shade infilling. One bush population of the shade plants should be infill at the place which is being rejuvenated. In widely spaced areas, spacing at side may be reduced by half, leaving one vacant space between two plants. Hegde-wise infilling is also quite useful.
- The plants should be healthy with good growth. The job of vacancy infilling may be started around the month of March in the first years, and may be continued till around May. Spacing of 4ft x 4ft or tea plants spaced wider than this should be infilled with double the plants' number.
- Infilling with inter-planting is advantageous for yield and it helps in reducing the recovery period to two-three years. In case of infilling alone, the crop loss consequent to rejuvenation pruning is recovered in four-five years. The in-fills should be examined and established if they may be centred in the month of July during the first year. They may be ready for tipping around September-October at a height of 16-18 inches.
- The plucking table of the in-fills should be brought up to the height of that of the old bushes during second year and this should be done step-wise. In rejuvenated area, tipping allowance over the general level of pruning varies. While it may be kept at 4 inches and 6 inches in cases of China and hybrid bushes, Assam bushes may be tipped at 8 inches. In the second year, the bushes should be plucked at skiffed level and raised around the middle of July.
- On getting new foliage after pruning, YTD mixture with a provision of 90/100 kgs N/ha should be scattered in the first year followed by YTD with a provision of 100 kgs Nitrogen per hectare in February or March of the second year. Based on soil analysis, *heavy potash doses may be given from the third year onwards for a few years.*
- Break all ant-hills and level the ground around February in the first year of rejuvenation. *Fill the depressions wherever found*

and check weeds in the rejuvenated area. While spraying weedicide, it is necessary to be extra careful to protect plants that have been planted to fill the vacancies.

- The areas can neither be uprooted and replanted nor rejuvenated in near future. *These can be replaced with planting on available land. Such replaced section should, however, be uprooted within the fourth year of replacement in case of gardens situated in plains and one more year in case of gardens in hilly areas.*

Role of Deep-rooting Grasses as Rehabilitation Crops

Out of 'Guinea', Pan-goal, 'Weeping Love' 'Elephant' and Guatemala grasses, Guatemala is most popular and useful followed by other grasses Pusa Giant Hybrid Napier. The latter is also a very nutritious food for the cattle. Deep rooting grasses such as Guatemala and Pusa *Giant Hybrid Napier* can be used as rehabilitation crop. *Mimosa invisa legume* is also useful. All these varieties grow quickly. Quite a good amount of organic matter is added to the soil by Guatemala roots and lopping. This native grass of Guatemala can be grown everywhere upto an altitude of about 3,300 feet for mulching and rehabilitating the soil. Moisture storage and good aeration due to improvement in soil structure by Guatemala's deep root system is made possible with the added advantage of nutrients' movement to root's top layer from deep layer. Pusa Giant Hybrid Napier grass can be grown on higher elevation upto an altitude of about 4000 ft for soil rehabilitation and mulch material. Following area is required to be re-looked:-

- *Mimosa invisa can be ussed as a green manure crop.* A thick-layered mulch is expected from it once it is established. One should not worry if it dries out in cold weather, as it re-generates again in spring. The brown seeds germinate well. The germination of yellow seeds is not good. The seeds should be drilled in rows 3.5 ft to 4 ft away from each other. For vigorous growth, some super-phosphate should be drilled in the rows. About 3.5 kg seeds can be sown for propagation in one hectare and re-seeding can easily be done.
- Before the rehabilitation crop is sown, the uprooted areas should *be prepared, levelled up, sub-soiled and provided with drainage.*

Before planting rehabilitation crop, thorough ploughing and proper levelling of soil are necessary to avoid the need of major ploughing and levelling before re-plantation once the rehabilitation crop is raised.

- While planting rehabilitation crop, *the slope of the land should be considered to decide the pattern of planting. Contour planting is required on uneven land having above two per cent slope.* On the other hand, the rehabilitation crop can be put out across the slope if it is within two per cent.
- Two-three noded stem cuttings of Guatemala and Pusa Giant Hybrid Napier grass can be used *for propagation*. Divding the root stocks can also propagate them. Cuttings can be planted ideally on the start of rains at 2ft x 2ft distance by their flat placing in furrows or by sticking them to the soil in such a way that an angle is provided. In latter case, one node should remain above the ground and the other one or two should *be buried*. March, April and May are the months when the rehabilitation crops can be planted or sown. By this time, some rain has already been received. They can be planted in the rains also.
- The soil should be tested and based on the report any of the N P K mixtures 10:5:15: or 10:15:10 may be applied at the time of rehabilitation crop's *plantation for more green matter. The rate of application may be kept at 600 kgs* for one hectare. Guatemala is ready for lopping in about six months time. Lopping should be done at about 12 inches from ground. Further lopping depends upon growth and can normally be done after two or two and a half months.
- In case of Pusa Giant Hybrid Napier Grass, first lopping at about 4-5 inches above ground may be done after about four months and subsequent lopping two months thereafter. After each lopping 300 kgs of 10:5:10 or 10:5:15 NPK mixture per hectare should ideally be applied to replenish the removed nutrients. Before re-plantation, the green crop litters should be mulched after cutting the rehabilitation crop at the level of ground. Guatemala and Pusa Hybrid Napier stumps require uprooting and removal.
- The re-plantation should not be done on when the soil is dry or

when it is very soft immediately after heavy rain. It is better to plant from about the middle of October to the middle of December in areas which are not drought-prone. In drought-prone areas, the period from the middle or last week of April when some rain moistens soil, the month of June is good for planting the grass. With right irrigation, autumn planting may, however, be done in drought areas.

- That *NPK* mixtures are applied to the *pits while planting is known to the planters*. However, for plants with broken *'bhetis' and those grown in sleeves, sterilized animal meal or oil cake should not be utilised* as their immediate contact with roots can kill the tender plants. For better success, robust and healthy plants having a collar diameter of 8 mm and a height of about 18 inches should be used for re-plantation.
- Different clones available are well known to the planting community. It will, however, not be out of place to mention here about the new standard drought tolerant clones TV 27 and 28. The leaf pose of TV 27 is semi-erect while that of TV 28 it is erect. As regards yield, TV 28 has been found to yield more than TV 27 in second and fourth years. But in third year it has been found yield less than TV 27. One the whole, yield-wise TV 28 has on edge over TV 27. Tocklai has released another vigorous and fast growing high yielding clone with average quality the TV 29. Its leaf pose is semi-erect. Excellent rooting and large shoot size are its characteristics.

Role of Green Crops in Young and Heavy Pruned Tea

Green crops are useful in young and heavy pruned tea. The trees and shrubs used for perennial manures are known as green manure plants. They are initially used as cover crops and later the crop or its lopping are either hoed into the soil or mulched to enrich the soil with available nitrogen for increase in fertility. The topsoil helps the ground cover crops in regaining the content of humus and fertility. The roots of young infilling in the rejuvenated area do not take the plant food. Young plants in the replanted area are taken up by ground cover plants retaining that on soil and returning some of it through leaf fall and finally through lopping. Crotalaria Anagyroides is most useful among Crotalarias. It grows rapidly and resists the drought well. Generally, root nematodes do not attack crotalarias. Following prescriptions are made for better growth of young and pruned plants:-

- *Careful control of green manure plants' competition with tea is necessary. Unmonitored green crops may cause Red Rust and Blister Blight. Lopping them is necessary, otherwise the tea growth is depressed and the luxuriant green crop growth misleads.* Unless properly and timely lopped, they cause not only poor flush of tea but the tea also loses its vigor and its upper portion becomes thin as a result of very thick shade.
- Lopping may be done just before *the green manure plants flower* because the lopped portions are richer in nitrogen by that time and there is the added benefit of getting more crop for lopping. The placing of the green crop lopping in one year and two-year old tea should be done near the collars. These loppings during decomposition generate heat and to avoid bark damage the placement of lopping should be about three inches away from the collars during the rains.
- *Normal pruning cycles*, based on different factors in individual gardens, *can be adopted in case of replanted teas also*. It may, however, be mentioned here that considering crop as well as the thickness of the wood, the replanted tea may be given the cycle of CA: DS: UP or CA: UP: DS. CA: UP: DS gives more yield compared to CA: DS: UP. Basically, wood thickness should be the main criterion in deciding a pruning cycle, which should be shorter in case of vigorous sections and longer in case of weak sections. The policy of the company is also considered while deciding a pruning cycle.
- *In replanted tea, Red Rust on young plants* should be watched and *timely treatment must be given*. As a matter of fact, it should be taken more as a *disorder than a disease*. An alga causes Red Rust, which mainly occurs on stems in the form of red hairs, small in size and ending as small knob of spores. On stems and upper surface of leaves the alga appears as patches which are somewhat circular in shape and orange-yellow in colour.
- The seed termed as spore, which is carried by air, *settles on*

stem or foliage and Red Rust is reproduced. Workers moving through affected plants also spread the spores to some extent. Irregular and uneven surfaces of new wood on stems provide the most suitable places for infection. Some planters believe that rain stops it but it is just opposite. *A gentle rain can help in spreading this disease and during the rains it grows quickly. The parasite is visible by naked eye only when it comes to fruiting stage after nearly one year from first infection.*

- *Due to Red Rust, the bushes appear thin and weak* as dropping of leaves and dying of stems takes place. *Branches affected by the disease find difficulty in throwing new shoots.* On side branches, shoots without leaf or with few leaves, that too variegated, are seen. Leaves become yellow. The tissues of stem die in patches and consequent 'die back' occurs. *The twigs become hard early.* Greenness of twigs does not continue and greyness sets in. Marked depredations on young tea stems occur. Mature bushes' top hamper becomes weak showing die back in season's latter part.
- In case of young teas, the branches die back and *the development of young bushes is obstructed.* The stem and the leaf's upper surface carry bodies, which are disc-shaped having projecting hairs minute. Red Rust causes loss in crop, as the affected bushes may not flush freely. Leaving young tea un-centered for two years after plantation means weakening the lower shoots and consequently inviting this disease during the third year especially in areas prone to it.
- *Shallow soil, inadequate manuring, poor drainage and weakness of bushes etc.* are some of the causes of this disease. A few cases of Red Rust on vigorous bushes may also be found, but only on into weak branches. The formation of Red Rust cankers is a very unpleasant development and chemical spray may, in that case, not be able to control the alga in the tissues. Replanted teas, in the absence of adequates rehabilitation attract more Red Rust.
- *Increasing the bush strength may prevent the parasite. Adequate manuring of potash helps in controlling it.* Soil samples from the affected areas should be tested and based on the report,

MOP should be applied to correct the poor status of potash. It is quite beneficial to spray MOP and urea. High pH causes weakness in bushes and creates an opportunity for Red Rust to set in. Soil samples from affected areas should be tested and aluminum sulphate or pyrites applied to correct the pH status, if found high. Maintaining suitable soil pH, good drainage, good shade and application of correct fertilizers at correct doses help in prevention of Red Rust.

- *Putting checks on the factors which debilitate the bushes is very essential:* Faulty plucking and low fertility in soil contribute to the condition suitable for this disease and taking care in these matters in imperative. Proper irrigation gives benefit. Plucking measure in infested young tea should be liberal. Irrespective of the age of bushes, plucking should be done over one leaf in case of severe infestation and weak top hamper.
- As a matter of fact, no *chemical can destroy the algae which is responsible for this disease*, as it remains underneath the bark. Spray of copper fungicide, however, destroys the fructification. It also reduces the infection in new wood.

Causes for Low Yield in Tea in Replanted Area- A case Study

Replanted tea normally yields lower crop than extension areas planted with the same cultivars. A possible reason for this is "soil sickness" due to physical, chemical or biological factors: the three are not mutually exclusive. A case study of an area replanted without rehabilitation is presented. Although soil physics and chemistry were poor in the entire area, this did not explain the differences observed between the good and bad fields within this area. The soil phenol profiles obtained by HPLC analyses, however, were different, with areas under Guatemala grass showing a phenol profile intermediate to that of the good and bad fields. An explanation for the tea replant problem is postulated along with the reasons for, and the necessity of re-plantation. Scope for future work for elucidating the role of the rehabilitation crop, and for alleviating the re-plant problem are also discussed.

Uprooting and replantation or irredeemably uneconomical sections of tea is essential for maintaining the productivity of tea gardens. However, the need for soil rehabilitation by a green crop for approximately two years delays the realisation of economic returns from the replanted teas. Poor yields in replanted areas could arise from many reasons (Table 2.1). Studies at Tocklai have shown the deterioration of soil nutrient status and soil structure that results from continued growth of tea. The beneficial effect of the green crop has also been demonstrated, but the exact mechanisms that are responsible for reconditioning soil have not been identified. The green crop can be used to rectify any of the problems listed in Table 2.1. However, if it is necessary to hasten the rehabilitation process, there is need to identify causes of the bottleneckes and thereby devise appropriate control measures. The various causes listed in Table 2.1 are obviously not mutually exclusive. Any or all of these could be operative in a particular replant situation. In fact, various experiments of Tocklai have shown that improving the soil nutritional status, soil physical condition, or fumigation of the soil all result in some improvement of yields in replanted areas. The possibility of (auto) toxins accumulating in old tea soils has not been previously studied. Some evidence for the presence of such compounds in old tea soils is presented here.

Table 2.1: Possible Causes for Poor Yield of Tea in Replanted Areas

Possible cause	Remedial action of green crop	Possible shortcuts
Nutrient depletion or other adverse changes in soil chemistry	Restoration to missing nutrients from decaying tissues	Fertilization of missing nutrients
Loss of soil	Improvement of soil through root growth	Mechanical impıovement of soil
Weak pathogens to which young tea is more susceptible than mature	Changes in the rhizosphere eco-system	Fumigation or other chemical treatment
Allelochemicals/toxins	Detoxification by plant or rhizoshpere-microbiota	Inoculation with appropriate micro-organisms

Source: Assam Review and Tea News August 1990

Materials and Methods

Soil chemical and physical characteristics, i.e. soil pH, organic carbon, potash, phosphate, moisture content, texture and bulk density were determined by using the standard methods.

Microbialcounts were determined by performing viable counts using the dilution plate method, with soil extract agar as medium. Glucose was used as the carbon source, ammonium nitrate as nitrogen source and the medium was adjusted to ph 5.0. Plates were adjusted at 30 degree C for 48 hours to determine the bacterial numbers and for five days to determine the fungal and actinomycete counts. These were also determined using specific media for these types or organisms, but higher counts were obtained in the soil extract medium.

Allelochemicals were isolated from soil using the method of Kaminski and Muller, except that the EDTA solution was adjusted to pH 12 rather than to neutrality, as this resulted in more efficient extraction of phenols. The extracts were evaporated to dryness and redissolved in methanol. HPLG analyses were carried out on a C-18 column using water methanol mixtures for eluction. Generally, a linear

Table 2.2: Ratio of Compounds "A" to "B" in Soil Extracts from Various Gardens

Garden	Section	Cover crop	A/B	A	B
1	10	G-Grass	0.7	3.9	5.8
1	11	G-Grass	0.7	2.9	4.2
1	25	100Y Tea	1.3	4.2	3.2
1	26	1Y Tea	0.9	3.4	3.7
11	8	Scrub	0.2	1.0	4.2
11	8	G-Grass	0.3	0.8	3.0
11	15	30 y Tea	3.8	6.8	1.8
11	14	2 y Tea	0.6	1.2	2.0
11	-	G-Grass	0.3	2.5	8.0
111	10	Y Tea	2.8	2.0	7.2
111	10*	Y Tea	1.0	3.1	3.0

* *Former nursery area*

Source : Same Assam Review and Tea News August 1990

gradient from 50 per cent to 100 per cent methanols was used, but occasionally the elution was carried out in an isocratic system using 50 per cent of each solvent. A spectrophotometric detector set to 280 nm was used for determining the HPLC profiles. Mustard seed hypocotyl bioassays were carried out as described by Das. The control consisted of methanol without dissolved soil extracts so as to allow for any toxic material that may have been present in the solvent.

Results and Discussion

In all the soil samples studied, two peaks, having retention times of 1.5 and 2.0 minutes respectively, were found to be universally present. However, it was noticed that the ratios of the two peaks were different in different samples. As shown in Table 2.2, samples from areas under tea generally had a higher proportion of the peak with a retention time of 1.5 min (peak A), whereas areas under green crop or scrub had a larger proportion of the peak eluting at 2.0 min (peak B). The profile obtained in the case of garden III was particularly interesting in this respect since this was from an extension area where the young tea was generally doing well except in the specific location that had been earlier used as a nursery. The various soil chemical factors were not significantly different in these two locations. Although it was not possible to test the toxicity of the soil extracts on tea plants, extracts obtained from garden 1 were tested using the mustard seed hypocotyls assay. The results, shown in Table 2.3 indicated that the

Table 2.3: Inhibition of Mustard Seed Hypocotyls Elongation by Extracts of Soil from Garden I

Section	Cover crop	Hypo cotyl	Length (mm)	Percentage of control
Control *	None	14.15	+3.13	100.00
10	G-Grass	12.40	+2.58	87.63
11	G-Grass	12.30	+3.28	86.93
25	100 y Tea	9.90	+2.38	69.96
26	1 y Tea	11.90	+2.38	84.10

* *Solvent control*

Source : Assam Review and Tea News, August 1990

extracts from the mature tea area was inhibitory to mustard seed hypocotyles growth than the extracts from other areas. While the results obtained with mustard cannot be directly extrapolated to tea, the possibility of toxic compounds that are inhibitory to plant growth accumulating in old tea soils is strengthened. At present analysts have been working on the methods of testing these compounds directly on tea plants.

Lettuces hypocotyles elongation has been used as a model system by many workers studying plant growth regulating compounds. Since the germination of lettuce seeds under conditions prevailing in Assam is highly variable, the mustard seed assay was devised instead.

Section 8 of garden IV was replanted without rehabilitation. As the tea developed two distinct areas within the section were observed: one, where the development of tea was reasonable (the good area) and another where the tea plants were weak and showed high mortality after pruning (the bad area). Within the bad areas, Guatemala grass had been planted around some of the surviving tea bushes (the G. Grass area). Investigation of the soil chemical and physical properties of this area shown in Tables 2.4 and 2.5 did not reveal any major differences between the two areas. As can be seen from Table 2.4 , the soil chemical condition was extremely poor and the areas should not have been replanted directly. However, since the soil is poor in both the good and the bad areas, it cannot be the direct cause of poor growth in the bad areas. Similarly, as Table 2.5 shows, there is little or no difference in the soil texture or bulk density of these areas. Similarly, there was no difference in the

Table-2.4: The Comparative Soil Chemistry of Different Areas of Section 8 of Garden IV

Area	Moisture content (%)	Soil pH	Organic Carbon (%)	Potash (ppm)	Phosphate (ppm)
Good	19.40	4.15	0.598	60	36.44
Bad	13.30	4.35	0.479	160	27.95
G-Grass	16.50	4.54	0894	69	36.44

Source : Same as Table 2.1

Table 2.5: Comparative soil textures from various areas in section 8 of Garden IV

Area Depth	Good			Bad			Green Grass		
	Sand (%)	Silt (%)	Clay (%)	Sand (%)	Silt (%)	Clay (%)	Sand (%)	Silt (%)	Clay (%)
Top	53.07	38.00	8.33	56.00	37.33	6.67	62.00	29.67	8.33
30	54.33	35.33	10.33	66.67	22.33	11.00	63.33	29.00	7.67
60	59.00	33.00	8.00	54.00	36.33	9.67	60.00	21.33	13.33
90	43.00	49.33	7.67	53.33	34.00	12.67	70.67	20.67	8.67

Source : Same as Table 2.1

microbial numbers between the good and the bad areas of this section (Table 2.6).

There was a significant difference between the Guatemala grass area and the good/the bad in terms of the soil organic matter (Table 2.4). There was also a small but consistently observed difference in the bacterial numbers in this area. The significance of this is not known at present. However, in gardens A the non-tea areas generally show higher, microbial counts than to sections under tea (un-published results).

Table 2.6: Perennial Crops in which the Replant Problem has been Attributed to Autotoxins\ Allelochemical in soil (11)

Crop	Chemicals implicated	Ref
Apple	Phloridzin, precursors and derivatives	(12)
Peach	Amglydin	(13)
Citrus	Not known	(11)
Grape	Not known	(14)
Asparagus	Not known	(15)
Coffee	Caffeine	(16)

Source : Same as Table 2.1

The only difference between the soils from various areas of section 8 that could be detected was the soil phenol profile. The phenol profiles were both quantitatively and qualitatively different in the good and the bad areas. Interestingly, the soil from the area under Guatemala showed a phenol profile somewhere intermediate between that of the bad and the good areas.

From the data presented above its appears plausible that phenol accumulates in old tea soils. One of the functions of the Guatemala grass or other rehabilitation crop that enable successful rehabilitation may be that either the plant itself, or the micro-biota associated with the roots detoxifies the soil by metabolizing these phenolics to less toxic products. Satyanarayana has shown that sections that had been thoroughly rehabilitated showed a lower incidence of red rust in the replanted tea than areas that had not been rehabilitated. This shows that the micro-biota of soils is altered, as would be expected, when the cover crop is changed. As stated earlier, there is every possibility that more than one cause may be responsible for poor performance of young tea in replant areas. The effectiveness of the green crop may be that it can rectify many problems in the soil simultaneously as has been shown in Table 2.1. Therefore, in general replant situations, it may be more efficient and effective to allow for proper growth of the green crop before replantation. Nevertheless, where there is pressure for quick replanting it may be possible to use more rapid soil improvement techniques, provided the exact reason for rehabilitation is known in that specific section. The process of extraction of the compounds from soil is of necessity a harsh process. Therefore, there is every possibility that the chemical structure of the compounds may be altered during extraction. To determine the native chemical structure of these phenolics and to determine whether the replant problem in tea is indeed a case of autointoxication, it is necessary to determine whether such autotoxins exist in tea root exudates. The present, studies isolated phenol from tea root extracts and determined their structure and the action on the tea plant itself.

Conclusion

India is primarily a tea-producing nation. Nowhere in the world has agricultural growth of the proportion seen in Indian tea has been achieved from so little by way of increment in area under cultivation. There are inherent dangers of *extracting too much from a stagnant area. Policy makers at the highest level must be forewarned of these dangers and there must be now clear thinking as to how the Central and state governments can cooperate and jointly author a dynamic policy for tea, which allows for significant increase of area under cultivation for achieving growth levels consistent with the demands of our internal markets.* While on the subject of production growth, one must also remain alive to the dangers of over-estimating the demand profile. In the euphoria of post-1983 resurgence of demand for tea particularly in the Indian market, Indian tea industry may have been lulled into a sense of complacency as regards the untrammeled purchasing power of the Indian consumer. There are, indeed, grey clouds on the horizon. General inflationary condition in economy has made several inroads into the purchasing power of the average citizen and it would be myopic to believe that strong demand for tea can be sustained indefinitely. Indian tea industry has, however, been sensitive particularly to government's concern over the inflationary pressures and as a measure of its commitment to the common consumer, re-introduced economy tea packets at a national level. The price situation has been closely monitored by Monitoring Committee, which has offered a unique brand of industry-government co-operation and allowed for informal but effective decision-making to keep matter on even keel.

Chapter 3

Management of Natural Resources for Sustainable Livelihood in Tea Industry

Introduction

Natural resource management is the felt need in our country for the sake of sustainable agriculture plantation and rural development. The maintenance of natural resources available in the part of ours country is known for its rich heritage of bio-diversity encompassing the flora and fauna. The natural resources, if managed and utilised must suit the need of small, marginal farmers (both agriculture and plantation sectors) and land less labourers. Tea Industry is endowed with natural resources. Hence attempt has been made outline the role of soil conservation tillage, canopy of tea bushes and mulching, shade trees weed control, soil conservation structure, non conventionla sources of energy - wind, solar energies etc, organic residance nature of perfect plucking, drainage system etc. All these help in attainment of livelihood for sustainable development.

Soil Conservation Tillage

The soil is a natural source and its loss should be minimised for sustainable tea production. In some region, wind erosion is too less due to low wind velocity. But erosion caused by water is severe as rainfall is high. However, there is technology available to check soil erosion. Land clearing, land levelling, bush uprooting, packing disturbed soil, making drains, etc., are practices performed on tea gardens. These should be carried out during period of minimum rainfall. While clearing land, all roots, stones, etc. (buried in subsoil) should be brought up and then land levelling and packing should be done. The sub soil is rightly implemented for opening sub-layer of soil. The pits formed due to uprooting of tea bushes should be filled with soil and then loose soil may be compacted. If there is any biomass left in soil, it may decompose in due course and after that sinking of soil may occur. The section of plantation may have vacancies due to death of tea bushes, *faulty agronomic practices, etc.* Those patches should be filled with tea plants, soil building crops, shade trees, grasses, etc. and there should not be any open land and exposed soil in any part of plantation. The sub-soiling, harrowing, inter-culture etc. are field practices carried out almost on all plantations, with the help of some implements, tools etc. These practices should be performed across slope of land, so that furrows and ridges formed by these practices may easily check velocity of flowing water and thereby conserve soil and water. The undulation of field surface should be told to tractor operators and other workers prior to commencement of these practices. The field supervisors should also check operations as to whether these are being carried out as per instructions given to workers.

Canopy of Tea Bushes and Mulching

The pruning of tea bushes and plucking of green tea leaves should continue in area as it increases canopy of tea bushes. The soil has to be covered with canopy of the bushes. *The population and canopy of tea bushes are factors responsible to check soil erosion.* The rain drops falling on soil surface should be intercepted by canopy of tea bushes so that soil erosion is minimised to a large extent. *The run-off and soil loss have inverse relationship with canopy of tea bushes. Pruning and plucking, in addition to gap filling or infilling tea plants, maintain the canopy of tea bushes.* The risk of soil erosion is enormous in newly-planted area as crop canopy cover is negligible. The mulching of soil with locally available plant residues and grasses like Guatemala etc. give protection against soil erosion and conserve oil moisture too, in addition to checking growth of weeds which enriches soil after decomposition. *The mulching should be done immediately after planting @ 5 tonne/ha. The run-off and soil loss are minimum with mulching.* Whenever mulching materials are scarce, intercrops or cover crops can be taken up effectively for first 3-4 years of planting.

Growing cover crops, preferably leguminous like mimosa invisa, beans, pea, etc., between rows of tea plants can check soil erosion. This would minimise impact of rainfall especially during first 3-4 years, when there is not much canopy and less competition for resources. The cover crops reduce weed growth and improve soil fertility apart from giving an additional monetary return. *After harvesting, pods of this leguminous crop, plants etc. can be pulled out and spread as mulch in the same field, which will decompose and add nutrients to soil after some time.*

Shade Trees

Tea is partially shade loving crop and planting of suitable shade tress is an essential practice fogetting maximum benefit. The shade tree should *be planted along tea rows at 6.0 m x 6.0 m spacing. However, spacing may be altered as per requirement.* The shade trees should be pruned periodically, keeping in view their growth status, soil fertility, age of plantation, rainfall distribution, etc.

Weed Control

Until tea is three years of age from time of planting in field, it is young. Weed growth in tea is very rapid, particularly during initial years as ground is not completely covered by bush canopy. The weeds should be controlled effectively with minimum or no soil disturbance in tea plantation by selecting suitable and effective weed control measures. *Manual weeding may accelerate soil erosion by disturbing soil and cause damages to surface roots. Besides, its cost is high. Herbicides are the most obvious alternative to manual weed control, as they cause little or no soil disturbance.* But excessive application of chemicals may pollute the soil and kill microorganisms engaged in building soil. In young tea, Simazin (1.5-2.0 kgs/ha) may be applied as pre-emergence after early rain between March and April, to keep soil surface free of most of annual brod-leaf weeds and grasses. Parquets is the most widely used herbicide in tea. It is a herbicide applied as post emergence @ 0.3-0.4 kgs/ha to control grasses. Glyphosate herbicide is most effective on perennial weeds, which have underground rhizomatious root system.

Soil Conservation Structure

The soil conservation structures suitable for tea plantation, include contour wall, boundary drain, contour drain, staggered contour trenches, etc. The contour wall is effective measure against soil erosion, if materials such as stones, logs, etc. are locally available. The drains can be constructed to take out excess rain-water from field and to minimise concentrated flow of run-off and soil loss. The drain should have quick growing and spreading type of grasses on bed so as to avoid any possible scoring of bed. On larger area, collective (leader) drain should be stone-pitched with suitable drops, if slope is higher. The outlet should also be constructed and maintained properly to prevent formation of gully due to concentrated flow at end. The staggered contour trenches are also effective measures to prevent soil erosion and conserve moisture. The dimension of trenches may be 2.0-3.0 m (length). These soil conservation measures, if strictly adopted, would certainly help in maintaining soil productivity and thereby sustainability of tea production could be enhanced.

Non-conventional Sources of Energy

Coal, diesel, electricity, oil, etc. are present energy sources for processing green tea leaves. There is scarcity of these sources at most of the tea estates. Besides the cost of these sources is high. The demand for energy is going to increase in coming years. The atmospheric pollution is also increasing and, therefore, appropriate measures are needed to arrest further deterioration. *The reserves of conventional fossil fulls may not be available after a few decades. The non-conventional energy sources are capable of meeting all energy demands of today and tomorrow. Hence, these sources need to be harnessed with full determination for having sustainable tea production.*

Wind Energy

The velocity of wind in the north-eastern region is low as compared to other parts of the country. *However, wind-mills could be easily installed on hill-tops or in open locations available in tea estates. In some region wind velocity is more during summer months than in winter months.* There is great potential of harnessing this energy throughout the year *for generation of mechanical and electrical power in most effective ways*, provided the site is selected rediciously. A minimum of 10 km per hour of wind speed is needed for running windmills, though optimum speed should be 12-15 kms per hour. Wind pumping is a well-established technology that offers an alternative to diesel, electricity etc. on farms. Different types of windmills are available today. *These include vertical axis and horizontal axis and also single blade and multi-blade systems. For water pumping generally multi-blade* windmills are used and they do not require high wind speed. In fact, they start operating at a wind speed of 10 km per hour and could be operated up to a wind speed of about 70 km. The wind pumps, working at wind velocity between 7 km and 30 km per hour are available at present. Wind machines used for power generation have two or three blades and their diameter is much more than diameter of windmills used for water pumping applications. Now, claims are being made that India happens to be third in world in area of power generation from wind energy. The wind generators erected in a large area are called wind farm. A wind generator with 5 KW capacity would be economical and viable. It can be installed in factory for lighting purpose. Wind energy battery chargers are also available the now-a-days in the country. They are wind machines generally with a rotor having diameter of 1 to 2.5 m and the outputs are 50-600 watt at 10m/s wind speed. The main components include a wind power generator, a converter and a container of batteries. Recently, a 4 KW, two bladed, horizontal axis permanent magnet generator for battery charging has been developed by BHEL and same may be adopted.

Solar Energy

The solar energy alone can provide required *electrical energy for whole world*. The intensity of *solar radiation is also much more on earth*. Solar thermal technology for meeting demand of energy for processing green tea leaves could be adopted. There are about 100 manufacturers of appliances based on solar energy in the country. In fact, solar energy has tremendous prospect in comparison with other energy sources. Many solar devices and applications are quite simple. *The solar energy can be utilised in a variety of ways such as for water heating, air heating, etc. needed for washing and cleaning processing utensils, equipment, floor of processing hall,* etc. It also could be used for drying fermented leaf-mass, lighting the area, etc. The technology for operating sprayers, while applying chemicals on tea *bushes and weeds is in existence in India for adoption*.

Now, solar lighting system is being propagated for street lighting, domestic lighting, and solar-lantern for light in community centers. About 30,000 stand-alone street light systems capable of providing light for whole night, have been installed in different states. Nearly 15,000 have been provided indoor light powered by a photovoltaic system on roof-tops. There are around 5000 portable solar lanterns, being used in the country as source of light.

Briquette of Organic Residues

The energy output per kg of biomass is more when it is dry, as some energy is wasted in removing water if biomass is wet. Therefore, in most cases, dry biomass is used. However, in processes like generation of combustible gas for use in biogas plant, presence of water in the biomass is essential. *Biomass has been in use as a source of energy since times immemorial and it will continue to be used as source in future also*. Earlier, firewood was used for generation of heat on tea gardens of north-eastern region. Later on, planters switched over to coal and now they are switching over to oil, while using modern equipment. These fuels are brought from long distances. If briquettes are made from locally available biomass, cost of tea production could be minimised. It was found during a survey that a lot of biomass of weeds of and grasses, while using shrup, master with tractor, is available on tea gardens. It is essential to make *briquettes from biomass as bulky organic residues have low thermal efficiency and their use is smoky*. The briquette of such residues will offer a promising alternative to costly fuels. The briquette of rice husk, saw dust, tree leaves, weeds, agricultural waste, etc. can easily be made. These smokeless briquette fuels could be used for operating boilers, furnaces etc. The main attraction of briquette lies in using agricultural residues, particularly of no value, such as weeds, grasses, etc. cut from road-side. The rice husk is also available in this region in plenty. The water hyacinth also could be used for making briquettes. It was found that water hyacinth, which is a weed, is found in waterlogged areas, lakes etc. in this region. While making briquettes, paddy straw, coal dust etc. may be added. Clay mixed with water may be used for binding and stabilising the mass. The most was briquettes may be sun-dried.

Briquettes are usually cylindrical in shape with diameter in range of 26-100 mm and length 10-400 mm. Their density varies from 0.45 to 1.20 mm and heating value from 2000 to 4800 k cal per kg. The briquettes could be an effective substitute for solid fuel like coal, etc. Coal produces sulphur-dioxide, which ultimately changes to sulphuric acid, an extremely corrosive chemical. On the other hand, briquettes do not corrode equipment and thus increase their life. The briquette processes may be of screw or piston type. In first case, biomass is screwed forward under high pressure through a nozzle (funnel) shaped component, in which, biomass gets its cylindrical shape. In the other case, some forward pressure is applied with a piston. These are two methods of making briquettes. One of them operates with a binding agent and other one without binder. The briquette without binding agent needs a raw material, with a maximum moisture content of 15 per cent and a briquette press, which can generate a pressure of a least 1000 kg/cm. The minimum pressure will vary depending upon nature of raw material. The briquette with binding agent does not require same moisture content. The stages involved in a briquette are collection of waste, storage and drying, size-reduction, mixing with binding agent, processing, cooling and storage.

Energy Plantation

Fire-wood and other biomass are cheap in our country. With growing awareness of fire wood scarcity, now considerable attention is being paid to production of fuel wood. *The total output from land is a function of initial investment on tree planting, irrigation and application of manure*. The productivity could be mixed by proper management. Irrigation is free in north-eastern region. Here, the concept is to raise quick growing species at intervals of 5-10 years. *The energy plantation has many advantages*. Some of them are: (a) *biomass can be generated at will*, (b) *it can be grown without help of outside agencies in own field*, (c) *several varieties are available*, which could be used to give fuel in different forms, (d) *integrated culture of growing* biomass, fodder, food crop, vegetable, etc. in same field could be adopted, and (e) *leaves of some plants could* be used as fodder for animals.

It is almost inexhaustibly renewable source of energy with flexible harvesting time. The ash obtained by use of this energy could be used as fertilizer. It is a non-hazardous mineral-rich ash. The energy plantation can create pleasant and beautiful surroundings with shade and shelter, which would maintain better ecological balance. The erosion-prone land of tea plantations could be easily covered with energy plantation and thereby soil erosion could be checked. There are various species of energy plantation which may be used depending upon condition of land such as water logged soils, highly sloping land, etc. There are multipurpose species too *for meeting different types of needs such as fuel, feed, erosion control, soil improvement, etc.*

Human Energy

Most of the operations of a tea plantation are human energy intensive and, therefore, there is *need to develop suitable devices and attachments* to convert muscle power to useful mechanical power. The productivity of workers could be enhanced by providing them *with tools and implements capable of operating in comfortable posture. The tools may be push and pull type weedier, trolley sprayers, etc. These mechanical devices generate less fatigue during operation and thus result in more work output. A man, on average spends 65 to 75 per cent of his working* time with manually operated devices. In conventional tools, time spent in their use is high in proportion to amount of work accomplished. During continuous work, a man can develop horse-power equivalent to about 1/10th of his own weight (0.5 hp). There is need to improve existing tools and devices for efficient utilization of energy. The desirable features of a good hand tool should be: (i) *ergonomic design* to enable operator to work in least tiring posture; (ii) *lightness of weight* of tool for easy transportation; (iii) *easy construction and comfortable operation* with tool; (iv) *high quality* of its components, (v) *low cost and facilities* for local production of tools.

The working part of a tool should be designed for efficient performance of job. The handle is important as it determines position of worker and method of doing work. It has been experienced that drudgery and physical exertion are main features of Indian agricultural practices, which affect adversely man's intelligence and ability. The manually operated machine should generate less vibration and noise.

The soil conservation measures would certainly provide sustainability to tea farming. The use of non-conventional/renewable sources of energy would save fossil fuel to large extent and provide sustainability to tea production. The ergonomically designed tools enhance productivity of workers and thereby provide sustainability to tea production.

Role of Perfect Plucking

Importance of Plucking : Good plucking is *necessary to harvest better crops*. Bad plucking neutralises all the constant good efforts made in grooming the tea for better productivity. Plucking must be given its due if the value of other efforts is to be realised. It is the final assault made cautiously by the planting soldier to hit the target and hoist the victory flag. Inefficient plucking causes big loss in crop. Damaged and uneven surface of bushes after plucking and unacceptable plucked shoots are most unpleasant consequences of bad plucking. Substantial crop increase can be there if plucking is proper. Correct plucking is very important both for quantity and quality. The system of plucking flat has been there for the last many years due to constant experiments and experiences of the dedicated old planters. The early planters probably used to take entire one flush growth together. During early stage of the history of plucking, it was done taking all growth without caring for maintenance foliage. Modern planters are indebted to George Williamson, the manager of Assam Company, who left maintenance foliage in 1858 before plucking. He lost early crop as a result, but made it up with progressive plucking and achieved remarkable crop by the end of the year. The foundation of modern plucking was, thus, laid in 1853 or 1854.

Several Flushes : There are several flushes in a year. Tentatively, the first flush continues till April. Second flush may start in late April and continue till June. Third flush may start in July and continue till September. The tentative period of fourth flush is around the last part of September to November. Fifth flush may start around the middle of November and it may be felt just before season's close on slight out-turn rise. The crop during different flushes depends upon the pruning. However, in all cases, maximum crop is harvested during rains followed by the second flush. The back-end crop from pruned sections is more than the skiffs and un-prune. While about three per cent of back-end crop is expected from un-prune, the pruned sections may give about fifteen per cent of crop during the same period. During the first flush, un-prune gives the highest crop to the tune of twelve-thirteen per cent compared to the minimum during the said period from light prune. The distribution of crop also depends upon the pruning cycle adopted and the proportion of different pruning in a particular garden. For example, a garden on three-year cycle of LP: UP: UP having one-third of each is expected to harvest about four per cent more in early season, three per cent less in main season and one per cent less in the back-end of the total crop compared to a garden on a four year pruning cycle of LP: UP: DS: UP having twenty-five per cent of each.

Tipping — Timely and Regular : When the bushes recover from pruning and come up with new foliage, the plucking in the beginning and several rounds thereafter is known as tipping, which must be done carefully for preparing the bushes to give better yield. Tipping stimulates the buds on leaf axils and lateral shoots are produced for plucking on their reaching above the level of tipping. New lateral shoots of higher order emerge after the laterals are plucked and this sequence goes on. The necessity of right tipping lies in the fact that it creates necessary maintenance foliage canopy and forms the surface of plucking. Apical domlnance ln checked and lateral growth is formed by it. Subsequent crop is limited due to reduction in first order laterals' basic number in case the tipping-round is extended beyond seven days. *Regular and timely tippings increase multiplication process and result in crop gain during main season.* Abnormal delay in tipping is bad, as it hardens up primaries, making it difficult for tippers to break with finger. Lack of smoothness in tipping the hardened primaries inflicts injuries, which disturb the process of recovery after pruning and their coming to bearing is delayed. One should not be misled by the logic of starting tipping only when a good number of tipable shoots show up at height for the sake of obtaining a better level. To obtain early density of plucking points for more harvest, it is advisable to start tipping early. About four weeks time is required in developing first flush after the start of tipping. The fixed tipping height should be measured over the central pruning or skiffing mark on vertical new growth and there after the other and the side branch flush should be tipped at the level of that height in horizontal plane to form the new surface of plucking. Although there are variations due to genotype, about 80 per cent shoots come to the height of plucking table after pruning.

Frame Forming and Re-centering : In bringing up the young tea, thumb or lung pruned young plants should be tipped at 24 inches. Frame forming prune at 14-16 inches should be tipped at 24-26 inches while final frame tipping at 26-28 inches should follow forming pruning done at a height of 16-18 inches. During the bringing up of young tea, whenever the un-prune year comes, the plants should be plucked to janam. While the main aim at bringing up the young tea is the establishment of permanent frame at a lower level, one must ensure that within three years of age, drought does not occur in full foliage. Considering these aspects, *the frame forming skiff and re-centering in third year should be followed by a tipping measure of 24 inches, raising it by another two inches during each season for about two years before final frame forming prune*. Before these, the first de-center should be followed by a tipping measure of 24 inches and stepping up based on necessity. De-centering after the middle of August does not require skiffing and in that case step-up plucking should be allowed to continue. Plants de-centered in April, May and given a skiff in December should again be followed by a tipping measure of 24 inches. Step-up for next year should also be given. *From the auxiliary buds new shoots arise after the tipping of primary shoots and the new shoots grown over tipping level are plucked.* Major portion of crop comes from the fourth order laterals out of eight orders of laterals produced in the span of one plucking season.

Primaries contribute to first flush and second flush contribution comes from primaries and first and second order to laterals. Third, fourth, fifth and sixth order laterals contribute to rain flush. The back-end flush comes from sixth, seventh and eighth order laterals. Below the fish leaf there is an oval leaf, which is malformed and small. When one fish leaf and three full leaves and a bud grow over it, normal plucking starts subsequent to the growth of the bud between the stalk, which is tipped with the first leaf. Out of some dormant primaries below the level of plucking, some grow and reach the level of plucking and are plucked. But a few of them remain permanently dormant. While plucking, leaving the fish leaf and one full leaf above it pays handsomely in terms of growth and bush health.

Tips for Plucking : *Janam plucking may be done in the areas where the rate of growth is quick*. From the janams new lateral shoots arise and the former should, therefore, be left while plucking. When plucking is done over fish leaf and not over janam it is called fish leaf plucking which causes lower yield. Good wither is not possible on fish leaf and flaky tea is produced from it. Bushes may be plucked over fish leaf in drought. In black plucking, only buds and janams are left on the plucking table. It is not advisable in general and in the drought prone areas and un prunes in particular. During drought it must never be done. Crop loss will definitely be there if black plucking is continued throughout the season. The bushes suffer due to continuous black plucking. It should be adopted only when compelled to do so when the infection of blister blight or trips is found, that too for one for two rounds only. Never be misled by more leaf in the beginning in plucking black on seven-eight days round, as overall crop loss will be there. One round of plucking may be done in an area where excessive manifestation of banjhiness is observed. If the bushes are healthy and vigorous, having sufficient maintenance foliage cover, black plucking, when necessary, can be done in unpruned LS and MS areas. It should, however, not be done in DS and pruned areas. It cannot be adopted as a long-term policy in any type of skiffing or pruning. Black plucking in second un-prune year may not be useful.

Hard plucking disturbs the constituents which form the wood as well as bushes' carbohydrate reserves causing weak and thin frame and general weakness; and initial crop increase is quite misleading. Branch die back also occurs during drought or after pruning on those bushes which are hard plucked.

Fine plucking means plucking only one and a bud, two and a bud and a single banjhis. Excellent quality is made from the leaf consisting of one and a bud and the buds. But such very fine plucking is not economical and practical.

Finely plucked shoots produce bright coppery infused leaves. The cup is brisk with good strength and colour in liquor. Stems of fine shoots contribute positively to the quality of liquor. If a planter wants to pluck fine, he can do so on seventh day from last plucking date in the gardens situated at medium elevations. At higher elevations, this can be done on ninth day. At low elevations, fine shoots can be plucked on fifth day.

Plucking two and a bud, three and a bud and single banjhis comes under medium plucking standard. Medium plucking produces fair color. Although infused leaf may be fairly bright, briskness is little and the cup is thin.

In *standard plucking,* small one and a bud, buds and janams are left and large one and a bud, two and a bud, three and a bud and single banjhis are plucked. Standard plucked leaf produces a cup, which is fairly brisk and bright. Some strength is also there. Infused leaf is bright with proper care. In coarse plucking, three and a bud and four and a bud are also plucked with two and a bud and double banjhis. In very coarse plucking, three and a bud, four and a bud and double banjhis are plucked and such harvest does not have any appreciable number of one and a bud, two and a bud, and single banjhis. When the stand of shade is very dense, the nature encourages the shoots to struggle to go upward in search of sunlight and in course of this struggle they develop longer internodes often becoming coarse in case of Assam bushes with large leaves. Nodes and leaves of shoots in fine plucking are succulent whereas big amount of cell wall is rigid and long inter-node in coarse plucking results in more fibers. Increased fibers and reduced water extractive result from coarse plucking.

Morning Hour Plucking : Compared to other hours (afternoon), the leaves plucked in the morning hours of the day produce superior strength and colour. Higher poly-phenol content and lower content of protein bestowed upon the morning leaf by the nature due to scientific reasons may be contributory factors for the superiority in the tea manufactured from the leaves plucked in morning hours. It is thus, logically suggested to pluck as much leaf in the morning hours as possible. Pluckers should always be motivated to start plucking at the earliest possible time in the morning. Further, the accumulation rate of dry matter in shoots which determines made tea recovery is more during morning hours due to more photosynthesis as a result of the temperature of leaf and intensity of light. As the hour advances in the morning, the dry matter keeps on increasing, not in the afternoon beyond 2 to 2.30 p.m. and some gain in annual crop can be there if everyday maximum leaf is plucked between 9 a.m and 1 p.m. As far as possible and practical, the plucking of those sections which are high-yielding may be monitored during this period of the working hour. Poor sections may be plucked before and after this period. As far as contribution of dry matter in pluck-able shoots is concerned, maxim, contribution comes from the leaf which is at the top. Fish leaf also contributes as much as any normal leaf. More absorption of atmospheric oxygen by the crushed leaf due to air exposure and its becoming red minimises its soluble tannin continuously finally resulting in dull infusions and thin liquors. It is, therefore, essential to ensure that the leaf is not packed tightly in the baskets. Neither it should be allowed to be packed tightly in bags for transportation to factory. Any other cause damaging the leaf must also be avoided. It would not be out of place to mention here that maximum location of tanning is in the bud and first leaf followed by second and third leaves.

Plucked Leaf Spread for Withering does not Require any Heating : Once the leaf is plucked, till it is spread over for withering in the factory, one should always be careful not to allow any heating otherwise it would result in quick increase in the number of bacteria, particularly when the surface moisture is there on the leaf, and consequently tea quality would suffer. Both harmless and harmful bacteria are carried by leaf on the plants, but they do not create any problem unless due to carelessness particularly wet leaf is pressed in the basket and left there to heat up. On a hot day, leaf moisture may be lost @ 0.50 per cent per hour. The leaf should be allowed to remain cool by light packing in bags or baskets. Leaf temperature rises quickly with tight packing. Damage of leaf cells takes place and fermentation initiates if the leaf temperature goes over 109-110 degree F. This results in red leaf. In hilly gardens where leaf is brought down to the factory with the help of ropeway, care is essential to ensure that the sacks full of leaves are not allowed to crash to the delivery platform with force to avoid bruising and damage to leaves inside the sacks. Discoloured leaf and brown tea are the consequences of damage in plucked leaf. If tearing damages the leaf, the damaged cells get exposure to atmosphere resulting in fermentation at faster rate and the harm of leaf damage by bruising is comparatively less. Damaged leaf results in uneven wither, as the damaged portions wither at faster rate than normal shoots. Damage to leaf is conducive to bacterial infection. *Care should always be taken in all stages to avoid heating of leaf, as the leaf heated in green stage produces dull liquors.*

Productivity of Plucker and Reduction in Plucking Cost : Plucking is a costly operation and *productivity should be increased to bring down the plucking cost, which constitutes 60 per cent of total labour cost and 15 per cent of total cost of production.* On an average, *about sixty per cent of the workers are engaged in plucking.* Plucking includes employment related important fringe benefits like medical, welfare, food subsidy, dry tea and fuel etc., and variable fringe benefits such as bonus, gratuity, provident fund and sick and earned leaves. The wages of sardars and their fringe benefits should also be taken in plucking cost, which is calculated per kg of saleable tea. The more green leaf is plucked, the more is the reduction in cost. *The gardens having an yield of above 1500 kgs per hectare with about 32-34 per cent un prune and on 7/8 day round in the beginning stretching to 8/9/10 days later, should have an annual average of 25-26 kgs of green leaf per day.*

The average will be higher, in the vicinity of 30-32 kgs per day, in case of gardens yielding above 2000 kgs per hectare. If land productivity is increased, the increase in output per labour result in cost reduction. On the other hand, other factors contributing to increase in productivity of labour on a particular estate should also be identified for improvement. The factors are given below.

Good Cultural Practice, Adequate Shade, Manuring, Less Vacancy and Moderate Height of Plants

Good cultural practices, adequate shade and required manuring, influence a plucker's productivity positively, as he or she harvests more leaf from vigorous bushes compared to weak ones abounding in banjhis and having less number of shoots, that too not heavy enough. Plucking cost is less in higher yielding gardens due to higher plucking averages there. *The areas which are high yielding, always help in achieving higher productivity for pluckers. The efficiency of a plucker suffers when he or she plucks in a section which have vacancies.* On the other hand, plucking efficiency gets a boost in *compact section*. Effective plucking time reduces with increase in vacancies. How the vacancies adversely affect can be well be imagined by the fact that if 180 bushes are plucked in one hour in a section without vacancy, in case of a section with 20 per cent vacancy, only 135 bushes will be plucked in one hour. For achieving higher productivity of pluckers, it is necessary to ensure that the height of plants are neither very high nor very low so that it results in difficult postures for workers engaged in plucking.

Time of Season, Plucking Management and Deployment of Plucker: Various times of the season have their own natural influence on plucking. For example, *from the sixth to the ninth months of the calendar year, average daily plucked leaf may be highest in August followed by September. In one hour, the highest number of bushes may by plucked in June followed by July. Highest number of shoots per bush may be plucked in September followed by August.* Deployment of pluckers should be judicious, avoiding the situations of both less pluckers in the areas where more leaf is there and overcrowding the areas where the leaf is less. Getting abnormally low quantity of leaf one-day and abnormally high another day reflects erratic management of plucking. Pluckers' deployment and areas to be plucked should be so organized that the quantity of green leaf is distributed in an even way throughout the week.

During the period of rapid growth, it is wise to arrange making more number of weightments than is normally done as otherwise, on seeing the baskets full, the pluckers soon slackken lowering their productivity or press the leaves in their baskets to prevent them from off, consequently damaging the leaves. For uniformity in wither, it is required to aim at plucking same type of leaf on one day as far as possible and practicable. Plucking unprunes and level off, light and medium skiffs should be organized together.

Avoidance of Wastage of Efforts and Time of Plucking : It is essential to identify and avoid the wastage of effort and time while plucking to increase productivity. The plucking challans should be organized line-wise and engaged in such a way that the pluckers of the challans reach the plucking sections in shortest possible time from their lime. It is necessary to ensure that off, time is not wasted in preparation after timely arrival of pluckers in changing the section and in first and other weighments before going back to plucking again. The alertness of assistants, field staff and sirdars is necessary in this respect. It should be ensured that productive time's wastage is not allowed and maximum utilisation of productive time is achieved by fixing weightment points near the plucking sections.

Right Motion for Right Plucking, Proper Training on the Spot and Strict Supervision etc. : Right motions are necessary for right plucking Plucker must never be allowed to use their palm to grab the shoots and detach them by pulling. Until it is done deliberately, a few casual pluckers do it due to ignorance. Proper training on the spot and strict supervisions thereafter are the answers to this defective way of plucking. Plucking is done with the help of different motions. Before grasping and detaching the shoots, the motions of looking at and selecting them come together for which better eyesight is necessary.

While recruiting new workers, the garden medical officers should make medical examination. During the medical examination, the eyesight should also be checked together with the nerves of the hand and the general health. Thumb and two fingers are vital organs in grasping the shoots before plucking them. Pluckers with weak thumbs and defective fingers cannot pluck efficiently, as their grasp on shoot and detaching them with wrist's turn cannot be efficient.

Use of Both Hands by Expert Pluckers : The expert pluckers pluck with both hands holding the plucked shoots in palm for about a minute. The pluckers should be trained to transfer the shoots to their baskets or jhulies as quickly as possible otherwise their productivity would slow down, since apart from tensed muscles their palms would not be able to hold beyond a capacity and they would be tempted to start plucking by one hand, holding the shoots beyond capacity in the other. The planters using jhulies should note that about one second more time is required each time the shoots from the palm is transferred.

Number of Shoots Plucked, Speed of Plucking and Shed : Fat pluckers are generally lazy and physically weak. Weak pluckers are poor in plucking. Healthy pluckers having a body weight of about 50 kg are the best. These things should be considered while recruiting the new workers. It is beneficial to choose taller pluckers as far as possible, as they can pluck more efficiently and at a faster rate, and increasing productivity. Efficient pluckers pluck more shoots per bush, as their efficiency leads them not to leave ready shoots on bushes. Number of shoots plucked and the speed of plucking play important role of plucker's productivity. In normal conditions the number of shoots plucked per bush is highest in Upper Assam followed by Dooars. Plucking speed contributes very positively in increasing the productivity of a plucker. The speed of plucking of a fast plucker is about ten per cent more than that of an average pluckers and the speed of a slow plucker is about 25 to 30 per cent less than that of a fast plucker. The speed of plucking increases with increase in the number of shoots progressively on plucking season's advancement contributing to increase in total quantity plucked by a plucker per day.

A good Short density Leads to Pluckers' Productivity : A good shoot density on the bush contributes positively to the increase in plucker's productivity. Compared to a fast plucker, a slow plucker plucks about 28 to 30 per cent less per day and compared to an average plucker, a fast plucker may pluck about 14 per cent more. If a slow plucker plucks 40 kg of green leaf per day, a fast plucker will pluck not less than 50 kg as a result of his efficiency in plucking more bushes per hour and more shoots per minute. Slow pluckers, seeing the fast ones moving ahead while plucking, try to keep pace and advance leaving some shoots unplucked. The plucking sardars must be alert not to allow their. For good plucking, a good training must be given to the pluckers by sardars. The supervisory staff and the assistants should train sardar, and the manager should also check whether all concerned are moving in right direction.

Jhapies and Shade enhance Pluckers Productivity : In inclement weather, the efficiency of pluckers drops. Increased heart-beat are not conducive to good and efficient performance. For normal heart-beat, curtailing solar radiation's impact is necessary for which old planters found "jhapies" useful. They were really very useful. Umbrella, which has already replaced jhapie, also contributes in minimising solar radiation's impact. But it is not as convenient in use as jhapie was. Productivity of the plucker decreases when he or she holds an umbrella.

Shade pays a positive role in plucker's productivity. This can be well imagined by realisation of the fact that shade trees contribute to improved thermal environment putting a check on development of fatigue in pluckers. It is an accepted fact that fatigue curtails productivity. In well-shaded sections more productivity per plucker can be achieved.

Role of Drainage in Sustainable Tea Production

The vigor and growth of tea is inhibited by poor drainage which affects soil aeration and rooting depth of the plant. Poor drainage limits the aerated soil's amount and development of plant system is halted. The plant does not get required food and production of crop suffers. The general health and yield potential plants are influenced tremendously by improvement in drainage. Improvement in drainage increases crop. But it is too much to expect the increase in crop immediately in the same year. The result of improvement really starts showing up in crop after a few years. No sizeable increase in crop is expected in the first year of improving drainage facilities. It starts showing up in the second year followed by further increase in third year. Without efficient drainage, no field management practice can give its full benefits. On tea estates, planned development drainage projects give quite a good cost benefit ratio. The investment may be realized in the very first year and maintenance expenses are minimal during the coming years. Crop increase and weed control become less expensive and there is better utilisation of nutrients. Forced economy of drainage should never be allowed. Piecemeal and haphazard works cause wastage of money. Money is lost due to reduction in crop as a result of inadequate drainage. Inadequate maintenance and faulty construction of drains cause unnecessary expenditure.

Surface Water, Central Subsoil and Denitrification: Drainage should not be confused with cutting of some ditches of a particular width and depth in a section unless the drains are cut considering the topography and the soil and its gradient so as to remove from root zone water which is in excess of plant requirement. The soil is drained for field capacity in root areas. Field capacity is the saturated equilibrium condition of the soil after losing excess water through drainage for a period of time on receipt of rainfall. All water cannot be held by the soil. Modern planters feel that drainage consciousness is prevalent now-a-days. But, the early planters too never lacked in it. Of course, drainage is posing problems now due to rising river-beds. Rise in Brahmaputra's bed in occurring as a result of salvation. The river-bed have, in course of time, been raised by earthquakes also. Storm and surface water cannot be dealt with without drainage and surface drainage is necessary in view of heavy rainfall. Surface drains down the slope work as receivers or water carriers. They control seepage and work as intercepting drains if laid across the slope. Drainage is required to remove excess water during high rainfall periods without excessively drying out the soil during low rainfall period. Seasonal water table's height should be kept within bounds and runoff water should be disposed of quickly to arrest the adverse effects of excess rainfall. What is "runoff"? It is precipitation's portion making way towards drainage line.

Drains Dispose of the Surface Water and Control Sub Soil Water : Drains dispose of the surface water and control sub-soil water. Excess of water on soil surface or beneath the surface in the root zone create problems. Standing water on soil surface causes flooding whereas excess of water beneath soil surface means high water table and consequent soil waterlogging. A good drainage system removes the surplus water from land and reduces moisture in soil, which is more than what the tea requires. The air spaces clogged with water cut off oxygen supply to roots in water logged and wet conditions. If water needed by the bushes or soil's field capacity, is not evacuated, waterlogging may result from any of flooding and run off, rain fall and seepage.

Water Logging Attributes to Out Fall Restriction : In several gardens water logging is blindly attributed to outfall restrictions without detailed examination of the grading adequacy of outlet channels. The problem of waterlogging will remain if the outlet channels are undersised. Waterlogging does not provide the nitrification conditions due to excessive moisture and lack of oxygen. This results in poor growth of tea. In such situation, root penetration is restricted and yield is reduced. The tea and the shade trees are attacked by violet root rot. The plucking points are reduced as a result of back off growth. The leaves become yellowish and leathery. Waterlogging is a contributory cause of greay and brown blights. If the ground surface is uneven, localised waterlogging can be removed by way of levelling the ground and filling the collar depressions. Shallow drains may be provided to dispose of surface water in case levelling the ground and filling the collar depressions are not possible immediately. For controlling the water table in waterlogged areas, Eucalyptus may be useful to some extent, as it may possibly increase transpiration.

Flood Weakens the Bushes : Further, the flood weakens the bushes and on such bushes light plucking is necessary. Rest is essential for the bushes show sings of wilting after the flood and after the rest, these bushes must be plucked light. Forking is useful in the area after flood for aeration. In such areas, scrapping off the silt from bush trunks and drains is advisable. Flood affected areas should be looked after for mites and, if found, proper spraying should be done. Three to four days' flooding may be tolerated by tea at a time on occasions but beyond this the bushes in general and their roots in particular get damaged seriously. In preventing waterlogging, removal of water from retentive soil is necessary for which drainage is required. Tea cannot obtain oxygen from water itself like a few other plants and inadequate oxygen owing to air spaces being filled up with excess water causes root's asphyxiation and the growth is adversely affected. If the soil is ill-drained, one cannot expect a good root development. The roots will be shallow and have lateral spread with upward twists. Good development of roots is essential for extracting more nutrients from the soil. Roots develop better in good soil environments, which can be created by controlling ground water level and draining out excess water during the monsoon.

Increase in Rooting Depth, Nitrogen Economy and Water Storage Capacity as Well as Reduction in Soil Erosion : For maximum growth, proper root environment is necessary which is possible only by providing proper drainage. Proper drainage increases rooting depth. Aeration is improved as a result of easy movement of water through soil. Shallow root system is bound to be there in badly aerated soil. When pore spaces are filled with water in the soil, the breathing pores, known as lenticels, are enlarged on teas in inadequately aerated soil. This is a sign of reduced oxygen uptake. The excessive water accumulated in soil results in decay of feeding roots, restricting thereby the absorption of nutrients and water. If the tender feeding roots continue to be destroyed, the root system becomes bunchy. Unless the drains function properly and the excess water is drained out, there is danger of reduced mineral elements, which may produce toxic effect. Excess water in soil facilitates the accumulation of gases and carbon dioxide, which also increase the probability of toxic effect. Soil structure and tilt are improved if drains function efficiently. Good drainage improves nitrogen economy in the soil. Full benefit of any fertilizer cannot be derived without a good drainage. Excess moisture in soil in nursery invites "damping" of seedling of tea within the age of six months. Green crops and young shade plants may also suffer. As far as tea is concerned, in case of very stiff clay soil, the suitable moisture content may be 24-25 per cent or higher than this, where as around 15 per cent may be the optimum moisture content in case of very sandy soil. In case of good loam, optimum moisture content may be somewhere between 18 to 20 per cent.

Availability of Soil Moisture of Increased Drainage : During day time, the soil moisture availability is increased by drainage as a result of root penetration and good drainage alleviates the drought effects to some extent. The benefit from mulching is increased by drainage. Root rot enlarged lenticles and sun scorch are minimised by good drainage. Reducing waterlogging and improving the drainage in red rust affected areas start showing results soon. As the water table lowers, the plants start gearing up to protect themselves from the infection. The aeration of soil impeded by waterlogging continuously invites red rust to tea and also some shades. Drainage reduces soil erosion. Water storage capacity is increased by it. Drainage and soil conservation are inter-related, as the downstream areas suffer due to soil wash. Contour drains help in erosion control. Soil is washed to the tune of nearly 150 tonnes on the erosion of one acreinch.

Leaves of Shade and Green Crop Plants Turn Yellowish: In absence of proper drainage, the excess water forces the leaves of shade and green crop plants turn yellowish. They may drop off thereafter. "Fusarium Wilt" may attack small shade plants as well as green crops in wet soil conditions. This attack may either be through stem at collar region or through the root. Due to transpiration through leaf the permanent shade trees help in maintaining low soil moisture to a considerable extent. The soil is also opened up through their roots, which helps proper aeration. A good shade, therefore, should also be maintained with a good drainage. The main drain discharges water into river or channel and the average level of water and highest level of flood there during the monsoon period should be known to design proper drainage system. The rainfall intensity and the area of catchments are the factors which influence the water discharge volume. Although visual inspection and reconnaissance give initial information for planning the drainage, competent surveyors and subsequent contour map should ideally base it on the topographic survey. While laying out tea topography natural drainage should be considered to avoid drainage problem later. Without topographical planning, planting is not considered in Malawi. Other countries also give topographical planning more consideration compared to our region of the tea world. The topography varies between Brahmaputra valley's flats and the foot-hills. The latter is undulating, while the former low-laying. Level survey and accurate contour map are very useful in knowing the depressions and basis of contour lines. Before laying drains and planting, level survey should be done and contour plans made to ensure an effective drainage. Knowledge of ground water flow helps in planning the drainage, as in that case the excess water can either be checked at source or the flow can be intercepted. Before digging the drains, the first exercise should be to set out drain lines on ground and walk over it. While walking over such lines, extra attention is required to find out possibilities of any further improvement.

Advantage of Planting in Water and Soil Environment

The practice to construct field, collector and main drains prior to the commencement of planting is essential for better water and soil environment. Subsidiary drains feeding into the primary drains should run across the slope. In the beginning, shallow drains may be dug and later deepened gradually as a measure against caving in of the sides. If the soil from drain excavation is not flattened, it will be washed into the drain. Its weight may also force caving in of drain sides. The nearby depressions may ideally be filled by the excavated soil. In absence of adequate outlets, main drains and their maintenance, even of the efficient field drains, cannot be effective. In spite of available outlets, if main drains are found undersized and choked up, it clearly indicates bad drainage. The main drains should be sited on the natural line of the lie of depression as the depressions collect underground and run off water. The field and main drains are interlinked, as the former discharge water to the latter. Field and main drains are, in fact, complementary to each other. Distance between lateral drains depends upon the lie of the land. For example, steeper terrain requires closer distance than the gently undulating ground and the flat land may have wider distance, Horizontal spacing of subsidiary drains cannot be the same in all the soils. Sand and loamy sand soils may have 100 feet and 80 feet spacing, respectively, on flat land and gentle slope, whereas sandy loam soil may have 60 feet spacing, loam soil may have 60 feet spacing, loam 40 feet spacing and heavy clay even a shorter spacing of 20 feet. Determining the spacing requires local practical experience.

Closure Spacing Required for Heavy Texture Soils

As saturation period is longer in heavy textured soil, closer spacing is better there. Silt-clay soil with fine texture may require the drains at 40 feet distance or even closer. However, wider spacing may drain the area having porous soil. The water level movement is rapid in sandy soil and the deep drains are not required to be close there. There may sbe 20 feet vertical interval between subsidiary drains in sand on a slope between 20 and 30 per cent. On such slope, loamy sand may have 16 feet interval, sandy soil may have 13 feet interval whereas loam and heavy clay may have 10 and 5 feet intervals, respectively. In case of more than 30 per cent slope, the sand may have 30 feet vertical interval between the subsidiary drains and an interval of 24 feet may do in loamy sand. Sandy loam, loam and heavy clay may have 18, 12 and 6 feet vertical intervals on such slope. During the period of short rainfall, too many close drains will cause drying out in sandy soil. Gravels and sands are highly permeable and they drain freely. In most cases, clay and clayey and silt-loam soils drain slowly. They are less pervious. In case of sand, very rapid draining should not be done. Neither should there be over draining.

Spacing Based on its Depeth of Drains

The spacing is also based on the depth of the drains. Deeper depth allows wider spacing, whereas the spacing will have to be closer if the depth is shallow. Over-drained or excessively wide-drained sandy soil faces reduced moisture during the dry weather. Practical experience on a particular estate plays a vital role in determination of depth. Mature tea's effective root zone and the permissible water table depth below the surface are the factors which govern the optimum depth of the drain. The depth also depends upon the type of soil, the spacing of the drain and the availability of outlet. The average depth of effective rooting can be taken to be upto about two feet. The roots of the tea can penetrate deep into soil upto about one meter. Drainage to a depth of three feet improves yield, as the vigor of the bushes is improved. A depth of at least 3 feet is required in field drains for a safe level of water table. For adequate soil moisture during drought, more rooting depth is better. This, coupled with more bush density now compared to what it used to be in past, requires controlling the water table to a depth of minimum three feet. Between the drains there is water table curvature and it is better to keep the depth of subsidiary drains at four feet if water table is to be ideally fixed at three feet. In those gardens, which have high water table, immediate action is required to carry off the excess water and lower the water table and under such circumstances, deep drains are required. If sub-surface drains are deeper, they help in achieving better crop. As already pointed out, as a general rule, field drains of deeper depth may have wider spacing whereas closer spacing is necessary with shallower drains. Main and collector drain should be at least five feet deep. A minimum of 4-5 feet depth is required in primary drains. The outfall should be below the tea area and at least 5 feet deep. A level deeper than this will be required in case the outfall's distance from the tea area is more.

Natural Sub Surface drain Age and Annual Rainfal

Towards nullahs and rivers, natural sub-surface drainage is found due to permeability of the soil. The law of gravity applies to water's movement on the surface of the soil. Underground water moves in run off's direction at a slower rate compared to surface water. During high flood time, gravity drainage may not work efficiently in the gardens with low gradients as a result of "jams", streams and "pathars" rising sometimes to the water table of garden lands. This problem has been experienced more due to rising levels of important river-beds like Brahmaputra in Assam.

Major portion of the total annual rainfall during this period is very important. In several gardens there is a practice to clean the drains only in dry season thereby restricting the operating efficiency. Proper maintenance during monsoon is also necessary. Before the monsoon sets, drains should be kept clean with wedeicide. The maintenance of drains is very important during the monsoon. However, during this period, the shortage of labour is experienced on the estates due to plucking, manufacturing and absenteeism resulting from the cultivation of paddy and a planter, who some how manages a good standard of maintenance of drains, gets good results.

Operation Capacity of Drain

To keep the maintenance cost down and to avoid costly reconditioning and repair, it is necessary to maintain the frequency of inspecting the drains. Blocking by slips and choking with weeds restrict the operating capacity of drains. While using weedicide to control the growth of weeds in drain beds, it is wise not to affect the grasses on drain sides where soil erosion is a problem. It should be ensured that the velocity of water flow is not reduced due to any resisting force in water movement. Partially closed, raised or narrow culverts are the bottlenecks, which must be removed for proper flow of water. The flow is obstructed when the workers make fish-traps in the garden drains and villagers in streams where the garden water goes. While controlling the workers is very easy, good public relation work well to ensure villagers' co-operation. Drain junctions should be watched. It is important to ensure that one drain's flow does not slow the flow of the other drain.

Corrective Measures in Cold Weather

To take up corrective measures in cold weather, the functioning of all drains must be inspected thoroughly in preceding October. The drains for carrying off surplus water should have minimal slope not more than 1 in 100, otherwise the problem of erosion sets in. Depending upon various factors, the gradients may differ. However, 1 in 300 may be considered to be suitable in case of subsidiary drain. Erosion of drains is common in sandy soil. These drains should be identified to reduce the gradient. They may be given "V" shape by widening the top.

Locating of Outlet for Defective Drainage

Cleaning of drain should start from the outlet. No drainage scheme will be successful without a good outlet. Satisfactory outlet is necessary. Gravity outflow into river of stream should not be interrupted. Restrictions of various magnitudes may be experienced in some gardens and this is an area where improvement results in definite gain. Sometimes, a single outlet does not work efficiently and this fact must receive due attention. Outlets and main drains should have sufficient size to facilitate the removal of about one and a half to two inches of rainfall in one day. Water brought to the outlet must be carried away quickly and keeping this in view, the outlet must be sufficiently large. For an effective drainage system, first the outlet should be located. In low-lying areas, pumping may be advantageous at a particular time during the monsoon.

Drain Beds, Once in Three Years be Regraded

At the time of cleaning, depressions should not be allowed to form near the collars, nor cleaning should be done on wet days to avoid paddling in clayey soil otherwise in spite of the well maintained drains the ghosts of waterlogging and inadequate aeration will follow. Local collection of run off water should be watched out after heavy rain and drained out by shallow drain to the nearest available permanent drains. At least once in three years, the drain beds should be re-graded. The level below soil's surface where complete saturation of soil with water is found is the water table, which is lowest at the close of dry weather and highest at the close of rains. During the rainy period, water table may be above the depth of the drain. It does not harm if it rises shallowly for short periods. During dry months, it is below the depth of the drain or at the level of drain depth. The yield depresses considerably, if after heavy rain the high ground water table persists for long. High water table creates drainage problem.

Ground Water Table and Surface Run offs'

If the ground water table remains high, even surface run off's efficient control will not be able to give result. Ground water flow may continue for about two-three days whereas the run off is discharged in about four-five hours' time after the rain. Due to high water table, upward growth of roots results. Thicker root laterals start dying back at the ends. Waterlogged or marshy areas, tea bushes with poor health and low harvest are indications of high water table. For measuring the water table, battery powered "water level indicator" is used in developed countries. Down the bore-hole on a cable, an electronic probe is lowered and on contact with the surface of water audible and visual signals emit from the unit above ground. An electronic probe attached to a cable is lowered down the bore hole. On coming into contact with the water surface the proble transmits acidio-visual signals which are recieved by a receives installed on the ground surface. The cable graduated in meters then determines the depth at which water is found. "Portable water level recorder" and "water level recorder and logging sytem" are used in those countries.

Groundwater Potential Probe Set

The measurements of water pressure difference at various positions at a particular depth providing potential difference pattern, which may help in planning drainage configuration, are taken by "ground water potential probe set" in sandy, sandy clay or peat soils. Water table levels can be observed by sinking shallow inspection pits. With the help of auger holes or inspection pits, the water table should be observed from July to August to work out the corrective measures required in drainage. It is beneficial to have a section-wise record of water table to rainfall. A "T" scale is quite suitable for measuring water table from ground level to water level's surface.

Middle of Two Sulsidiary Drains

In the middle of two subsidiary drains in sections lowest area, one-fourth feet hole should be made for about forty/fifty acres. This hole should be encircled by a three inch bund and no "jabra" etc. should be allowed to enter therein. Before putting the "T" scate in the hole for recording the measurement, the scale should be cleaned and any water stain found on it should be wiped. Daily recordings of standing water's level should be taken in the pits during the wet period. Below the ground surface, water table should not be allowed above three feet in the centre between drains. After heavy rain starts, control of ground water table in the centre of secondary drains should ideally be achieved below the ground surface within a day at more than two feet within two days this control should be achieved at three feet and more. Saturation should not be allowed in the top three feet of soil in tea. Shallow run off drains across main slope and interceptor drains are able to control the water table on the slopes of Darjeeling.

Pipe Drain

Sufficient fall is necessary for gravity drainage and where the fall lacks in gardens situated in low lying areas, pumped drainage can be tried during the monsoon. In flat land with restricted outfall, the ground water table can be stabilized and the level of channel water controlled efficiently by pumping, which is economical. This, however, does not mean that it would remain economical even in the area where the necessity of pumping is felt during the whole monsoon period. Pumping should be considered on the basis of the area to be benefited and the cost of the operation and overall possible gain. During the period, wherever there is no possibility of the accumulated water being drained out by normal gravity, and the water level rises to a few feet above sluice, pumped drainage may be opted for, using low-head, high discharge mixed flow or axial pumps.

Considering the high maintenance cost, erosion of drain bank and land loss etc. in case of deep open drains and pipe drains are now-a-days being discussed which involve high initial cost. But this system may be found economical in the long run if PVC pipes and concrete tiles etc. are used. In this system, coping with the surface run off will require shallow and narrow contour drains, the width, depth and spacing of which will naturally depend upon the characteristics of the soil and the slope. Laying of pipe drains must be done after due consultations with TRA experts. Pipe diameters will depend upon the peak discharge, which depends on the proposed drained area. Planters fear that the roots might clog the pipes. The pipes can be cleaned by flushing water and covered by an envelope material which does not allow the roots to enter into them. In unstable soil, it is difficult to maintain the requsired depth of open trenches. Pipe drains are suitable under such conditions. Drain laying and making functions, if necessary, require utmost care. The flow inside the pipe should have self-cleaning velocity, Fine sand and silt particles must be filtered out for which a gravel enveloped layer can be provided around the pipe drain. It should be well understood that open drains can control water table as effectively as pipe drains, provided the former are maintained well.

With proper drainage the quantity of stored water available during dry spells increases due to more depth of rooting. Root development of less than two and half/three feet indicates inadequacy of drainage. Inadequate drainage results in depletion of plant's stored reserves. Mottling-greenish grey or bluish grey colloured sub-soil may be found in poorly drained area.

Role of Foliar Fertilizer and Point Injector Fertilizer Applicator for Sustainable Tea Plantation Management

Plants need different kinds of nutrients like iron, sulphur, potassium, nitrogen, etc. for growth and healthier crops. Fertilizer provides these nutrients to the plants. The conventional application of fertilizer is either in soil or on fields and the plants collect their requirement through the roots. But there is also an unconventional and less known fertilizer, which is neither applied in soil nor on fields but sprayed on leaves of the plants. This fertilizer is called 'foliar' fertilizer. In this case, the plant collects the required nutrients through the stomata, without much difficulties, foliar fertilizer can be made in abundance. Leaves of local plants may usefully serve as the source of raw materials, suggested Mr. Pedro Rene Chalco Lopez of the department of Solola, Guatemala. The process of making foliar fertilizer is also simple as it requires boiling ½ kg of plants leaves in 4 lits of water for about fifteen minutes. The mixture is then filtered and the pure liquid thus obtained is added with eight parts of water to make the solution really fit for spraying and congenial to plants' health.

Time and Duration of Application of Foliar Fertilisation

In making foliar fertilizer, Mr. Lopez used black nightshade (solanum nigrum). In course of this study, he observed that late afternoon was the ideal time to spray this solution as the possibility of unwanted evaporation was almost nil or negligible at that time. Nevertheless, satisfactory results can be achieved if foliar fertilizer is applied 'every five days from flowering until harvest'. But at the same time, he cautioned against the application of strong concentrated solution, which, instead of fostering growth, may severely injure the delicate leaves of the plants. However, the process of preparing foliar fertilizer and the study of its effect on different kinds of plants are at a nascent stage.

Developing Ecofriendly and Less Costly of Foliar Fertilisation

Agriculture research institutes, CSIR complexes, tea research centres in India should, as such, carry on strengthen to further intensive research with a view to developing fertilizer which congenial to the health of tea bushes. This will, moreover, be eco-friendly and less costly. Fertility of the soil will also be protected, no doubt. Well-distributed rainfall throughout the year is essential for the cultivation. But tea is also grown in some areas where rain is not well distributed. In India, rainfall varies between 125 cm to 750 cm in tea growing areas. The friable loamy soil is available in these areas and due to that probability of excessive N transfer to outgoing water is more. Several studies have been conducted which indicate that yield could be almost double by placing fertilizer in soil layer at depths ranging from 5 to 15 cm. The conventional methods of fertilizer use efficiencies have been reported to be 50 per cent to 60 per cent, and under wetland farming conditions it is 30per cent to 50 per cent only. In fact, point injection can only provide increased use of nutrition by reducing fertilizer losses and this technique can favourably influence yield. The old method of broadcasting fertilizer normally result in loss, while point injections give satisfactory performance in application of various types of fertilizer.

Point Injection Fertilisation Application

The point injector fertilizer applicator is now under development. It offers economy in energy conservation and provides advantages over the current methods of application, particularly with the increasing use of conservation tillage system. Use of knife-type subsoil fertilizer applicator is not much suited to apply fertilizer in standing crops like tea, as it is likely to cause injury to roots, disturbance to soil, in addition to greater energy requirement while opening subsurface of soil. Any type of disturbance to soil is harmful in high rainfall areas. Point injector fertilizer applicator aims at removing the disadvantages of conventional type of applicator. On observation, the salient features of applicator are (i) fertilizer can be injected with conservation tillage to reduce NI_3 volatilization, without destroying soil protecting crop residues, (ii) power, fuel and fertilizer needs for application are less than other methods, (iii) very little or no root disturbance occurs with fertilizer placement close to growing plant, (iv) more accurate placement and potentially improved plant uptake efficiency can be achieved.

Hence, a first generation point injector fertilizer applicator, suitable for soil condition of North East India, can be fabricated and tried in this region.

Avoiding sickness for sustainable tea cultivation

The problem of sickness in the tea industry has been claiming serious attention of Government since 1973/74. Sickness is generally identified by low productivity, loss in annual operations and failure to pay statutory dues for a number of years. It is due to a combination of factors in varying degrees e.g. unsuitability of land for tea cultivation, low productivity, poor quality, drought, lack of proper upkeep and maintenance of tea bushes and machinery, absence of replanting and extension, insufficient use of fertilizers, diversion of profits from tea industry to other industries and or misappropriation of funds, lack of proper cost control and general mismanagement, including willful neglect of the tea estates by owners who have no lasting interest in the tea industry but had purchased tea estates only with the object of making quick profits for a few years thereby making the estates uneconomic and inefficient beyond repair. Luckily, the number of tea estates which have become so sick that they cannot be rehabilitated with some enlightened attention, adoption of modern methods of agriculture and better management is not large and their production constitutes a very small proportion of total tea production.

Remedial Measures for Marginal Incidence of Sickness

The problem so far as it concerns tea estates which have already become sick is, therefore, not so important as it may appear at first sight and is, therefore, not a matter for serious concern. However, to remedy the marginal incidence of sickness, the industry had at one stage put up a scheme for the tea estates which were already sick, or were approaching sickness, to be nursed back to health by an association of tea producers to be set up by the industry for the purpose. The proposal was, however, not accepted by the Government of India. On the other hand, the Government assumed powers by making suitable amendments in Tea Act on the lines of the Industries (Development and Regulation) Act for taking over of management of tea estates which are found to be in default in certain respects and whose performance is considered unsatisfactory, according to certain criteria, and also to issue directives to delinquent estates for taking such steps and measures as may be considered necessary. Since these amendments were made in 1976, a few tea estates have already been taken over by the Government.

Sick Estates are Put Back on the Rail for Use of Productive Resources etc.

Experience so far with the tea estates taken over has, however, not been very happy. Apart from the fact that almost in every case there has been litigation followed by judgement in favour of the former owners of the tea estates there is nothing to indicate that there has been any worthwhile improvement in the economic conditions or profitability of tea estates since they were taken over the Government. The available balance sheets and P & L accounts of the taken-over tea estates do not perhaps reveal the correct position taking into account all the liabilities of the estates. As a matter of fact, if is not unlikely that under the high cost government management, the taken-over tea estates will become more and more sick particularly because the government does not clearly have the machinery with adequate experience, expertise and managerial abilities necessary for running a large number of tea estates. There is no valid reason why the losses of tea estates belonging to inefficient or negligent owners should be transferred to the public exchequer. Sick tea estates no doubt constitute a valuable national asset and it should be the earnest endeavour of everybody concerned to see that they are put back on the rails so that productive resources may not be wasted and workers employed in the estates concerned may not be thrown out of employment. However, it would be in nobody's interest to envisage a system that would merely transfer the losses of individual tea estates belonging to unscrupulous and inefficient companies or owners to the national exchequer with the possibility that such losses will mount from year to year unless the successor management possesses more than usual technical and professional expertise.

The Problem of Sickenss Calls for Fresh and Careful Look

Although the problem of sickness in the tea industry is not yet large, one cannot lose sight of the fact that in both 1980 and 1981 a large number of tea estates had to suffer losses because of sharp escalation in cost of production and less than commensurate increase in prices. Since the escalation in costs is likely to continue and no adequate and sustained improvement in prices can be envisaged in the near future, the entire tea industry is now on the verge of becoming sick. The problem of sickness in the tea industry, therefore, calls for a fresh and careful look not so much in the context of the isolated cases of sickness that have already arisen or been identified as in the larger context of the growing tendency for more and more tea estates becoming sick in the near future unless preventive measures are taken well in time. Take-over of management is, as stated earlier, not a satisfactory or desirable solution.

Amalgammation of Sick Units with Healtheir Units

A fundamental policy decision regarding take-over of tea estates is, therefore, necessary. The rationale and justification for take-over of tea estates should be critically reviewed and the circumstances under which it should be resorted to, if at all, should be clearly laid down. Take–over should, however, be the exception and the last resort rather than the rule. As a rule, efforts should be made to attach sick tea estates to other well managed and prosperous tea estates in the locality solely for the purpose of management without involving formal amalgamation. The managing companies may look after all aspects of production, marketing, export as well as various statutory functions on a reasonable remuneration. The principle of amalgamation of sick *units with healthier units has already gained recognition in India* in respect of other industries. There is no reason why the same principle should not be applied in the case of the tea industry. It is also hoped that efficient tea companies will gladly respond to a call to take up the responsibility for management of sick tea estates. It is suggested that the *Tea Act should be suitably amended to vest the Government with the power to appoint efficient and willing tea companies to manage sick tea estates without involving any transfer of ownership*. If this means revival of the Managing Agency system in a limited sense, we should not fight shy of it. *Enlightened pragmatism rather than fanatic dogmatism is necessary for tackling the important question of rehabilitation of sick tea estates as also for preventing sickness.*

Improvement in Tea Prices and Reduction in the Incidence in Cost Components

In this context, preventive measures for avoiding sickness are highly necessary. While for meeting the larger question of growing sickness in the industry the remedy lies only in *improvement in tea prices on the one hand, and reduction in the incidence of cost components* e.g. excise duty, sales tax, rural employment, cess, cost of various inputs, etc., and on the other, there is scope for certain other actions at the micro-level by individual estates. The macro-economic issues are, no doubt, very important and efforts to rectify the situation at the macro level should be continued by the industry in consultation with the Tea Board. It would, however, be idle to expect that any relief that may eventually be granted or any improvement in prices that may take place at the macro-economic level will offer a complete solution to the problems of all individual tea estates. Actions at the micro level are, therefore, highly necessary for reducing cost, increasing productivity and improving price realisation under any given set of conditions.

Cost Control

The main difficulty about adoption of cost control *measures is the lack of detailed information on various components of cost of production*. Some information at the macro level is collected from time to time by the Tea Associations or the Tea Board on a sample basis mainly for the purpose of arriving at a general appreciation of the cost of production of tea in different tea growing districts. Even this *information is not very accurate. For adoption of cost control measures, however, it would be necessary for every tea estate to compile detailed cost data and compare the same with item-wise standard costs in the same locality.* It is clearly not possible for the Tea Board to undertake this micro level work. Every tea estate must, therefore, in its own interest, regularly compile cost data and critically examine them in comparison with available standard costs so as to locate scope for reduction in cost of production. For this purpose, it may also be necessary for the Tea Associations to prescribe a standard proforma for computing costs as also a cell for assisting the member tea estates so that they may undertake necessary cost control measures. The cell may also review the progress or benefit achieved from adoption of such measures at regular intervals and may give further advice to concerned tea estates on the basis of such review.

Management

Quality of management is highly important for increasing productivity, improving quality and obtaining better prices. It is common knowledge that many tea estates do not have managers possessing the required abilities and this shortcoming is the largest single factor because of which many tea estates are not doing so well as other estates with similar agro economic conditions. Improvement in the quality of management in such cases is essential even under present conditions. The need will be all the greater in view of the anticipated increase of production to about 1100 million kg by 2000. A.D. Tea companies will, in future, have to play a more important role in marketing both for domestic consumption as also for export specially for an increase in export of blended and other value-added forms rather than confining their activities mainly to production and sale through auctions as at present. Tea garden managers will, therefore, have to have more varied skills than at present. Apart from being experts in tea cultivation and manufacture, they will have to possess adequate skills in financial management and cost control methods and techniques of marketing, maintenance, repair and installation of machinery and a variety of other skills to cope with the complex nature of their future responsibilities. It would, therefore, be necessary to recruit adequate number of agricultural graduates and engineers who should be trained to acquire a thorough knowledge about all aspects of their manifold duties, including marketing, accounting, costing, human relations etc.

Conclusion

A well conceived scheme for training of would-be managers through a multi-disciplinary programme should, therefore, be strengthened and put into effecgive operation as early as possible. The scheme should include pre-posting training for about six months, refresher courses for about three months, opportunity to acquire a reasonable period of experience and other refresher course of shorter duration at regular intervals so that there is adequate opportunity for the managers not only to acquire the basic skills required but also to improve their skills by exposure to latest developments in different fields. The younger generation of managers already in employment who are still young and have many years to work, should also be exposed to such training. The setting up of an Institute of Plantation Management has taken desirable step in this direction and the industry has taken concrete steps in the matter. It is worth while to mention here that more and more training programme that suit the needs of the manáge rare being in implemented on a regular basis.

Side by side with training of managerial personnel, arrangement is being made for social and vocational training of workers to make them better citizens conscious of their responsibilities and duties to the country and the tea industry as also to enable them to acquire the skills necessary for performing their duties more *efficiently and improving their productivity. It is, therefore, suggested that more workers' education centres specifically meant for tea garden workers may be set up by the Government of India in consultation with the industry and the Tea Board.* To start with additional four such centres in Assam Valley, two in West Bengal, one in Tripura, one in Cachar and two in South India would be enough though more centres may have to be opened in future.

The industry should wholeheartedly cooperate in the matter since a more *responsible and more efficient worker will contribute substantially in increasing productivity, improving quality and promoting industrial peace.* Once we have a fully responsible community of tea garden workers guided by trade unions which are free from political domination and are solely concerned with improving the conditions of workers in sympathy and consonance with the conditions of the industry, the next step would obviously be to *arrange for workers' participation in management which will undoubtedly be a step in the right direction that should be taken as early as possible.*

Reference

1. Tea Board, Kolkata, Annual Reports 1991-2002
2. Tea Association of India, Annual Reports 1987-2006
3. India Tea Association, annual Reports 1995-2003
4. Assam Review and Tea News, Various Issues, 1987-2002
5. Indian Institute of Plantation Management, Bangalore, Various issues, Tea in India
6. Tea Board, Kolkata, Various Issues of Tea Statistics
7. Tea Research Association, Tocklai, Jorhat, Annual Reports, 1999-2002
8. J. Thomas, Nilhata House Annual Reports, 2000-03
9. Calcutta Tea Traders Association, Annual Reports, 1998-2000
10. Barua, D.N. (1989). Science and Practices in Tea Culture, Tea Research Association, Jorhat
11. Mahaswani, S.K. and Singh B. (1987). Analysis of Repairs of Cost of Various Systems of Indigenous Agricultural Tractors, JNKVV, Jabalpur
12. Singh, B. and Singh K.N. (1991). Utilisation of Different Models of Traders on Large mechanised Forms
13. Banerjee, G.D. Economics of Tea Cultivation in India, Financial Express, 24 June, (1993)
14. Banerjee, G.D., Problems and Prospects of Assam Tea industry, Tripura Tea Industry, Nilgiris Tea Industry, Darjeeling Tea Industry Coimbatore Tea industry Published in Assam Review and Tea News during January-December 2000
15. Baneejee, G.D. Tea marketing A no longer Fashionable Slogan, IASSI Journal, January-March, (2001)
16. Banerjee G.D., Major Thrust of Tea Industry Published by Assam Review and Tea News in Six Instalments from June-November 2002

17. Banerjee, G.D. Sustainable Tea Plantation Management, IASSI Journal January-March, (2005)

18. Banerjee, G.D. and Karmakar K.J., The Tea Industry - A Survery (2005).

19. Banerjee, G.D. Pue'r Tea in China - Miraculous Functions, IASSI Journal, October-December, 2006.

20. Banerjee, G.D. and Banerjee Srijeet, (2007), Darjeeling Tea Industry - The Golden Brew.

21. Banerjee, G.D. and Banerjee Srijeet, Tea Plantation Industry - A Road Map Ahead, 2008, Abhijeet Publication, New Delhi.

22. Banerjee, G.D. and Banerjee Srijeet, Expot Potentials of Indian Tea, 2008, Abhijeet Publication, New Delhi.

23. Banerjee, G.D. and Banerjee Srijeet, Global Tea Trade - Dimensions and Dynamics, Abhijeet Publications, New Delhi.

Chapter 4

Quality and Performance of Tea Management Dimensions and Dynamics

An attempt has been made in this chapter to deal with dimensions and dynamics relating to quality and performance of tea management which include administrative setup, stages of tea development, management a social process, middle class temparament, preformance and productivity use of linear programming model in production planning and tea management. Labour productivity and plucking management of tea, dimension of low productivity, cost effective strategies in tea production have also been dealt with. Role of management in tea estates as well as cost and quality control of tea through improved methods of management have also been discussed.

Backdrop

Tea industry plays an important role in our national economy by way of earning foreign exchange, providing employment to around one million workers, supporting a number of ancillary industries and services and contributing significantly to state and Central exchequers. Tea is largely grown in Assam, West Bengal, Tamil Nadu and Kerala. It is also planted in Tripura, Himachal Pradesh, Karantaka and Uttaranchal in small scale. Tea cultivation in North India and South India differs on certain points. The productivity is somewhat higher in South owing to some climatic and environmental factors. An important difference in the process of cultivation is that in the South, plucking of tea leaves is carried out throughout the year, while in North it is seasonal. Tea industry's performance, which causes concern, is the gradual decline in the share of India's exports as per centage to world exports. During recent years, domestic consumption of tea has been rising faster than increase in output. The sharp growth in internal demand is overshadowing the already formidable growth rate in overall production. It has a dwindling effect on the export of Indian tea. However, our national interest requires that export earnings must be maintained adequately. Restricting the level of internal consumption can do this. But internal market provides the vital base upon which tea industry's flourishment depends greatly. There is thus a growing contradiction in the tea industry, which can only be resolved by accelerating the growth of tea production in India. The Lamond Committee in 1971, had stressed the need for setting up the annual growth rate of output from 1.9 per cent to at least 3.0 per cent within a decade for fulfilling the increasing requirement of domestic consumption as well as for maintaining the required level of export. But a good part of tea bushes in Indian garden has probably crossed their peak stage. So an increase in productivity needs an expansion in area under tea, replanting, replacement and improvement of yield through intensive cultivation. Development requires the provision of adequate finance. But an increase in the supply of finance does not necessarily result in an increase in productivity. The concomitant factors behind optimum results are good management and planning, financial discipline on the part on the industry and co-operation of labour.

Quality and Performance of Tea Management

In the context of competitive economy and ever changing environment, the quality and performance of management determines both the survival as well as success of any enterprise. The same holds good for the industry as well. But what does good management mean? Experts agree that management is a distinct type of *activity primarily responsible for getting things done through other people*. Similarly, they also agree that all *managerial functions are universal and all managers in any field of human efforts perform those typical managerial functions irrespective of what they are managing*. However, we do not have *any unified view on what are the managerial functions and what is management precisely.* Hence it seems difficult to get full hold of the term good management.

Let us now concentrate attention on tea management. The Indian tea industry has built up a crop, which in number and quality far exceeds that of any other producing country. This is not unusual since the industry has a glorious existence of 150 years to its credit. The first recorded mention of tea in India was in 1780 when a few bushes from Canton were planted in Kolkata which did not survive long. Serious thoughts were, however, given in 1788 for the culture of tea as a commercial proposition in India. It was not until 1830 that sincere attention was focused on this direction and a real progress was made in 1834 through the establishment of a "Tea Committee" by the British Government for investigating the possibilities of tea cultivation in India. Experimental tea gardens were opened during this era. It is thus found that the government of that day were the pioneers of an industry that has been instrumental in opening up large areas of jungles for the cultivation of tea. A report of a special committee, appointed on 1.2.1834, was submitted on 24.12.1834. It stated that "the tea plant which has been brought to light, will be found capable, under 'Last century' was 20th. It is 19th or 20th management, of being cultivated with complete success for commercial purpose".

Administrative Set-up

With the development of administrative set-up, British national took up the pioneering work in this regard and the Assam Company, the first tea company in India, took over part of Government experimental areas in 1839. The modern tea industry then began, although it was only around 1860 that it was firmly established. The formation of limited liability companies either to take over tea estates or to open new ones in North-East India had proceeded in the normal manner of business. However, Agency House System has also developed, whereby one agency may look after the affairs of several companies dealing with such diverse operations as tea estates, jute mills, coal mines, shipping, insurance etc.. Hence, the history of tea planting in India has a direct bearing on the corporate structure of the industry. Although tea has been known since 2737 B.C and has been consumed as a beverage for over the past twelve centuries, its cultivation in India commenced only in 1834 it and was initially scattered on small proprietary holdings. In the last century, at least until the 80's investments were mainly in coffee. Following the deadly incursion of coffee leaf rust disease, which wiped out the coffee industry in an era when fungicides were unknown, there was a definite swing to the investment. This was reflected by the progressive increase in the planted acreage. In this phase of expensive of industry, much of the initiative came from business houses in Great Britain and herein lies the explanation to the corporate structure the industry attained.

Stages of Tea Development

Tea industry in India, Sri Lanka, Indonesia and East Africa is based on four pivotal factors. They are *field technology, management, marketing and organisation*. Any discussion on future development of tea in India must take note of the significance of all these four factors. Tea is a permanent crop with an economic life span of 50 years with wide variations from this norm depending upon the location, terrain, type of plants and sustained cultural care. The product of commerce is the processed leaf of the plant features, which make it dependent upon large scale of green leaf and its timely manufacture. These two basic features of tea largely condition the organisation of production system most advantageous for commercial exploitation of the plant. The shift from peasant cultivation on which China depended, to large-scale plantation system which evolved in India, Indonesia and Sri Lanak and later in East Africa, brought about the complementary rise of large-scale mechanical process Grower-supported agriculture and product research structured management system and controled organisation and utilisation of resident labour of more or less a permanent character. These achievements were undoubtedly the result of colonial encouragement and support. The compact management process of the Indian tea industry probably has only one draw back against its name. There is no distinction between *the technical funcitions and managerial functions in the present system*. There is no need to dispute over the *quality and performance of the tea management in executing its technical functions*. The technical expertise of our tea management is the best in the world. But the same appreciation is, perhaps not similarly applicable to the other half or, at least, to a part of the same. Before chalking out some aspects of this unexpected lacuna there is need of good definition of management as an yardstick.

Management is a Social Process

Management is a social process involving co-ordination of human and material resources through the functions of *planning, organising, staffing, leading and controlling in order to accomplish the objectives like*: (i) management is a *social process*; (ii) it is in-charge of *allocation, utilisation and co-ordination* of all human and material resources; (iii) the resources are *co-ordinated and integrated by the management* through typical managerial functions of planning, organising, staffing, directing, motivating, controlling, etc., which constitute the process of management; and (iv) *management process is necessary to determine the objectives and goals* and to take necessary actions to achieve them.

It is known that the control function closes the management functions by providing adequate and accurate feedback or significant deviation from planned performance in time. Feedback can affect the inputs or any of the managerial functions or the process so that deviations may be removed and the goals achieved, As the tea management operates within the social environment, apart from its own business environment, it cannot deny its responsibility to the society. The Tea Board asked the National Council of Applied Economics Research in 1959 to conduct a survey of the *economically week tea gardens in North-East India*. The Tea Board is the organisation through which the Central Government exercise control over tea industry. The original intention of the Government was that the survey would be made if garden asked for an *investigation of its affairs*. It could be expected that an offer of this type would evoke interest of the managements in many gardens *facing financial and economic reforms*. But in fact, *none of the gardens put forth any request for the survey, which was thus entirely planned on the initiative of the Government*. Such an attitude *indicating lack of enthusiasm on the part of the management of the gardens may have been the result of several factors*. Some of them probably did not even know that the Government had made such an offer. Those among the management who knew about it might have been reluctant to let their affairs be scrutinised in detail lest some undesirable features were brought to light. Some of them might not be so sure of the strength of the case. A poor standard of maintenance of their record and accountants might have discouraged some. Also, it appeared that not many gardens expected quick and concrete results from such an investigation.

Middle Class Temperament of Tea Management

Middle class temperament of the tea management is really unsuitable for its hard earned good name even after conceding the fact that the remoteness of tea industry's location from easy accessibility and communication places this industry under considerable handicap. This, surely is not a fitting tribute to otherwise most eminent batch of management personnel. What is lacking then *in this outstanding managerial class*? The answer is certainly the *absence of flexibility in their outlook*, which is a must for any type of present day management in a world of competitive economy. This lack of flexible attitude has made them neglect the important aspect of supervisory management and when supervisory management is underestimated or neglected, organisations themselves face problems even if they have capable people at the top and a skilled labour force. *In the tea industry, only 7-10 per cent of supervisory staff has had formal training in supervision and existing training facilities cover no more than 1-2 per cent of the annual requirement.* Many supervisors do not receive training in the key aspects of supervision such as (i) operation, scheduling, and control; (ii) work organisation and rationalisation; (iii) communication; (iv) motivation; (v) team work; (vi) maintenance of records and; (vii) cost analysis. This only shows that management practices in some of the gardens are not satisfactory. It is only through better management at the financial, technological and administrative levels that yield growth potential of the tea industry can be realised.

The Lamond Committee also observed that *capable management is the first essential from which all other developments flow*. These assessments seem to run in the line of *goal models where an organisation is measured against* its goal or goals and the question most commonly asked it is : How close did it come to achieving its assignments? This approach defines success as a complete, or at least substantial, realisation of organisational goal. This approach has two potential pitfalls. *First, it tends to give organisational studies a tone of social criticism rather than a scientific analysis. Second, organisational monographs are frequently detoured into the lengthy discussion about this lack of success to the exclusion of more penetrating type of analysis.*

Tea management's Performance and Productivity

The tea management's performance should be measured not only in terms of the present organisational goal of the tea industry i.e. productivity. One should, instead, turn one's attention to the system model, which constitutes a statement about relationships, which must exist for the tea industry to operate. Research conducted on the basis of the system model requires more efforts than a study following the goal model, even when the latter focuses on real goals. *The system model requires that the analyst determine what he considers to be a highly effective allocation of means. This requires sufficient knowledge of the way the organisation of the tea industry functions*. Acquiring such knowledge is quite demanding, as (i) efforts made in getting the information required for the systems model will not be wasted, since the information gathered in the process of developing model will be of most of the value for the study of much organisational problems and (ii) theoretical considerations will serve as the basis for constructing a system model.

Now, a *well- developed organisational theory of the tea industry will include statements of the functional requirements it must meet. An awareness of these requirements will guide the researchers in formulating a system model for the study of tea industry. No such model for tea industry exists at present to indicate its organisational effectiveness, there by making the terms "good management" or "capable management"* sound meaningless. The question, which may arises now is: Is it possible to formulate and affect a system model for the tea management as well as for the whole industry? May be the best support for the idea that a system model can be formulated and fruitfully applied is found in a *study of organisational effectiveness by B.S. Georgopoulos and AS Tahenbaum, one of the few studies that distinguish explicitly between the goal and system approach to the study of effectiveness*. Instead of focusing on the goals of the delivery service organisations under the study, the researchers built up three *indices, each measuring one basic element* of the system. These were: (i) *station productivity*, (ii) *inter-organisational strains* as indicated by incidence of tension and conflict among organisational subgroups, and (iii) *organisational flexibility*, defined as the ability to adjust to external or internal change. The total score of effectiveness thus produced was significantly correlated with the ratings on effectiveness which various experts and insiders gave to the concerned stations. The stations were compared with one another on these dimensions rather than with an idealised picture of what a delivery station should be.

Operational Research in Tea Management

The availability of better management methods during the first half of the present century brought profound changes in functional specialisation in both technical and managerial fields to the business world. It facilitated the means and scope of achieving further economies of scale in production process. The result was that business enterprises grew phenomenally in size. This state of affairs presented the so called "executive type problem" which include certain management devices like mathematical tools, techniques and decision models. Linear programming is only one part of this model, which is known as operational research. Linear programming is a recently developed technique for providing specific numerical solutions of problems, which earlier were solved only in qualitative terms and helped to bridge the gap between abstract economic theory and managerial decision-making in practice. One can consider facilitating an operational method *for dealing with economic relationship, which involves discontinuities*. It has, thus, greater scope *of application within the tea industry especially where managerial decision-makings is asked for. Any linear programming problem* may formally be stated as follows:-

Maximise objective function subject to technical and non-negativity constraints.

Scope of Application Within the Tea Industry

In the context of Indian tea management, functional specialistion in managerial field is not sufficient, although it is more than adequate in the field of technical development. It implies that there is a vast scope for development in these regards. The first sign of awareness in this connection was noted in 1982 when the committees on work on plantations brought the subject of training of management personnel as a specific item of agenda. The committe report, therefore, represented the first attempt to ascertain the "*state of the art*" *of training for and within the plantation sector*. But definition of training given in the report was incomplete as it gave a narrow concept of training and tended to look upon it from a purely utilitarian point of view. It was also stressed that new methods of strategies should be used and both managers and workers should be given opportunity for study in the interest of the sector as a whole. Thus, *it was found that systematic training and retraining of personnel is a relatively new phenomenon in operation of plantation enterprises. Operations research can provide strong instruments in the hands of people.*

Meaning of Operations (OR)

There are a number of definitions of ORs in management literatures. *A descriptive definition says that OR is a scientific method of providing executive departments with a quantitative basis for decisions under their control. The types of decisions can be identified namely* (i) decisions made when future can be predicted with certainty, (ii) decisions made under conditions of risks and (iii) decisions made with uncertainty. Of these three types of decisions, *linear programming problems come in the first category.*

Models and Developing the Problem

The logical analysis of all decision problems is made on the concept of models and model-building. *The model represents reality. To build a model one has to use some device to represent an object on subject of inquiry.* This device may be schematic, physical, symbolic or a combination of these. The *term linear implies that all relationships involved in the specific problem which can be solved by this method are linear. The term programming indicates the process of determining a particular programme of action. A linear programming model arises when two or more candidates or activities are competing for limited resources and when it can be assumed that all relationships with problems are problems. Let us consider that we are to determine a Production Programme in Tea Factory involving three different grades,* say P, Q and R, each providing a separate profit contribution per unit. Let us assume further that manufacture of each grade requires some given processing time in each of, say, three processing operations. The product P, Q and R here are the candidates and three operations are the resources. Obviously, we want to design the programme, which will maximise contribution to profit. This type of objective is usually quantified as an **objective function**. Assumption of linearity implies that it is a linear objective function. The number of processing operations is taken as three only for the sake of simplification. In so far as it is assumed that the present capacity of three operations is not to be increased or decreased during a given time period, the capacity of the resources, although known, is limited. This type of limitation is expressed by saying that a set of **structural constraints** is given in the problem.

Production Planning

Let us now come back to our production problem. The times (in minutes) required per unit of each grade, the daily capacity of operations (in minutes per day) and the profit per unit sold of each product (in Rs) are assumed as follows :-

Table 4.1

Operations	Time per unit (Minutes)			Operation Capacity
	Grade-P	Grade-Q	Grade-R	
1	10	20	10	430
2	30	0	20	460
3	10	40	0	420
Per unit (Rs)	10	40	0	-

The zero time indicates that the product does not need the given operation. It is assumed that all units produced are sold. Moreover, the given profits units are not values which result after all pertinent expenses are deducted. The goal of the model represented here is to find out the optimum daily production for the three grades that maximise profit.

Let X_1, X_2,X_3 be the number of daily units produced of grades P,Q and R. As we have assumed that all units produced are sold, the total profit X_0 (in Rs) for three grades is $X_0=3X_1+12X_2+15X_3$. The constraints of the problem must ensure that the total processing time required by all produced units does not supersede the daily capacity of each operation. We can express these as follows:-

Table 4.2

A1 Operation 1	$10X_{13} + 20\ X_2 + 10$ X_3		> 430		
Operation 2		$30\ X_1 + 0X_2 + 20\ X_3$		>460	
Operation 3		$10\ X_1 + 40X_2\ 0X_3$		>420	

Since it is nonsensical to produce negative quantities, the additional non-negativity constraints $X_1 \geq 0$, $X_2 \geq 0$ and $X_3 \geq 0$ must be added. A some operations, research users have a tendency to replace the inequality (>) in operation constraints by a strict equation (=). The justification is that it is better to use all available resources than to waste a part of it. This reasoning does not hold good since use of (<) automatically implies (=). Thus, if the optimum solution requires that all the constraints be satisfied exactly, the inequalities '<' still allow this. In other words, the strict availabilities should not be imposed unless the problem requires that all operations must work to full capacity. This is completely different from simply stipulating that the capacity of each operation should not be exceeded.

The linear programming model is now summarised below:-

Productivity of Labour and Productivity of Tea Estate

Maximise	$X_0 = 3X_1 + 12X_2 + 15X_3$
Subject	$10X_1 + 20X_2 + 10X_3 < 430$ $30X_1 + 0X_2 + 20X_3 < 460$ $10X_1 + 40X_2 + 0X_3 < 420$ $X_1, X_2, X_3 < 0$

Tea industry in North-East India today accounts for 40 to 42 per cent of total cost of production to pay labour wages besides the additional expenditure of Provident Fund and Bonus and the fringe benefits like food subsidy, protective clothing, housing, medical expenses, fire wood, dry tea, welfare expenses etc. The cost structure of garden in Assam is shown below:-

	Composition of cost	Percentage of total
1.	Labour cost	44
2.	Manufacturing including packing, despatch, and sale charges	18
3.	Excise duty and Cess	07
4.	Establishment	15
5.	Others	04
6.	Agricutural inputs	06
7.	Provident Fund and Others	06
	Total	100

Source: Field investigation, 2005

Each labour tripartite agreement has resulted in wage hike, which varied from 7 to 14 per cent per year in the last five years, adding to the already increasing costs. Keeping this trend in view, it, therefore, appears almost certain that future increase in labour wages have to be accepted, more or less as a norm in future, irrespective of whether the productivity of labour increases in the same proportion or not. And this remains the chief concern of the industry. The problem of low productivity of labour acquires serious dimensions when viewed in the context of galloping costs, vis-a-vis increased cost of production.

Dimension of Low Productivity

The industry has been paying increased labour wages and providing the entitled benefits to its labour, irrepsective of the fact that prices of food stuff have escalated by 80 per cent during the last 10 years. The estates have been bearing additional costs on *"loss of food stuff" as subsidy. Price realisable from the worker has remained static between 40 and 45 paise per kilo of wheat and rice for a long time.* How can the labourers and labour unions be made conscions *of their duties as well, instead of thikinking of their right alone. It therfore, remains a vital issue before the tea estates and the industry at large, which is confornted with the problem of increasing labour productivity to the desired level. Thus the common concern of the estate management is to improve the output of his worker and control the cost of production.* But a garden labour remains essentially *'Ticca'-oriented worker, seldom having to exert himself beyond 5 or 6 hours a day to complete the task-based works.* Under the changed economic conditions, when 8 hours' work a day is obligatory in other industries, It is now high time that the present low *'ticca rates' are reviewed and revised to get 8 hours work a days from the labour.* These issues should provide adequate food for all concerned with the need to improve the productivity of labour vis-a-vis productivity of estate.

Need for a Sound Programme

Easier said than done' –as the age goes, till the time honoured 'ticca-system' changes, the estates perhaps have no choice but to function under this system. In the circumstances, programming each seasonal work gains major significance. The estate's works-programme must be chalked out on absolute time bound *schedules co-ordinated with the exact number of labour on roll and the actual number available for each type of work, for maximisation of labour contributing to productive work and minimisation of labour on unproductive work in an estate with labour to acre ratio of 1:1 the labour on unproductive work* (e.g. cowherds, painwala, waterman, malies, sweepers, chowkidars, creche attendant, etc.) should be restricted to about 8 to 10 per cent (maximum). Detailed programming for each and every item of work may seem a tall order but if done correctly, it would ensure timely completion of the seasonal cultivation works and most essentially, ensure timely availability of labour for the most important of all operations–plucking–during the season. Scientific planning of labour-deployment for each department of work–whether it is cold-weather work, development work, spraying or manuring–would entail detailed calculation of manday requirements for each type of work well in advance, linking the labour requirement for the programmed works with the monthly budget estimates, for effective control on costs.

Plucking & Labour Deployment in Plucking

With noticeable shift from 2/3–year pruning cycle to relatively longer cycles of about four or even five years by many estates in N.E. India, it becomes essential that minimum *55-58 per cent (approximately) of the total man days utilised in an estate, are on plucking–essential for controlling the cost of production.*

Production of maximum yield with minimum acceptable standard of leaf with quality remains an estate's main objective. Approaches to achieve this 'noble' objective could, however, vary and could be defeating if *'plucking' management is not understood in its correct perspective.* An estate programming high per cent of unprune/or lighter forms of skills with the aim of harvesting a 'big crop' could well lose on both the fronts–quality and quantity. This is simply because of its inability to provide requisite labour to pluck on regulated plucking rounds. An estate, with a more balanced pruning programme could also lose out on crop and quality. This attributes to the foot the estate is unable regulate plucking rounds and maintain the consistency in the standard of leaf during the flushing periods owing to incorrect planning of both plucking rounds and labour–deployment, in both cases. These phenomena not are uncommon in tea estates– where a somewhat ad hoc system of labour deployment is in vogue by way of increasing the number of labour on plucking as and when faced with the problem of tackling irregular plucking rounds, particularly long plucking rounds owing to holidays or high rates of absenteeism, or shortage of labour. The 'ad hoc system' of plucking vis-a-vis labour deployment on plucking, would have to be done away with in our quest for higher/improved productivity. Instead, a more pragmatic approach would be required, which would entail meticulous planning of man days for plucking, with the aim of maximising productivity of both labour and estate. A few petty jottings could be considered for effective planning of plucking in relation to labour in modern management. These are as follows:-

(i) Decide first the standard of green leaf an Estate desires to pluck at each stage of growing season. The standard of leaf to be plucked must be on a feasible/realistic scale. The percentage of fine leaf by weight should not be aimed at uneconomical level with the object of producing a standard of tea which is remunerative without affecting quantity, i.e. cost of production must not be allowed to exceed sale price, at all time.

(ii) Decide there after on the pruning programme— calculating the requirement of pluckers for each type of prune and skiff, and the feasibility of plucking to obtain both the desired standard of leaf and the quantity of crop, labour to the deployed for plucking must be worked out in advance for the plucking rounds programmed, for the entire 250 (approximately) plucking days available in North-East India.

(iii) Decide on the intervals at which each type of skiff and prune would be plucked at each stage of growing period.

Considering that the growth of shoots in each type of skiff/prune is never uniform plucking *rounds would have to be planned in relation to growth rates*. On practical level, it would be necessary, therefore, to pluck on shorter rounds. In the initial growing period. The tipping-varies, from 5 to 5-6 days (during February-March in North East India to 7 days plucking rounds during the active flushing period, till slower growth rates of shoots permit plucking on extended rounds of 8 days from mid-August to 9 days during October, and to about 9/10 days during November/December. The growth rates of shoots would largely depend on the length of sunlight hours, and movement of direction of photosynthesis in a bush with seasonal changes. It also nests more especially on severity of each type of prune or skiff programmed, and the health and vigour of a bush. Alternatively, an estate may choose to continue to pick on strict 7 days (or 8 days) plucking rounds, even during the comparatively slower growing period of September to November. This would mean adopting lighter forms of plucking during the back end-flushing period. Whatever may be the plucking policy an estate chooses to adopt, it must be based on sound economic considerations of requirements of pluckers and the feasibility of implementation of the policy–cost of production should not override sale price. While the pattern of growth of shoots during the season should be the basis of planning plucking rounds and labour deployment, the more specific part of planning (and also perhaps not appreciated fully) would be to consider the vital factor– the growing habits of each type of bush, and each clone–each with its own individual growing characteristics. The knowledge of the growing patterns would enable detailed planning for plucking each section on merit e.g. a UP section yielding 3000 kgs/ha (M. Tea) or above could be programmed to be plucked 40 times in a year while a lower yielding UP section of, say 1500 kgs/ha or so, may be required to be plucked 32–33 times in a year. Similarly, DS and pruned sections could be programmed to the plucked on an average 32–35 and 25–30 rounds in a year depending on the vigour of the bushes and the growing patterns. After all, it is an established fact that the more the number of plucking rounds higher is the total crop. Therefore, plucking rounds for each section could be planned in advance on merit basis.

Correlation Between Plucking Round and Requirement of Labour

The plucking rounds programmed would have to be correlated with the requirement of labour for each round and the problems likely to arise during the seasons, which could hamper plucking, must be anticipated in advance at the time of planning itself. This would mean taking into account the following factors:-

a) Weekly, national and festival holidays in a calendar year for programming plucking round.

b) Absenteeism/general rates of monthly absenteeism and unusually high rates of absenteeism; after pay days.

The objective would be to get the required coverage under plucking without losing control of the programmed plucking round (for each section). It involves calculating the likely losses coverage because of holidays or high absenteeism in advance and as a precautionary measure deploying additional pluckers to cover the additional areas before the unproductive day arrives. Alternatively 'ticca' plucking on these days could be programmed and organised. This would mean working out the economics and feasibility of the suggested measures and planning out the requirement of casuals or temporaries before the season begins. In case the requirement of pluckers so warrants, the shortage of garden pluckers must be anticipated in advance. The next task would be to decide the number *of pluckers for each day for each section. It is this area of day to day planning that a planter has to truly involve himself in not without some degree of flexibility. 'Planter's eye' (with frequent visits to the sections) and timely decision could only make plucking economical.* Engagement of too high a percentage of pluckers, or too low a percentage of pluckers, could both the disastrous and could lead to failing back on plucking rounds and to 'square-one': the age old ad-hoc system.

Considering the ever-increasing costs of labour wages and inputs, and the variable factors like fluctuating tea markets, climatic conditions, when the very viability of an estate could be at stake, it is deemed essential that productivity increases with improved productivity of labour. This is possible with a more scientific approach to labour deployment, based on meticulous planning at each stage. Plucking management with correct deployment of labour would, therefore, be one major step towards this planning for improving labour productivity, labour productivity being an effective tool for cost control measure.

Planning for Plucking Productivity

The single largest item of expenditure in a tea garden in plucking cost. *The productivity of the plucker is the vital factor of this cost. The blame for high costs or low productivity is always squarely put on plucker*. All over the North East the complaint of labour shortage during the peak season is increasing every year. Yields are going up but rise of plucker's productivity has not been proportionate and with further increase in yield in the coming years this shortage will increase. Mechanical plucking aids have been talked about and some experiments have already been made. However, this will have detrimental effect on quality. While these developments go on, it is also essential to direct concentrated efforts in increasing the plucker's productivity. Research on study of techniques, time and motion, psychology and strategies, are now vitally important for the future.

The Role of Management in Plucking Productivity

The role of management in plucking productivity is as important as pucker's efforts lays down *"plucking strategy" for pluckers*. Wrong planning can lead to low efficiency. Facilities provided by the management to enable a plucker to perform at his or her optimum are equally important. This happens when plucking strategies and planning are often left to supervisors or even sarders to work out and implement. More often than not, a certain block or section is plucked in a particular fashion as it has been "customary" to do so for the last 80 years. *Plucking is field operation very much a kin to what an army does in battle. The target area to be captured has to be first identified, manpower and support requirements estimated, the attack and strategy planned and then implemented so as to give the best results in the quickest time*. At the garden level too, the management approach to plucking should be similar from day to day. The attack on a single front, twin pronged or multi pronged, depends on a commander or management's decision, which has to taken based on the condition prevailing, the terrain and the shape of the target area. Psychological and human angles of the attack or plucking force are very important aspects and have also to be considered when planning the attack. For example, on a hot sunny day, any human being would prefer to walk or even stand, with his\her back to the sun rather than face it; so it is during plucking too. Efficiency is higher when plucking force has the sun at the back, particularly in the mornings and late afternoon when the sun is low. This is a fact of human nature but something that affects the cost of production.

The following area's few points, which the management should remember, when planning plucking :-

(i) The plucking round should be designed so that the previous day "left over" are not too far away from the current day's area. A circular movement around the whole garden or division is generally the most efficient.

(ii) Only sufficient pluckers should be allocated for the "left over" which should be finished by the 1st or 2nd weightiest time. This reduces time wastage through "movement" to the next and also, restricts to the wastage to a limited number of worker.

(iii) The work fore should not be divided into small groups and scattered i.e. there may be several "challans" but these should be grouped together and plucking concentrated. This has two advantages :-

(a) Supervision is better; (b) the momentum of the better pluckers pulls the slower pluckers along.

(iv) Movement should be planned ahead. When a movement is required from one block to another, sufficient number of pluckers should be put in, so that movement and weighment can be combined.

(v) Continuous weightment saves plucking time and gives better quality, though requiring more staff and transport. The cost benefit rates should be looked into.

(vi) Saving in the number of weighment sheds are not a saving. There should be a weighment shed available within twenty metres of the plucking area, so that to and fro walking time is reduced.

(vii) In the old days it was said that a section should be plucked from a different section each week as it helped to keep the table level. This is now no longer applicable with hedge planted tea and is also not economical. The most convenient and labour efficient direction should be worked out and the section plucked from that direction only.

(viii) Plucking should start from the furthest point and mode towards the weightment shed. The pluckers do not like carrying heavy basket over long distances and if the movement is away from the weightment shed, then the tendency is to leave the basket near the weightment shed and walk to the basket each time the plucking cloth is full. With movement towards the weightment shed the basket moves with the plucker.

(ix) Big drains should have adequate number of footbridges to reduce crossing time.

(x) Access roads to the "back" of the section are very important, as it is here that plucking should start.

(xi) Plucking should be in one direction only. In hedge planted tea, there should be a "plucking path" about 30 cm wide across the hedge every 130 to 150 metres. In square or triangular planted tea there should be 30 cm wide "plucking path" every 25 metres along the direction of plucking and 130 to 150 metres across the direction of plucking.

Anyone who has tried to walk 50 metres in a section of compact high yielding tea would know that one has to struggle and leap over drains to cover tis distance. A plucker, who has moved 50 metres in a section has to struggle his way back to empty the plucking cloth and then retrace his steps to resume plucking. This goes on throughout the day, and if the plucking is full, say 30 minutes before weightment or quitting time, the normal human reaction is:-

(a) The plucker will slow down his or her rate of plucking.

(b) Come out and go in again.

This is more likely to happen on hot and humid days or when it is raining, which happens quite frequenty. Plucking paths, as suggested, makes going in or out easier, thereby saving time and increasing efficiency. Looping the sides of the bushes every 25 metres may make the plucking paths. In hedge planted tea, one row across has to be taken out every 150 metres. In practice, it has been found this looping, or removal of bushes, does not reduce crop. In fact, crop increases through better plucking, supervision and these paths also help in improving maturing, spraying etc. In new plantings, attention to planning of paths and roads is thus, very important.

(xii) Height of the bushes being plucked is another important factor affecting to plucking productivity. This aspect again is a management decision, which has to be taken in advance, and height reduction has to be pre–planned on a long-term basis. The height of the planning table should not exceed 42 inches (107cm). The garden workers in general, are of short stature, but as usual, men are taller than women. In high tea areas, therefore, productivity of male plucker is better. The saying in old planter's jargon "if you can see their, use men' remain true till today."

(xiii) The advantage of good shade on a hot day is obvious. Areas having adequate shade, are plucked, if its fit in with the overall strategy for the day, in early morning.

(xiv) A good table leads to faster plucking. The basis of a good table is formed during pruning, thus once again, past "mistakes" can lead to fall of current productivity. In addition to the aforesaid, there are many more social and economic factors that affect productivity of the pluckers. A study by Shri B. Srinivasan of UPASI on the subject is highly enlightening. This paper, "Profile of a Good Plucker" 'was published in a recent edition of Tea Today. The time has, therefore, has come to take a more scientific approach to plucking.

Cost Effective Strategies in Tea Production

Cost effectiveness of strategies in tea production were stressed in the 31st UPASI scientific conference held at Coonoor in 1994. *These strategies included painstaking research coupled with constant evaluation of the long-term needs of the industry by Tea Research Institute (TRI)*. Nutrition of potassium and zinc, control of fertiliser blight by protecting the plants by application of eradicate fungicides, mid–cycle application of shoot-hole borer, rejuvenation for pruning and no-tillage replanting were some of the time tested practices being adopted in tea eastes in South India. Among the more important recommendations of recent origin were rooting parmonal formulation, nursery grafting of fresh cuttings, biconal seed stock for partial mechanisation of harvesting, leaf expansion concept in programming plucking intervals, organic, systematic fungicides,'use of coal as additive to glyphsate, use of VLV nozzles and integrated pest management have been widely accepted by industry elsewhere also and researched upon by Tea Research Institutions (TRIs) in other tea growing areas as well. The TRI has been working on partial mechanisation of certain field operations such as pruning and harvesting since mid seventies. While pruning aid could not be developed in India, plucking aids, both mechanical and materialised, were developed in the country. Intensive and extensive investigations carried out on the effect of partial mechanisation of harvesting on the productivity of both the bush and the worker have helped in refining the techniques. Tea Estates India, which not only adopted shear harvesting but also integrated it with leaf expansion concept in programming their harvesting intervals discussed how productivity of their workers increased considerably by adoption of the technology.

Patter on Nutrition the Chief Concern of the Social Chemistry Division

The pattern of nutrition, particularly of the major nutrients, is the chief concern of the Soil Chemistry Division that issues recommendations from time to time. Steep successive hikes in the fertilizer prices have necessitated a review of the recommendations released in 1987. A review of the existing literature, emerging trends in ongoing experiments, survey of the existing manurial practices and response thereon facilitated the formulation of ad-hoc suggestions to tide over the present crisis. This introspection has assisted in evolving recommendations of interim nature, till such time that firm recommendations are evolved on the conclusion of the experiments in progress. The details of these interim recommendations were discussed. *The stringent residue limits imposed, arbitrarily, by the European Economic Community recently have been causing serious concern to the tea industry in India. The TRI has initiated extensive basket surveys on ethion and dicofol in different tea districts.* It is gratifying to note that most of the samples tested were well within the limits prescribed even by the EEC countries.

The collaborative study on ethion being carried out with Tocklai Experimental Station and Rallis Agrochemical Research Stations is very encouraging. The nature of the raw material and its influence on the made tea, the need to optimise withering even in the manufacture of residual teas, the advantage of steam based drier technology for drying tea were some of the cost effective strategies in tea production. *A comparative study of the raw material used for tea manufacture and processing technology in both North and South India offered guidelines for future manufacturing strategy in South*

India. The following are some of the more important points that emerged out of the presentations and discussions at the conference.

1. It was brought out that the schedule of shearing had a bearing on yield whereas quality was not adversely affected by shearing. The findings and opinions were unanimous in respect of an increase in plucking average and reduction in the requirement of pluckers under shear harvesting.
2. The importance of containing pesticide residues in tea to conform to the legislative requirements of importing countries was stressed. It was also stressed that producers should seriously consider the use of natural products for controlling pests and diseases.
3. Ad hoc changes to the existing manurial practices were suggested to minimise the effect of low returns in the tea industry. With the same objective, interim recommendations were also made till firm recommendations were evolved on the conclusion of the ongoing experiments.
4. Marketing of our teas in newer markets should be attempted to improve the overall profitability. South India has to adopt medium plucking to increase production and overcome the high cost of labour and slow growth.

Role of Management in Tea Estate

The manager, a key person in the management of tea estate, is like the axle of a wheel around which everything revolves in the life and activities of a tea estate. He is like the key stone in an arch, the element that connects both sides the higher management and the operating employees within the organisation of a tea estate - and makes it possible for each to perform its respective functions effectively. *A manager stands as the linking pin only.* A successful tea estate manager has to keep complete supervision over the internal organisation and management of tea estate. A typical tea estate manager is considered to be a friend, philosopher and guide by his work. He has to know each plant of tea bushes and forest trees of his estate, each house of employees and each chest of tea manufactured in his estate. The job of an estate manager is very much demanding in nature. But there is no specific job description of a manager in a tea estate. Thus an attempt has been made here to understand the role of a tea estate manager in the sphere of duties and responsibilities by way of personal interviews and discussions with tea planters/retired tea executives/trade union leaders. Henry Mintzberg, in 1975, identified that a tea estate manager must perform three managerial roles.

Definition of a Role Played by an Actor

The term role is defined as being *like a role played by an actor. In the management studies, one defines the role as the behaviourial pattern expected of a manager within a functional unit*. Role is inherent in function. Mintzberg, in his treatise, has highlighted ten roles of managers that can be grouped into three categories like (a) interpersonal, (b) information and (c) decisional. A manager derives his status from his formal authority as an incumbent and by virtue of his authority as a manager he plays:-

(I) Interpersonal rules, (II) Informational roles and (III) Decisional roles

1. Interpersonal Roles

In interpersonal roles, a manager means figurehead, leader and liaison office. As a figurehead, a manager performs routine legal and social functions. As a leader, he leads his subordinates and as a liaison person, he deals with people who are neither his superiors nor his subordinates.

2. Informational Roles

Informational roles of a manager are to work as monitor, disseminator and spokesman. As a monitor, he constantly seeks information; as a dissemiantor he transmits information to others and as spokesman, the manager communicates with outside agencies like press, government etc.

3. Decisional Roles

In this category, a manager plays four roles ie.that of negotiator, resource allocator, disturbance handler and entrepreneur. He negotiates with his suppliers, creditors etc. in his role of a negotiator.

Table 4.3: Role of Managers in Tea Estates

Role	Description	Identifiable Action
1.	**2.**	**3.**
Figurehead	Performance of a few social duties	Welcoming visitors; attending subordinates' marriages; attending social and cultural gatherings in the neighbourhood community; arranging week-end parties for other tea executives; taking customers and guests to luneh.
Leader	Personnel managerial functions	Hiring, training, motivating and encouraging subordinates.
Liaison	Maintenance of contacts with outside agencies and informers providing information	Receiving letters, telephones, telegrams etc. replying incoming communications; courtesy visits to local government officers, police stations, etc.
Monitor	To act as nerve centre of internal and external information of the organisation.	Receiving notices, instructions, circulars etc. from higher management; listing the subordinates on affairs on tea estates; meetings with Sirdars and Muris; visiting plantation sites.
Disseminator	Transmission of information to other members of the organisation	Issuance of letter, reports etc. to higher management, instructions to subordinates; interpretation of government communications and court order.
Spokesman	Inform outsiders on the plan and policies of organisation	Attending board meeting; issuance of press reports; talking of representatives of neighbourhood community.
Entrepreneur	Searches organisation and its environment for opportunities to improve	Designing of improvement of projects e.g. introducing new variety of tea saplings
Distubrance handler	Responsible for corrective action in the event of disturbances	Dealing with strikes, grivance handling; and enforcing discilie among subordinates

Resource allocator	Responsible for the allocation of organisation resources of all kinds	Preparation of budget; determination of costs and expenditure of all items; scheduling of planting, plucking etc., programing of subordinates' work.
Negotiator	Representing the organisations at major negotiations	Negotiations with trade assocations, creditors, bulk buyers, transports, local community leaders, law enforing agenceis

He deals with disciplinary matters relating to his workers as a disturbance handler. He decides how the resource made available to him can be distributed for the attainment of the organisational goal in his role of a resource allocator. It has been observed, however; that tea estate managers play all ten roles as indicated by Mintzberg. There cannot be any difference of opinion in this matter if one looks at Table No 3. produced below.

Cost and Quality Control of Tea Through Introduction of Improved Methods of Management

India enjoys a unique position in the world being the major produces, consumer and exporter of tea, the world's most populas non-alcoholic beverage. Over the years the Indian tea industry has been making significant progress in terms of employment and output. But improvement in production is considered inadequate to cope with rapid increase in domestic consumption of tea. The domestic demand, which is assessed, to be rising at the rate of 5 to 6 per cent per annum, is affecting the country's exportable surplus. Unless a high rate of growth in production is achieved, India may be forced to import tea to meet its domestic demands. We are in the 3rd year of 21st C.

Tea Board Ambitious Plan

The Tea Board prepared an ambitious plan to reach the production target of 1000 million kgs of tea by 2000 with a total financial investment of Rs. 3300 crore. It was rightly understood that neither the tea industry nor the Tea Board nor even the financial institutions engaged in tea finance alone was able to generate such a massive fund needed by the industry. Therefore, a package programme launched, in which the tea industry, the Tea Board, the financial institutions, the commercial banks and the State Financial Corporations are equal partners. Greater emphasis was laid on the tea industry's internal generation of funds (a minimum of Rs. 300 crore). For this a minimum of Rs. 2.50 post tax profit per kilogram of tea on an average was to be earned by the tea industry.

Assam, which is the major tea prodcuing state in the North East India, fulfils 80% of the financial and physical targets of the Tea Board's plan set for the region. However, the performance of other sections of tea estates is not encouraging and unless their present standard of efficiency is improved not only the financial obligation but also the production targets will be difficult to meet and achieve.

All these imply that the Tea Board has vested greater responsibility on the tea industry itself. It is expected that all tea estates in the country, irrespective of their size, ownership and location, must contribute their share of funds and help in the realisation of production targets. For this they must improve their present profitability rate through the improvement of estates' management, both general and financial. In the tea auction market there is no system of minimum support price, and therefore, a fall in the world demand for it may sometimes result in the fall in the price level below the cost of production of per kilogram of tea. However, the quality tea produced by a tea estate always has a good demand and fetches remunerative price under all market situations. To generate adequate surplus, therefore, all the tea estates, in addition to their efforts for the realisation of their production targets with the aid *of intensive and extensive cultivation, will have to lay emphasis on cost and quality control through the introduction of improved methods of management. In this respect, the following areas are required to be re-looked.*

1. Improvement in Estate's General Management

Competence in estate's management is the king-pin of success in tea cultivation and manufacture. *The only permanent assets in a tea estate are the tea bushes, which demand maintenance and upkeep like all other fixed and variable assets*. Thus, the estate's manager must maintain and upkeep this *permanent asset by way of acquiring knowledge of scienstific and up to-date methods of tea culture and manufacture. The scientific experiments in the field a of tea cultivation and manufacture have invented different methods with their own advantages and disadvantages.* For instance, intensive tea plantation from clones adds to the increase in productivity within a short span than from tea saplings, but when one considers the involvement of heavy expenditure in new plantations and the lifecycle and economic age of tea bushes, the latter method is found to be superior. Similarly, coarse plucking results in higher yield per hectare than finer plucking, but when one considers the stable and remunerative price of quality tea in the market, then the latter method is more commendable. The same can be said about pruned and unpruned sections of tea bushes. Unpruned section can result in higher production in the short run, but from the point of view of long term increase in production of tea, the pruned sections always produce better results.

(i) Maintenance of Reasonable Productivity and Quality of Tea

A tea estate's manager aiming at maintaining reasonable productivity and quality of tea at the lowest possible cost should make the best combination of different methods of tea culture and manufacture. The estate's manager must be well acquainted with the scientific techniques of tea cultivation, nursing or tending of tea bushes, pruning cycles, methods of plucking and manufacture. For this, all tea estates, irrespective of their size and types of management, should lay emphasis on the appointment of their estates' managers from that section of managerial personnel, who not only have the needed educational qualification, but also receive necessary training on tea culture and manufacture from recognised institutions, such as the Tea Research Association and India Institute of Plantation Management. It has been found that the tea estates of smaller sizes owned by private limited companies, partnership and proprietor firms are either managed by the owners themselves or by managers, who hardly have adequate knowledge of the scientific methods of tea culture and manufacture. In addition, most of these tea estates also decline to be a member of the Tea Research Association on the pretext of its higher membership fee. As a result of this, the benefits of scientific research are not available to these tea estates. Both these factors limit the managerial competence of most of the managers of all such tea estates in terms of quality and quantity of teas made by them.

(ii) Maintenance of Higher Productivity and Quality of Tea at Lowest Possible Cost

In order to survive in a seasonal industry such as tea, there is no alternative to the maintenance of higher productivity and quality of tea at the lowest possible cost. So, all tea estates should appoint skilled managers who are not only capable of making the best and the fullest utilisation of all fixed and variable factors at their disposal, but also prove their competence in maintaining higher productivity and quality at the lowest possible cost. The smaller tea estates, in particular, should give up the tendency to appoint unskilled managers, as this results in greater losses in production against some marginal gains on the payment of lower salaries to them. If the owners themselves bear the responsibility of management of their tea estates, then they should receive necessary training on tea culture and manufacture under the guidance of a recognised training institute. Further, to reap the benefits of scientific research in the field of tea culture and manufacture, they should also acquire the membership of Tea Research Association.

2. Better Financial Management

The basic objective of financial management is *to ensure adequate flow of funds to a tea estate through the attainment of the condition of wealth maximisation*. The maintenance of adequate flow of fund to a tea estate is most significant, *because in its absence, even a competent manager would fail to realise the triple objectives of success in the tea plantation and manufacture, namely, maximisation of productivity per hectare of area under tea, minimisation of the cost of production per kg. of made tea and the improvement of its quality. In the same way, he will also find it difficult to prepare and execute planning for the sustained growth of his tea estate*. The preparation of a realistic plan requires some basic information on estate's production and costing and its execution requires adequate flow of funds. A tea estate not equipped with a system of standard financial management is neither able to provide needed information to its planners nor finds enough resources for its execution. The success achieved by the tea estates under public limited companies in attaining a definite standard of financial management and the benefits derived therefrom would provide enough evidence to support such a conclusion. So all tea estate's, irrespective of their size and management, should lay maximum emphasis on the attainment of the required standard of their system of financial management.

(i) Generation of Own Cash to Meet Financial Obligation

It is true that being a unit of cyclical industry, it would not be wise on the part of a tea estate to depend entirely on *its own generation of cash needed to meet its entire financial obligation*. But at the same time one cannot ignore that as a unit of the most organised industry of the country, a part of the estate's financial requirements, both short term and long term, should always *come from internal generation of funds*. In fact, csommercial banks and the term lending institutions, which are responsible for the flow of external resources to the tea industry, set the condition of *"margin money" as an eligible* criterion to attract funds from them.

Working on the Principle of Sound Finance

In order to fulfil the norm of margin money, there is no alternative to generation of internal surplus, and a tea estate achieving this conditions will always have assured flow of funds from outside. To fulfil the objectives of internal generation and assured funds from outside, a tea estate under all circumstances will have to work on the principle of sound finance. The concept of sound finance applicable to a business unit does not imploy avoidance of deficit. To a business unit it has two implications, the proper utilisation of funds at its disposal and the promptness in meeting its obligations of debt, interest, sundry creditors, and the likes, as and when there is a generation of its own cash.

Not Likely to Loosen Credit Worthiness

A tea estate can work on the principle of sound finance by making earnest and constant efforts to bring all round development through proper utilisation of funds at its disposal on are hand and by laying prima-foci importance on maintaining its "credit worthiness" through prompt payments of its debts and interest as well as meeting the other market obligations, on the other. A tea estates working on the principle of sound finance rarely faces the problem of internal generation of funds even under unfavourable agro climatic conditions. It may fail to create surpluses in some years due to unfavourable working of some factors beyond its control, but it is not likely to lose its credit worthiness in the financial sector, if it works on the principle of sound finance.

But a slight deviation from the same principle will have disastrous consequence on the estate's eligibility criteria for the flow of funds, and if proper care is not taken to resort to the principle of sound finance before it is too late, the very existence of tea estate may be at stake.

3. Basic Requirements of Sound Financial Management

(a) Financial planning

Financial management is not a process, but processes involved in maintaining the flow of funds may be broadly classified as financial planning, co-ordination, control and replanning. The introduction of financial planning involves three fundamental steps, *first, determining both long-term and short-term financial objectives; second, formulating and promulgating financial policies*; and third, developing procedures that aid in promulgation of farm's policies. The significance of financial planning in a tea estate of any size and under any type of management cannot be overlooked. Absence of financial planning not only results in paucity of funds in times of need, but also results in the large-scale diversion of funds for purposes other than maintenance and development of tea estate. Such paucity and diversion of funds are mainly responsible for the sickness of a considerable number of tea estates in tea growing region of Assam.

So, by taking maintenance and growth as the primary objectives, all tea estates should set up the short-run and long run objectives of their financial planning. Appropriate policies are to be formulated to assess the exact amount of capital required and sources from which it should be raised. Financial planning in a tea estate is generally done in two ways, - short term and long term. Short term planning aims at maintenance and upkeep of the existing assets of a tea estate while the long term planning is undertaken with the basic intention of achieving success in its policy of growth through addition of new assets.

(i) Short Term Planning

A tea estate can not only maximise its profits *in good years but also minimise losses in bad years by distributing it over a large scale of output.* The tea bushes are depreciating assets. After the expiry of their economic age, they require replacement . So, short term planning is to be introduced for proper upkeep and maintenance of young and matured tea bushes and replacement of old tea bushes by new ones through replacement, infilling, rejuvenation etc. At the same time such short term planning should also aim at upkeep, maintenance, and necessary replacement of the other fixed and variable assets of a tea estate.

A tea estate with the help of its annual budget executes short term planning. To a tea estate, *budgeting implies item-wise determination of its expenditure, both revenue and capital for the current year.* A tea estate equipped with a system of scientific budgeting can not only lay out plans and programmes for raising *necessary resources and undertake investment plan on items of revenue and capital expenditure by taking full account of changes in input cost and their supply position*, but also go ahead with the state-wise implementation of long term or perspective plan introduced for its future growth. However, in order to achieve success in tea plantation, budgeting is not an end in itself; equal emphasis must be laid on the item wise balancing of actual expenditure with the budgeted ones.

Scientific budgeting also helps a tea estate or a company in making the best use of its surplus resource. With the help of proper budgeting it can use its surplus resources for the improvement and addition to its permanent assets. This improves its liquidity position, which is not only the *sine qua non* of its higher profitability rate and more solvencies but also an eligibility criterion for the easy flow of outside resources to it.

(ii) Long Term Planning

It has been found that due to cyclical nature of tea industry most of the tea estates prefer to execute and realise the objectives of long planning through short term capital budgeting. But, what ever is the procedure of its execution, no tea estate should ignore the significance of long term planning. Because in the face of ever increasing competition among tea producing countries the existence of individual tea estate and company is solely dependent on their competence in the production of adequate quantity of tea at reasonably lower cost. For this, long term planning for improvement and addition to their fixed and depreciating assets is to be undertaken. *Such long term planning should include replanting of existing tea area, where tea bushes prove uneconomic and the extension of tea plantation in new areas as well as addition and improvement of the techniques of manufacture, transportation and other allied activities related to development of tea industry.* The extension of tea cultivation in fallow areas is a must because such fallow areas constitute an overhead cost.

(b) Financial Control and Co-ordination

The second step in financial management is financial control and co-ordination, which consists of two steps developing standard performances and comparing activities with these standards. The significance *of this process lies in the maintenance of adequate flow of funds through the fulfilment of the objective of maximising output or maximising returns from the factors employed by the firms. In the tea industry, due to cyclical nature of performance, the development of standard performances and comparing the ongoing activities with these performances, have immense value.* Of course, in our country, the rate of utilisation of funds by a tea estate is mostly influenced by factors that are outside human control and, therefore, its standard performance is not easy to determine. Further, uneconomic size of a large number of tea estates pose a problem in the establishment of basic infrastructure needed to determine their respective standard performance. In spite of such limitations, some standard performance is to be worked out by a tea estate on the basis of certain scientific principles that suit the conditions of tea industry. One such principle may be like this: a tea estate, in order to determine its standard of performance, will take into account its performance for a period ranging from five to ten years and compare the same with the performance of the same period of some tea estate within the same area enjoying identical agro-climatic conditions. On the basis of such comparisons, a common performance can be found out which can be regarded as the standard performance. If some internal barriers prevent a tea estate to adopt such a procedure then it can seek the help of the Tea Research Association of find out the standard a performance for its locality.

(i) Proper System of Accountancy and Costing

The achievement of standard performance should be the basic objective for all tea estates and for this they must utilise the resources at their disposal in the best possible manner. In order to ensure the best utilisation of resources, the introduction *of proper systems of Accountancy and Costing are must for all tea estates*. Estate Accountancy is the most important asset and valuable qualification of the young tea planter who is aspiring to be incharge of the property. He should be able to discern the meaning of each and every entry made in the books of account without any doubt whatsoever, and so be in a position to check the correctness of such entries. This most useful knowledge will not only help him to see how the finance of the estate stands, but he will also have a clear command over expenditure which is vital for working to one's estimates. In order to have success in accountancy, adequate knowledge of book keeping is required on the part of the estate manager. The introduction of proper methods of book keeping will help him in obtaining results, which will be absolutely accurate. Because books of accounts can be proved with same ease as one can prove an addition by subtraction or multiplication by division.

Costing helps a tea estate to assess the rate of utilisation of monetary resources in quantitative terms. A tea estate generally adopts costing in two different ways, namely cost of production of per kilogram of made tea and cost per hectare or acre of cultivated area. In the estate's monthly report form, in the statement of analysis of expenditure, there are usually three columns of statistics, namely cost per kilogram of made tea for the month, to date for the year. Such costing is done to ensure that the resources are properly utilised for purpose for which they'are allocated or granted. So, all tea estates should lay emphasis on the use of such a method of costing.

(ii) Intergarden Comparison of Cost Figures

Of course, such a type of costing *within the estate cannot give a correct picture about the best utilisation of resources employed in it. For this*, inter-garden comparison of cost figures, as done by the tea estates under public limited companies, is necessary. These tea estates can undertake such a type of costing due to the practice of *appointing one Visiting Agent for a large number of tea estates under different tea companies*. But in tea estates owned by other types of management such a system of appointing Visiting Agent is not found. So, for them, a system of *inter-garden information is to be built up in each tea growing area. The 'Area Scientific Committee' existing in some tea growing areas can take necessary steps to build up a system of inter-garden information in their respective area.* If such a system is built up, tea estates of the same area would be able to make comparison of cost and productivity of their estates. This could help the tea estates to find out their deficiencies in maintaining the standard cost and productivity of their respective area, and to take up corrective measures accordingly.

(iii) System of Appointing Experts in Accountancy and Costing

For the introduction and maintenance of such effective system of accountancy and costing, an adequate knowledge of these subjects on the part of estate's manager or superintendent is required. But in case of the majority of the managerial personnel there is limited knowledge of estates' accountancy and costing. Therefore, they resort to the system of appointing experts in the said field. There is nothing wrong in appointment of experts in accountancy and costing, since their expertise could help the management to place the estates' accountancy on healthy footing. But, as the risk of investment in a tea estate always lies with its owners or management, a system of checking accounts for them is to be built up to ascertain the correctness of entries made in the books of accounts and other registers. For this, the following steps will be very useful.

1. Checking of Accounts and Stocks

In order to ascertain the correctness of entries in the books of accounts and stocks, the management must introduce the following system.

(a) Cash Book balance must be checked with actual cash in hand in each month.

(b) Bank balance as per cash book must be checked with a certificate from the bank and verified subject to reconciliation statement.

(c) Stocks must be checked with the stock book and all stores with relevant inventories.

2. Verification of Stores Received

In order to ascertain that the resources meant for the estate are duly received and properly utilised, the management must have the system of verification of stores. For this, the following methods are very useful.

(a) Vouchers should support all stores received in the estate. All local purchases should be in the form of invoices and bills. Their memos should support the supplies received from one's agent.

(b) All invoices and agent's memos should be scrutinised carefully by the management to make sure that nothing described therein has failed to arrive.

(c) Issue notes of a responsible member of the staff must support all issues of stores.

3. Verification of Check Roll

In order to ascertain the correctness of entries in the check roll, the management must satisfy itself that there are no fictitious names on the rolls. For this, the undermentioned system of verification of the check roll must be introduced.

(a) The check roll made by the clerical staff must be test checked with the pocket check roll.

(b) The check roll weight of green leaf plucked should be roughly checked with the factory weight as appearing in the Tea Book. This means that when payment is made on a kilogram basis, it must be ascertained that the green leaf for which payment is to be made has actually been received in the factory.

The system of accountancy and costing described above would ensure the best utilization of resources of a tea estate. No one can ignore the significance of proper methods of accountancy and costing in the generation of internal surplus. In fact, a tea estate equipped with a system of proper accountancy and costing rarely fails to generate internal surplus. With the help of such a system of accountancy and costing it is in a position to prepare improved balance sheet showing higher ratios of profitability, liquidity and debt to its equity. With such improved ratios the development efforts of the estate will not suffer for want of funds. Therefore, all tea estates, irrespective of their size, location and management should lay emphasis on the introduction of standard system accountancy and costing. The tea estatis of smaller sizes, in particular, need a lot to improve in this respect. They should give up their practice of appointing unskilled accountants and appoint those who have fair knowledge of accountancy and costing.

(c) The Process of Replanning

The replanning process is the last function performed by the financial managers and is of vital significance for the ultimate success of the business firms. If the evaluation of the performance reveals that the end results of the firm's activities will not meet predetermined standards, it may be assumed that either the firm's policies or personnel are not effective. If it is the former, the management must first ascertain which of the policies it is so that the firm can achieve its goals. This process of replanning has its significance to a tea estate. A tea estate requires constant vigilance and evaluation of its performance to achieve success in tea business. If some defects are detected in its policies then corrective measures must be introduced or new ones must replace such policies. Otherwise, its chances of success in tea business will be dim.

Conclusion

The tea industry is more or less contended with a small margin of profit and superlative quality production. The emphasis is more on quality than on quantity. Further, there was some parity in production and consumption with established tea growing nations. Since 1950's, however, the situation has been fast changing due to various political, social and economic factors and we now come to the phase where we are. Of late, our slogan has been 'Quality tea'. It is surprising that we are yet to take positive steps in shaping the fiture of tea industry. The banner, slogans and square pegs in or round holes must be avoided forthwith to overcome disasters. If we wish to identify what we were, what we are and what we want to be, it would be worthy to remember the age old saying, "Prevention is better than cure".

In order to survive in a cyclical industry like tea, one has to achieve the objective of *wealth maximisation through productivity maximisation of tea estates*. Thus, tea estates, whether sick, small or prosperous, should make constant efforts to improve their standard of management both general and financial. Tea, basically an agro-based industry hence the management of all tea estates must always bear in mind the two basic requisites for success in tea cultivation. Firstly, tea plants require utmost care and attention to bear their fruits and it is neither over-investment nor under-investment but only adequate and right type of investment at appropriate time that helps to achieve such a goal. Secondly, being subjected to the law of variable proportions, the achievement of higher productivity is possible only at a higher rate of investment on tea culture and this may result in a fall in a rate of yield per rupee of revenue expenditure at estate's head. Thus it should not be cause of concern for the estates and companies, which have introduced planning to raise their productivity.

References

1. United Planters Association of Southern India (UPASI), Annual General Meetings 1995-2002,1
2. Tea Association of India (TAI), Annual General Meetings 1995-1995
3. Indian Tea Association (ITA), Annual General Meetings 1985-1990
4. Chaki Bat, Bharatiya Cha Parishad, Various Issue, 1985-1990
5. Tata Tea, Annual Reports, Various Issues
6. Kolkata Tea Traders Association, Various Memorandums Submitted to Government.
7. Small Tea Grovier's Association, Annual Reports, Various Issues.
8. Tea Research Association, Tocklai, Annual Reports, 1980-85
9. Indian Institute of Plantation Management, Banglaore, Tea in India, Various Issues
10. Tea Board India, Unpublished Materials
11. Tea Board India, Tea Directory
12. Tea Board India, Various Development Schemes
13. Ministry of Agriculture, Plant Documents
14. Tea Board, perspective Plan for Tea
15. NABARD, Annual Reports
16. Green Page, Various Issues
17. G.D. Banerjee and Srijeet Banerjee, Darjeeling Tea - The Golden Brew, 2007.
18. G.D. Banerjee and Srijeet Banerjee, Global Tea Trade - Dimension and Dynamics, 2005, Abhijeet Publication.

19. G.D. Banerjee, and Srijeet Banerjee, Export Potentials of Indian Tea, 2008, Abijeet Publication.
20. G.D. Banerjee, Tea Plantation Industry in India - Structural changes between 1950 and 1992.
21. G.D. Banerjee and Srijeet Banerjee, Tea Plantation Industry - A Road Map Ahead, 2008.

Chapter 5

Sustainable Development of Tea Industry in National Perspective

Tea : Agriculture as well as Industry

Tea can be placed both under agriculture and industry. It is industry in the sense that tea is a processed commodity which is subject to excise duty and cess. It is also agriculture crop becausal it is grown on land and thus agricultural income tax is also levied on it. Moreover, a tea plantation is governed by both agriculture and industrial rules and regulation. The tea crop involves both agricultural and industrial operations. Agricultural operations like cultivation, plucking, manufacturing, irrigation, weed control, disease control, pest control, transportation of green leaf and uprooting are undertaken for growing tea. The final product of tea goes through various processing and manufacturing stages like withering, rolling, fermenting, drying, weighing, sorting, cutting, that place it under industry. Thus tea plantation is a big agricultural enterprise that has also some characteristies of industry. Tea industry employs large amount of labour force which mainly resides in the estate and is under more or less elaborate management. The establishment of operation requires massive investment of capital. Modern technical equipment is also necessary for processing the product. The outstanding feature of tea plantation economy is that a large portion of tea has been consulted by the internal market from the very inception of this industry. This has, therefore, made it necessary to have well organised marketing services. The requirement of capital, technical know-how and organised marketing services explain why the unit of production of tea has taken the shape of a large industrial establishment. Tea is thus both industral and agricultural activity. Keeping in view the importance of tea there is need for detailed discussions in respect of the various developments that took place over a period of time. The development of the tea industry, as it emerged over the periods is discussed below.

Development initiatives of Tea Industry

1. UBI Expanding Business in Southern Region: The UBI, popularly known as Tea Bank of India by virtue of its expanding almost 50% of tea finance, is actively considering ways and means to expand its tea business in South India, which, after Assam and West Bengal, is the largest tea growing region in the country. Thus the experience gained by UBI in tea has been of immense benefit to the growers in the South. At the same time the UBI widened its presence in the North-East. It had already very impressive presence in the North-East.

2. Pioneer Business in Tripura and Manipur etc.: It is quite possible that with successful experiments in tea in new areas within the same geoclimatic region, the UBI launched pioneer business in Tripura and Manipur besides Arunachal and Orissa which had already sent their first flush tea for auction in Kolkata and Gauhati. In Arunachal, UBI has two gardens and 4 more are likely to be extended within be few years.

3. Top Tea Companies Asked to Raise Output : The then Addl. Secretary in the Union Commerce Ministry, Shri R.Sivraman, wrote to 225 top tea companies, which accounted for 35% of national production in the country, to take effective measures to raise tea production. Another step increase tea production was taken by the Tea Board which on its part had concentrated its attention only on sick, weak and marginal gardens estimated to number 145. In separate letters to the owners of these gardens, the Tea Board asked for relevant information about their rehabilitation and development plan progress as also the kind of assistance they would like the authorities to render. Accordingly the Union Commerce Ministry and the Tea Board, as part of integral exercise, monitor use of various loan and subsidy schemes for development programme initiated by the tea companies. The research and development establishment of the UPASI and the Tea Research Association catering to the needs of North Indian gardens were also being asked by the Ministry to furnish details of R&D inputs to be made available to gardens to supplement their efforts to raise tea production.

4. Tea Industry's Process for Tax Review: A representative delegation of the Tea Industry called on the then Chief Minister of Assam and urged him to re-examine the taxation proposals. A memorandum detailing the hardships caused to the industry as a result of new tax proposals of Assam government was submitted to him. The memorandum pointed out that the tea industry was the highest taxed industry in India. It felt that the new tax proposal would arrest the tempo of development. The memorandum further stressed that the cost of production, on an average, was worked out at Rs. 75 per kg and price realisation was Rs. 74.05 a kg. This situation would not only wipe out profit but also would result in net loss.

The delegation met the Home Minister and submitted the copy of the memorandum and requested him to setting up of a joint body of representatives of the Central and State governments to take decisions on tea industry's development co-ordinately. The memorandum also hinted at retention of tea in domestic market so as to keep a share of 28 per cent of global trade.

5. Tea bushes and Depreciation : There is a continuous demand from the association that tea bushes, which constitute the major assets of the tea industry, should be considered for depreciation. The absence of a provision for depreciation does not allow the industry to generate internal funds.

6. Revision of Replantation Subsidy rates: The association pointed out that the replantation subsidy rate had not been revised for many years. The enhancement of subsidy in the context of cost up-swing will encourage the companies to quicken the pace of replantation to the targeted 2 per cent per annum from the current 0.5 per cent per annum.

7. Arunachal Tea Auctioned : Orthodox tea from Sreenanda Tea Estate set up in Arunachal Pradesh came under the hammer at Kolkota auction. This estate was the second tea estate from Arunachal Pradesh to bring its produce to Kolkata. The first was Donytpoloo.

8. Uplift of UP Tea Industry : The Union Commerce Ministry sponsored a two-pronged strategy for development of tea industry in UP. It included rejuvenation of existing tea gardens and identification of new area in the hilly districts of the state including the terai region. With this overall aim in-view, Tea Board had prepared the cost of development and rehabilitation schemes for sixty units for submission to financial institutions.

9. Fixation of Unit Cost of Production : With a view to providing a guideline to assess the performance of tea gardens, the committee for fixation of area-wise standard unit cost of production convenes meetings on a regular basis.

10. Russia to Buy from India : The then Union Minister of State for Non-conventional Energy at the inaugural ceremony of 101 Annual Conference of UPASI said that Russia would start buying tea from India. The Russia government had designated two of its companies to buy against the credit extended to India.

11. Vietnam for India's Expertise in Tea Industry : At a recent meeting with the representatives of the Federation of Indian Chambers of Commerce and Industry (FICCI) the visiting Vietnamese delegation sought India's expertise in planting and processing of tea. It was emphasised that India's 100 year's of experience in this sector would be of importance to Vietnam which is presently drawing up an action plan for becoming one of the major tea producers and exporters in

Asia pacafic region.

12. Study by Multi-agency Research Group (MARG) : In view of dwindling exports and fall in overall growth of domestic consumption of tea, the industry has employed MARG, a research organisation to make a comprehensive study of the Indian tea market. The research group has been assigned the task of finding out demand and consumer preferences based on which new marketing strategies will be evolved.

13. Disputed Land under Tea Cultivation : It was reported that tea gardens had mushroomed on unauthorised land throughout North Bengal. According to official statements, there are 105 estates in Uttar Dinajpur covering more than 30,000 hectares, 80 in Jalpaiguri with 16,000 hectares, 15 in Darjeeling having 16,000 hectares and 8 in Coochbehar owning 2000 hectares. These gardens were set up in 1988-89 when tea prices were abnormally high. Of the total land that was purchased for the purpose, 60 per cent is taxed under agricultural income tax of the state government and balance 40 per cent is taxed under the Income Tax Act. A scheme in line of Kerala model was advocated for a 20 per cent reduction in taxes for contributions made to plantation development fund.

19. Politics has Over Ruled Economics : The Indian planning has been so lop sided that neither in production nor in consumption has there been any appropriate development. What is more, politics has over ruled economics, even in the latter's sphere. The tea industry, busy to meet Russia's demand at the behest of the Government, did not have enough to time look for a balanced export market. Now that the export market of India is strictly limited, the domestic market which had so long been neglected as a residual market, will hardly be able to absorb the surplus.

20. No Deeper Study on Tea Consumption : Lately there has been a lot of discussion about generic promotion of tea in India, which is the same as growth of consumption of tea. The need for such promotion was felt because we had left behind the idea of fixing the annual target plan or even the five-yearly one. The industry was merely given to understand so long that a target for production fixed at 1000 million kgs was to be reached by the turn of the century. The call was thus for stepping up production. But no action plan was started to find out what would be the distinct consumption pattern in quality by that year. No deeper study was made. Perhape one should not be so harsh for an intra-country default when the international efforts (International Tea Promotion Association) with governmental assistance could not sustain a generic promotion programme which broke down. If the different countries co-operated then, the industry as a whole would be taught with demand and tremendous R and D activities taken up to match production.

21. CCPA's and Tea Board Initiatives for Promotion of Tea Consumption : The CCPA arranged a thorough study on the current situation and future possibilities through professionals. The study team was advised to probe the drinking habits and consumption pattern in particular. The professional team should find out actual consumption and possible drawal from the market. Tea Board has reportedly also commissioned a survey for estimating the domestic consumption between the period 1995 and 2000. It has already become too late for the study. Let there be no further delay.

22. India Blends Projects : The Chairman of Indian tea industry association (CCPA) observed that (i) a record 1993 crop combined with sharp fall in the export to major markets (Russia, Iran, Egypt had led to significant supply-demand imbalance throwing prices in disarray, and (ii) given that the 1994 crop was also surging ahead the oversupply was likely to persist. Based on these views, the industry sought to wipe out surplus and correct the imbalances. To look for a nieche in the market to boost exports and try to regain the lost markets in erstwhile USSR, the tea industry sought to build a brand equity for Indian teas' including formation of a consort under an Indian Blend project. More specifically the idea was to prepare the industry to face the intrusion of multinationals and recover the Rusian market. The project has been under discussion for some time and it appears that an earlier plan to appoint the Tata Tea as the nodal agency for routing the tea of 25 companies has now been shut down. Earlier the industry had decided to focus on a blend of quality, the Broken Orange Pekoe (BOP) out of orthodox Assam category. The project did not take off as some tea majors apprehended a common blend as such would cut into their own market while others did not want one company to build up its presence in Russia. Indications are that now the Indian lend export will be limited to 500,000 kgs. in the first phase and a team of tea industry leaders will shortly visit Russia to find out ways to set up either a fully Indian owned company or one in collaboration with Russian firm. If the project succeeds, Russian market can be salvaged. If the market imbalance can then be corrected, it will be another instance of the industry's buoyance.

23. How the Wheels of Fortune Move : According to late tea export statistics, China became the largest supplier of the commodity to the USA, leaving behind Sri Lanka, Indonesia, Argentina and India. India had hardly ever a mentionable position as exporter of tea to the USA. It had, however, been associated since long in popular stories with the greatest ever public consumption of tea in the states namely the Boston Tea party. The Boston Tea party was, however, not a tea party in the conventional sense but was a great historical occasion adding a new dimension to the American way of Independence. It was connected with tea, no doubt but that was not Indian tea at all. Tea for the party was exported by the East India Company and the consumer might have imagined the tea to have been procured from India, the company's main area of operation. The trouble really started with the enactment of Townshed Act, 1767 which sought over the huge expenses incurred by England in the seven years' war, imposed a tax on some items, including tea and taxed tea was forced on the colonial people by the East India Company which was granted the monopoly right to procure and export those items by Queen Elizabeth under the Royal Charter of 1600. The colonist raised serious objection : "No taxation without representation". When the East India company's ship carrying the cargo of tea entered the part of Boston, it was considered a deliberate insult of the popular will the some Americans as Mohawks got into the ship and threw the entire cargo over board. This was known in history as the Boston Tea Party and India was held a captive of deep misunderstanding. Political and economic situations changed since then and China lost contact with the Freeworld. Till a few decades back, Chinese tea was almost unknown in America, its share of the US tea market was only about 1 per cent. Srilankan tea became their favourite and its share rose to 24 per cent with Indonesia following closely with about 16 per cent of share of the market. With small beginning in 1974, Argentina, almost a non-entity among producers, has now become the second largest exporter to USA accounting for 27 percent of the market there.

24. No Honours, no Dollars : Poor India, producing best of tea in the world, and the largest quantum too, has no way with America, the richest country. In 1983, India's percentage share of US imports of tea was minimal. The largest importer of Indian tea was United Kingdom and then the USSR. Consumers of India's best tea are Japan and Germany. Being the world's largest producer too, India now looks about for safe foothold after the dismemberment of Soviet Russai. No honours, no dollars.

25. Tea Security Force : The doubt and uncertainty surrounding the formation of Assam tea plantation security force against terrorist assaults was finally dispensed with the signing of memorandum of understanding between the Government of Assam and the Indian Tea Association which controls the gardens involved. The first batch of 600 members representing the tea security force could undergo training for six weeks beginning on November 30, 1996. This force was be deployed from end of January 1997 in 75 vulnerable ITA gardens in the BODO-infested northern Assam. Each garden will eventually have 20 personnel for its protection. Out of which 17 will be security-men and rest will be supervisors. Each garden has spent Rs.3 lakh for the entire exercise, the recurring monthly expenditure apart. The security force will be equipped with weapons 75 per cent of which will be conventional and the rest sophisticated. It would be under the control of Director General of Police, Assam and shall be used exclusively for the security of the tea gardens and their personnel against the threat from insurgents. The formation of such a security force has been as timely as its has been morale boosting for its harassed personnel. Such a positive measure is surely worth trying out and will go a long way in providing strength and protection to the insecure planting communities. They are no longer at the mercy of a gang of savage extortionists. It is also remarkable that tea security force is the first of its kind organised by private sector industry in the country to contend terrorism. No other industry has organised such resistance ever.

26. Research Is Sine Qua Non for Progress : The policy of economic liberalisation provided the Indian tea industry to enjoy some benefits of protection round about way in view of its largeness and expanded home market. Under the scheme competition is inevitable but any attempt at import of tea in India is looked upon as unpatriotic. It was therefore tried by mainly some tea multinational companies inspite of criticism. Thanks to the MNCs who do not take failure once or twice, at the end of it all a new line of thinking a consumer prone approach-is now developing. Indian producers are also aware of the trend. A higher price charged by them consequent on higher cost of production had been questioned. If Kenya, with higher productivity and lesser cost of production, today sells at Rs.50 per kg against India retailing at Rs.100 to Rs. 130 per kg., how long *will Indian consumer resist or the government of the country is expected to look at the possibility of import. Obviously, the only way to stall imports is to improve productivity and reduce cost of production. That again can be done by effective R&D work . Nobody denies that research is sine qua non for progress and development of an industry. And tea industry is no exception.* The tea industry is well aware of the importance of research as evidenced by the formation of Tea Research Association and United Planters' Association of South India. The level of performance of the laboratories established in such units is yet to be assessed. But none of us brought the matter to the notice of research bodies. It is necessary that in such a situation a central body of producers like CCPA should ask its members to state their problems and CCPA would collate issues and urge various research bodies in the country to address themselve to the urgent task of finding out the solution. Workshops, seminars would be useful not if held once in blue moon but when they are held frequently in different selected locations. Also, it may be noted that *research is now dimensional job. One is to improve upon the methods already in practice and the other is to develop newer lines of approach a break—through as it were*. Then, substantial investment, necessary for sustained research even though some producers say finance would not be a problem. Some laboratories appear to have been hamstrung for want to adequate resourcs. Sometime ago, the CSIR allocated funds for tea research which were not niggardly but discriminatory as well. In a recent study of 250 tea companies, it has been found that Indian private companies spend very little on research and development. *In fact R&D expenditure as a percentage of gross sales came down, though marginally, from 0.47% in 1993-94 to 0.45% in 1994-95. Here, both the public and private sector should cooperate*. For years industries did not care much for research. Now suddenly, with the liberalisation of economy, the system is sought to be changed. Some are of the view that the government should offer incentives and indeed some sops have been given for R&D expenditure. The Department of Scientific and Industrial Research had offered to centrally fund and proposed a five-year tax holiday for new category of commercial R&D companies. Research should be, rather must be, carried on and adequate finance must be arranged. It must not be forgotten that what is at stake is future of Indian Tea Industry.

27. Sri Lanka Scientists Bit Tea Cola : Sri Lanka produced a quality tea and its production is copious. Moreover, scientists of Sri Lanka's Tea Research Institute (TRI) *are now developing a sort of a ready-to-drink tea beverage as have done by beverage* giants such as Coca-Cola and Pipsi Co. Recently TRI director Wester Moddar said Sri Lanka is being left behind in the scramble to cater to the tastes of new generation looking for conveinent health beverages. Press reports state that current research mostly on green teas has *properties that can fight cancer and cardio-vascular diseases. However, the great bulk of world tea trade is in black tea. That does not matter. "Traditionally, we have been exporting bulk tea to Western markets, he said in an interview with the Reuter.* "If we make the value addition here, we will have an instant take off he added. TRI came to it in the 1960's but could not patent an instant new product. Shortage of finance as a factor stood in the way. A liquid tea concentrate perfected by the TRI's biochemistry division is now available for commercial exploitation. The concentrate, precursor for the preparation of carbonated tea comes with a range of flavour like apple, pineapple and strawberry. The patent is offered for sale on the condition that only Sri Lanka tea be used in making the tea concentrate and the plant be located on the asland. It is a pity for the Indian scientists that with so much of knowledge and resources they had to step back in such an important matter. Possibly because they did not take interest in diversification.

28. Tea Producers of the World Unite : While the world market of tea remained low during 1994, the consumer prices remained high and the producers received only a fraction of the price paid by the consumers. Naturally many producers became anxious and producers particularly of Sri Lanka and India have been in communication for quite some time. Colombo convened an international conference in April 1995 to check the trend. It was meant not merely for a short term action but also for a lasting solution. It sought consideration for forming an association to launch united action. Sri Lanka's the then Deputy Plantation Minister hoped other tea producing countries would join the proposed association so that some concrete steps could be taken for betterment of the industry. It was observed at the Conference that though tea trade accounted for more than $ 1,300 million annually, the producing nations had so far not been able to establish their own inter-Governmental organisations. The Sri Lankan miniiter called for generic promotion of tea to increase consumption of the beverage. Even a marginal increase in consumption, he said, would have a salutary effect in enhancing the prices. Other representatives attending the conference must have shared his views. Individual countries have their plans for generic promotion of tea. The Tea Board of India as well as the Consultative Committee of Plantation Associations, the apex body of Indian planters is going ahead with the projects for promotion of tea consumption. But only that cannot achieve the purpose. They must keep in view that solution to the present international crisis could be found through "collaborative approach by the producers". The objective should be to encourage remunerative prices for the product not only to sustain the tea industry but to ensure continued supply of tea to the consumers around the world. Already besides India and Sri Lanka the other producing countries participating are China, Indonesia, Bangladesh and Malawi, while Iran participated as net importing nation. Let those falling behind come up and participate. It is a common cause.

29. Crisis in Tea Industry : The then ITA Chairman pointed out that although cost of production of tea is high and productivity per worker is low, he asserted that 'managements' duty was to see that man productivity was improved to the extent that we *remain not only the producer of best tea, but the producer of the most cost-effective tea*". Meanwhile Indian newspapers report that auction prices have sharply fallen in all centres. Nearly 80 per cent of the tea companies in the country are reportedly operating below the cost of production as no alternative avenues seem to be available to revamp their exports after the Russian market had been lost. Some producers in North India fear that they may have to suspend production if the down-turn continues till September. Some gardens in South India have also threatened to shut down unless the government announces support price of tea. Producers have complained about wage hike. Also about increase in input cost. The acquisition cost of urea and other fertilisers, they said, had gone up as those have to be procured from the blackmarket, sufficient quantities not being available in the normal market. It is the duty of the Government to stand by the tea industry at such a critical point of time.

30. Funds Crunch Stalls Tea Export to Iran : Tea exporters, who had contracted with the State Tea Organisation of Iran for supply of bulk and packet teas some time in August 1993. ran into a major problem. The buyer was unable to open letters of credit for the full quantity in view of paucity of funds. During December 1993, after repeated follow-up, a few exporters were asked to bifurcate their contracts into two and LCs for part quantities were opened. In March 1994, a few other exporters, who had contracted for relatively smaller quantities, received their LCs. and were able to complete their shipments shortly thereafter. Two major exporters. however, have not receive, an LC for even part quantity till date. During the visit of the Iranian Deputy Minister of Agriculture and the Chairman of STO to Calcutta in March 1994, the exporters were assured that the balance LCs would be opened within a month or two. Unfortunately, this has not happened. Initially, these contracts had been negotiated at highly competitive prices with low margins. The exporters are now facing serious problems in holding such large stocks of tea, namely by way of high interest costs. What next?

31. Tea coffee Acts to be Damended Soon: Tea Act and Coffee Act were amended. Though very little changes were incorporated in the Tea Act, changes in Coffee Act was an indication of the straw in case of Tea Act. It was reported that the export cess on coffee was raised while import duty was retained at 20 per cent. These changes were introduced in view of the new coffee policy which abolished the pooling mechanism announced by the them Commerce Minister, Shri B.K. Ramaiah. It was, however, anticipated that removal of pooling would lead to higher prices of coffee. Earlier when prices rose, the Coffee Board was advised to release more coffee to its retail outlets to moderate the high prices. The ministry intended to continue monitoring coffee prices and proposed to intervene through STC and the Coffee Board to curb speculation. The coffee was sold at cost plus price and would be distributed through outlets of the Coffee Board in branded packets.

32. Tea Board Strategies to Enter US Market : The Tea Board of India, that has been eying the rapidly growing demand for iced tea in the US, chalked out the strategy to enter the market in a big way. The then Tea Board Chairman, Shri S.S. Ahuja, said that the Board had already worked out a strategy to enter the sizeable iced tea market in the US. The Board Director in New York said that the US market was growing rapidly and was maintaining a steady growth rate of over 20 per cent. Mr. Ahuja said that the Board had collaborated more closely with the Tea Council of US and realised the fruitfulness of the association of the Tea Council. The US market had undergone vast changes in the last decade but India had positioned at a strategic supply of special teas. 'We will continue to cater to the high yield market which is growing rapidly.' India had not wished to compete with such countries as Argentina that had captured the market segment which was known as superior market variety.

Mr. Ahuja admitted that the iced tea market had great potential in the US and India now had varieties of tea that were suitable to the brewing of iced tea. Previously India lacked varieties of tea that were fast in colour so they were though unsuitable of for iced tea, he said. 'Now, we have developed newer varieties of tea (Nilgiris) which are also suitably priced'. Mr. Ahuja said that Tea Board rejoined the Tea Council of US as a fullfledged member on the concil rather than observer member. India also worked closely with the Council's Speciality Tea Registrar.

33. Indian Tea Industry shifting from Loose to Packaged Tea : Tea traders and growers of South India shifted the trend of marketing tea to packaged tea from the traditional loose variety in response to changing demand. Loose tea production increased by 5 per cent while packaged tea by 20 per cent during the last 5 years. Domestic consumption of loose tea jumped by 48 per cent and packaged tea consumption by 140 per cent during the last 5 years. Traders said that more than three quarters of export were in value added forms like tea packets and tea bags. The then Tea exporter Shri Nanda Kumar said that even when we export in loose form, the importer package them and brand them with their own trademarks. Instead of losing our identity, we can brand them ourselves. Dealer Ramchandra Nair stated that in the domestic market, quality consciousness is picking up. Traders say that packed tea was more profitable than lose category, as consumers were becoming increasingly brand loyal. Organisation and modernisation affect consumer preferences. Loose tea consumption is disappearing fast. Brook Bond India Ltd., with its 17 brands accounted for 60 per cent of domestic packaged tea market. The company spent nearly 600 million rupees a year on marketing its different brands both overseas and at home. Tata Tea Ltd., accounted for 25 per cent of the domestic market and Duncan 10 per cent. Packet tea were exempted from Tea Marketing Control Order of 1984. The order, promulgated under the Tea Act of 1953, requires all manufacturers to sell 75 per cent of their production.

34. Tea Marketing : Indian Delegation to Pakistan : Pakistan, the largest importer of tea in Asia, was overlooked by the industry, for long because political relations between India and Pakistan were not satisfactory. After a long period, a deputation of the Indian tea industry representatives visited Pakistan to study the market situation there.

The Pak market is divided into three distinct groups, CTC is most popular and particularly Fannings. The loose tea retail market is situated mainly in Karachi. Packed brown paper bags, loose tea is offered in an unblend form and is of average quality. As far as packet tea is concerned, well known international brand names hold the majority percentage share but in recent times local packegers have succeeded in making inroads into these sales and it is understood that the balance is now in favour of these brands. Tea bags constitutes a small portion of the market and sales are confined mainly to the higher social groups. Green tea is sold mainly in Peshawar and consumed largely by Afghan refugees.

Though there are provincial variations in consumption, the overall Pakistan market is discerning and quality-conscious. Price factor does not appear to restrain consumption and there is no evidence as to the sensitivity of tea prices. This is attributed to the raising standard of living and to the fact that per cup of tea still remains cheaper in relation to other beverages. All in all, proximity is a plus factor for the Indian tea industry in relation to export to Pakistan Old guards will remember how at one time there was practically a scramble for licences at the Amritsar office of the Tea Board for export through land routes. The delegation was sure to strengthen many opportunities for trade.

35. Strategy of stabilisation of tea prices :

a) Value Addition through Brands : India had a price lead in international trade but she was unable to hold on to that lead for some times. With erstwhile Russia buying more of Sri Lankan tea, prices had dipped. Sri Lanka offered cash credit where has India did not offer. When prices had fallen substantially in Cochin auction against Colombo sometimes back Sri Lanka jumped into the fray and quickly bought some teas there, for certain South Indian varieties are much in demand in Sri Lanka also.

To get out of the morars, the Indian Government has been looking for various options. Experts reckon, the thrust has to be on value addition through brands. It was interesting to note that the then Indian Minister, Dr. Ramaiya, on his tour to China in 1996 was offered some Darjeeling tea. Brand name made for value-addition. Dr. Ramaiya took decision for setting up of a 'Brand-Equity Fund'. The trustee for this fund was appointed.

b) Support Prices : The then honorable Union Minister for Public Grievances and Parliamentary Affairs, Shri S.R. Balasubramanian mooted that support prices be announced for tea as in the case of some agricultural commodities. This would ensure remunerative prices for tea growers. The same idea was projected by the United Planters' Association of South India (UPASI). The then Vice-President, Shri Vadera, stressed that 50,000 small growers in Nilgiris who accounted for 40 million kgs of made tea must ensure remunerative prices. The Minister could hardly war off the pressure

36. Populist measures against unlawful activities of tea farms:

Tiger Is Out of The Cage : Though it was not exactly against the tea industry as such, that the apex bodies of all chambers of commerce in the country had raised objectives for severe stepdown on Indian corporate sector for alleged irregularities and violation of revenue laws. The leaders felt the need of conducting investigation against corporation. One cannot deny that present actions of investigation agencies are detrimental to industrial growth and could deter planned foreign investment. The spectre is haunting corporate circles and they said that while stringent laws should be taken in dealing with any breach of law, the present actions of the investigating agencies could be detrimental.

Industry houses did not minimise the magnitude of unlawful practices in Virginia Honse. In fact, under-invoicing and over-invoicing in export-import trade are not new phenomenon in business community and this has been going on for years together with a devasting effect on national image and morale. What is more depressing and damaging is unrestrained temptation of the reporting authority and agencies to sensationalise every trivial detail in deference to populist instinct. The most unfortunate part being that while some of the reports are not quite based on facts, they do irreparable damage to individuals and institutions. The tiger is out of the cage and only hopes that at this critical stage of globalisation, the overseas investors would not be scared.

37. CIS and India be partners in tea trade

Market Economy and Democracy Require a Different Approach : Although despatch of some consignment of tea of indifferent quality to CIS countries during the later part of 1993 caused a great concern to tea circle, the Tea Board brought to book the delinquents. India has been trade partners for many years both before the USSR broke down any after the restructuring of the state. There were hardly and complaint against Indian tea so far. After the Chernobyl disaster, it was because of India the tea drinkers of Russia could sip at the beverage leisurely. No other countries could have supplied so much of tea and in required quantity. Then, at a time when CIS countries could hardly have foreign exchange to buy tea, India offered a technical credit not once, as a token only, but lent several times as a friend in need would do to the other. In the face of all these services the behaviour of CIS administrators in vilifying campaign against Indian tea in media—print and electronic could not be called friendly. CIS and India shall have to be in business hereafter. Let them be friendly and both exercise modernisation.

38. Replantation Is a Time Bound and Cold Weather Based Programme

a) Replantation Is a Cold Weather job : In winter, tea bushes generally depend on replantation work which is undertaken to achieve production and export targets under the Five Year Plan. The reason for carrying out such operation during cold season is that the workers thereby get the fire wood both for warmth and cooking.

b) Replantation is a Time Bound Programme : Replantation of uneconomic tea areas with newly developed planting material is a time bound programme. The tea industry understands that once uprooting operation of tea bushes is delayed, the rehabilitation period also gets delayed; and the entire process as well. As a measure of assistance to undertake such work, *the Replantation Subsidy Scheme* *was introduced as early as in October 1968*. The objective of the scheme had been to achieve an annual replantation rate of 2 per cent of total areas under tea in India with newly developed planting materials giving higher yields, better quality and other desirable characteristics. It has been found that approval is generally accorded unless or until contribution to National Tea Research Foundation is fully paid. But as hinted above, uprooting of bushes is time bound and cold weather based programme.

Approval up rooting should, therefore, be accorded duly. Bharatiya Cha Parishad has suggested this *sometimes back. Tea estates should, therefore, be allowed to uproot the bushes as per their programme and they should be allowed.*

39. Development of Tea :

a) Reorientation of Regulatory Laws an Immediate Necessity : Liberalisation is there in Indian Economy except in its tea industry. This industry still suffers from various controls, un warranted under the existing circumstances. Most important among these controlling regulation is the Tea Act 1953, which says: provide for the control by the union of tea industry, including the control, in pursuance of the international agreement now in force, of the cultivation of tea in, and of the export of tea from India and for that purpose to establish Tea Board and levy a duty of excise on tea produced in India". The international agreement was signed about 40 years ago. Obviously, the scenario has since changed, if not completely, at least, substantially. Neither this agreement is there nor the levy of excise on tea. The Ramakrishnaya Committee studied the working of the Commodity Board and made certain recommendations diversiting the Board of certain powers. Basically the Board should stress on *development rather than regulation*.

Then again, with the increasing consumption of tea in India and abroad, more production is urgently needed. A plantation being land based, opportunities must be provided to bring more land under cultivation. Restriction on use of agricultural land should be withdrawn. The Ramakrishnaya Committee suggested how more land could be brought under plantation.

b) Land Ceiling Acts Not Socio-economic in Contents but Political objectives too : The Government had distributed lands to landless people but the move became far from helpful. Parent and child theory of big tea estates helping these smaller land holders as proposed by the tea industry has not been fully tried. The point is that growers should be encouraged. Chapter II of the Tea Act hamstrings one to do so unless prior permission of the Tea Board is taken. On the other hand, the regulation should be so amended as to allow to grow tea without prior permission also. Only a person must register himself with the Board for identification and statistical purposes. All the State Governments have laws against alienation of land. It was therefore, not necessary for the Tea Act to repeat the restrictions.

c) Several Control Orders Aggravating Actions of Tea Act : Section 16 C of the Act allows Central Government to control prices or regulate distribution of tea produced or manufactured by tea unit. Tea Marketing Control further aggravates the action of Tea Act. The order sought to chammeise late of tea through auction. While it had its uses at a point of time it has ceased to do so now. Unless these are reviewed they may become in the long run self-perpetuating and prevent free marketing. It has also been noted that many producers are interested in directly marketing teas in value added form. That trend is essential keeping with the liberalised policy of the economy and desirable too, but the order thwarts the trend.

It is full of anomalies such as that it is not possible to go into third party packaging and marketing under the order or for producers having a number of gardens to bucket and market their teas in a suitable central unit. The order is required to be repealed. Tea is an item also under Essential Commodities Act, a stringent regulation, but it remain a dead letter so far as this commodity is concerned. Actually the item sold through public auctions has had no occasion to have the price restricted further. Moreover, when necessary the industry in its own sense of social responsibility sold directly to consumer at a rate even cheaper than the auction prices and distributed through various centres so that bottlenecks at any point could be got over.

On restrictions on export of tea and tea seeds the Tea (Regulation of Export Licensing) Order, 1984 came into force; lately it has been replaced by the Tea (Regulation of Export Licensing) (Repeal) Order 1993. The only original order still in vogue is the Tea (Distribution and Export) Contract Order which requires a licence for every consignment of tea shipped from Tea Board on JCCI&E though the item is not in the negative list of export under the Exim policy. A similar anomaly is noticeable in respect of renewal of annual licence. While the government has abolished Central excise licensing and periodical renewal, a tea exporter is required to obtain a licence from Tea Board and renew it regularly under the Tea (Distribution and Export) Control Order.

Not only this but there are Tea Waste (Control) Order 1958 and the Ware-housing Order which are anomalous too. While the latter is an unnecessary burden put on the Tea Board, over the years tea manufacturer has shifted to CTC production where "tea waste" becomes negligible. Yet the system of taking out licence every year by producer and buyer continues. A reorientation of the regulatory laws is, therefore, an immediate necessity.

40. Core Committee for Tea Industry Constituted:

In order to look into the major problems of tea industry, the Ministry of Commerce constituted a core committee with the following persons:

1. Commerce Secretary - Chairman
2. Chairman, Indian Tea Association - Member
3. Chairman, Tea Association of India - Member
4. Finance and Taxation Member of ITA - Member

5. Chairman, UPASI - Member
6. Chairman, Bharatiya Cha Parishad - Member
7. Chairman Tea Board Member
8. Joint Secretary (Plantations), Ministry of Commerce Member

The Order dated 22nd November, 1993 stated further that members from trade and other spheres might be co-opted by the Committee as and when necessary.

41. Distribution Policy on Economy packs of Tea

The Monitoring Committee of Tea Prices at its meeting decided that distribution on economy packs of tea should be followed up with vigour and scope extended to rural areas. Accordingly, Mr. P.K. Bora, the then Chairman, Tea Board, sent a telex message, as under, to all Tea Associations : "Ministry of Commerce has noticed that the availability of economy packs of tea at Rs. 40/- per kg. has declined over the past few weeks. The Government is seriously concerned at this development and desires suitable remedial action immediately, Unless substantial quantities are pumped in immediately, Tea Board may be constrained to recommend to the Ministry drastic control measures to keep the prices under control. Please therefore, take immediate action for stepping up supply of economy packs in the market. Please also advise your constituents to take suitable measures to bring down the prices to the level of Rs. 40/- per kg."

It is learnt that each company will have to complete its quota by March 1990 and that if consumer off-take be slow in certain areas, the economy packs can be distributed anywhere in India."

42. Neem Oil Cake as Goat Repellent

Tea bushes very often bear the invasion by cattle, particularly the goat. During winter when there is scarcity of grass, goats chew the bark of tea, thus inflicting serious injuries. Such debarking may lead to die back of smaller branches. The plant tries to recover the injury by callusing. In such cases, death of the bush may not occur immediately but certainly there will be some loss of vigour leading to less yield in subsequent harvests.

Repelling goats from tea areas had remained an unsolved problem because there was no chemical available with the industry which could take care of this. Neem seed kernels and the oil have found their ways in pest control. Use of neem products in the war against pests is not a new concept. But in tea, it was never used before. Neem cake mixed with a spreader/sticker in a section of tea which was badly damaged by goats was experimented upon at Tocklai Experimental Station.

Results show that neem cake can reduce the change by damage of goats. Neem cake at 100 gm with 4 ml Triton and 200 g with 2 and 4 ml Triton per litre of water gave good results. 100 gram cake with 3 ml Triton failed to check the damage, there was 11% increase of damage within three months. The oil emulsion too showed less effect. One kilogram neem cake and 40 ml. Triton mixed with 10 litres of water could be used esconomically as a repellent for goats.

43. Minimum Break Sizes

In consonance with the Tea Board directives relating to the Ahuja Committee recommendations which are to be strictly adhered to, estates manufacturing 2 lakh kgs. or more should not pack breaks of less than 20 chests/bags during the manufacturing period 1st July to 30th November. This is applicable to all grades except the following:

CTC : BPS, Small Dusts and Secondaries

Orthodox : Tippy teas, BPS, Fanning, Dusts and Secondaries.

The above stipulations are, however, not applicable to Darjeeling gardens.

44. Restrictions in US on Goods Produced by Child Labour

The Ministry of Commerce, Govt. of India, stated that a legislation was introduced by the United States to prohibit the importation of goods produced abroad by child labour. This was aimed at prohibiting US trade with countries that permitted children under the age of 15 to work in industry or mining where the risk of exposure to injury or occupational disease is highest. As a condition for bringing of manufactured product into the American market place, importers would be required to certify in writing that the product they handle are not made by children.

The report on tea labour engaged in tea plantation received directly from different tea estates each year indicated the utilisation of child labour in Tea Plantation Industry. It was also learnt that child labour are also engaged in the packaging industry on tea.

45. Managerial Pay & Perks Ceiling up

The Union Government scrapped several regulatory provisions governing remuneration of managerial personnel and made an upward revision of maximum admissible salary from Rs. 15,000 to 50,000 per month. The decision to amend the relevant Schedule XIII to the Companies Act, 1956, followed persistent demands from trade and industry. The amendment gave necessary freedom to companies to appoint managerial personnel and fix their salaries and perquisites in accordance with the higher revised ceilings. Several procedural requirements were also done away with. Earlier, all companies were required to obtain government approval for appointment of managing director, whole time directors and managers. No such permission will be required now, except in the case of sick companies.

46. Ensuring Availability of Packets Tea at Uniform Prices : The PHD Chamber of Commerce and Industry (PHDCCI) urged the government to postpone the implementation of the recent notification making it obligatory to indicate the maximum retail price, inclusive of all taxes, on all packaged commodities. Differences in freight costs were due to the distances involved, rates of local taxes and levies, etc. These made it difficult for producers to mark a uniform retail price on packets. If the manufacturer took into consideration the maximum rates of freight, which might be payable if the product was transported to a remote place and the maximum local taxes which might be leviable on the product, the price so arrived at would be unduly high and unfair to the consumers living in the state where the goods were manufactured defeating the purpose of this amendment. PHDCCI, while appreciating the government gesture to protect consumers' interest and also the endeavours to ensure availability of packaged commodities at uniform end-prices all over India, stated that unless party is brought about in tax rates and provisions of the regulations, the implementation of the amended rules would not serve the interest of consumers.

47. Bush Teas Tie Up with Twinings : R. Twining and Company Ltd., UK in collaboration with Bush Tea Co. Pvt. Ltd. a Kolkata based recognised trading house, set up dehumidifying plant at the latter's warehouse in the city. This plant enhanced the quality of the speciality teas which are brought by Twinings for the speciality and quality segments of the UK tea market. The cost of the plant and the related infrastructure is around Rs. 15 lakh. Twinings had a substantaial financial involvement in this quality enhancement exercise. It was out however pointed by their commodities director that speciality and quality tea market in the UK has been growing at an impressive rate even though the overall market size may have shrunken little. He assured UK buying from India went down in the last decade for a number of reasons, one reason being the ban on CTC tea some year back by the Indian Government. Naturally UK buyers, who have to supply to the popular market had to look elsewhere. Kenya because of its climatic conditions, has been able to provide teas of more or less uniform quality round the year and has now emerged as a major supplier of popular teas to the UK. However, there is still no substitute for the first and second flush Assam and Darjeeling teas and their demands cannot go down.

48. Tea Not Free But Closely Guarded Market

During the year 1994 there was an attempt to cut in tea production to bring balance between cost of production and price realisation. But no endeavour was initiated to explore the possibility of new market and improve the quality of tea. This would have prevented the producers being saddled with surplus stock. Loose tea should be auctioned because it fetches higher prices and hence higher profit margins. It was also argued that there should be direct sale of tea by plantation. The market could have been retained by evolving strategy for global export and continuous process of upgradation. It is not a free market. It is a closely guarded market with fierce competition among, India, Sri Lanka and Kenya, ot only the CIS but the European market is quality conscious. Emphasising the need for sophisticated tea tasting procedures and proper scientific and technological back drop to boost tea trade, there is a need for synchronized efforts by the Ministry of Agriculture, Science and Technology as well as Commerce and Industry to develop the export market.

49. Tea industry Drew a Blank from the Budget of 1999

The Central Budget of 1991 proposed appropriate modification in Sections 33AB of 91 as well as in Rule 8(2) of IT Rules, 1962 and provide declarifications in respect of Section 80 HHC of the IT Act. The modifications in Rule 8(2) are intended to extend the benefit of deduction to tea plantation in new and abandoned areas as also to infilling and inter-planting in the existing tea gardens. In other words, the modified Rule 8(2) allows tea companies to charge expenditure on those counts top revenue.

As of now, under Rule 8(2), tea companies are allowed only replanting expenditure as full charge to revenue. But doubts persisted over the extent of benefit that the tea companies would be able to derive from the proposed modifications in Rule 8(2). This was because land for extension planting in the traditional tea-growing areas was just not available and the state governments were chary to commit to suggestions for restoration of ceiling-surplus land to tea companies. As for Section 80 HHC, the proposed clarifications are intended to ensure inclusion also of the proportion of export income apportioned to state income slab. As is known, under Rule 8 of IT Rules, 40 per cent of the income of a tea company is subject to central corporate income tax and the remaining 60 per cent is subject to agricultural income tax levied by state governments.

The Central Board of Direct Taxes is of the view that the deduction under Section 80 HHC is available only on 40 per cent of the income, which is subject to central corporate income tax. The industry knows this already and that is why it suggested transfer of the provisions of Section 80 HHC from Chapter VI-A where they belong to Chapter-IV. But now nothing has been done that way. And though certain clarifications have been made in the Budget, those are of little avail to the tea industry as such. The Commerce Ministry had reportedly taken note of the fact that even with due allowance for admissible deductions under Section 33 AB of IT Act to facilitate plough-back for long-term development, the tea industry will be subject to a higher incidence of taxation than other industries, for whom the effective rate of taxation including surcharge works out to only 46 per cent.

50. Land Transfer for Tea Stopped in West Bengal

The then West Bengal Land and Revenue Minister Shri Binoy Choudhury was determined to stop illegal transfer of land for tea plantation. On his instructions, the Land and Revenue department suspended issuing "no objection certificates" for transfer of land for tea cultivation until it was satisfied that it not violate the guidelines set down by the State Government. The government had issued guidelines on land use in North Bengal for tea plantation. But the guidelines had been violated with impunity. In the process number of a tea companies—big and small are taking away Testee command area land, prime agricultural land as well as inalienable land. Under the guidelines, tea is not allowed to be grown on such lands. A committee was set up to identify persons affected by illegal transfer of land and to ascertain the extent to which this has taken place.

Illegal transfers of land have taken place secretly. Many had secured government seed money and bank finance with the stated purpose of setting up new industry but used it to buy land for tea. Many such people are now raising green leaf and selling them to tea firms which have processing factories.

51. Ahuja Committee Recommendations on Tea Trade Accepted

A committee was set up in 1986 headed by Mr. S.S. Ahuja, the then Deputy Chairman of Tea Board to consider various matters relating to the Tea (Marketing) Control Order, 1984. The report of the committee was accepted by the Licensing Authority under the Marketing Control Order. In July 1992, a meeting of the Calcutta Tea Traders' Association was held under the directions of the Tea Board Chairman to decide on the adoption, or disposal otherwise of the recommendations in the final report excluding those on warehouse rent and insurance, the last issue being sub-judice. The CTTA meeting reportedly approved the recommendations for due implementation.

52. Round table Conference with CSIR Scientists

The tea industry is in urgent need of the technological break to the yield barrier. The Association had already initiated research work in some of the advanced areas. The hi-tech research capabilities were established in several areas of CSIR laboratories and CSIR provided technologies to other countries. It was, therefore, felt that instead of duplicating efforts and getting delayed results, it was worthwhile to collaborate with the CSIR laboratories to facilitate faster accomplishment of modern technologies for the tea industry. With this objective, the Tea Research Association organised a round table Conference with the Directors of CSIR laboratories interested in tea research sometimes in 1990.

53. Renewal of Field Assets : The issue relation to the need for increasing the rate of renewal of field assets (including replantation) was discussed in broad based meeting held in Kolkata on 18th April 1994 at the instance of the Tea Research Association. The meeting ended with the following recommendations:

i) The criterion for replantation shall be yield or land productivity, and not the age for any section of tea.

ii) Tea gardens should undertake replantation to the extent of a minimum of 0.5% mandatorily within the overall new plant input of 3% to 5% and a production growth rate of about 3% should be aimed at.

iii) The subsidy to the extent of 40% of the cost of replanting as settled by NABARD should be introduced without any further delay. Simultaneously the NABARD should be advised to estimate the current cost level since the earlier costing was carried out a fee years back.

iv) Withdrawal of Section 32AB and 33A from the Finance Bill 1990 was being viewed by the industry as a grant disincentive to under take replantation and further developmental work. These incentives for plough back should be restored.

v) The concept of the tea plantation fund should be explained to the producers associations by outlining the scheme envisaged by the Committee. A final decision would be taken by the producers after studying the scheme.

54. Global symbol for Tea Proposed

The health-related tea project started by the eighth session of the inter-governmental group considered the ways on launching international test marketing and a number of measures were identified. The executive director of the UK Tea Council suggested the creation of a universal symbol and trade mark for tea, that would highlight the fact that tea is a user-friendly drink. He observed that the appeal of this beverage lies in the fact that it is a natural product without any additives or preservatives, and is interprered during the process of production. The importance of generic promotion of tea was seriously felt at the inter-governmental group meet in 1989 because the glut in the global tea market had been continuing for some years. Even though the group had considered generic promotion, a firm decision was taken as large funds were required and the mid-term return could not be forecast.

His approach was devised at modest cost based on the premise that it is known as the world's most-used drink but was not fully appreciated for its values as a healthy drink. The message would reach the industry and percolate to trade, distribution, retail, catering and finally consumer channels.

The symbol, which would probably incorporate a copy phrase, satisfied national and international legal requirements. The aim was to create a frame work and establish guidelines logical enough to make it popular quickly without recourse to any major advertising efforts.

55. Demand for Tea Transhipment at Singapore by European buyers

Buyers of Indian tea in Britain and the Continent urged Eropean shipping lines like P & OCL, CGM. Hapag Lloyd and Nedlloyd to abandon Colombo as the transhipment port in favour of Singapore in the tea season. British and Continental tea buyers made it clear that they do not want a repetition of the unhappy experience of the past few years when the ethnic violence that rocked the island nation of Sri Lanka also affected operations at Colombo Port. Shipping lines operating through the port were hard hit.

56. Thomas Plans Output hike with Tissue-cultured tea

The AV Thomas group, a major player in the commodity market, used its advanced tissue culture techniques to cultivate tea on its plantations. The group proposed to plant tissue cultured tea plants on 500 hectares. At present the group is producing 150 tonnes on 1,800 hectares. The use of biotechnology revolutionised tea yield which reached an astronomical 400 tonnes per 5000 hectares in just three years from the day of planting.

57. Cash Credit to Tea Companies

The Reserve Bank of India (RBI) advised the leading commercial banks to keep a close chéck on tea account and make assessment and monitoring of working capital finance of the tea industry as per the guidelines of the apex bank. As regards tea industry, the RBI permits banks to extend cash credit to the companies of the basis of their cash budgets prepared on a year-to-year basis. RBI, however, changed the norms from the so called 25 per cent margin concept of "total drawing limit" to "peak deficit" for the tea companies. Since the cash budget method is being followed for financing working capital requirement of the tea companies, the cash balance in the beginning of the calendar year and the end of the period should be either zero or positive after being in the negative zone during most producing months, attaining the peak deficit level in October. A close scrutiny of some of the tea accounts with leading banks in the eastern region revealed that the tea companies had received higher cash credit limits than what was due to them on the basis of their inflated cash budget figures.

Prudential lending norms suggested the bank to extend support to a level, which is the gap between the peak deficit and cash margin available within the company. Thus, to that extent the net cash credit level was required to have been pruned to meet the exact amount. However, this has not happened. A question may arise here as to what happens to the cash generated in the business? If there is no generation of funds, then on what basis has the company submitted its cash budget to the lending institution? Further, on what basis has the bank continued to lend, when year after year the gap between current assets and current liabilities has existed in favour of liabilities?

58. Introduction of Bar Code Technology

The concept of automatic product identification system through bar code technology is now well established in most of the developed and developing parts of the world. Indian exports are adopting such system in line with the international marketing practices. The Ministry of Commerce, Government of India had identified the Indian Institute of Packaging as the Nodal Agency to set up an organisation for promotion of this concept in the country. The local body is known as EAN India which has now taken up the membership of EAN-International, Brussels, the country code allowed is 990.

The establishment of EAN India is fully supported by the trade apex bodes that include C11, FICCI, FIEO, ASSOCHAM, besides BIS, PICES, Board and APEDA. Exporters of tea from India, particularly the manufacturer exporters who intended to adopt the Bar Code Technology were advised to contact the Institute/EAN-India at the address noted below for any further assistance they need besides taking up membership of EAN India.

Indian Institute of Packaging,

E-2, MIDC Area, P. BNo. 94444432

Andheri (East), Mumbai 400 093

59. Certification for Tea Board schemes

The issue of extension of Tea Board's Tea Area Rejuvenation and Consolidation Subsidy Scheme to the Plain tea gardens of Assam and North Bengal; and enhancement in rates of subsidy had been reconsidered for administrative action. To facilitate submission of application under the scheme, Board's field officers were empowered to issue fitness certificate for rejuvenation, pruning and infilling with or without inter-planting at the time of carrying out of pre-approval inspection. Such certificates were issued by the Board's officers only in respect of fields having the level of vacancy not exceeding 25%. Wherever the vacancy level exceeds 25% the fitness certificate shall be issued by TRA/UPASI-TRI, stated a Tea Board circular.

60. India Blend Ltd ad. Campaign Gets Going

India Blend Ltd., company set up by some major companies to help create a sustained market for Indian packet teas in Russia and other

CIS countries, reportedly approached the Union Ministry of Commerce for grant of funds to undertake the required advertising campaign there. The grant was sought from the Brand Equity Fund set up recently by the ministry. The ministry, however, offered a promotional incentive to this unique exercise being carried out for the first time.

India Blend also marketed the "Nargis" brand in the CIS nations over the past couple of months with some success. The brand was accepted and now requires a proper campaign to spread awareness among the tea drinkers there. The initial blending was done with Assam teas only. The first few consignments were largely confined to orthodox varieties. Later, some of the South Indian varieties under the Nargis brand were marketed.

61. Export of Flavoured Tea from Terai Co EOU

Terai Tea Co Ltd. finalised an export order worth Rs. 10.2 crore from JSC Soyuztrade International of Russia. The order was completed by November 30, 1995. During the fiscal year (1995-96) the company already achieved an export turnover of Rs. 16.2crore as of September 30,1995. The company had planned manufacture of flavoured teas in tea bags, tin caddies and chestlets for export to the US, Germany and South Africa.

62. Tea Estates in Bengal up for Sale

Growing pressure from the West Bengal Government to clear outstanding tea cess payments by March 31 1996 forced several tea gardens in the Darjeeling and Dooars region to put themselves up for sale. The Darjeeling gardens and Dooars gardens which formed a group of 180 gardens in the state, accumulated cess and other liabilities of Rs. 100 crore over the past few years. There were, however, no takers for these gardens. The going price for a Dooars gardens was Rs. 100 per kg. For Darjeeling gardens the asking price was Rs. 300 per kg.

The decision to sell came at a time when the companies with these gardens found it increasing liabilities and other duties because they lacked reserve funds and liquidity. They did not also make any provision for cess in their balance-sheets all these years. In West Bengal, cess was levied on green leaf production at the rate of 15 paise per kg. This worked out to Rs. 70 per kg (4.5 kg of green leaf makes one kg of processed tea).

63. Crisis Hits Sri Lankan Tea Industry

The Sri Lankan tea industry, which brings in a substantial foreign exchange for the island nation, headed for a major crisis when with more than half-a-million plantation workers went on strike from April 22, 1996. Sixteen organisations belonging to the Joint Plantations Trade Union Centre joined the seven-day strike organised by the Ceylon Workers' Congress, a trade union outfit of plantation workers. The strike call was first given by the ceylon Workers Congress (CWC) president, Mr. S. Thondaman, a member of the Chandrika Kumaratunga cabinet. According to rough estimates, there are more than a million Tamils of Indian origin working in the plantations. The week-long strike hit the plantations very badly. It had a disastrous effect on the tea industry. As of now, the tea price reached an all time high but the strike brought it down very badly.

Sri Lanka earned foreign exchange worth Rs. 2 billion (US $ 4 million) last year from tea exports. "This year, we will be hit because the strike will affect the tea factories, producers of green tea and also the rubber production," Mr. Seneviratne said.

64. Tata Tea's Presence in Jorhat

The Tata Tea acquired a small garden, Konikar Dallim, based in Jorhat. Subsequently Konikar purchased was gardens like Borjan Tea Estate in Assam and Badabari Tea Estate in Dooars in West Bengal. While Borjan produced about 6.5 lakh kg. of green leaf, Badabari had a production capacity of seven lakh kg. Konikar Dallim added another four lakh kg to Tata Tea's overall production. Mr.

R.K. Krishna Kumar, the then managing director of Tata Tea confirmed that the acquisition of the estate helped the company to increase the production of tea from Teok. Since Konikar Dallim did not have any tea factory the entire green leaf production was transported to Teok for tea production.

Teok at present manufactures around 5.5 to 6 lakh kg. and is also embarking on an expansion plan. The Konikar acquisition added to Teok's production. The managing director said the Tata group was extremely committed to Assam and took a policy decision to buy as many properties as possible in that state. He said the company was also offered other properties in other regions, but barring Badabari, it turned down that other offers. About the cost of acquisition, the company paid price of about Rs. 105 per kg. considering the fact that Konikar Dallim produced about four lakh kg. the price was a little over Rs. 4 crore. For Borjan, acquired last year Tata Tea paid a price of Rs. 110 kg. of tea.

65. Additional Scheme for Deposit by Tea producers

The Centre notified a new scheme for development of tea gardens and also to improve their liquidity. Tea growers and manufacturers could now set aside 20 per cent of their pre-tax profits in an account maintained in any nationalised bank. Such amounts will qualify for deduction under Section 33AB of the Income tax Act. The money can be spent on development schemes approved by the Tea Board. The amendment to the section proposed in the 1994 Finance Bill stated that the amount could be made available by the Board without the stipulated lock-in period of one year. This new facility for the tea industry took effect from April 1, 1995. However, the one-year lock-in period clause was applicable only to existing schemes covered by Section 33AB. For existing schemes, the 20 per cent pre-tax profits or any amount earmarked by tea companies were to be deposited with the National Bank for Agriculture and Rural Development (NABARD). The amount could be released by the Board for development. An authoritative note on the subject stated in the memorandum explaining the provisions in the Finance Bill, 1994 is appended below:

Section 33AB of the Income-tax Act, provides that where a person who carries on the business of growing the manufacturing tea in India has during the previous year, deposited with National Bank for Agriculture and Rural Development (NABARD) any amount in a Tea Deposit Account maintained by such person with the Bank in accordance with the scheme approved in this behalf by the Tea Board, such person shall be allowed a deduction of the amount so deposited during the previous year, or twenty per cent of the profits from the business of growing or manufacturing tea in India, whichever is less. It is proposed to extend the benefit of Section 33AB also to such tea growers and manufacturers who make deposits in the Tea Deposit Account in accordance with, and for the purposes specified in another scheme framed by the Tea Board and approved by the Central Government. The proposed amendment will take effect from 1st April, 1995 and will, accordingly, apply in relation to assessment year 1995-96 and subsequent years.

66. Critical Review of World Bank-aided Schemes

Serious problems plaguing a Rs.43 crore World Bank financed scheme for increasing tea production in the Darjeeling gardens were identified by a Tea Board team following a recent tour of the plantations The five-member team of the board's technoeconomic cell underline two principal defects of the scheme after surverying 46 gardens, 33 of which were the borrowers of the scheme. According to a senior board official, major research and development programmes in tea cultivation were not done since the Darjeeling Tea Research Centre did not function well. The 1983 World Bank scheme received Union Government clearance two years later.

The Interest Subsidy Scheme (ISS) for the tea in Darjeeling gardens, which is famous the world over, represents only two per cent of the national tea production. The average productivity is only 650 kgs a hectare while the national average is 1500 kgs. The main reasons for the low productivity, the scheme noted, were agro-economic factors neligence of the gardens situation, high costs of production and low returns. The ISS noted that the estimated selling price in the past three years was lower than the cost of production, leading to a loss of about Rs. 2 per kg. Besides, export earnings from Darjeeling tea is only 4.3 per cent. Extension of the areas under tea cultivation and replanting of the uneconomic area were suggested by the scheme.

To carry out the project, the expenses were to be spread over 10 years. The investments were to be made under a composite scheme to be executed through institutional banks with the help of Agricultural Refinance Development Corporation. The Tea Board study states that the loan giving was initiated at the height of the Gorkhaland agitation. The resultant turmoil made the planters chary of availing the loan, Many garden owners, the recent survey said, felt they would not be able to repay the loan. A team member said that the owners felt an infusion of investment was necessary. However, they apprehended that the unrest would inhibit the flow of investments. As a result, only about Rs. 7 crore were advanced as loan while the remaining amount lay with the disbursing banks. However, many of the planters did not know of the scheme. Cumbersome procedures shifted the borrowers' interest.

67. Japan Switches over to Back Tea

Japan, a quality conscious market, has been purchasing the most expensive teas from India and Sri Lanka. Barring West Germany, Japan pays the highest prices for Darjeeling teas. At present the Japanese are switching over from the traditional green Teas to black Tea. John Keells quoting Tea & Coffee Trade Journal, indicated that of the black tea consumption, Ready-to-Drink-Tea (RTD) such as canned tea showed a sharp increase.

68. Destruction of Tea Wastes

In a circular issued on 3rd March 1994 the Central Excise notified that the Central Board of Excise and Customs are now aware that the tea waste has been piling up due to unwillingness of the Excise authorities to supervise destruction of tea waste. The matter was examined by the Board. It was decided that Central Excise Department, the Central Excise officers may continue the supervision of destruction of tea and issue certificate of destruction of tea waste. The procedure laid down in Circular No. 16/89999999-C.X. 6 dated 7th March, 1989 is again reiterated.

69. Andrew Yule's Memsahib Tea

Andrew Yule and Company Ltd. launched a super-premium tea in the Indian market. Priced at nearly Rs. 600 per kg the "rare Darjeeling tea" was available at select outlets largely in northern India. It was packaged in caddies (tin boxes) of 100 grams and 250 grams each. Each caddy uses photographs of the estate from where the tea comes. Called "Garden of Mim", the tea is name after the legend of Mim sahib (the lock version for memsahib). The publicity material for the product drew a parallel between the dedicate tastes and strength of character of Mim Sahib and that of the tea and traced the history behind the tea garden.

Andrew Yule looked at India Tourism Development Corporation (ITDC) outlets, duty free shops, select supermarkets, five-star hotels and some tourist destinations to stock the product. It put out a total of 2000 kgs of the tea in the country by March 1995. Garden of Mim was the first super-premium variety marketed by Yule, which started pushing packaged teas in the Indian market recently, despite having been in the tea business for nearly 150 years.

70. TTCI to Enter Domestic Pocket Tea Market

The Tea Trading Corporation of India (TTCI) is making a last-ditch bid to stay above water by planning to enter the domestic packet tea market for the first time. Though the corporation has a couple of gardens under its management, precious little has been done in the last few years to make the gardens viable. TTCI had been mostly buying teas for the export market. Recently, however, the company is making a concerted bid to buy teas and packet them for the market.

71. Multi-pronged Strategy for Meeting Tea Output Target

The Union Government, along with Tea Board, adopted a multi pronged strategy for taking ways and means of increasing per hectare yield of the crop, and initiating proposals to bring in more areas under tea cultivation. This, besides financial support, was provided through NABARD to "weak' tea estates so that they could improve productivity. Accordingly, a special committee was set up to explore the possibility of converting about 50,000 hectares of land under coffee plantation in South India into tea and rubber cultivation. Efforts were also made to bring in more areas under tea cultivation, since an industry survey revealed that while 23,000 hectares of land was readily available, another 24,000 hectares could be made available after reclamation and rehabilitation. Talks with various state governments on the issue were held. The Environment and Forest ministries dwere approached for securing some denuded forest land for tea plantation. Pointing out the wide gap between the per hectare yield of different tea estates in the same agro-climatic zones, it was said that an additional 500 million kg of tea could be available if efforts were made to minimise the vast gap in per-hectare yield of tea estates in the same area.

72. CCPA Condemns Extremist Attact on Tea Planters

The Consultative Committee of Plantation Associations condemned the attack by a group of suspected extremists on tea planters and their families at Bosola Planters' Club in Sonitpur, Assam and described it as most heinous. The Assam Government and the Union ministries of Home Affairs and Commerce were once again urged by the CCPA to ensure that stern steps could be taken to curb disruptive activity in Assam where the tea industry, among others, has a major stake. Recurrence of such incidents would further demoralise the plantation community which, in turn, would cause serious setback to the tea industry's efforts to maximise production and exports and thereby contribute to the growth of Assam's economy.

73. Registration of Forward Contracts for Tea Produced Till End-November

In accordance with the Tea (Regulation of Export Licensing) Order, 1984, the Tea Board, acting on the recommendations of the Panel of Experts for North India, announced that from mid-October 1990 onward, applications for registration of forward contracts (concluded on and after 9.10.90) covering tea production upto 30th November 1990, would be accepted by the Tea Board for the purpose of registration for exports to all countries except Iraq and Kuwait.

74. Tea Industry Meets the Tenth Finance Commission

Some Tea Industry experts appeared before the Tenth Finance Commission at Guwahati on the 7th of October, 1993, and they apprised the commission on the incidence of taxes not only for Assam but for tea industry of the entire country. The subject covered were:

1. The incidence of tax on the tea industry -
   a) Agricultural Income Tax
   b) Corporate Tax under the Income Tax Act.
2. Section 80 HHC under the Income Tax Act.
3. Consignment Tax.

In addition, the attention of the Commission was drawn to the following subject in line with the write-up entitled, 'Tea Industry—some Issues'.

1) Apportionment of income of tea industry between agricultural and non-agriculture.
2) Tea cess.
3) Extension and Replanting : Allowance under Section 33A.
4) Loss due to calamity such as floods and compensation thereof.
5) Additional land.

75. Pakistan Plans Tea Cultivation : Pakistan, which imported 170 million dolar worth of tea annually earmarked 150,000 acres in the country's mountainous north for tea cultivation. A board was set up to develop plantation on the specified land within two years and work was progressing in the research centre near Mansehra in North West Frontier Province. It was promised to provide adequate loans and incentives to tea growers. Chinese experts assited the experimental tea cultivation at the research centre.

76. Tea Cess Upped by 75 Percent in Sri Lanka

The tea cess was increased in mid-April 1990 from Rs.2.00 to Rs. 3.50 per kg, a Sri Lanka Tea Board spokesman said. He said that the Rs.1.50 per kg, increase generated a revenue of Rs. 300 million for the Board. Of this sum Rs.100 million was utilised mainly to provide fertiliser to tea small holders on credit on an interest free basis. This fund was established to assist tea producers, particularly smallholders if there was a downturn in tea prices below the cost of production. A total of 55 per cent of the country's tea holdings were in the state-owned plantation sector while the balance 45 per cent was smallholder owned.

77. Assam Tea Industry to Create 12,000 More jobs

The Assam tea industry agreed to create 12,000 jobs for unemployed youths in the state in pursuance of the Government's efforts to generate fresh employment. The Governor reportedly agreed to provide 7,000 skilled jobs while the remaining would be created in the class IV, clerks, accountants categories within two months. This was in addition to the 16,000 unskilled jobs already created by the Government.

78. Export Enquiry for Kangra Valley Tea

Good export enquiry for Kangra Valley tear the highlight of the tea auction, held in Kolkata. The first invoices of the Kangra Valley tea evinced keen competition from exporters and six lines of whole leaf sold at prices above Rs. 100 per kg. These teas, which had won high acclaim in the Amsterdam and London markets way back in 1952, later lost their quality and flavour which have now been restored. With the Himachal Government, the Counsil of Scientific and Industrial Research (CSIR) and the Agricultural University at Palampur taking a keen interest, the Kangra Valley tea industry is regaining its popularity.

79. Review of Tea Prices : Since tea comes under items included under essential commodities, its prices were being monitored at the highest level. A cabinet committee has been constantly reviewing the price trends in order to evolve measures for bringing down the price line to the levels of consumer interest. A big disparity existed between auction and consumer prices of tea, any correlation could be established between auction and consumer price. Consumer price does not fall even the he auction price declines. It is appealed to the industry to bring down the tea prices as it is a common man's drink.

80. Goodricks Revives Iran Deal : The Goodricke Group Ltd. revived a controversial Iranian order for 25 million kgs of tea which was disallowed by the Tea Board July 1992 on the ground that the tea producer was undercutting other exporters. The order was revived at the earlier prices, after the Commerce Ministry, overruling the Tea Board, agreed to Iran's demand that the contract be honoured. Goodricke had booked the order at Rs.51.9 a kg, for the Assam orthodox whole-leaf component and Rs. 51.7 for the brokens. The Tea Board had withheld registration of the Goodricke export order on the ground that the prices struck were below the broker valuation. Other producers and merchant exporters who got 13.5 million kgs of the Iranian bulk tea orders bagged prices which were about 20 per cent higher than the Goodricke price. The system of brokers' valuation was introduced after it was seen that exporters were undercutting each other. But the ministry felt that auction prices had not fallen to a level near Goodricke's original quotation, so the deal can be cleared.

81. Nestle and Coca-cola in Joint Tea-coffee Venture : Nestle SA and Coca-Cola, two of the world's biggest food and drink companies, negotiated a joint venture contract to manufacture and market concentrates and beverage bases for ready-to-drink coffee and tea, under the Nestea brand names. The new company, with an initial capitalisation of US$ 100 million, was owned and funded equally by the two giants. Its products were marketed world wide with the exception of Japan, since both companies separately offered canned coffee in that country. Robert C. Goizueta, Chairman and CEO of Coca-Cola, say, "The joint venture has the potential to combine some of the world's most admired and recognised trademarks with a distribution system of uparalleled reach and efficiency. According to Helmut Maucher, Chairman and CEO of Nestle SA, ready to drink tea and coffee is one of the most rapidly growing segments of the world's beverage market.

82. The Rs. 5,000.00 Sip : A line of tea from Castleton, a garden in Darjeeling, sold at Rs.5,000.00 per kg at the auctions in Kolkata. This was the highest ever price paid for first flush. It was said that earlier sales of first flush tee from Darjeelings had, on an average, fetched prices below Rs. 1,000.00 per kg. It was the second flush which generally commanded fancy prices. Castleton but the headlines for the last couple of years for such record-breaking prices for its tea. The garden is owned by Tiru Tea Ltd.

83. Tea Auction in Georgia : Sri Lanka's tea broker, John Keells, purveyed the interesting news that the first tea auction for the year 1993-94 was held in Georgia in the middle of July 1993. It was expected that tea grown in the Commonwealth of Independent States (CIS) was sold at this auction centre.

84. Fresh Export Sops for Value-Added Tea : The Commerce Ministry drew up a list of what it called 'extreme focus' sectors to provide them more incentives to boost exports. Only value-added items with the premise of generating an additional 30 per cent earning in foreign exchange in dollar terms a year got a place in the list.

Value-added tea items like instant tea, tea bags, packed tea, tea caddies and chests had already been identified for inclusion in the list. All these items were eligible for getting exim series at 40 per cent of the f.o.b. value under the supplementary trade policy announced recently by the Commerce Ministry. Additional incentives to step up tea exports included allowing these items the full benefit of Section 80 HHC of the Income Tax Act like other. However, the tea industry put up a stiff resistance, forcing the ministry to postpone implementation of the proposal. The proposed "tea fund" is of the nature of a corpus, the interest accrued on which will be utilised to finance infilling replantation export products and abolishing the double excise duty on packet tea. The Commerce Ministry had shelved a proposal to raise the cess on tea and used the additional collection to set up a fund to help the gardens meet infilling and replantation costs. The Planning Commission approved a few months ago a hike in cess by seven paise per kg activities. The cess, which is the main source of revenue for the Tea Board, is levied under Section 25 of the Tea Act. The last increase in cess on all varieties except Darjeeling tea, by seven paise to 15 paise a kg was effected on August 15, 1986.

85. Tea Seminar Urges More Employment for Local People : Inaugurating a seminar on Tea in Guwahati, Assam, on 28th March 1992, the then Assam Governor Loknath Misra, called upon the tea industry to take a rational approach in view of the current situation in the state. In order to meet the challenges, the industry needed to improve its employment generation activity by absorbing more local people and helping young entrepreneurs with their technical expertise and machinery back up. Stating the tea industry, on an average, exported 65 per cent of its output and there was need for preserving the country's position of being the largest tea exporter by improving the product quality. Mr. Misra said the tea industry should not be complacent but find other markets for exports to retain its place in the world. The then managing director of Tata Tea, Mr. R.K. Krishna Kumar said Indian tea industry should carry out a detailed appraisal of its production techniques with particular refinance to its cost structure. Mr. H.P. Barooah, the then chairman, ITA, of said that there should be a rational and factural appreciation of the industry's role in the socio-economic shpere. It should be understood that production growth can only be there when there is a commensurate profitable market growth. Among other, non-availability of land and exporprietary taxation are the two major constrains that affected production growth of tea.

86. Reliable Telecommunication Link for Tea Industry : The North East region and remote area people particularly associated with tea industry in India are facing hardship due to limited telecommunication facilities. Telecommunications Consultants India Ltd, a Govt. of India enterprise under the Ministry of Communication, Department of Telecommunication, was set up to render consultancy services and to undertake turn-key jobs from concept to completion in all fields of telecommunication in India and abroad. TCIL introduced the Remote Area Business Message Network (RABMN) a Public message/data transmission facility offered by Department of Telecommunication (DOT), to meet the growing demand of public/ private sector undertakings, industrial establishment and other users from any location in the country, including remote places. RABNM provided a highly reliable and versatile service employing state of the art technology which was already well proven internationally. To started operation of Network in March 1990.

87. Packing of Tea Chests for A.R.E. : The famous broker, J. Thomas, advised that buying from the auctisns for the A.R.E. was more regular. The A.R.E. supported teas packed in ISI (BIS) chests lined only with APL (Aluminium Paper Lining) and they did not accept any other packaging material. Their inquiry was towards orthodox fanning and orthodox dusts, as well as CTC fannings and CTCPDs. Their preference was well sized, clean and brackish teas in the plain and medium range. In view of the uncertain market the broker considered it advisable to pack teas, which were suitable for their requirements, in ISI (BIS) chests line with APL to get their support.

88. Restricted Use of Darjeeling Tea Logo Soon : The Darjeeling tea logo, which proved very successful in expanding the market for quality Darjeeling tea abroad, was reserved for packets containing only 100 per cent Darjeeling tea. While for the domestic market the logo was used only on packets of 100 per cent Darjeeling tea, in the export market it was used on packets containing blends with a minimum of 60 per cent Darjeeling tea. Giving this information at the fifth annual general meeting of the Darjeeling Planters' Association (DPA) in 1992, the then Tea Board Chairman, Mr. P.K. Bora, said the Board had decided to restrict the use of the logo as the mark was being increasingly identified with very high quality teas. Now the decision was taken and the modalities for implementing the new policy were worked out.

While Darjeeling tea planters had been supporting the move, Mr. Bora said importers from Japan, Germany and other countries were of the view that restricting the logo to only 100 per cent Darjeeling tea would enhance the perception of quality and help expand the market for Darjeeling tea. The Tea Board chairman said the time had come for the tea industry to look ahead. While mentioning that the disintegration of the Soviet Union had affected Indian tea exports, he felt that the situation was not depressing as there had been a perceptible increase in exports to general currency areas. Referring to Darjeeling in particular, he said extensive R&D should be undertaken to improve productivity without sacrificing quality.

89. Training in Plantation Management : Vijay Dudeja+, the then Chairman of Paramount Academy of Technology, proposed to set up a college of plantation management in Kolkata to offer specialised education in various plantation crops like tea, coffee, rubber, spices and floriculture. The state government was requested to allot land for this. The college also proposed to introduce a six-month course in tea tasting. To ensure effective technology transfer, the academy proposed to establish research centres in Calcutta, Delhi and Bangalore besides Coimbator where it has established an R&D unit and laboratory.

90. TRA to Admit Tea Machinery Makers : The Tea Research Association (TRA) has, for the first time, opened the door for associate membership to tea machinery manufacturers. So far only planters and certain agro-chemical manufacturers were admitted to the TRA. It was believed that a direct interaction between TRA and the tea machinery industry paved the way for faster development of sophistication.

91. Floods Affect Tea Arrivals : Tea arrivals in Kolkata fell sharply because of the floods in North Bengal and Assam. Both the modes of transport—road and rail—were affected. Even the movement from ICD Amingao came to a halt. The fourth rakes' arrival was anyone's guess. Under the circumstance the shipping companies were reallocating the containers earlier earmarked for tea for general cargo.

92. India May Buy Tea From Vietnam : India is exploring the possibility of importing tea from Vietnam against export of machinery in a sort of barter deal to help Vietnam overcome its 'hard currency' shortage. Disclosing this at a recent meeting convened by the Indian Merchants Chamber (IMC) the then Indian ambassador to Vietnam, Mr. J.C. Sharma, said the imported tea could be blended with varieties and re-exported to other countries. Though the quality of tea produced in Vietnam was poor, Indian exporters selling blended tea abroad could use them for getting a better mix, he said. Mr. Sharma, however, said the idea was still at a formative stage.

93. Assam Logo Formalities : The Chief Executive of the U.K. Tea Council met the Tea Board Chairman to discuss the formalities preceding the final launch of the Assam logo in the UK. The Tea Board announced shortly the formation of a tea testing panel in the UK. The panel was responsible for monitoring the quality of tea packets bearing the Assam logo.

The Board's London office wrote to leading UK packers, who have agreed to display the logo on packs of Assam tea, asking them to nominate their representatives of the tea testing panel. The packers submitted their blends for approval to the Tea Board.

94. Tea Retention Trend in India on the Increase : Tea retention in India had been increasing very rapidly during the past few years and the trend is affected to continue in the years to come according to trade circles. To meet domestic demand, estimated to be growing at 10 to 15 per cent annually, and to increase export earning, the Tea Board suggested a two-pronged strategy with a time-bound research plan with emphasis on its application . It was apprehended that if this trend continued, India, which is present the world's largest producer, might have to turn importer in the near future. The urgent need of the country was, therefore, to increase production since the present rate of production is less than that of the domestic consumption.

95. New Tea Gardens in Terai region : The Bihar government evinced interest in new tea plantation in areas contiguous to the Terai region of West Bengal, according to H.P. Barooah, the then Chairman of the Indian Tea Association. He said the West Bengal government promised to return lands which had been taken away from the gardens and given to the forest department in the past. The challenge before the industry was to maintain India's share of 18 per cent in the global tea trade while catering to the phenomenal rise in domestic demand. The ITA chief called upon the government to remove all the controls over the industry. He said the task of raising production to 1000 million kgs by the turn of the century was achievable provided the government was more generous in allocating additional stretches of land. He cautioned the planters about a possible clampdown by the government in respect of the use of firewood and environment norms. He urged use of coal briquettes as cooking fuel for workers.

96. Tea Gardens put N. Bengal flood loss at Rs. 15 cores : Devastating floods in Jalpaiguri, the worst since 1952, had wreaked havoc on the tea industry in the region. Tea gardens stretching from Banarhat to Jainti Sankos were indated and as many as 40 estates were seriously damaged. Total damages in the flood-hit gardens was not less than Rs.15 crore in the year 1994.

97. Indo-Rumanian Trade Plan for 1992 : The Annual Trade Plan with Rumania for Calendar year 1992 was concluded between the Government of India and Government of Romania. As per the sai trade plan, the provision of export of tea to Romania during the calender year 1992 was Rs. 5 million of packaged tea and bulk tea combined, stated a Tea Board Note.

98. Joint Venture with Singapore : The Indian Commerce Minister visited Singapore in October 1991, and met Mr. Lim Boon Hann, Senior Minister of State, Ministry of Trade and Industry, Singapore. It was agreed in their meeting that joint ventures between the two countries for the marketing/exports offered potentials. And this was explored by the Trade in the two countries.

99. To Get Back the European Market : Aware of its slipping share, the Indian tea industry had identified the UK market along with four others as one that needed attention and further servicing. A high-level delegation visited London, Dublin, Warsaw and Hamburg in 1991. The team, led by the then Tea Board Chairman Mr. P.K. Bora, sought to assure importers that India had shifted its policy of tea exports from a hitherto conservative "residual" approach to a stance of production for export. The industry members who accompanied the delegation tried to reaffirm its resolve to prospective tea buyers to ensure uninterrupted availability of a wide range of tea catering to diverse taste.

100. Exports to the CIS : The Tea Board discussed the strategy for export of Indian teas to Russia and other members of the Confederation of Independent States (CIS). The Board also discussed the reintroduction of the practice of granting approvals for tea packets meant for export. This will go a long way not only in assuring the quality of Indian teas, but also enable the Tea Board to specify checks and controls. Further, the export strategy included the suggestion that tea packets produced in export processing zones should carry the Tea Board logo for easier identification of Indian tea in overseas markets as also to ensure their quality. Tea Board sources say that Board may also consider the possible reintroduction of the Tea (Regulation of Export Licensing Order, 1984) that has been repealed recently. Such a measure, they aver, could check under-invoicing and, thus, help curtail possible loss in foreign exchange.

101. Tata Tea's Hospital Chabua : At a cost of Rs.7 crores the Tata Tea Company set up a 55-bed sophisticated hospital at Chabua, in Upper Assam, know, as the Tata Referral Hospital and Research Centre with a primary aim of catering to the needs of Tata Tea's 25,000 employees and their families in the state, it is kept open for the economically weaker sections of the local population free of cost. This hospital with a broad-based out patient wing has well-established radiology, pathology, physiotherapy, anesthesiology, intensive care unit with cardiac monitors, ventilators, defibrillators, piped oxygen and suction arrangements.

102. CTC Factories of Harrison Malayalm Ltd. : Two CTC factories were set up at Munnar and Vandiperiyar by the Harrison Malayalam Ltd. Tea from these factories were sold mainly through auctions. The said company introduced in the market two new varieties also.

103. India's Green Tea Manufacture : What makes the Amritsar city of Punjab unique to the tea industry is the handling of 10 million kgs of a scarcely known commodity green tea. Amritsar, with its 50-odd factories, is the only distribution centre for green tea in the country. Since this city also possesses the technical know-how for sifting and grading the product, tea is pouring in Amritsar from the hills of Dehradun. Kangra, Tamil Nadu and North Bengal. Meating-eating countries are the eager take of green tea due to the digestic properties. In India the green tea is consumed mainly in Kashmir. The big buyers till recently, however, were the Afghans, followed by Pankistanis.

104. Tea in Arunachal Pradesh : Arunachal Pradesh initiated a massive programme to go in for tea cultivation. The Government and banks assisted the villagers interested to take up tea planting as a source of income. Private sector tea estates, as such, came up in Chalang, Tirap, Lohit, Siang and Dibang districts. Apart from this the Arunachal Pradesh Forest Corporation undertook tea plantation in some parts of the state. But is has yet to set up factories for the made tea.

105. What Kerala Thinks Today : The Indian Tea Association urged the West Bengal Government to introduce an investment deposit scheme under the prevailing Agricultural Income Tax Act as such a scheme introduced by the Kerala Government is functioning well. Under the scheme, tea plantations in Kerala are allowed deduction of upto 20 per cent from thier pre-tax agricultural income for the purpose of rejuvenating and modernisation of both field and factory. It helps better plough back of profits for the best interest, if tea industry, says ITA.

106. ABITA's Welfare Programme : For the welfare of small and marginal farmers, the ABITA initiated a few agricultural development projects in collaboration with Hindustan Fertilizer Corporation. The farmers trained in lined transplanting and technical details of paddy varieties and application of fertilisers. This agricultural development programme immensely helped them to raise production from 2 quintals to 8.4 quintals per bigha.

107. Farmer Participatory Research Project by ABITA : An agricultural development project in technical collaboration with Assam Agriculture University included planting of saplings in the Hari Mandir premises and laying the foundation stone of an agricultural library. The main objective was to utilise the fallow land after 'Sali' harvest to enhance cropping. Keeping the objective in view a Farmer Participatory Research Project (FPRP) was inaugurated with sowing of seeds of wheat, rape seed, lentil, rejmah, French bean of high yield variety type.

108. "INDIAN GOLD" : A new TEA PACKED :Tea Board convened a meeting to discuss various aspects of introducing a new tea brand under the name "Indian Gold" in the premium markets. The blue print of this premium market worked out by the Tea Board.

109. Plans to Increase Production Level : Production of '888 million kgs of tea by 2000 A.D. at least Rs.2, 228 crores would be required to finance different plans. The sources saw non-availability of suitable land for tea as a major impediment, that extension of planting, in about 30,000 hectares in the traditional area was essential. Referring to the requirement of huge funds, the sources maintained that the industry could arrange for nearly Rs.800 cores from its own resources and hoped that Tea Board and the National Bank for Agriculture and Rural Development would also chip in. The industry wanted to bring in 5,000 hectares under new plantation in the non-traditional areas, and replantation in 20,000 hectares. And also as a part of the plan it intended to ensure irrigational facilities in 64,000 hectares and drainage system in around 50,000 hectares.

110. Assam Supports I.T. Relief for Tea : The Assam Governments supported the tea industry's demand to 88 HC of Income Tax Act. The government opined that infrastructure support would received top priority.

111. ABITA's Agricultural Development Programme : Assam Branch of the Indian Tea Association launched a scheme of potato cultivation in North Lakhimpur at the initiative of Ananda Tea Estate. Around 600 poor rural people in the area were benefited from the project, it was estimated. Necessary guidance in implementing the scheme was provided jointly by the Hindustan Fertilizer Corporation and District Agriculture Department.

112. Goodricke Banned Chemical Pesticides use in Darjeeling Tea : Chairman of Goodricke Group Limited banned the use of any chemical pesticide in its Darjeeling gardens, making the German European buyers free from the fears of any consumer reaction.

113. Memorandum of Understanding on Cess Signed by the Assam Government : Assam Government signed a memorandum of understanding with tea companies on the question of cess on green leaf. The memorandum provided for cess on green leaf at 18 paise per kg as against 50 paised per kg. earlier demanded by the State Government and contested by the industry. The industry circle observed that the 18 paise cess on green leaf would mean an extra provision of 5.5 paise per kg of leaf, since tea producing companies have already provided for cess at the rate of 12.5 paise per kg in terms of The Supreme Court's interim order. The extra burden would work out to roughly 22 paise per kg of made tea.

114. 106th Annual General Meeting of Calcutta Tea Trades Association : The then Chairman of the Tea Board, Mr. P.K. Bora, said that opening of an office in Moscow would help the Tea Board to regulate Indian exports, and the exports of sub-standard teas more effectively. Shri Giridhar Gomango, the then Minister of State for Planning and Programme Implementation, observed that increased production was being consumed by the rising domestic demand, leaving very little exportable surplus. India's export stagnated at around 200 million kgs. He, however, expressed his satisfaction for the plan drawn up by the Tea Board to produce 1000 million kgs by 2000 A.D.

115. Co-operation is an Era of Genuine Partnership Between Industry and Governments : The tea industry in India which received so far a stepmotherly treatment from the State Government, is now being offered close co-operation. Indian Government had appreciated need for vigorous action for industrial development and there was a joint sector to operate under a planned programme. Government was at best to position itself equidistant between industry and labour. Rather a tilt towards labour was openly indulged in. As regards tea industry, politicians of the generation grew up on Mulk Raj Anand's "Two leaves and a bud" for socio-economic background of the industry. The politicians learnt to look upon labour as oppressed and management as oppressor. With political power in hand the oppressed willnow turn on the oppressor. The governments in Kerala and West Bengal squeezed the tea industry by imposition of higher agricultural income tax at the expropriatory rate of 100 per cent and even more. However, Supreme Court declared the legislations in both the states ultra virus. In view of this there is a need for close understanding between industry and states. The Chairman, ITA, had rightly said in his 112th Annual Meeting that "But more important than what has been specifically done by the government, is the fact that for the first time in history, an era of genuine partnership between the industry and the government has been ushered in".

116. Tea Under Central Budget :The Central budget of 1996 disappointed the industry by not considering Development Allowances under Section 33A of Income Tax Act and deduction in respect of export project under Section 80 HHC. Development allowance earlier available for extension/new planting of tea bushes had been withdrawn following the withdrawal of investment allowance in respect of other industries. Withdrawl of this allowance was a negative step and the same should be reintroduced in the interest of improving productivity and exports. The Section 80 HHC of Income Tax Act 1961 suggests that deduction in export profit to be allowed from business income. The Central Board of Direct Taxs had, however, directed a few years back that deduction under Section HHC would only be allowed against 40 per cent of total income in respect of tea companies. This direction grossly discriminates, against the tea companies vis-avis other indutries because tea companies are hereby liable to pay higher tax as compared to others.

117. Planning for Aftermath of Production cut : Consultative Committee on Plantation Activitiy (CCPA) action may send wrong signal. It was given to understand that CCPA's directive relating to suspension of production during early part of December were aimed at creating a shortage and pushing up prices. Thus it was thought that CCPA was sending wrong signal to outside tea world. However, both Forbes and Walker from Ceylon and African Tea broken from

Kenya commented in their weekly review that Indian producers had taken steps to further up grade quality.

118. Domestic Tea Demand Growth Higher Than Estimates : While addressing the 108th Annual General Meeting of the Calcutta Tea Traders' Association in Kolkata in August 1996. Dr. Asim Dass Gupta, the West Bengal Finance Minister said the growth in the domestic consumption of tea was higher than what was indicated by study conducted on behalf of the tea growers. Dr. Dass Gupta said the growth would be around 5 per cent and not 3 per cent as stated in the report. He said the projections were mechanical and did not consider the increase in income level of rural sector which has direct relationship with the consumption of tea. Dr. Dass Gupta pointed out that the growth of each of the factors which influence tea consumption need to be projected, the effects ascertained and then these added up to finally arrive at the growth consumption pattern.

He said it was important to look at the behaviour of income growth in rural areas. Dr. Dass Gupta felt that since tea is superior commodity, growth in income does generally elicit a greater demand for tea. He said that he could not vouch for the income growth in other states, but in West Bengal, the average income growth in rural areas has been 10 per cent, which is significantly enough to trigger the increase in tea drinking habits in these areas. He urged the tea industry to respond to demand growth through adequate preparation. In this context, he pointed out that even now almost 50 per cent of tea bushes was over 50 years old. Planters need to address this problem and make every effort to increase productivity. Dr. Dass Gupta also asked the Tea Board to explore the possibility of assessing developmental finance from the newly-constituted Rural Infrastructural Development Fund (RIDF).

Earlier, Welcoming the Finance Minister, CTTA the then Chairman D.K. Ghosh congratulated the state government for taking a very keen interest in the development of the tea industry. He also thanked the Finance Minister for responding positively to a CTTA suggestion for dispensing with the system of declaration forms in respect of teas sold in Kolkata auctions for resale.

Mr. Ghosh further complimented the government for reducing the rate of central sales tax on teas purchased in Kolkata auctions for sale to other states from three to two percent. He also expressed his gratitude to the minister on behalf of the plantation industry for the reduction in agricultural income tax from 70 percent to 50 percent. The CTTA Chairman, however, hoped that the state would consider a request for exempting levy of sales tax on teas purchased privately for export after blending. He said such exemption would encourage exporters to carry out value addition in a more aggressive manner.

119. Tea Produced in Kangra Valley - High Aroma and Flavour: The tea grown in the Kangra Valley in general and Palampur in particular is of the rare Chain hybrid leaf variety. The local tea reportedly acquires unique characteristics unmatched by any other orthodox tea in the country. The high aroma and the flavour of the tea is fast gaining popularity both in India and abroad. The tea plantations there were owned originally by Europeans who later sold them to the locals after a devastating earthquake decimated the crop in 1905. The tea was traditionally manufactured by tea planters themselves in their 'power-driven' factories while other small growers made mostly green teas with manually operated equipment. The tea went to Amritsar (known traditionally to be the big market for green tea), as well as to Kashmir and Afghanistan.

120. Utility of Cooperative Institutions : A sales office on behalf of the Kangra tea growers was also set up in Amritsar and the gains were almost doubled for the growers in the next open auction. The growers realised the utility of a co-operative institution and since then the marketing society in Amristar has been functioning with success. Later, the need to extend the benefits of the co-operative approach to the process of manufacturing was also felt and the humble green tea leaf of the marginal tea growers was combined with the luxurious produce of the bigger growers.

The Palampur co-operative factory was registered in 1970 with just 11 members. The membership subsequently increased to 279 and the Himachal Pradesh government too became a shareholder. The green tea, which is roasted right away and then rolled and dried, could not gain acceptance in the Kolkata auctions so the factory began to manufacture black tea (for which, the leaf is never roasted but withered, rolled and then dried).

Kangra tea, 85 percent of which si grown in Palampur tehsil only, is now being exported to Germany, Japan and Iran among other countries. Beautiful packs name after various ragas like Darbari, Malhar, Bahaar and Baageshwari have found eager takers everywhere. The black tea did get good response at the initial auctions in Kolkata but, due to poor maintenance of the tea gardens, inadequate technical knowledge and lack of financial resources, the subsequent consignments could not attract good prices, until in 1994.

121. Plough Back of Profits : Tea industry in India hardly had any opportunity of mobilise internal resources because of high taxation. The dual taxation (agriculture and industry pursuit) caused heavy burden on the industry. The Central Government, appreciating the cause of erosion of internal resource, devised the deposit scheme by an amendment first of Section 32 and then of Section 33 of Income Tax Act. It allowed incomes of the industry to the extent of not below 20 per cent deposited with NABARD to get exemption from income tax. The change, though a mere palliative, retained some irritants. These were : firstly, a lock-in-period during which the deposit could not be withdrawn, and secondly, the purpose for which the deposit could be with drawn were to relate to some technical or agricultural improvements needed on the estate, as detailed in the Tea Deposit Account brought out by the Tea Board. When the industry chafed under these restrictions, its main difficulties related to State Government's agricultural income tax rates, State Government imposed taxes and conditions as they pleased.

122. Second Meet of the Core Committee : A Core Committee was set up in 1994 with the Union Commerce Secretary at the head and select representatives of the tea industry as members. The objective of the Committee was to study regularly the problems of the industry on a regular basis. However, the Committee's advice was not available when some problems were most keenly felt. The second meet was held in December 1995 when some of the pressing issues such as cut-back of production, search for ex-post avenue were discussed. The industry demanded that the centre should deduct all expenditure made on raising and maintaining the special protection force for the Assam Garden from the computed income tax. Another demand was made by industry to amend Section 80 HHC of Income Tax Act for removing the discrimination against producer/exporter of tea. Finance Ministry rejected both the requests. On the issue of export, the ITA & CCPA pleaded for sovereign guarantee and ECGC cover to regain export market in CIS countries. Commerce Ministry officials, however, made it clear that ECGC cover would be available only on selective basis for companies with good track record. They also suggested exports could be organised through third parties with good track record.

123. Let Not Too Many Cooks Spoil the Broth : Lately there has been a lot of discussion about generic promotion of tea in India which is same as growth of consumption of tea. The industry only gave a call to step up production at 1000 m kgs by 2000 AD and implemented the action points of this Perspective Planning (1995-2000 AD). Unfortunately no action plan was started to find out the distinct consumption pattern in quality by the year. No deeper study was made. The CCPA finally had arranged a thorough study of the current situation and future possibilities through professionals. The study team was advised to probe the drinking habits and consumption pattern in particular. Tea Board has reportedly commissioned a survey for estimating the domestic consumption between the period 1995 and 2000. It has already become too late for the study. Let us wait for its findings.

124. Indian Tea is Gold but Gold can be Better Too : To stop glut in tea production during 1995 fetching low price per kg, the industry stopped plucking in all gardens of Assma and Dooars from 3 December 1994 and Terai and Cachar from 10 December 1994 till the first flash production in mid-March 1995. In South India, the cut was in operation after the second week of February because quality teas were produced at that time. This situation created a problem for fulfilling the target 1000 million kgs by 2000 AD. Therefore, the decision did not take into account the realistic growth rate of domestic demand the structuring of international market for absorption of surplus tea and indifferent quality of tea produced.

125. Demand for Tea is Elastic to a Point and its Demand Cannot be Stretched Farther : Although demand for tea is elastic to a point, quality is an important factor. It is possible and reasonable too for the consumers to resist buying teas that are not satisfied with the quality offered at the prevailing rate. India tea is good but gold can be better too. The cut, though not an unusual/unknown weapon, was the latest weapon to be used for correcting the market deviations. Tea industry and Government should take care that wrong signal is not given in future.

Organic Tea to Boost Exports : According to tea industry pundits and experts the demand for organic tea has surged in the global market. In their opinion, the growing demand of organic tea in Europe, united States and Japan is not just a craze now but has really caught on with health-conscious consumers. In the near future, it will get good reception from Australia, New Zealand and other developing countries also where the demand of organic agricultural products is on the rise. This was confirmed from a report of the International Trade Centre, which indicated that the demand of organic products is fast expanding due to growing awareness of the people against harmful effect of fertilizer and chemicals. Naturally, it would not be misleading to infer that organic tea has also a bright market. Indian tea industry should capitalize this opportunity to boost its sluggish exports. In this context it may be mentioned that while in the last couple of years exports and prices of our conventional teas fell severely, organic tea commanded premium, demand in the market as well.

Currently, the world demand for organic tea is about 3 million kg a year. The growth rate is 10 per cent per annum. But with the consumers' growing preference for organic tea to conventional tea, it is likely to be increased phenomenally. So the industry should be wiser to avail the advantage of a market at its nascent stage. It will enable the industry to secure a strong foothold before competition intensifies, which will occur over the next few years. However, organic tea production on a large scale should be launched only after building up adequate knowledge on foreign market. The industry should not overlook the necessity of viability study, such as collecting sufficient information on potential demand, the strength of other suppliers and the prices offered future competitors, distribution channel available and the right importers of such product. The Tea Board and the tea associations should not target just for the export market and without formulating supportive marketing strategies one more point, production of organic tea. It has to be popularized in the domestic market also so that the producers do not depend on export market only. This will serve as a shield to the producers against possible catastrophe in export demand

Report on Bulk Packaging : The Report of the Expert Group, comprising representatives of the Indian Tea Association, Consultative Committee of Plantation Associations and others concerned, on the existing bulk packaging norms with recommendation for an alternative and effective system is ready to reach to the Tea Board. After examining various alternatives such as Jute Bag-laminated with LOPE, Multi-wall paper sacks, HOPE-woven bags, the expert group recommended Polythene-lined jute bags as suitable for bulk packaging in North India. This Expert Group was set up by the Tea Board.

Tea from Coca - Cola

In the hot beverage market of the country, Coca-Cola presented soon with tea. Coke's hot beverage is available through vending machines in Delhi and Kolkata. Announcing this, Mr. Sanjiv Gupta, the then Deputy President of the Coca Cola India said, "Indians do not drink anyone kind of tea. We have kept regional tastes in mind while developing the products." The company, however, declined to mention the launch site in Kolkata but said that for opening of retail spots this town was chosen next to Delhi on the basis of a study carried by the company. "Kolkata has a strong tea culture," the study reported.

UBKV Introduces Diploma Course on Tea : The Centre for Advanced Studies under the Uttar Banga Krishi Vishwavidyalaya (UBKV) introduces a Post-Graduate Diploma Course on Tea Science and Technology. This is a I8-month course which would cost RS.30,000. The curriculum was drawn up after taking into consideration the suggestion of the professors from Jorhat University - the only varsity in the country that offers tea science at the postgraduate level. UBKV was accorded the status of a separate university in May 2002 earlier it was the North Bengal campus of the Bidhan Chandra Krishi Viswavidyalaya.

Major Initiatives that took place during 2003-04 have been highlighted:

News Highlights

The World Bank informed that the tea estates in the country interested to change over from conventional to unconventional energy sources for their power requirement will be assisted financially .

Dooars Branch Indian Tea Planters Association, started at Banarhat in the Dooars and later shifted to Birpara in the Dooars, West Bengal, celebrated its Golden Jubilee .

The North Bengal national Chamber of Commerce initiated a signature campaign for a tea auction center at Jalpaiguri, West Bengal.

In a press meet held at Nagon, Assam, the President and the General Secretary of All Assam Tea Tribe Students' Association alleged that the tea industry in Assam did not take up any constructive work for the economic development in the State other than providing arms and ammunition to the militant outfits active here, and air ticket for the leaders of some organizations .

The then Arunachal Finance Minister, Mr. L Wanglet announced on February 23, 2003 a RS.500 crore scheme for tea cultivation by small and medium growers to better the lot of the poor, particularly in insurgency-affected Tirap, Lohit, and Changlang districts .

The Sang Martam Tea Growers' Cooperative Society, Sikkim, had initiated the cultivation of tea in a virgin land measures 1000 acres. The land is located at the height of 3500 feet and 30 km away from the state capital.

The Makaibari Tea Estate in Darjeeling signed MoU with the society to set up a tea processing plant with 50 per cent equity participation.

The noted Assamese writer, Mr. Mahim Bora, was conferred the Assam Valley Literary Award for 1998, instituted by Magor Educational Trust.

The then Minister for Municipal Affairs, Government of West Bengal, Mr. Ashoke Bhattacharya, ruled out the possibility of setting up another auction center in Jalpaiguri .

The Manipur Government launched a campaign to popularize tea as a horticultural product.

Under an arrangement with RPG Group Company Spencers Ltd., Harrisons Malayalam got the right to use Spencers name to its latest brand of tea that was launched in Chennai.

The Assam unit of the Bhartiya Janata Party appealed the Central Government for granting 'Scheduled Tribe Status' to the tea garden workers in Assam. The party also demanded a minimum daily wage of RS.50/- for the workers and paid holiday every week.

The Tea Board sanctioned RS.32.47 lakh for the development of Tripura Tea Industry .

Darjeeling Planters Association urged the Tea Board to expedite the process of registration of 'Darjeeling' Trademark at London. The Association stated that as the first flush crop in Darjeeling was badly effected due to adverse climatic condition, the overseas market may be flooded by spurious tea marked 'Darjeeling' which will blacken the image of Darjeeling tea .

Abrupt change of course by the river Dima was threatening the existence of Atiabari Tea Estate at Kalchine in the Dooars region of North Bengal. According to a report the river had already swallowed a vast tract of land of the garden .

The promoters of Project India Blend, comprising Tata Tea, Williamson Magor, Rossell Industries Ltd., Warren Tea, and Goodricke Group, decided at a meeting to set up their packaging unit in Russia in view of the hurdles against export to that country. The Bureau of Indian Standards decided to bring a good number of tea companies under the Hazard Analysis Critical Control Point Certification. Accordingly, an apex Committee under the Secretary, Ministry of Food Processing, Government of India, was set up to implement this measure .

At the Annual General Meeting, Tata Tea's plant 0 acquire major shareholding and management control in the UK based Tetley Limited, a global player in the tea industry, was approved. The meeting also approved Tata's plan to float a 'Special Purpose Vehicle' for funding controlling stakes in the UK based company .

In order to massively campaign for the tea brand "Taj Mahal", Hindustan Level Ltd. brought out a commercial feature wherein Ustad Zakir Hussain, the renowned Tabla maestro, and TV personality Ruby Bhatia shown associated with Taj Mahal tea .

Allaying the fears of the Russian buyers on the quality front, the then Tea Board Chairman, Mr. S S Ahuja assured that consignments marked for Russia would be inspected by competent authorities .

The Darjeeling planters decided to initiate plans for marketing and promotion of Darjeeling tea for arousing consciousness of the consumers in both domestic and overseas market.

According to Horticulture Station, Udhagemandalam, Tamil Nadu, spraying of Bordeax mixture (1 %) or Copper Oxychloride (0.25%) at 7 -10 days interval prevents

Blister Blight. Nickel Chloride and Biteranol also contain the preventive properties against this disease .

Hindustan Level Ltd., formulated a plan to relaunch Lipton's 'Taaza' brand tea, largest brand in India, to reach to 50,000 villages across the country .

The National Dairy Development Board has decided to sell both tea and coffee as Amul product to be marketed by the Gujarat Cooperative Milk Marketing Federation of India .

The new tea gardens, particularly in Raiganj, Sadar Kotawali, and Maynaguri, complained to the local police station of uprooting and cutting of tea bushes .

Tea Research Association, the research and development outfit sponsored jointly by the Central Government and the tea plantation industry again in fresh trouble. The Tocklai Employees Union demanded nationalization of the association because of mismanagement of the unit.

The India International Millennium Tea Convention will be held from 22nd to 24th March 2000 in New Delhi. The inaugural Session at Vigyan Bhawan and other functions at the Taj Palace Hotel, New Delhi. The Convention is a joint effort by the Consultative Committee of Plantation Associations and the Tea Board .

The Rossell Tea acquired the Nagrijuli Tea Estate in Nalbari, Assam, from Derby Tea & Industrial Ltd .

The members of Dibrugarh, Moran, and Naharkatia circles under Zone-I, Assam Branch Indian Tea Association donated a sum of RS.l ,00,000 to the Assam Chief Minister's Army Welfare Fund in aid of the Kargil martyrs .

The Teesta Tea and Tourism Festival, inaugurated by the West Bengal Tourism Development Minister, was held at Kanchenjhanga Stadium, Siliguri, West Bengal. Warren Tea Ltd's associate, the Darjeeling Plantation Industries Ltd. acquired the controlling stake of the Kathalguri Tea Estate in Dooars, West Bengal.

Terai Branch Indian Tea Association on behalf of member tea gardens in Terai, West Bengal contributed Rs.2,02,251 towards Central Army Welfare Fund.

At the initiative of the National Bank for Agriculture and Rural Development, various banks agreed to finance the small tea growers in West Bengal.

There are about 600 small tea growers in the region and a potential 24,000 hectares of land under small scale tea plantation.

The Expert Group, constituted by the Tea Board, comprising representatives of the Indian Tea Association, Consultative Committee of Plantation Associations and others concerned, to review the existing bulk packaging norms and to forward its recommendation for an alternative and effective system has examined the plus and minus points of Jute Bag-laminated with LDPE, Multi-wall paper sacks, HDPE woven bags. The Report of the group awaiting discussion .

Hindustan Level Limited introducing tea containing Vitamin A, Niacin, and Vitamin B2 with the object of giving 10 per cent of the recommended dietary allowance in each cup of tea .

Hindustan Lever will be the first company in the country to open the market for micronutrient fortified tea .

According to a recent notification of the Union Ministry of Agriculture, tea plantation units in West Bengal and Assam came under respective state's agricultural sector for the allocation of Urea, a government-controlled input for which this sector was previously enjoying a separate quota .

The Manipur Plantation Corporation, a Manipur Government Undertaking established in 1981, is set to manufacture tea at its own factory .

The Indian Tea Association advocated the repeal of the Tea Marketing Control Order 1984, since the tea industry, on one hand, is being asked to gear up for free trade and imports while, on the other, the industry is being fettered with internal control.

Micronutrients Fortified Tea by HLL: The Hindustan Level Limited (HLL) introduced tea containing Vitamin A, Niacin and Vitamin B2 with the object of giving 10 per cent of the recommended dietary allowance (RDA) in each cup. Hindustan Level was the first to open the market for micronutrient fortified tea. Tea will be the third move of the company towards capitalization of the market for fortified goods and commodities after salt and atta (flour).

Tea from Manipur Plantation Corporation: According to an official report, the Manipur Plantation Corporation, a State Government undertaking established in 1981, produced tea during 2000 with the commissioning of its own factory. The corporation constructed tea factory at Jiribam based Manipur Tea Estate on a turn-key basis in three phases to produce around 3 lakh kg of tea at the first phase, 6 lakh kg at the second phase, and 10 lakh kg at the last phase. In 1982, the corporation took up tea cultivation on commercial basis. The garden started selling of green leaves to Jhirighat Tea Estate in Assam from 1985.

DBITA's Health and Safety Programme: Dooars Branch Indian Tea Association (DBIT A), in collaboration with the West Bengal Chapter of the National Safety Council and Directorate of Factories, Government of West Bengal, organized one-day Seminar on the "Executive Development Programme on Health and Safety" on

September 1, 1999. It was attended by 40 participants from neighbouring member tea estates. Issues connected with health and safety were discussed.

Small Tea Gardens Growing Fast in North Bengal: On the strength of 'No Objection Certificate" (NOC) issued liberally by the Land and Land Revenue Department Government of West Bengal, small tea gardens have flourished in North Bengal. The District Magistrate of Cooch Behar said recently that the State Government had asked the Land and Land Revenue department to issue NOCs to small land holders without delay. However, the detail survey of land schedule submitted by the big tea cultivators is yet to be completed, the official source added.

Single Yardstick Needed to Define Small Growers in Assam: There is no agreed yardstick in Assam to define 'small tea growers'. While according to the Tea Board a small tea grower is he whose land under tea cultivation does not exceed 75 bighas (l0 hectares), the State Government recognizes those as small tea growers whose area under tea cultivation does not exceed 30 bighas. However, the All Assam Tea Growers' Association has demanded that the area under cultivation for recognition as small tea growers be increased from 30 and 75 bighas to 250 bighas.

New Periodical from North-East: Assam Tea Planters' Cooperative Society is bringing out a new periodical, North East Tea News. It will be a quarterly and will aim at covering various issues connected with tea plantation, cultivation, marketing and futures.

Tea Control Order be Revoked : ITA: Recently the Indian Tea Association (ITA) has strongly asserted that the Tea Marketing Control Order 1984 (TMCO) be scrapped. The ITA said the TMCO is an "anachronism" since the tea industry, on one hand, is being asked to gear up for free trade and imports while, on the other, the industry is being fettered with internal control. ITA felt it was imperative for the tea industry to have the flexibility to determine the method of sale of its own product. Expressing concern over the decline in tea prices ITA said that the All India Average Price up to October 1999 remained lower by Rs. 5/per kg and in South India the price were down by *RS.12/-* per kg. "The decline in prices is of serious concern to the tea industry. The lower crop has had a serious impact on unit cost of production by way of labour wages, higher food grains subsidy and major export costs on account of fertilizer, fuel and transportation."

Mushrooming of Tea Factories: To combat the spiraling costs of production, a few tea estate owners and some newcomers set up bought leaf factories which mushroomed all over the tea producing regions in India. With lower overheads/expenses and little statutory commitments, owners of bought leaf factories were able to sell 'made tea' below RsAO per kg which is below cost of production of over 95 per cent of the established tea estates in India. These teas despite being devoid of quality attracted the price-conscious Indian consumer to the detriment of common and medium tea estates. Although official figures of production from bought tea leaf factories are not available, reliable sources indicate this to be in excess of 100 million kgs.

Adulteration Racket: Although tea is known as a health drink, it could not escape the target of adulteration racket. Adulteration of tea had taken a new dimension from 2000 onwards. These unholy practices in the trade front not only rocked the growers' sentiments but also sent a shivering feeler to the consumers. The West Godavari Police unearthed a tea racket by seizing 59,950 kgs of fake tea made of cashew nut rind mixed with betonies powder and edible soda. The seizure of 54,000 kgs of spurious tea from four rice mills of Andhra Pradesh had revealed that it was difficult to differentiate spurious tea from genuine tea as both the colour, the smell and the granular finish were almost identical. Such fake tea could lead to health hazards including blindness and irrevocable damage to the digestive system. In North Bengal, consecutive raids in a few bought leaf factories confirmed that adulteration racket is active in this region too. Seizure of 200 gunny bags containing a non-tea, tea like material, from a factory of Jalpaiguri district was indeed shocking news.

No one can deny that tea is in a disastrous condition at the auction centers and ex-factory outlets. There is hardly any reflection of this gloom at the consumer outlet. It is difficult to buy an average quality tea below RS.120 a kg. This riddle is a difficult to unfurl. There is hardly any answer to the question, why there is a gulf of difference between ex-factory and consumer retail outlets. This is the high time when all efforts to be made to improve both productivity and quality for the survival of Indian tea. Let us pin point a few scientific problems in the tea field and suggest measures to partially or fully overcome those problems:

Organic Food Festival in New Delhi: A week long International Organic Food Festival was held in New Delhi, starting from November 28, 2002. The festival has been arranged by the Biodynamic Association of India in collaboration with the Union Commerce Ministry. Jaswant Purohit of the Tea Association said, "the festival will show-case India's organic teas and food grown the way nature intended. We are expecting a lot of foreign buyers."

Organic Tea to Increase Exports: In order to increase exports of tea from the country, the Indian tea industry is now giving more attention to organically grown teas. According to information available from the Ministry of Commerce, India exported 1.9 million kgs (4.1 million pounds) of organic tea in 1999-2000 fiscal and the plan was to double the export quantum in 2000-01. Fragrant organic tea from Darjeeling commands premium. During 2006-07, the annual export of organic tea would be around 12 million kgs. Growers believe, health-consciousness of consumers in Europe, USA and Japan has enhanced the demand of organic tea comparing to that of a decade ago. The industry is convinced that in coming years the demand will increase phenomenally in view of growing popularity of organic tea. And hence, the tea growers have been advised to take this opportunity to boost exports.

Tea Board to Launch Web Site: The Tea Board of India launched a web site as its strategy to boost the demand of Indian tea in international market. The site provides inforn1ation relating to production capacity of gardens, market prices, quality of Indian teas and also techniques of preparing good tea. In this regard, however, Mr. Basudeb Banerjee, Chainnan of the Tea Board said, "in any effort to boost demand of tea in the international market there is no alternative but utilizing information technology.". In the setting up of the web site the Tea Board took help of IBM.

Government Considering ISI Mark for Tea: The Ministry of Commerce, Government of India introduced ISI certification for tea. Mr. Sharad Yadav, the then Consumer Affairs Minister, said, for this purpose "the Indian Standard for tea has been revised by the Bureau of India Standards (BIS) in consultation with the Ministry which will be published shortly". Ministry officials thought that the move helped improving realization for tea growers and companies as the consumers are provided with high quality certified produce.

ITA's Sales Promotion Campaign for Tea: In order to expand the domestic market of tea, the Indian Tea Association (ITA) has been advertising tea through TV and other publicity media. On the basis of the observation of the Director of American Health Foundation, the advertisement says that tea contains al the nutrients necessary for good health and regular drinking of tea reduces the risk of heart stroke, tumour, some types of cancer and many other diseases. Meanwhile, the impact of the advertisement on the viewers has been studied which indicated 70 per cent of them considers tea not only as a temporary stimulant but a beverage providing vigour and vitality.

Flavoured Tea Market in The Country: Tea majors namely Tata Tea and Hindustan Level Limited (HLL) have been exploring untapped flavoured tea market in the country. They wanted the Indian Tea Association to persuade the Government for allowing the use of natural identical flavours in black tea. Other leading tea manufacturers also 'supported this proposal.

Orthodox Production Necessary In South India : At a seminar on Orthodox tea manufacture, organized by the Tea Board and the United Planters' Association of Southern India, Mr. Vikram Kapoor, Executive Director of the Tea Board suggested the tea growers in South India to switch over to Orthodox manufacture from CTC. In his opinion, this could salvage the southern tea growers from the continuing dull situation. The Tea Board had sanctioned RS.5 crore to 45 producers for the switchover to Orthodox tea production. He advised the planters to learn from Sri Lanka where 98 per cent of the produce was Orthodox and 68 per cent of the small growers engaged in the production of the same. Mr. Kapur said, the soil and weather in South India were ideally suited for the production of Orthodox tea.

Sanjiwani Rehabilitation Centre Inaugurated: In the third quarter of 2002, the pern1anent building of Sanjiwani Rehabilitation Centre for spastic children was inaugurated by Mr. Sanjoy Lohia, Deputy Commissioner, Sonitpur, Assam. Amongst others, the ABITA Chairn1an, Mr N N Sharma, ABITA Chairman (Zone 3), Mr. A Singh, ABITA Secretary and offices of ABITA (Zone 3) attended the function. For the construction of the building the Assam Branch, Indian Tea Association (ABITA) Headquarters and the Zonal Office jointly contributed Rs.2.5 lakh.

North Bengal University started Soil Testing Laboratory for Tea Gardens : The Department of Tea Management under the University of North Bengal has started a Soil Testing Laboratory for the benefit of the tea plantation units of North Bengal, Bihar and Sikkim. Estimation of Organic Carbon, pH, Nitrogen, available Potassium and Phosphorus, Electrical conductivity costs only RS.50 per sample. That besides, estimation of Sulphur and soil texture is also undertaken at reasonable cost.

WB Government to Survey Tea Industry : On 23rd October, 2002, Mr. Nirupam Sen, Commerce and Industry Minister, Government of

West Bengal, said in Kolkata that the government along with the Tea Board had conducted a survey and prepared a situation report on tea industry in the state. The survey covered and recorded the number of tea gardens, area of the gardens, and so on. The report was submitted in December 31,2002.

Tea Board to Monitor Organic Tea Production: Following the commerce ministry's decision to appoint the Tea Board of India as a 'National Accreditation Agency' for the national programme on organic tea production the Board has formed a sub-committee and fixed the terms and conditions for detailing the rules on organic tea production, accreditation and certification. The commerce ministry assigned the Tea Board four major tasks prescribing the package of practices for organic production of the product; undertaking inspection and certifying product as having been produced in accordance with national standard for organic product; monitor inspection by the accredited inspection agencies; and laying down of the inspection procedures.

Study of Benchmarking by Tea Board : Tea Board of India conducted a study on benchmarking for the Indian tea industry by the Indian Instituted of Plantation Management (IIPM) at an estimated cost of RS.6.00 lakh. The objectives of the study were (i) to suggest ways to strengthen the tea industry at the enterprise level and (ii) to develop data for enabling benchmarking at the operating unit level i.e. the estate level so as to have improved performance vis-a.-vis other estates in the district and region.

Employment of Additional Workers in Gardens: The Consultative Committee of Planters' Association (CCPA) recruited 10,000 additional workers to the tea industry. The distribution of the new workforce currently remained confined in the 194 tea plantations of the Dooars and the Terai though it is uncertain whether the West Bengal Tea Development Corporation or the Tea Trading Corporation of India Plantations will absorb new workers. According to CCPA sources, however, Darjeeling tea estates might be excluded for the moment. The employment issue is an overriding one in the tea industry since July 21, 1999. This could not be solved due to Coordination and Defense Committees charge in on the one hand, and on the other tea associations' failure to establish a distribution formula of new workforce acceptable to the gardens. The employment issue was virtually settled.

Certification of Darjeeling Tea The advent of 'Certification' pursuant to the Geographical Indication of Goods (Registration and Protection) Act, 1999 and the post WTO scenario will ensure that only 100 per cent Darjeeling will get certification and no tea without certification can be sold as Darjeeling. According to industry sources, the volume of teas sold annually in the name of Darjeeling is about five times the actual production in 80 gardens that produce champagne teas in the hills of North Bengal. Thus, while an often fake or adulterated Darjeeling tea commands a fabulous price at domestic and international outlets, Darjeeling gardens are in a state of perpetual penury. The industry circle feels, however, certification of Darjeeling tea is a welcome move to protect Darjeeling teas.

Orthodox Tea Manufacture: With the globalisation and free market economy the scope of export and import has been widened. This has resulted in increase awareness among the consumers and bulk buyers for quality and price. It is, therefore, imperative to produce value added and quality products for the survival of any unit. Good Olihodox tea production can add value to teas provided standard is maintained at all stages of harvesting and manufacturing.

Indian Tea Industry under Threat: Kenya and China are emerging as a threat to the Indian tea industry and these countries are capturing more and more of the export market at the cost of India. Unless Indian exporters gear up to face the challenge, there will be surplus in the domestic market, said analysts.

Push for Tea Exports: A 19-member Committee comprising representatives of the government and the tea industry has suggested that Indian tea exports could be increased provided the industry adopts a strategic perspective of efforts rather than viewing it as a domestic surplus. It targets export volume of 240 million kgs by the year 2006. The Committee's Report is an outcome of four months of rigorous assessment of the country's relative competitiveness in the world trade, according to Mr. Anup K Matilal, Secretary, Tea Board of India. It calls for a differential approach to various markets, based on a specific assessment of the overall market attractiveness.

ITA Plans for Afghan Exports: Indian Tea Association (ITA) sent a delegation to Afghanistan to revive India's export to that country. "Apart from a tea delegation comprising the Union Commerce Ministry, Tea Board officials and industry people, permission to export tea to Afghanistan as part of credit to that country helped the industry". The ITA Chairman, Mr Bharat Bajoria said. He told to the press that the association impressed upon the Commerce Ministry for sending a delegation to Afghanistan.

Duncan Establishing Tea Boutique Chain: Duncan's Industries Ltd (DIL) sat up a chain of tea boutiques in select areas. The stores were established under the Duncan's brand name and logo. "After extensive research into tea purchase habits and sales pattern, we have identified 10 locations where outlets will come up in four months", said Mr Gauri Prasad Goenka. The group collected data from actual visits to markets and buyers feedback from popular tea selling shops in the unorganized sector. The boutiques firmly focused on tea because "that is the business we understand the best", said Mr. Goenka. He added, "I am convinced that retail will be a good experience for us, given the strong data-based approach that we have taken and the direct retail model we have adopted". The first shop came up in B B D Bag. This is the central business area in Kolkata, where several popular tea retailers already were located.

AASTGA Steps to Check Price Fall: The All Assam Small Tea Growers' Association (AASTGA) took steps to ensure reasonable return for the small growers. Accordingly, Mr. Hemanta Kumar Gohain, Secretary of the AASTGA requested the bought leaf factories and the organized sector to buy quality green leaf from the small growers on an area to area basis. The association also wants to get rid of the intermediaries, who were eating away into the profits of the tea growers. Mr Gohain remarked that these intermediaries are a major cause of concern to the association. They are making money while the growers are left with almost no return on their investment. He said, the mushroom growth of brought leaf factories in upper Assam has not contributed to the making of quality tea, and that these have led to the growth of the nuisance of green leaf theft and dubious tea making processes. He named a factory, which "does nothing but reprocess worst quality tea dust with some fresh made tea". For such unscrupulous tea makers, quality is the last concern and ill-gotten profits the primary concern, Mr. Gohain said.

TAI's Supervisory Development Programme: National Productivity Council (NPC) arranged a 6-day "Supervisory Development Programme for Plantation Supervisors" on request of the Tea Association of India (TAI), Barak Valley branch sometimes in February 2002. The main objective of the programme was to sensitise the sardars regarding various aspects of tea manufacturing and processing, basic productivity concept, supervisory skills, teamwork and kaizen activities, discipline and motivation. The experts suggested the supervisors to keep a check on alcholism and absenteeism as the habits are barrier to quality tea production. 70 supervisors participated and exchanged opinion. 5 supervisors were selected for further training under the 'Training for Trainers' scheme.

TBITA on Tea Industry Crisis: Admittedly "pushed to the wall", the tea industry is considering to take up drastic measures. While addressing the 40th Annual General Meeting of the Terai Branch Indian Tea Association (TBITA), Mr A Bhagat, Chairman, said: "It's time we discard our grandmother's regulation. Children must be introduced to tea at an early age. He proposed a turn-around measure for the crisis - ridden tea industry by "repositioning" tea as a "health drink". The health properties of tea, backed by scientific evidence, can be a powerful platform for this campaign", he said. Mr A K Matilal, Secretary, Tea Board of India asked the tea industry to be "competitive" and emphasized for improvement quality.

Cachar to Improve Quality of Tea: At the 101 Annual General Meeting of the Surma Valley Branch, Indian Tea Association, the Chairman of the Association in his written address laid overwhelming emphasis on the need to bring about substantial improvement in the quality of tea for the long term revival of the Cachar tea industry. He said that the time has come for Cachar to explore all avenues of marketing its tea and one such is to search overseas markets. Cachar producers can directly target markets such as Pakistan, which is an exclusive CTC market.

ASPEE's Farmer of the Year Award: At a function held on 23rd March, 2002 in Mumbai the "ASPEE L M Patel Farmer of the Year Award 2001" was given. The awardees were Mr Chandrashekar Haribhau Bhadsavle for Rainfed Farming Category - Rice Crop, Mr Subhash Dattatraya Arve for Horticulture Category - Grape Cultivation, Smt Maltiben Joitaram Chaudhary for Women Farnler Category - Dariy Farming and Smt Padmaja Parshuram Chitala for Horticulture Category - Grape Cultivation.

Government Assistance for Tea Exports: To make Indian tea more competitive in the global market, the Government has prepared a plan for meeting miscellaneous expenditure of tea exporters. "A RS.5.25 crore package has been finalized for reimbursing the expenditure tea exporters incur in value addition, handling, packaging, transport and freight to boost the sagging exports of the commodity", official sources said. "Basically, the idea is to encourage exporters to move from bulk trade to value - added segments without totally neglecting the former", the official added it. Exporters of tea bags, packet tea, orthodox, bulk tea and tea directly purchased from the bought leaf factories could now take the benefit of the assistance package. The break up is in favour of value-added product. The reimbursement rates are Rs.10 per kg for tea bag; Rs. 2.5 per kg for packet tea; Ra.2 per kg for Orthodox and bulk tea; and RS.2 per kg for Orthodox and CTC tea from bought leaf factories.

Diatea for Diabetics: The Boulevard Agro Services of Guwahati, Assam, has recently launched a new tea "Diatea", exclusively for the diabetic patients. This tea is a blend of pure Darjeeling tea and three Himalayan herbs. The tea was originally manufactured by Makaibari Tea & Trading Co(P) Ltd., of Kolkata, the expertise came from Mr P N Banerjee, a renowned tea planter of West Bengal. However, the entire bulk of this herbal tea was exported to Japan, said Mr. Raj Kamal Choudhury, Director of Boulevard Agro Services. According to Mr Choudhury, a diabetic patient can take diatea without sugar and milk three to four times a day along with antidiabetic regimen. This tea stimulates insulin secretion by pancreas, stimulates heart and circulatory system, increases the volume of urine and activates uterus in case of women, without influencing the carbohydrate metabolism. The diatea not only controls blood sugar but also obesity. Diatea is a pure herbal tea that has no side effect. Evidences reveal that sugar problem is under control who takes diatea regularly, added Mr. Choudhury. It has tremendous prospects, he said.

Tata Tea Relaunched Kanan Devan: On 17 March, 2002 Tata Tea relaunched its popular South India-based tea brand Kanan Dean in a new package. Commencing on the launch Mr P Siganporia, Deputy Managing Director of Tata Tea said, "the new packaging has been developed after intensive consumer research and embodies Kanan Devan's attributes of being a tea blended by nature. The company's investments in Kanan Devan's new packaging and production processes are in keeping with our commitment to bringing the best cup of tea to consumers".Kannan Devan derives its taste from combination of natural elements present in the Kanan Devan hills in Kerala. The forthcoming advertising campaign of Kanan Devan aims to capture the essence of the brans in its strap line, "blended by nature for that unique taste". Apart from Kanan Devan, Tata Tea's portfolio of brands include Tata Tea, Tetley, Agni, Chakra Gold and Gemini, With 55 tea estates across India and an area of 26,500 hectares under cultivation, Tata Tea produces over 60 million kgs of tea accounting for 21 percent share (in volume terms) of the

Indian packet tea market.

Goodricke Launching Sub-economy Brand: In May 2002, Goodricke Group Ltd. has launched a sub-economy tea brand in the face of increasing competition from unorganized regional packeters. The brand will be sold at the same price as the regional brands.

At the Annual General meeting of the company held in Kolkata, Mr P A Leggatt, Chairman, said : "The recently launched economy brand, Zabardast was well received and the current year should see a substantial increase in sales. There are plans to give packet tea sales a further boost by introducing new brands and other campaigns to increase sales." Mr. K S David, Managing Director said that the company's gardens in Darjeeling is facing competition from highgrown teas from Nepal. Over the years, tea growing areas in Nepal, adjacent to Darjeeling, have been steadily improving their production using clones brought over from Darjeeling. With lower production costs and negligible statutory overheads, ssuch teas produced by Nepal are being sold to overseas buyers, especially Japan and Gernlany at one-third of the sale price.

Futures Trading in Tea Beginning Shortly: Futures Trading in Tea will start in India by the end of 2002 .. "This will break new ground in tea trading. For the first time, all Indian teas, irrespective of their origin, will be traded under one roof', said Mr. Karan Paul, Director of AFT Industries. He said that "Ideally the catalogue of the futures exchange should include teas of foreign origin. But Kenyan and Sri Lankan producers and foreign trading houses will watch the progress of the exchange for the time before they join it". The likely locations for the exchange are Kolkata and Cochin, which boast good infrastructure and very old auction centers. The Indian Forward Markets Commission (IFMC) insists that futures trading in tea will have to be screen-based from the beginning.

UP ASI Seeks Import Duty Hike on Tea and Coffee: United Planters'

Association of Southern India (UPASI) has urged the Union finance minister to increase the basic import duty on tea and coffee to 35 per cent from the current 15 per cent to ensure adequate tariff protection, as provided in the WTO stipulations. The apex association has also demanded a retrospective amendment of Sub-Section 4(B), incorporated in the last Budget, by virtue of which a tea producer-exporter was made eligible to get export profit exemptions to the extent of 40 per cent only. In a representation made to the finance minister, UPASI said several hundred items likely to be placed on the free list of imports, effective April 1, 2000, had been pegged at the peak rate of 35 per cent plus surcharge. But the basic import duty for tea and coffee remained unchanged at 15 per cent.

Such low levels of import duties would, the association said, lead to the import of cheap tea from various other countries and ring the death knell of both the tea and coffee industries in India. With the progressive dismantling of QRs in regard to imports, it was becoming essential that tea and coffee be given adequate tariff protection (like other agricultural commodities) by increasing the basic import duty to 35 per cent, UPASI said. The association added: "If the import duty (in the light of QR removals) is a new problem for the plantation industry, excise duties in the case of the tea industry is an old issue that needs to be sorted out. The revenue implication of the total withdrawal of excise duty on bulk tea would not be significant if one were to take into account factors like excise exemptions already granted to cooperatives and bought-leaf tea factories, the refund on exports, the revenue loss to central and state governments by way of lower income tax and no agricultural income tax and the infrastructural costs of collecting all these taxes".

Distressed Small Tea Growers: Due to severe fall of the prices in the last two years the small growers in the country suffered most. The misery of small growers in both south and north India was of same magnitude. According to available reports, their produce could not be sold to the bought leaf factories and to other regular buyers even at a price of Rs.6/- per kg throughout the last year. This low price, in turn, crippled the normal functioning of many business units. And finding hardly any possibility to get remunerative price the small growers became frustrated and restive. They demanded the government of respective tea growing states to share their pains. The governments should come forward immediately with a package of relief to rescue them from the strangulating market condition. Hence, they urged to set a floor price of their produce, a subsidy as well. And to mak~ their demand forceful the small growers frequently resorted to road blockade, various forms of movement in front of assembly house of the tea growing states. But fulfillment of their demand is in no way the remedy of present maladies. Relief package would not prevent recurrence of the situation. Rather the small growers would be judicious if they remember that those remained consistent in quality and supply did not suffer much due to price fall. The low price in the market was not too low to shake the confidence of quality tea producers in their business. It is imperative for the small tea growers to put their home in order. For higher price realization all they have to do is to see across the fence to realize that quality tea producers get better return in terms of prices. World's demand is now only for quality tea. In coming years the survival of tea units will virtually depend on this slogan - quality first, quality second, quality last. This is the only "mantra" for their survival. Small tea growers alongwith their different associations shall have to take do or die resolution for achieving this "mantra and should leave no stone unturned to upgrade the quality of teas.

Dandi Salt and Tea: The Board after long duration was able to stop the negative publicity the manufacturer of a table salt which is giving in TV commercials in Hindi and regional languages. This advertisement from the manufacturer of Dandi triple refined salt was telecast over Doordarshan and private channels. In the course of the commercial, a doctor was shown to be advising the people to stop drinking tea and save RS.2 a cup which could be spent on consuming the Dandi salt. The stress was that Dandi salt helps people gain mental and physical health. It was not for anyone in the tea industry to waste time, effort, money and other resources to test the veracity of this claim by the Dandi salt manufacturer about the product. But, a question that remains unanswered is : why should the tea industry allow a negative publicity of tea by a salt manufacturer just to promote his brand?

Positive Health Effects of Tea - Research: More so, now that researchers from all over the world have proved the positive health effects of tea. They have repeatedly stressed that tea drinking can help fight cancer, common cold, flu, cholesterol and heart ailments. This is in addition to stimulating mental ability. On the contrary, the general feeling is that the intake of salt leads to blood pressure, heart ailments and even obesity. So, many a doctor for many a patient advises less salt intake. Whether the Dandi brand is above such ill effects of salt consumption in general is a different question. But, in promoting this brand what is the sanctity for lowering the health effects of tea ? In fact, it is only recently that the Government, through the Tea Board, has shown interest to promote tea consumption based on the positive health effects proved by the scientific community at large. On a day in September 2001, the Government released an advertisement through the Tea Board covering full pages in some select newspapers with the title : "Live life healthy way - Piyo more chai every day".

Murasoli Maran Released Accenture's Report on Tea Export Strategy: The then Union Minister of Commerce and Industry, Mr. Murasoli Maran, was in Kolkata on January 21, 2002 to formally release Accenture's Report on medium term tea export strategy for the country in a meeting held with members of the Consultative Committee of Plantation Associations (CCPA) and Tea Board officials. Mr. Maran suggested the tea industry to submit proposals for stepping up exports immediately to countries like Afghanistan, Iraq and Iran. He urged the industry to chalk out a comprehensive action plan for quality upgradation and quality assurance particularly for the bought leaf sector. The key elements of the Accenture's recommendations revolve around market portfolio diversification, differentiated market development activities including a focused effort at developing and promoting the "India" brand, a comprehensive exporter rating system, export quality and reliability management programme, building up of a robust industry-wide information backbone for greater transparency and dissemination of price and market-related information, and value addition opportunities in specific market economies. The back-end recommendation included realignment of production in line with demand in key high value markets. This envisages a shift of part of the production base to quality Orthodox tea.

FAITTA against Dandi Campaign: The Chairman of the Federation of All India Tea Traders' Association (FAITTA), Mr. P O Desai, strongly criticized the 'Dandi Namak' campaign which discourages tea consumption. The campaign sends out the message that, if need be, a cup of tea can be sacrificed for the sake of iodised salt which is more expensive. Mr. Desai pointed out that the Tea Board has also raised the issue with the company.

FAITTA Pushes Sports Sponsorship for Tea Promotion: The Federation of All India Tea Traders' Association (FAITTA) suggested to push the idea of generic tea promotion through sports sponsorship. Mr. P O Desai, Chairman of FAITTA, said: "We will discuss the issue with Tea Board. Producers, packet tea companies and buyers' associations must come together and contribute towards this generic promotion. If all producers contribute around Re.l per kg of tea produced, then given the fact that total production is around 850 million kgs. the budget will be as good as that of the colas". Mr. Desai further pointed out that the exercise would lift the image oflndian tea in the global market. "Exports will increase by 20 per cent and prices fetched by producers at the auction will also increase substantially."

Export Increase in Afghanistan Likely: The fall of the Taliban brought a ray of hope for the crisis ridden Indian tea industry. Officials of tea associations hoped on a boost in exports of Afghanistan. The country used to import tea regularly before the Taliban took over, officials said. In 1998, Indian tea exported to Afghanistan amounted to 55 million kg. Afghans lost their interest in Indian tea under the Taliban regime and exported in 2001 came down to just 0.20 million kg. Traditionally, Afghanistan and other Central Asian countries imported Greed Tea, most of it from India. Aerated drinks as alternatives to tea are yet to gain popularity in Afghanistan. Seniors in the industry believe that the demand for Indian tea in that country has not decreased. Now, with the defeat of the militia, the industry took all effort to regain its market in Afghanistan.

Tea Campaign through New Year Cards : As the tea industry has been trying to bolster generic promotion of tea within the country through different ways, a unique experiment was carried out this year by Warren Tea Limited, a tea giant, and J Thomas & Co., the country's largest tea broking firm. Warren Tea has come out with two types of cards. One wishes friends and associates and says : "This year drink four cups of tea everyday". The other hopes that "every cup of tea will bring cheer to those who drink tea". The cards also harp on the many health aspects of tea : "Tea refreshes and relieves tension" and "Tea reduces the risk of cancer, heart attacks and strokes", say the cards. J Thomas greeting cards have been highlighting the antioxidant qualities of the early morning beverage. What is more interesting that a New Year Greeting Card (2002) of the German company, Kloth and Kohnken Teehandel GmbH depicted the goodness of tea thus: "Tea for two-thousand two ! One for me. One for you".

Vikram's Products & Services Bulletin: Vikaram India Limited, which has a track record of rendering services to the Tea Industry for over 27 years, has brought out a Bulletin. The newsletter presents a summary of the nature and development of activities of the company, Range of Products for Withering, Rolling, Fermenting, Drying, Sorting and Packing, Workshop equipment, etc. with a few colour photographs. Paper and printing of the Bulleting are of very good standards though, of course, a few mistakes cannot escape from the eyes of a meticulous reader. All said and done, it is a respectable publication.

Eveready's PBT Sharply Declinedm : In the three months ended December 31, 200], the Tea division of Eveready Industries, engaged in cultivation, manufacture and sale of tea posted a Loss Before Tax and Interest amounting to RS.l1.37 crore. In contrast, the FMCG division, operating in dry cell batteries, flashlights and packet tea, posted a Profit before Tax and Interest from the two divisions amounted to RS.I0.46 lakh. Sale/income from FMCG division stood at RS.145.04 crore and that from the tea division at RS.81.01 crore. Combined sales income from operation in the same period last year was RS.263.38 crore.

Loan Sought to Improve Soil Structure : The Darjeeling tea planters have requested the Tea Board to introduce a 'Scheme of Loan and Subsidy' for improving the soil stmcture of tea gardens in the hill district. According to Mr. R K Dixit, former Chairman of the Darjeeling Planters Association, the top soil of the Darjeeling tea gardens has been washed away during the lat 150 years. As a result, carbon content in the top soil has fallen drastically. "Unless we improve, the soil stmcture and increase the carbon percentage to the required minimum level of four per cent, the desired result of uprooting and replanting will not be achieved which is evident from the existing yield of young tea areas," Mr. Dixit added.

Assam Trade 'Body Urges Lower Tax Rates : There is an urgent need for a better relationship between the trading community and the Government for a congenial business climate in Assam. This is the view of Kamrup Chamber of Commerce President, Mr. M P Jain. The Chamber is the premium body of traders in the state. Mr. Jain said, members of the Chamber feel that increasing tax rates in the State will not help the government improve its financial condition. Rather, whatis required is a better monitoring and collection system to check leakages in tax collection which take place at various check gates.

Assam Agricultural University Tea Industrial Work Experience Programme: Since 1968 the Tea Husbandry & Technology Department of the Assam Agricultural University (AU) has been imparting education leading to graduate and post-graduate degree in Agriculture with specialization in Tea Husbandary and Technology (in undergraduate) and on single crop i.e. Tea on post-graduate curriculum. Each student taking up the discipline as elective in under-graduate course gets first hand knowledge of commercial tea estate where a student has to undergo practical garden training as a partial requirement for fulfillment of B.Sc.(Agri) degree. Rural Agricultural Work Experience Programme (RAWEP) now finds its place in the B.Sc (Agri) degree programme of the AAD. Moreover, in view of the emergence of small tea cultivation in North East region, the department has decided to revamp the course curriculum of Practical Garden Training. A Memorandum of Understanding (MoU) between Assam Agricultural University and All Assam Small Tea Growers' Association was signed on January 9, 2002 to extend full co-operation in conducting intensive training, henceforth be termed as Tea Industrial Work Experience Programme. The Department has launched the programme and it is expected to take off with its first batch in February 2002.

Tantea's Auction Arrangement Criticised : Tea planters in South India criticized the Tamil Nadu Tea Plantation Corporation's (Tantea) decision to allot its eight factories to only three auctioneers for selling tea. It was alleged that norms were violated and hence investigation was demanded that why the selling arrangement of around 10 million kg of tea was changed when auction through seven brokers earlier had ensured all India sales of the Corporation's tea. The planters said, often seven at least four auctioneers operating in all six auction centers in the country, three each in north and south. This facilitated Tantea to sell its teas through any of the centers.

ITA's Tea Promotional Campaign: The tea industry of the country is under recessionary pressure even today. While production of tea has continued to increase regularly, exports from the country has fallen drastically in the last couple of years. Domestic demand of tea did not increase also. This situation has led to over-supply of tea in the market resulting in sagging prices at all the auction centers in the country. Obviously, to alleviate the suffering of the tea plantation units, the need is to increase demand commensurate with growing production. Although increasing the demand of our tea in the global market is an Herculean task, which, however, is not impossible. In this regard, the tea industry is required to identify the strategic and structural issues, immediate and remote, and then to formulate a comprehensive plan of action. For, the global market is now highly competitive with the presence of other tea exporting countries as Kenya, Sri Lanka, China, Indonesia and Vietnam. Prices of their teas are not only lower to that of ours, they are conscious of quality and the demand pattern of the buyers. Naturally, the expected result from an endeavour to boost exports is unlikely to come immediately. It is a must, therefore, to substantially improve the domestic demand of tea. Indian Tea Association (ITA) has realized it. The Association, besides taking up some other measures, already launched a tea promotional campaign through the TV and other media. The opinion of the viewers reported, 70 per cent of them favoured drinking of tea regularly. They were convinced that it should not only be considered as a temporary stimulant but a beverage that could keep a person energetic and healthy, far way from some deadly diseases. All said and done. It is point to ponder that ITA along with other promotional bodies have failed to facelift the reputation of the Indian Tea damaged by the unscrupulous exporters. They have not succeeded in moulding the importers to start buying the Indian Tea by assuring them that the unethical an irreligious doings of exporters would not occur again.

Tea Board to Launch Web Site: The Tea Board oflndia launched a web site as its strategy to boost the demand of Indian tea in international market. The site provides information relating to production capacity of gardens, market prices, quality of Indian teas and also techniques of preparing good tea. In this regard, however, Mr. Basudeb Banerjee, Chainnan of the Tea Board said, "in any effort to boost demand of tea in the international market there is no alternative but utilizing information technology". In the setting up of the web site the Tea Board took help ofIBM.

Government Considering ISI Mark for Tea: The Ministry of Commerce, Government of India introduced ISI certification for tea. Mr. Sharad Yadav, the then Consumer Affairs Minister, said, for this purpose "the Indian Standard for tea has been revised by the Bureau of Indian Standards (HIS) in consultation with the Ministry which will be published shortly". Ministry officials thought tha~ the move helped improving realization for tea growers and companies as the consumers are provided with high quality certified produce.

ITA's Sales Promotion Campaign for Tea: In order to expand the domestic market of tea, the Indian Tea Association (ITA) has been advertising tea through TV and other publicity media. On the basis of the observation of the Director of American Health Foundation, the advertisement says that tea contains all the nutrients necessary for good health and regular drinking of tea reduces the risk of heart stroke, tumour, some types of cancer and many other diseases. Meanwhile, the impact of the advertisement on the viewers has been studied which indicated 70 per cent of them considers tea not only as a temporary stimulant but a beverage providing vigour and vitality.

Flavoured Tea Market in The Country: Tea majors namely Tata Tea and Hindustan Lever Limited (HLL) have been exploring untapped flavoured tea market in the country. They wanted the Indian Tea Association to persuade the Government for allowing the use of natural identical flavours in black tea. Other leading tea manufacturers also supported this proposal.

Export of Tea Declined : At the 119th Annual General Meeting of the Indian Tea Association (ITA), held in first half of 2001, Mr. Bharat Bajoria, Chairman of the Association, expressed grave concern for the declining trend of exports in the last couple of years. Mr. Bajoria pointed out, the quantum of total export in 2001 was the minimum in the last five years. Russia's curtailment of tea imports from India, ban on Indian tea imports in Iran and Libya, lower prices of tea produced in Kenya, China, Indonesia and Vietnam have pulled down Indian exports, Mr. Bajoria added.

Orthodox Production Necessary in South India : At a seminar on Orthodox tea manufacture organized by the Tea Board and the United Planters' Association of Southern India, Mr. Vikram Kapoor, Executive Director of the Tea Board suggested the tea growers in South India to switch over to Orthodox manufacture from CTC. In his opinion, this could salvage the southern tea growers from the continuing dull situation. The Tea Board had sanctioned RS.5 crore to 45 producers for the switchover to Orthodox tea production. He advised the planters to learn from Sri Lanka where 98 per cent of the produce ·was Orthodox and 68 per cent of the small growers engaged in the production of the same. Mr. Kapur said, the soil and weather in South India were ideally suited for the production of Orthodox tea.

Sanjiwani Rehabilitation Centre Inaugurated: In the third quarter of 2002, the permanent building of Sanjiwani Rehabilitation Centre. for spastic children was inaugurated by Mr. Sanjoy Lohia, Deputy Commissioner, Sonitpur, Assam. Amongst others, the ABITA Chairman, Mr. N N Sharma, ABITA Chairman (Zone 3), Mr. A Singh, ABITA Secretary and officers of ABITA (Zone 3) attended the function. For the construction of the building the Assam Branch, Indian Tea Association (ABITA) the headquarters and the Zonal Office jointly contributed RS.2.5 lakh.

North Bengal University Started Soil Testing Laboratory for Tea Gardens : The Department of Tea Management under the University of North Bengal has started a Soil Testing Laboratory for the benefit of the tea plantation units of North Bengal, Bihar and Sikkim. Estimation of Organic Carbon, pH, Nitrogen, available Potassium and Phosphorous, Electrical conductivity costs only RS.50 per sample. That besides, estimation of Sulphur and soil texture is also undertaken at reasonable cost.

WB Government to Survey Tea Industry: On 23rd October, 2002, Mr. Nirupam Sen, Commerce and Industry Minister, Government of West Bengal, said in Kolkata that the government along with the Tea Board had conducted a survey and prepared a situation report on tea industry in the State. The survey covered and recorded the number of tea gardens, area of the gardens, and so on. The report was submitted in December 31, 2002.

Godrej in Tea Business: Godrej Group recently entered in tea business through a new company, Godrej Tea Limited. This new company was established in September 2002 in which the Group have 65 per cent shares.

Excise Duty on Tea Waste : Excise authorities in South India have been insisting that Excise Duty should be paid on 'tea waste', even if it is destroyed at the garden level. It is understood that there has been similar demand in North India. Since tea waste destroyed at the garden level does not have any commercial value, the United Planters' Association of Southern India (UP ASI) has sought total exemption of Excise Duty on tea waste.

Pesticide Effect on Tea Workers' Health: With chronic ailments on the rise among tea workers and their families, especially children, a BBC team visited in second half of 2003, Kurseong, Darjeeling District, West Bengal, to conduct a survey on the effect of pesticides on the health of workers. The survey reported more severe impact on the second generation. Dr. Sujit Chakraborty, Director of the Centre for Sustainable Living (CSL) said, "most of the cases are found in the slums where tea garden workers live. The graph has become steeper since the mid Eighties. Uncontrolled use of pesticides started in the country in the early Seventies. Pesticides need some time to accumulate in the body, only then we see how it affect. The disorders are carried on to the next generation."

Sick Tea Estates - An Investigation

Generally sickness in tea estates stems initially from mismanagement, and a low non-viable yields, and usually a mis-guided, lazy indisciplined work force. This finally leads to annual losses and ever rising liabilities. Sufficient funds are therefore not available for upkeep and necessary development. Often these estates tend to be attracted to bank schemes in an effort to improve and develop, which is all well and good, if the managerial structure is capable of proper utilization of the loans sanctioned.

Factors Affecting Sickness

However, sickness is usually caused by mis-management over a long term and unless the entire managerial infrastructure is not first corrected, then the utilization of loan funds will prove to be of little value, and indeed the repayment of the principal with interest can lead the sick estates into further financial problems. At the risk of sparking off a controversy, one would caution, any board of directors of a sick estate from taking any loans for improvement unless the entire project has been studied by an expert, who would advise the estate management at every step regularly. The expert would see that sufficient planting materials, and all other aspects would also be available in time to effect proper utilisation of the loan funds to render the programmed scheme effective. For example, it is often the case that the planting schemes programmed under the loan cannot be properly implemented to cover the extension hectarage, or replanting schemes, envisaged under the project. This then leads to areas planted out not being consolidated by infilling of mortalities, thereby rendering new young tea areas full of vacancies. Having worked in the industry for a longer period and gained some experience of the weaker tea sector, it is advised that one may avoid any loans of any kind, until and unless the estate viability creates the possibility for further development in field and factory.

Quite often sick estates have a permanent labour force too large for the small yield per hectare of tea to maintain effectively. This only aggravates the sickness, and coupled with unskilled managerial expertise, really renders the position bleak.

What is the remedy?

The first step is to recruit better experienced experts in the managerial cadre, and believe in general that estates workers can be quite quickly trained in better all round practices. Sick estates usually have most of the following defects:

1. Absence of proper drainage over several years.
2. Existence of vacancies in the sections, along with sporadic lack of shade tree canopy.
3. Poor or inadequate fencing and large scale entry of cattle in the estate.
4. Prevalence of general water logging and local water logging in bush collars.
5. Dearth of proper phased prune cycle.
6. Negligence of medium and other height reduction prunes and necessary knife clean out of knots in the frame.
7. Persistence of general poor standard of pruning followed by poor plucking standard.
8. Insufficient crop protection and weed control spraying.
9. Poor weed control in general.
10. Non balanced managing and poor supervision of the same

Expert Management of the Available Workers

Assuming that most of these factors, do exist, can see no remedy in taking loans to rectify the situation. Rather, again assuming that permanent and casual workers are available, the situation can be vastly corrected in a span of about 6 years, by better expert management of the available workers, based mainly on the prune cycle adopted, and remember that the permanent workers have to be paid in any case. Thus, it is believed that the first thing is to fix a prune cycle either 3 or 4 years cycle, dependent on type of manufacture and availability of pluckers, viz. L.P. - UP-UP OR LP-UP-DS-UP. Normally sick estates neglect to provide proper tools and implements such as pruning knives, hoes etc., so that workers engaged can do a decent job. Height reduction prunes and knot clean out are usually neglected on poor estates. It is wise to check each section for height of the bushes at the last light prune (or cut across prune). Sections at or above 32" (or 82 cm) must be medium pruned or lowered as soon as possible. At the same time all knots in the bush frame should be removed. Therefore, to perform this proper implements are required. Initially during the cold weather the drains can be redug and repaired only over the light pruned sections as a start to reinvigoration of the sections, so that in 3 or 4 years, depending on the prune cycle selected, the entire estate drainage structure can be initially corrected.

Repaired/Deepened Drainage in Old Tea Section and Supervision of Fertilizer Application etc.: It should however be noted that repaired, deepened drainage does not give a quick and miraculous response in old tea sections if drainage has been neglected over a long period. The bushes tend to seek new root level of water availability. Therefore shoot growth is initially affected. The new rooting leads to better shooting only after a year or two. Fertilizers are expensive, and scarce. One can use Urea and Muriate of Potash only at rates selected according to standard. Yields of the sections of the estate becomes more viable. Strict supervision of fertilizer application is essential and where weed control is ot possible, a single dose on damp soil in April is the best bet.

Maintain Well Control Plucking Round: Having covered drainage, pruning and fertilizer application, one must ensure that plucking is well supervised, and if possible maintained on a well controlled plucking round. Although expensive, new planting and infilling can also be carried out with the estates' own labour force available with surpisingly little difficulty in actual practice. The Tea Board has some good schemes for replanting, extension and hire purchase, for irrigation and factory machinery etc. however, one would be inclined to avoid even these facilities until the estate becomes more viable and better organized, and one agrees and knows that one views on this aspect will not be supported my many, however one stick to his guns so to speak !

Tea Section be level Cheeled During Cold Weather: During the cold weather as many sections as possible should be level cheeled with filling of soil in bush collars to check local water logging, and in light pruned section where drains have been attended to, all drain soil must be leveled up. Crop protection can be handled with some economy if pests are controlled on appearance and not sprayed on a prophylactic or palliative basis. Of course a water tanker and some decent hand sprayers are a must and probably the hypothecating bank would probably offer a term loan for this purpose for this smaller capital outlay. This would obviate the usual sick estate from resorting to "more praying than real spraying".!

Having dealt with some of the problems usually faced by sick or semi-sick estates it is summarized as follows:

1. Properly teach and guide the work force.
2. Provide proper implements so that the workers can do a better job.
3. Estate workers do have an Inherent capacity to pick up better practices for the wellbeing of the estate and for themselves eventually, if properly taught and guided.
4. In a fairly short span of time, by utilization of the basic resources available at the estate level, the estate can be made more viable, and can earn a surplus of funds and a degree of availability.

Assam Delegation Met Murasoli Maran: An all-party delegation from Assam met the then Union Commerce Minister, Mr. Murasoli Maran, on April 29, 2002 to communicate its concern over the fall in export of tea and increased competition from smaller countries such as Kenya, reported PTI from New Delhi.

Lower-end Product from Tata Tea : In keeping with the strategy to offer packaged tea across all price points, Tata Tea has entered the fast growing lower-end economy segment with Agni Sholay. "Agni Sholay will be our vehicle to complete in the fast growing low-end category which has traditionally been dominated by regional players. Market size of this category is 80-90 million kg", said Mr P Siganporia, Managing Director of Tata Tea. Initially the product will be available in North and East India.

Duncans in Retail Tea Market: In a significant shift from its earlier policies, the Kolkatabased Duncans Industries Limited (DIL) has entered the retail tea market. On April 5, 2002 the company opened its first outlet for premium quality tea at Lalbazar, Kolkata. Mr. J K Mazumdar, Senior Vice-President, said the company will initially focus on West Bengal, a major tea consuming state. The company, however, intending to set up 30 outlets across the state in the next few months. DIL also plans a "Duncans self-dependence programme" whereby the company would sponsor retail centers by small entrepreneurs under the Duncans umbrella. The company has 13 tea estates, located in the Doors, Terai region and Darjeeling.

Eveready Promoters Raise Stake : The promoters of Eveready Industries India, the tea and battery maker of the Brij Mohan Khaitan Group, have enhanced their holding in the company to 61.1 per cent, an increase of 6.68 per cent in the last one year, from 54.42 per cent as on March 31, 2001. Eveready sources said, part of the increase is through the creeping acquisition route, while part is a reflection of the merger with Bishnauth Tea Company. "The shares acquired through creeping acquisition were bought at market rate", sources said. Bishnauth was merged into Eveready to ensure a better focus on the tea business and also rationalize and streamline the management of the company. The initial plan after the separation with Magors was to bring the tea business under the Eveready fold and then demerge the battery business.

Government Considering FDI in Tea Planatations : The government is planning to make an exception in its "Foreign Direct Investment (FDI) policy for the plantation sector, and allow fresh foreign investment in tea plantation companies. According to an official of the Union Commerce Ministry, "there is an increasing feeling today that if we do not allow foreign investment, the tea plantation companies will find it difficult to grow". This will not apply to other plantation sector, growing rubber and coffee as most of the companies are Indian owned and smaller in size. They could raise money from the domestic market to expand their business, the official added. The Commerce Ministry has recommended that FDI of up to 75 per cent be allowed in tea plantations. However, the final decision on the issue has not been taken over the government yet.

Southern Tea Planters Worried over China CTC Tea: While global tea experts advise the South Indian tea sector to focus on newer areas to establish comfortable market, majority of the tea plantation in the South India are yet to reorient their manufacturing practices to suit the market requirements. The South, in particular, has until recently been exporting a substantial chunk of the produce to Russia. The setting was perfect until other tea producing countries emerged and India lost its place in terms of export to Russia. China has entered the scene and has started to produce CTC grades similar to that of South India. These teas, according to market sources, are available in Russia at 50 cents per kg.

Conclusion

Plantation industry which developed over 150 years has a colonial origin. It is now a valuable asset to the nation. Plantation is that branch of agriculture which, in the broad sense, demands separate study and classification. In other words, the organisation of modern plantation relates more to the factory than to the farm. Generally there is specialisation in one crop which is produced in a large scale for export and for maintenance work. The output is continuous throughout the year. The major plantation crops like tea, coffee, rubber and cardamom have now developed to a large extent. Coffee is probably the oldest plantation in the country. It came to India via Arabia in the early part of 17th Century but the systematic cultivation started in the hills of Karnataka state during the last part of 19th century. Tea was found widely growing in the hills of Assam in 1823 and its large-scale cultivation started around the same time as of coffee in Karnataka. Rubber came late from Brazil and commercial cultivation of this crop was not undertaken till the beginning of the 20th century. Cardamom, the ancient spice of Indian economy developed as plantation crop only about few decades back.

In India, plantation accounts for 0.9% of the total cultivated land. It also contributes 7% of the total national income in agriculture. Besides, provides more employment per rupee of investment in the country than either in agriculture or in industry. Compared to agriculture, tea industry alone employees per acre about 5 times mandays. Thus plantation industry employs large amount of labour force. It accounts highest percentage of human workers compared to any industry. Moreover, this industry helps in development of other industries.

Among the different plantation crops tea is considered to be the most important crop in our country. It is the second biggest foreign exchange earner and is exported to about 90 countries. It also contributes a sizeable amount to national income of the economy. Moreover, it provides direct employment to a large number of people and helps in providing indirect employment in various sectors like road construction, transportation, building of warehouses, manufacture of plywood tea chest, aluminium foil, templates, metal fillings, paper cardboards, fertilisers, insecticis, pesticides, coal, iron, steel, etc. Apart from its contribution to the economy of India, tea today provides the common man a pleasant and stimulating non-alcoholic beverage. Thus, there is need to improve production and productivity. To accelerate the process various developement initiatives were taken.

Chapter 6

Some Aspects of Green Tea

Early experiments on the drying of tea leaf had shown that tea leaf undergoes major changed in physical and chemical characteristics in the absence of proper precaution resulting in differences in taste between the brew prepared from the dried leaf and fresh green leaf. With the variation in the conditions of drying, two kinds of products are finally evolved, namely, the black tea and green tea.

The preparation of green tea is by and large, similar to black tea, a significant departure being the avoidance of milk. Besides the brew of green tea is lighter and consumers patronising green tea in North African countries have a strong preference for sugar and flavour.

The preparation of green tea is by the large, similar to black tea, a significant departure being the avoidance of milk. Besides, the brew of green tea is lighter and consumers patronising green tea in North African countries have a strong preference for sugar and flavour.

There are plenty of literatures dealing with the various aspects of black tea but those on green tea are comparatively few. A brief account on some of the aspects of green tea such as the method of processing, the type of manufacturing, bio-chemical control, grading, etc and also of green are presented in this chapter.

Method of Processing

The plucked young shoots of tea are the raw materials for the manufacture of black tea and green tea. The main difference in the method of processing of tea of the above two types of explained below. In case of green tea every care is taken to retain the green colour and the chemical make-up of the tea leaf. As regards manufacture of black tea, conditions are regulated to encourage the change of the colour of leaf to blackish brown.

The chemical reactions for browning of tea leaf take place with the help of group of biological catalysts called the enzymes present in the tea leaf. These catalysts become completely inoperative by application of heat. By heating the tea leaf to the desired temperature for sufficient time the browning reactions re completely removed and the resultant product obtained at the end of subsequent processing is 'green tea'. In the early days of tea cultivation, the initial heat treatment of the leaf was the basic step in the manufacture of green tea. With the advancement of technology, the method of heat treatment underwent several changes like cooking in open pan, application of dry heat in a closed vessel, dipping in boiling water and exposure of the leaf to free flowing steam. The quality of final product, however, depends on the nature of initial heat treatment and the method of production.

Type of Manufacture

The method of manufacture of green tea can be grouped into two main heads namely the Japanese method and the Chinese method. Irrespective of the method, the raw materials utilised for production of quality green tea are the tender leaves and buds from the tea bushed of the China type. The fresh green appearance of manufactured tea can be preserved only if pure China jat leaf is used. Assam jat leaf always tends to give a brownish product. Production of high quality green tea involved proper care in the plucking of leaf and its transportation to the factory. Prior to manufacture, the green leaf requires careful handling, transportation and storage as bruising and excessive heating of the leaf immediately cause fermentation and encouraged microbial infection.

The various steps of manufacturing under Japanese, Chinese, Soviet, Indian and other methods are shown below:-

1. Japanese Technology

The details of technology adopted by the Japanese in preparation of tea are described as follows:-

(a) Steaming - Steaming machine of various designs are used. One of the popular type is cylindrical drum - 2 meters long and 1 metre in diameter. Fresh leaf is fed through upper end and the steam leaf is discharged from the other end. Slight steam (pressure around 1.5 kg. per sq. m) is injected into the drum at the feed end. The passage of leaf through the steaming drum is regulated in such a way that leaf is in contact with the steam for at least two minutes. This heat treatment inactivates the oxidising enzymes of the leaf, fixes the green colour, eliminates its raw smell and gives the leaf the elasticity required for the subsequent step or rolling. Once the leaf is properly steamed it becomes firm.

(b) Cooling - The Steamed-up leaf should be spread in a thin layer and cooled by a fan. This reduces the surplus moisture acquired from steam.

(c) Rolling/Drying - The equipment includes a rotating wooden box with arrangements for heating by oil or gas burner. A rotating shaft attached with sweeper and forks runs through the centre of the drum. The shaft and the drum rotate in the opposite directions. The leaf kept in the rolling drier for about half an hour to ensure partial drying and partial rolling. The loss in weight reaches about 48 percent.

(d) Rolling - Rolling of the partially dried leaf is undertaken in orthodox rollers. The rolling time is about 5 minutes of which 3 minutes is spent in rolling under light pressure followed by 2 minutes without pressure.

(e) Rotary Drying - The rolled leaf is fed into rotary drier which is a horizontally rotating drum-through which hot air is blown. Once the level of moisture content in the rotary drier can be kept reduced for about half an hour, the material is ready for treatment in a twisting machine. The temperature that prevails in the rotary drier is about 45°C.

(f) Twisting - It provides the product a flattened and polished appearance. The rolled and partially dried material is rubbed against a hot plate which gives the product a flat, smooth and silky texture. The plate is heated either by electricity or charcoal fire and is maintained at a temperature around 90°C.

(g) Final Drying - This is carried out in chain drier at a temperature around 60°. Drying is completed in about 20-25 minutes time and the moisture content is kept around 3-4 percent.

2. Chinese Technology

China adopts the following procedures in the manufacture of the Green Tea:-

(a) Primary Panning - The equipment comprises a cast iron pan, turning forks, steel sheet cover, steel frame with gears and pulleys and a furnace built of bricks. The pan is heated to 280°C by using wood/ coal as fuel. Green leaf is put in and held in the pan for about 10 minutes to destroy the oxidising enzymes. When the weight is reduced to 35 percent due to drying, the leaves are taken out quickly from the pan.

(b) Rolling - Conventional rollers are used. Rolling is done for about 15 minutes.

(c) Rotary Panning - The equipment includes a rotary drum with frame and smoke cover placed on a brick furnace.

The rotary pan is heated to 170°C., rolled leaf is put in and dried to reduce 55 percent weight of green leaf. A second drying which reduces 65 percent weight is done by using twice the quantity of leaf used in the first drying. The dried leaves come out when the pan is rotated in the opposite direction.

(d) Final Panning - The pan is heated to 90°C.. Partially dried material is inserted in the final panning machine to get them fully dried.

3. Soviet Technology

With the passage of time, some modifications have taken place in the manufacture of green tea. In the erst-while Union of Soviet Socialist Republic the following steps were being adopted.

(a) Steaming - This was done in steaming machine by injecting steam under pressure. Steaming of leaf is effected in 2 minutes.

(b) Slight (preliminary) Drying - The process is akin to mechanical withering of leaf as in black tea manufacture and is undertaken in drying machine at 110oC., for 12 to 15 minutes. The product retains a residual moisture of around 60 percent.

(c) Re-rolling and Sorting of Rolled Leaf - Open type rollers are used. Double rolling each of 40 minutes duration with 50 revolutions of roller per minute is applied with slight or no application or pressure, special type of ball breakers are used for sorting of rolled leaf.

(d) Firing (Drying) - The rolled leaf immediately requires double firing at the same temperature as similar to drying of black tea.

(e) Sorting - This is done in the conventional type of sorting machines (cylindrical and flat) with all precautions in order to minimise the production of broken tea.

4. Indian Practice

In India, green tea is manufactured through rolling and drying operations in stages by using orthodox rollers and conventional tea driers. The roller receives wet leaf and the first roll is usually for 10 minutes with rolling table moving about 30 r.p.m.. Any juice that is excreted during the first 10 minutes of rolling is discharged. At the end of 10 minutes' period a light pressure is applied and the juice is retained for use later in the manufacturing processes. At the end of the second period of 10 minutes, the pressure is raised and the roller allowed to continue for further 5 minutes with pressure. The extent and the duration of rolling have to be carefully controlled to achieve larger leaf grades. After the first roll, the leaf is ready for first the carried out in a conventional drier using an inlet temperature of 80°C., and an exhaust temperature of about 48°C..

The semi-dried leaf is then spread on the floor to a depth of about 2.5 cm. and allowed to cool for about 15 minutes. The product after the first fire is gummy and flaccid. It should normally be olive green in colour. The second roll is for about 30 minutes without pressure and this gives the leaf an attractive twist. After the second roll the leaf goes for the final drying in a conventional drier. An inlet temperature of 100°C. and exhaust temperature of about 50°C. are used. Drying time is usually 18 minutes after which the leaf is spread out to cool and is not sorted for 24 hours.

5. Other Technology

The basic step in the manufacture of green tea is the heat treatment of the freshly plucked leaf to activate the enzyme system responsible for fermentation which results in browning of the leaf. In case of non-availability of steaming drum the activation of enzyme may be done by putting the leaf in boiling water. A popular method is wire baskets which fit into a drum or a tank containing water. The water in the tank is then brought to boiling point by employing a suitable method of heating. The wire basket filled with freshly plucked tea leaves is then immersed in boiling water and held there for two minutes. After removal from the boiling tank the surplus moisture in the leaf can be removed in a centrifuge. Centrifugation also helps in cooling of the leaf and makes it ready for rolling.

Biochemical Control - Soviet Approach

In the green tea factories of formerly Soviet Russia a routine laboratory test is made in order to ensure that heat treatment of the leaf has been sufficient to inactivate the enzymes. After steaming two or three shoots are taken and pounded in a porcelain mortar. Then 0.2gm. of the paste and 3ml. of water are put into a test tube into which 2-3 ml. of a 1 percent alcoholic solution of quatreoil and 2-3 ml. of a 1 percent alcoholic solution of quatrefoil and 2-3 ml. of a 1 percent hydrogen peroxide are poured. If the enzymes are inactivated the pounded leaves will have a green shade. The colour of the leaves with partially inactivated enzymes is light brown and leaves with active enzymes acquire a dark brown. On the basis of the shade or colour obtained it is possible to judge the degree of steaming of the leaf and the residual activity of the enzymes.

The Chinese Polishing and Dyeing

Sorting and grading of green tea are done in a conventional manner. The Chinese type of green tea is generally soft after polishing and colouring. The polishing is done in a revolving polishing drum of hexagonal cross section of about 120 cm. in diametre and 120 cm. in length, lined inside with zinc sheets. The rate of revolution of the drum is kept below 20 rpm to minimise breakage of leaf in the drum. The polishing in the drum can be carried out with or without the addition of polishing agents like french chalk or gypsum. Colouring is usually done with indigo.

Grades

There are various grades of green tea and these vary from country to country. The main grades of Chinese green tea and their characteristics are described below :-

a) Special Chum Mee : Small, twisted leaf; excellent liquor

b) Chum Mee : Leaf larger than (a); average to poor liquor

c) Special Hyson : Big, uneven, rolled leaf, good liquor

d) Hyson : Uneven rolled leaf, larger than (e) good to average liquor

e) Young Hyson : Small, even twisted leaf, excellent to good liquor

f) Special gun powder : Very fine leaf, perfectly rolled, excellent lilquor

g) Gurn powder : Well rolled leaf, good liquor

h) Sow Mee extract : Fine leaf, very good liquor

i) Sow Mee : Uneven leaf, average liquor

j) Fannings : Open leaf, poor liquor

Japanese Grade

In Japan, green tea is classified into following five kinds :-

(a) Gyokuro or 'Pearl Dew' is the finest tea in Japan. It is made of the leaves grown under shade which (i) reduces the tannin content, (ii) increases caffeine and amino acids, (iii) brightens the colour of the leaf and (iv) sweetens its flavours.

(b) Matcha or Ceremonial Tea : It is made of leaves from shaded bushes. Manufacturing process is similar to that of Gyokuro but without rolling. After drying the product is pulverised.

(c) Sencha : Made of young tender leaves and is well twisted. It is the popular grade for domestic consumption.

(d) Kamairicha : Made in Kyushu district. The raw material is same as in Sencha, but the first process is parching in place of steaming. It has a curly appearance.

(e) Banch : A coarse tea, made of coarser leaves, or by separating from raw sencha in the refining process.

Indonesian Grade

In Indonesia green tea is sorted into four basic grades which are as follows :-

(a) Peku - This is the main leaf grade and accounts for 60 to 70 percent of total leaf grades. Has good colour and appearance.

(b) Djikeng - This is the second leaf grade and is about 20 percent of the total.

(c) Tulang - Mainly stalk and about 5 percent of total production.

(d) Bubuk - Dust and fine particles accounting for 5 percent of total production.

A fair portion of Indonesian green tea is reprocessed into scented tea using various types of flowers such as jasmin and red gambir. The process involves watering of graded green tea followed by slow drying of the mixture over charcoal fire which helps the transfer of scent from the flowers to the tea. After heating for about 2 hours the mass is cooled and the flowers are picked out manually. The process can be repeated with second and a third lot of flowers for obtaining highly scented teas.

Production of Green Tea

The word 'tea' is always regarded as being synonymous with black tea or fermented tea. The green leaf plucked form the China jat tea bush is manufactured in another way to produce green tea or unfermented tea. The major producers of green tea are China, Japan, India and USSR. The main consumers are Morocco, Algeria, Afghanistan, Japan, U.S.A. and Canada. India is a traditional producer of green tea. The bulk of the green tea produced in India come from some parts of West Bengal, Assam, Himachal Pradesh, Uttar Pradesh etc. Similarly, sizeable quantity of green tea is also produced mainly in Nilgiris of South India. Production of green tea in India is shown in the Table 6.1.

Data presented in the Table 6.2 above revealed the fact that share of West Bengal to All India reached maximum at 71 percent in 1971 while it was minimum at 42.19 percent in 1990. Assam's percent (in 1961) which enhanced to 21.14 percent in 2005. Tripura's share to total was 4.91 percent in 1961 and 1.22 percent in 2005. Tripura did not produce green tea from 1971 to 1986. Uttar Pradesh accounted for about 12 percent of total production while it was about 17 percent in case of Himachal Pradesh in 1961. Except 1961, the share of North India declined and the share of South India increased. In Assam, the districts of Darrang, Goalpara, Dibrugarh and Sibsagar produce green tea. A small quantity of green tea is produced in Karimpur, Lakhimpur and Cachar also. In West Bengal, Terai and Dooars are the main producers of green tea while small quantities are also manufactured in Darjeeling. In South India Nilgiris produces green tea. It's share increased and the years.

World Production

No reliable data are available on world production of green tea. Attempt has, however been made to arrive at an estimated figure. It is a fact that nearly the entire quantity of Japan's present annual production (in 2005) is about 107 million kgs. of tea is of the green variety. In 2005. Taiwan produced about 40 million kgs. of green tea. The main green tea producing area is mainland China. She produced about 712 million kgs. of tea of which accounts for 50 percent of green tea. Thus, China produced nearly 353 million kgs. of green tea. In USSR annual production of green tea is about 18 million kgs. The total world trade of green tea at present is estimated 530 million kgs. The details are given in Table 2.3.

It may be observed from the table above that China accounted for about 67 percent of world production of green tea, while Japan accounted for about 20 percent. Taiwan, USSR and India jointly produced about 11 percent of the total world production of green tea.

It was revealed from the data that India produced 5.56 million kgs. of green tea in 1961. This was, however, increased to 9.84 million kgs. in 1992. It again d 5.31 million kgs. On an average. India has been producing 7 million kgs. of green tea annually.

Share of green tea

Region-wise. North India, on an average produced about 78 percent of total green tea in 1992 as compared to 22 percent by South India. Among the other States of India. West Bengal is the major producer followed by Assam and Himachal Pradesh. In case of South India. Nilgiris is the only tea producing district. The state-wise share of green tea is exhibited in the table given below:

The total world trade in green tea was restricted to 530 million kgs. in 2005 compared to the volume of trade in black tea of 3294 million kgs. in 2005. That is green tea accounts for about 17 percent of total black tea. Amongst the tea producing countries Japan imports some quantities of green tea mainly from Taiwan and partly from Mainland China while her exports are mainly to U.S.A. and other countries like Canada, U.K., Germany, Libiya etc.. More than 50 percent of total production of green tea in India is consumed internally. Afganistan has

Table 6.1 Production of Green Tea in India during 1961 to 2005.

(quantity in thousand kgs.)

District	1961	1971	1973	1977	1981	1983	1985	1986	1987	1988	1989	1990	1991	1992	1995	2000	2001	2002	2003	2004	2005
1	2	3	4	5	6	7	8	9	10	11	12	13	14	15	16	17	18	19	20	21	22
Darrang	314	528	548	373	666	688	768	828	364	331	480	318	301	320	270	249	217	212	205	201	205
Goalpara	–	–	841	457	238	133	219	230	260	292	215	172	265	310	244	170	153	148	139	133	140
Kamrup	176	–	146	–	–	10	–	–	–	–	60	18	22	24	18	8	–	–	–	–	–
Dibrugarh		70		338	274	325	336	343	340	371	329	197	229	231	357	395	203	215	220	219	215
Sibsagar (b)	43	62	108	99	259	78	189	228	322	593	295	163	–	–	498	490	372	382	387	387	390
Cachar	–	–	–	–	–	–	–	–	655	619	512	370	505	457	135	190	188	169	174	163	172
Total	533	660	1643	1267	1437	1234	1519	1629	1941	2206	1891	1238	1322	1342	1552	1402	1133	1110	1141	1103	1122
Darjeeling	69	–	–	–	–	37	–	–	–	–	591	329	409	419	37	–	–	–	–	–	–
Terai (b)	984	1117	1159	1150	1870	1331	1635	1937	2485	3043	1674	1245	2411	2401	2901	1458	1132	1162	1043	972	1245
Dooars (c)	2089	4110	5476	2294	2899	2081	2638	2626	2136	3075	2490	1905	2052	2042	1899	1932	1552	1012	1188	898	1050
Total W. Bengal	3139	5227	6634	3444	4769	3449	4237	4563	4621	6118	4727	3479	4872	4862	4837	3390	2684	2174	2231	1870	2295
Tripura	273	103	66	–	–	–	–	–	589	346	481	256	230	240	89	72	71	46	70	60	65
Bihar	51	40	22	–	–	–	–	–	–	–	–	–	–	–	–	–	–	–	–	–	–
Uttar Pradesh	632	420	333	24	262	208	208	208	208	208	208	484	471	482	250	105	95	79	201	189	192
Himachal Pradesh	934	274	763	610	567	334	295	261	301	301	104	463	722	742	682	670	560	265	278	267	290
Total North India	5562	6684	9461	5345	7035	5225	6295	6661	7660	9179	7412	5920	7617	7688	7411	5639	4527	3762	3833	3489	3964
Nilgiris	–	683	626	182	560	1926	2171	1362	2685	4257	2467	2243	2158	2169	466	577	938	958	947	1328	1350
Total Tamil Nadu	–	683	626	182	560	1926	2171	1362	2685	4257	2467	2243	2158	2169	466	577	938	958	947	1328	1350
TOTAL ALL INDIA	5562	7347	10087	5527	7595	7151	8466	8026	10345	13436	9879	8163	9775	98837	7877	6216	5465	4720	4780	4817	5314

Sources : Various Issues of Tea Statistics Tea Plantation Industry in India- Structural changes between 185 and 1992 by Dr. G.D. Banerjee

Note : (a) Including Mikir Hills of North Cachhar, (b) West Dinajpur and (c) Coochbehar

Table 6.2 Share of Green Tae in India during 1961 to 2005

(Percentage)

State	1961	1971	1977	1981	1985	1986	1987	1988	1989	1990	1991	1992	1995	2000	2001	2002	2003	2004	2005
1	2	3	4	5	6	7	8	9	10	11	12	13	14	15	16	17	18	19	20
Assam	9.58	8.98	22.92	18.92	17.94	20.28	18.76	20.89	19.15	15.16	13.52	13.62	29.15	22.51	26.73	33.52	33.50	20.03	20.14
West Bengal	56.43	71.14	62.32	62.79	50.47	56.85	44.68	46.97	47.86	42.19	49.84	49.42	51.86	54.53	49.16	46.05	46.05	43.07	43.17
Tripura	4.91	1.39	–	–	–	–	5.69	6.16	4.86	3.36	2.35	2.44	1.12	1.15	1.31	0.97	0.96	1.25	1.22
Bihar	0.92	0.54	–	–	–	–	–	–	–	–	–	–	–	–	–	–	–	–	–
Uttar Pradesh	11.36	5.72	0.44	3.44	2.47	2.59	2.01	2.12	2.10	5.93	4.27	4.89	3.17	1.68	1.92	1.67	1.75	3.92	3.61
Himachal Pradesh	16.79	3.73	11.04	7.47	3.78	3.25	2.90	3.09	1.05	5.67	7.34	7.54	8.18	10.84	10.24	9.49		5.54	5.46
North India	00.00	91.50	96.52	92.63	74.36	82.97	74.04	79.23	75.02	72.31	77.32	77.91	94.08	89.66	87.44	96.70	89.85	72.44	74.60
Nilgiris	–	8.50	3.48	7.37	25.64	17.03	25.96	20.77	24.98	27.69	77.32	77.91	5.92	10.34	12.56	9.30		27.56	25.40
South India	–	8.50	3.48	7.37	25.64	17.03	25.96	20.77	24.98	27.69	77.32	77.91	5.92	10.34	12.56	9.30		27.56	25.40
All India	100.00	100.00	100.00	100.00	100.00	100.00	100.00	100.00	100.00	100.00	100.00	100.00	100.00	100.00	100.00	100.00	100.00	100.00	100.00

Source : (i) Various Issues of Tea Statistics & (ii) Tea Plantation Industry in India- Structural changes between 185 and 1992 by Dr. G.D. Banerjee

Table 6.3 World Production of green Tea during 1988 to 2005

(Quantity in million Kg)

	1988		1989		1995		2000		2005	
Name of the Country	Quantity	Percentage to total	Quantity	Percentage to total	Quantity	Percentage to total	Qty	Percentage to total	Qty	Percentage to total
China	273	68.08	300	69.90	336	69.77	340	68.89	350	68.76
Japan	90	22.44	92	21.26	95	21.16	100	21.05	105	21.13
Taiwan	16	3.99	18	4.15	26	4.19	28	4.35	35	4.94
U.S.S.R.	12	2.99	13	3.00	15	3.02	15	3.43	20	2.92
India	10	2.49	10	2.30	12	1.86	13	2.28	15	2.25
Total	401	100.00	433	100.00	484	100.00	437	100.00	445	100.00

Source - Internation Tea Committee. Annual Bulletin of Statistics.

	1995		2000		2001		2002		2003		2004		2005	
	Quantity	P.C. to total	Quantity	P.C. to total	Quantity	P.C. to total	Quantity	P.C. to total	Quantity	P.C. to total	Quantity	P.C. to total	Quantity	P.C. to total
China	336	70.14	340	68.54	340	68.14	335	66.37	342	66.40	350	67.41	353	66.60
Japan	95	19.82	100	20.16	102	20.45	100	19.80	102	19.80	103	19.12	107	2018
Taiwan	22	4.60	28	5.65	29	5.82	35	69.30	38	7.38	38	7.42	40	7.57
U.S.S.R.	18	3.76	15	3.03	15	3.02	20	3.96	19	3.70	17	3.32	18	3.40
India	8	1.68	13	2.62	13	2.57	15	2.97	14	2.72	14	2.73	12	3.40
Total	479	100.00	496	100.00	499	100.00	505	100.00	515	100.00	522	100.00	530	100.00

all along been the largest market for India's green tea and until 1982-83 it was practically the only market.

Exports from India

India has now been exporting green tea to other countries, the main amongst which are Morocco, Pakistan, U.S.A. etc.. Data relating to quantity of green tea exported from India to various countries during 1960-61 to 2004-05 are furnished below :-

Others include Australia, Italy, Kuwait, Muscat, Nepal, Singapore, Saudi Arabia, Netherlands, Syria, Qatar, A.R.E., Saudan, U.A.E., U.K., Germany, Ireland, USSR.

One of the most interesting fact is that Pakistan, USA and Japan are

Table 6.4 Export of green tea form India during 1960-61 to 2004-05

Year Countries (quantity in th.Kgs.)

	Afghanistan	Japan	Morocco	Pakistan	USA	Others	Total
1	2	3	4	5	6	7	8
1960-61	1,823	–	–	15	–	2	1840
1970-71	3,187	20	1,760	–	28	1	4996
1976-77	3,029	–	–	8	118	2	3157
1982-83	1,811	2	666	–	30	201	2710
1983-84	744	–	524	203	15	192	3468
1984-85	73	1	730	227	21	61	1113
1985-86	159	–	927	490	2	51	1629
1986-87	805	0	417	559	33	47	1861
1987-88	1,395	0	1748	537	12	478	4710
1988-89	1,226	5	1168	1099	17	1020	4535
1989-90	616	0	2089	870	20	102	3697
1990-91	416	4	1937	186	44	682	3269
1991-92	353	3	1,798	220	29	1813	4216
1992-93	358	4	1,813	240	32	1,952	4,399
1995-96	170	4	590	180	35	471	1450
2000-01	172	3	560	181	34	450	1400
2002-03	165	4	550	179	33	445	1335
2003-04	160	4	545	179	33	444	1365
2004-05	162	5	555	180	34	464	1400
2005-06	165	5	575	187	35	484	1451

Source : (i) Various Issues of Tea Statistics & (ii) Tea Plantation Industry in India- Structural changes between 185 and 1992 by Dr. G.D. Banerjee

Note : 'O' (zero) and '–' 'dash' indicate below 500 kgs. and nil respectively.

the consumers of Indian green tea. Besides, other countries particularly USSR, U.K., Sudan, Canada, Netherlands have also come in contact with green tea market of India. On an average, India exports 60 thousand kgs. of green tea annually to these countries.

Consumer's Preference

Like black tea, the consumers' preference for green tea also differs in different countries. There is general belief that in dry leaf the green tea should have a bright olive green colour with no trace of brown or red. The Japanese green tea, preferred in Japan and USA, provides lemon yellow or greenish yellow liquor without any tinge of brown which is liked by consumers in China and North African countries.

Consumers in many countries want their green tea in the natural or 'unfaced' form while others like a faced product which is polished and coloured. The Food Laws of many countries, however, prohibit the sale of green tea coloured and polished with artificial dyeing and polishing agents.

Afghanistan prefer green tea liquor of Chinese type rather than Japanese type. Unlike the Moroccan consumers, the Afghans are not, however, fastidious about dry leaf appearance.

Green tea of various kinds to suit the requirements of three main groups of importers like Japan; USA; Morocco; North African countries and Afghanistan, are being produced in India.

Nutritional and Medicinal Values

Fresh tea leaf contains Vitamin C. The significant Vitamin 'C' is however, reduced during the manufacture of black tea. The loss is considerably less for green tea. The comparative figures for Vitamin C content of green and black tea are reproduced below :-

Type of tea	Vitamin C (mg./gm.)
Japanese Black Tea	Nil
Japanese Green Tea	0.02 to 6.33

Indian Black Tea	0.002 to 0.03
Indian Green Tea	0.07

Like black tea, green tea is also rich is some of the Vitamin contents of Group 'B' particularly thiamin and riboflavin.

The polyphenols (so called tanin) existing is fresh tea leaf posses Vitamin B activity which is property which helps in reduction of capillary fragility of the blood vessels. Comparative studies have shown that tannin preparation of green tea is much more active than that of black tea in strengthening the walls of capillaries. This highest B Vitamin activity of green tea is attributed to its manufacture of black tea there is a considerable loss of polyphenols present in the fresh tea leaf.

Besides the tannin, green tea has other important biological and medicinal values, such as its ability to stabilise Vitamin C in the body and the ability to normalise the hyper-function of the thyroid glands. A strong infusion of green tea also possesses significant antibacterial activity. This was first demonstrated in 1951 in the large scale use of green tea infusion in combating plague in Japan. Subsequent clinical trials carried out in Russia demonstrated that a strong infusion of green tea is useful in the treatment of bacillary dysentery. These biological and antibacterial qualities have contributed to the popularity for green tea among the consumers.

Chapter 7
Sustainable Tea Plantation Management

Efforts have been made in this chapter to define sustainable plantation and its management, explore scope for intervention in such management, maintain natural resources and improve property on sustainable basis, identify natural factors and their contribution in tea production and suggest indicators of sustainable plantation management. In the process, field management with particular focus on land preparation, transplantation and cultural practices, pruning young in-fills, manuring, pest and diseases, soil-water-nutrient management, organic matter management, soil conservation, human resource management, crisis management, environmental hygiene and sanitation, management of cost of production, productivity of land and labour management, ecology management, faith and dependence management, employer-employee relation, training, safety of workers, monitoring and control of processing variable in tea manufacture etc., have been discussed threadbare.

Tea as a drink in India

Indeed, no record is available as to when tea as a drink was first consumed in India, So far it is known that as early as in 1662, tea as a drink found place at a social function. And as tea harvesting was not in vogue in those years, it may be very safely assumed that for the function, tea obviously came from abroad. In fact, tea cultivation in India was first started by Warren Hastings, them Governor General of India. He took initiative in planting and production of tea in 1774, though it is not something very noteworthy. It was Sir Joseph Banks, a renowned botanist and one of the directors of the East India Company, who took keen interest in this matter. To observe the conditions of growth and development, he planted tea buses at the

Botanical Garden at Howrah. Credit also goes to him for bringing to the knowledge of the then government that soil and climatic conditions at the foothills of Himalayas perfectly suited tea harvesting. In 1823, Major Robert Bruce went to Assam and found to his surprise the existence of tea bush there. He collected and brought a few samples to the plains, which encouraged the British Government to initiate tea harvesting in Assam. Lord Bentinck was administering the country at that time. He constituted a "Tea Committee" in 1834 to look after the production of tea in India. Raja Radhakanta Dev and Ramkamal Sen were taken as two Indian members of this committee. It seems that their inclusion as members was motivated by two factors–hope of receiving business support from them, on the one of hand, and of getting wide recognition from Indians as a regular drink, on the other. Since then tea cultivation on commercial basis was started in Assam and was continued there since then. The first Indian who cultivated tea is the last king of Assam, Dewan Maniaram Dutta Barua. He cultivated tea in his own garden and sent it to Robert Bruce as a token of his compliments. For the first time in India, export of tea took place in 1838, simultaneously with harvesting of tea commercially. And to manage this affair effectively from business point of view, on February 12, 1839, a tea company was set up with the name "The Assam Company" the first such company in the world. Prince Dwarakanath Thakur and Motilal Seal were the two directors of the company. Thus, tea entered the market to occupy a place in the list of daily beverage items of the households. And during the last years of nineteenth century only tea consumption became popular among the people (see table of Appendix).

Sustainable Plantation

Over the years the plantation industry has been facing the problem of environmental deterioration. Such deterioration has been drawing increasing attention of the media. The issues of pollution, fast depleting soil and forest cover did not succeed in transmitting the right message to the industry until 1992. The question, therefore, necessarily arises as to why the industry is concerned about environmental disorder. If the pace of environmental disorders continues the industry will dig its own grave through a process of ruining its sustenance base. Hence, the significance of the goal of sustainable development for industry in the 21st century is important. The World Commission on *Environment and Development* of 1987 defines sustainable development as "*development that meets the needs of the present without comprising the ability of the future generations to meet their needs*". The operational essence of sustainable development summarized by the well-known environmental scientist *Dr Barbier is involvement of simultaneous maximization of biological system goals* (genetic diversity, biological productivity) economic system goals (satisfaction of basic needs, increasing production of useful goods and services) and *social system goals* (cultural diversity, institutional sustainability, social justice participation). It indicates that equal focus on three factors will enable natural and biological resources to be utilized operationally and for an enterprise to continue or sustain its activities for the benefits of future generations. *Plantation enterprises take into account both natural and human resources. Human resources play a valuable role both as managers and workers. The tea industry is unique as it combines the task of natural resources based production with industrial activities like processing of the produce cultivated and harvested viz green tea. The framework of plantation management outlines the principal issues in relation to the manager.*

Sustainable Plantation Management (SPM) — an Approach

Sustainable plantation management, a new approach, has gained momentum in plantation industry especially in tea. In wider perspective, sustainable plantation management (SPM) means an *integration of different factors of plantation activities to meet the present needs of production, productivity, quality and profits without compromising on the ability of future generation of plantation managers in meeting these needs.* In other words, sustainable plantation–management ensures that the *goals of production* "productivity", "quality", and "*profits*" are *achieved in perpetuity.* Contrary to the general notion, human resource are an integral part of the plantation eco-system and require to be managed on a sustainable basis along with land, natural biomass, cultivated biomass, water sources and capital equipment. In practical terms, "sustainable plantation management" would not just view natural, *human and other biological resources from the point of view of their contribution to production, quality and productivity on a sustained basis*. It see whether these factors of management are by themselves sustaining. Sustainable plantation management is summed up in the Table 7.1. The enlarged scope of management intervention entailed by sustainable plantation management is summed up in Table 7.2. Viewed in the context of the tea industry, the sustainable development framework requires plantation enterprise, which necessarily consider production and productivity as long-term objectives. Further, it takes into account economic performance of the enterprise with reference to the type, make and quality of the assets they leave with their succeeding generation. Consequently, sustainable plantation management removes the dichotomy between short-term and long–term objectives by progressively adjusting short-term measures in a manner that does not harm sustainability of the enterprise in the long term.

Table 7.1: Sustainable Plantation Management

Traditional management focus	Sustainable plantation management focus
Land, human resources, capital	Land, biological resources, created resources
Maximise production and productivity	Maximise biological, economic and social output
Indicators of progress are output/factors of production	Indicators of sustainable development include: Input to output ratio for individual factors, output per unit of factor or productivity per unit of factor
Health of tea bush and factory output determines enterprise health	Optimise in perpetuity, the health of all factors of production and resultant productivity levels

Source: Damodaran, A (1988), Working paper No. 9803, IIPM, Bangalore

Sustainable Natural Resources and Property Improvements

The history of tea plantation industry testifies the fact that clearings were made in jungles and forests for carrying out planting of tea,

Table 7.2: Sustainable Plantation Management-Scope for Intervention

- Tea planted area-field management
- Tea Bush management
- Labour relations management
- Intra-corporate relation
- Non-planted areas or natural area management
- Energy management (Estate/factory)
- Environmental hygiene and sanitation
- Management of health delivery services
- Waste management
- Management of interface ecology
- Natural risk management and factory safety
- Management of training to field and factory staff/officers
- Management of infrastructural support
- Education management of staff children
- Management of tea production with minimum residual level of pesticides
- Management of living standard of the people of tea estates

Source: Same as Table 7.1 and personal field visit of the author in Assam

coffee, rubber and spices crops. This was done keeping in view *the ecology of plantation crop. The ecological attributes assess the properties on which plantation crop is cultivated on a sustainable basis*. Plantations are generally undertaken in habitats not suitable for crop production. Crop damages arising out of natural factors such as wind, hails or pests and diseases have been a pervasive problem. To get over such problems, planters resort to application of pesticides and chemicals to prevent or reduce the incidence of pests of diseases. With growing green movements and consumer health awareness in India and abroad, the issue before tea industry is no *longer one of optimising production but also of ensuring that crops which are produced are "safe" from the health point of view of the consumers*. The raw material for manufacturing made tea should be free *from physical impurities, microbial contamination and pesticide residues*. In case of Indian tea exported to Germany and other European Community countries, these elements have been under scored.

Environmental Consciousness in Europe and the USA

Field trial data relating to *pesticide residue collected and analyzed in Indian Institute of Management (IIPM), Bangalore and in Tea Research Association, Tocklai, Assam revealed the fact that minimum residual limit (MRL) levels of pesticides in India tea could be set up at far higher levels than what the European Community (EC) prescribes*. The attitudes of the EC member-countries towards the pesticide residue are not likely to be liberal in the coming years. The growing environmental consciousness in Europe and the USA poses a more fundamental problem. Importing countries in Europe and the USA are under pressure from *green lobbies to view beverages such as tea and coffee not only from the safety angle, but also in terms of their environmental impact in the producing countries*. Tea cultivation practices, which cause "pesticide" related water pollution in watersheds, may not be considered to be environmentally-friendly. A tea estate factory, which has been dumping tea wastes in nearby streams and destroying nearby forests for timber and fuel wood may produce excellent "made tea" from an "organoleptic" perspective. However, this would still be considered as unsustainable plantation management practice. Indeed, on the basis of proposed life-cycle assessment standards under the ISO 4000 series, environmental audit of estates exporting tea could well be insisted upon by importing countries. Consequently, sustainable plantation management practices are a sine qua non for running successful plantation enterprises in the 21st century in India.

Parameters of Sustainable Plantation Management

It is not possible to categorise plantation managers into those following "*sustainable*" and those following "*unsustainable*" *management practices*. This is because there are many elements or parameters for judging "sustainability". One manager may score high in respect of some elements while scoring less with regard to certain other elements. To understand the relative strength and weaknesses of management practices from the point of view of sustainability, *one may list the following operational parameters relating to tea estate operations with corresponding indicators of sustainability.*

1) Natural vegetation type in clearing area.
2) Planting density of tea/ha, density of non-tea plants/ha.
3) Percentage of undisturbed natural area in the garden.
4) Types of natural areas in garden: – jungles, ponds/lakes lands.
5) Percentage of shade tree/ha – Permanent and temporary
6) Soil works undertaken – Mechanical and natural
7) Wind breaks – Reliance on artificial wind-breaks involving exotic species – Reliance on natural vegetation
8) Mulching and organic manuring – Area covered
   - Mature tea fields
   - Non mature tea fields
   - Frequency of mulching/application of organic manure
   - Ratio of organic to in-organic fertilizer use/ha
9) Frequency of shade tree pruning per annum
10) Shade tree falling cycle/rotation (No. of years)
11) Use of shade tree lops/tops – Firewood (%)
    - Disposed outside or used in tea factory (%)
    - Other forms of disposal
12) Frequency of pesticide application (No. of rounds/year)
    - Stem disease
    - Leaf related diseases
13) Crop diversity in garden – Area under other agricultural crops cultivated
    - Names and details of other crops
14) Yield/ha of green tea
15) Cost of cultivation/ha of green tea

The underlying purpose of these indicators or parameters is to gauge the degree of natural resource conservation and use of ecologically sound estate operations by plantation manager. The above parameters can be utilized not only as diagnostic tools but also to serve as indicator points for adopting corrective actions. It would be also useful to compare economic implications of adopting ecologically sound practices. If uneconomic results emerge from a "cleaner" and "ecologically" sound estate operations, the solution is not to abandon the concert of sustainable plantation management but to strive towards sustainable management "practices" which are economically feasible.

Sustainable Plantation Field Management

Modern management means rigorous analysis of input, output and cost. It demands meticulous planning and systematic execution. Yield of a section declines, if there are vacancies. Our prime object should, therefore, be to *consolidate such areas by in–filling with healthy and robust plants*. We must be able to pluck a hectare of plucking surface in a hectare of land. Side by side, with increase in yield the cost of weed control becomes less and pluckers' productivity increases. The following points must be given due consideration prior to infilling.

- The old bushes must remain free from root diseases, termites, and parias.
- Sections due for uprooting within next 10 years should not be in-filled.
- Drainage conditions must be improved.
- Sections having more than 25 per cent vacancies should not be in-filled in plain areas.
- It is essential to trace out the reason of mortalities of old bushes to check future deterioration.

Land Preparation

In pruned year of the section due for in-filling, all the dead and moribund bushes should be uprooted, drains should be thoroughly repaired and the soil levelled. Saucer or depression should be top-dressed with drain soil, and if the drain soil is in-sufficient then porous soil may be brought from the adjacent virgin land for filling the depressions. Light hoeing can be done to break the hard pan in case the soil surface is hard. After completion of the said operation in cold weather, green crop should be sown in alternate rows of the in-fills, as soon as the rain wets the soil.

Planting of Guatemala, lemon grass or Napier in the vacant patches will add organic matter and rehabilitate the soil, besides checking weed growth. But planting of these cover crops are done in the last pruning cycle, not in the year of medium prune and infilling.

Periodically, the cover crops must be lopped and trimmed and the leaves mulched. Land preparation should be completed in the pruned area and obviously in cold weather.

Transplanting and Cultural Practices

Infilling the section should commence in *May, June, or even early,* if there is sufficient moisture in soil, or if there is irrigation facility. *Planting pits should have a depth of 18 inches and the bottom should be further loosened to a depth of about 6 inches.* While infilling, care is taken so that the bheti remains intact without any damage. Breaking of bheti usually occurs due to transportation and rough handling. Proper ramming ensures firm establishment of plants in the soil. Any depression around the collar, if left, will cause waterlogging in rain and the young plants will die. *Tall plants above 18 inches of height with girth of about pencil thickness is ideal for infilling.* The plant is manured with 30 gms Reck phosphate, 30 gms Superphosphate, 200 gms Celrich and 2.5 gms Thiemet. If cattle manure is available then 2 to 3 kgs are applied per pit. Single vacancy is infilled by planting three plants, one in the middle and two on both sides of it, i.e. 2x vacancy+1. Also inter-planting by putting a new plant in between the row can be done in case of wider spacing of old bushes. To establish good stand of shade trees, for example, Odorattissima, Lenticularis, Lebek is necessary. The sections must be kept free from weeds by collar weeding and spraying Glyphsate periodically. Mulching the section with ideal mulching material as water hyacinth, ageratums, will add organic manure suppress weed and also retain moisture in dry season.

Clones like TV3, 22, 25 and 19 can be used as in fills. The sides of the old bushes are periodically lopped to allow free access to sunlight and air to the in fills.

Pruning Young in Fills

0 YEAR

Medium-prune the old bushes at 20-22 inches and tip 10-12 inches above prune mark. Transplant young in fills in March/April when soil moisture is sufficient, or it can be delayed to April/May in droughty condition. In January/February, when there is sufficient starch reserve in the root, centre out the plants at 6-9 inches and head back the laterals at 14 inches. Tip at 24 inches from the ground level.

1st YEAR

Medium–prune bushes are kept untouched and tipped at the same level. Selective re-centring is done in young infills, and tipped at 24 inches.

2nd YEAR

Young in fills are pruned at 16 inches and tipped at 26 inches from the ground level. Old bushes are light medium skiffed at 8 inches above prune mark and tipped over one leaf.

3rd YEAR

Young in fills and old bushes are kept untouched and plucked to the janam.

4th YEAR

Final frame forming prune is done in young in fills at 18 inches from the ground level and tipped at 26 inches. Old bushes are light pruned above 1.5 inches of prune mark and tipped at 8 inches above prune mark.

Manuring

Manure the in fills with Y.T.D. mixture at the ratio of 2:1:2 or 2:1:3 in ring method. In 0 year 30 g ms/plant in two splits, in 1st year 80 gms/plant in four splits, in 2nd year 100 gms/plant in four splits, in 3rd year 120 gms/plant in four applications. From 4th year onwards broadcast the manure as in old bushes in three splits.

Pest and Disease

Young in fills are susceptible to pest attacks as it shares the room with the old bushes. Hence much care has to be taken against Red spider, Helopeltis, Loppers, Trip, Green flies, Termites, Stem borers etc. Spraying with systemic contact insecticides as per requirement is essential. Disease like Blister blight, Red rust, Black rot, Porias may damage the young plants, hence spraying of copper fungicide is equally important.

New Technological Development

Technological developments are taking place at a breathtaking pace. Today's knowledge gets obsolete tomorrow. Advent of new technologies, new clones, seed stocks, chemicals etc. has improved the old practices. Long-term planning should aim at anticipating broadly the effects of action at the outset of every productive programme. Moreover, aftercare, followup actions, vigilant and expert supervision with strong administration will take care of the prospect of in fills.

Soil, Water and Nutrient Management

Tea, being a perennial crop, survives for more than 50 years economically, Hence all our efforts to improve yield would go in vain if the soil conditions are not improved. Tea is a Mesophyllic plant which can neither stand waterlogging conditions nor drought. In waterlogging condition, hydrogen sulphide accumulates, which is toxic to the plants. If water remains for more than 72 hours in the root zone, then the roots of the plant tend to turn in a horizontal direction, and sometimes even upwards, in search of oxygen. The roots are severely damaged under waterlogging conditions. Water table below the root zone must be 45 cm to 60 cm in young teas and 90 cm in case of mature tea root. In drought condition, transpiration and evaporation takes off all the available moisture from the soil and the plants start wilting and shedding leaves and finally die. In fact, both the conditions are detrimental to plant growth and are directly related to soil moisture content.

Changes in Carbohydrand Nitrogen Metabolism

Water stress condition produces important changes in carbohydrate and nitrogen metabolism of plants. Water stress at the stage of fuel break causes more injury to plant than at any other time. Young teas are also simultaneously affected. It is observed that NPK content of the plant is higher under moisture stress conditions. But potassium, calcium, magnesium content is decreased under moisture stress. Potash content is relatively low, as the rate of entry of K decreases to a great extent. Under such conditions, foliar application of potash is considered helpful. During cold weather, moisture stress condition is observed for five months and during that period for young tea 300 mm and for mature tea 500 mm irrigation per season of five months is required. Total water loss through evaporation comes to 0.60 mm over a period of five months. The average rate of evaporation is 3 mm to 6 mm.

Tea Plants Must Have a Healthy Root System

Tea plants must have a healthy root system, because without increasing the volume of roots, smooth growth cannot be expected. So, to ensure a healthy root growth, soil must be fertile, porous, well aerated and in good tilth, so that the roots may penetrate and extend deep in the soil for easy absorption of minerals and water. Soil water content should be in between field capacity and permanent wilting point. Soil having grittiness and some cohesion, is sandy loamy soil. This type of soils have 70-90 per cent sand and 15-30 per cent silt and clay. It is a light textured soil having pores, and in this pores chemical and biological process occur. Capillarity, infiltration and air movement is easy in sandy loam type of soil. Roots of the tea plant require fresh and continuous supply of oxygen for better root respiration. Soil aerobic microbes take oxygen and give off carbon dioxide. There is an inverse relation between soil and water. Excessive water reduces air movement in soil. Lack of sufficient air prevents oxidation of nitrogen and sulphur into forms that plant can readily utilize while high carbon dioxide content increases the solubility of phosphorus and sulphur. Physical and chemical nature of soil plays an important role in productivity, and is brought about by soil microbial activity.

Soils Have Many Living Components

Soils have many living components as algae, plant roots a small invertebrate and micro–organism. The micro–organism help in mineralization. Microbial activities in soil require a high temperature. Activities of soil micro–organism are much faster, in 105° C and get restricted at temperatures below 10°C. Besides, soil role as a reservoir important element for plant growth. Soils must be given periodically inorganic and organic manures to replenish the soil nutrient removed by harvest, mulching and erosions. It takes more than 50 years to build up the top six inches of fertile soil. This top soils is composed a decayed vegetation, animal residues and is known as humus. Waste vegetable matter and animal residue decomposition is accelerated by micro-organism present in the soil. In waterlogged condition of soils, decomposition is slow and nitrogen remains locked up in carbohydrate; acidity is more in this type of situations. Hence, soil maintenance and proper drainage results in breaking down of the complex organic matter and releasing soluble nitrate which is readily absorbed by the roots of the plant. Organic matter is as important to plant, as milk is to human beings. Organic matter also serves as food to the micro-organisms present in the soil and increases their activity. To maintain the fertility of soil, organic carbon should be 1 per cent in soil. If it is below 0.60 per cent then the soil is unsuitable for tea cultivation.

Soil pH A Power of Active Hydrogen Lone

The next important aspect is soil pH. It is the power of active hydrogen ione is soil. Ions are electrically charged particles formed by the loss or gain of electrons. The pH is the measure of soil acidity. If the plants do not grow well, the necessity of checking soil pH is essential as it indicates the position of soil chemical. In North East India, the soil pH for successful tea growth should be 4.5 to 5.5. Below 4 indicates high acidity, above 6 indicates low acidity and above 7 indicates alkalinity. When pH is 4 it means there are 1000 molecules of hydrogen ions (H^+) per liter of solution. A change of 1 unit of pH equals to ten-fold change in hydrogen lons (H^+) concentration. The acidity and alkalinity of soil is determined by its content of Hydrogen lons (H^+) and hydroxyl ions (OH) ions, the soil is said to acidic. The

H^+ ions and OH ions come from the breakdown or ionization of water molecules when there is more (H^+) ions than (OH) ions i.e., H_20=H+OH. Soil can be grouped in three parts as acid, base, calcareous. In calcareous soil, calcium carb onate reacts with soil to release hydroxyl ions. Availability of nutrient is related to soil pH. Under extremely low pH nitrogen availability increases while availability of K, Ca, Mg, S decreases with decrease in pH. Hence, before applying any nutrient to the soil, pH of soil must be checked.

Building up Soil Nutrient Status Requirement of Sound Culture Practices

To build up soil nutrient status, rather to make it a more wind blown soil, sound cultural practice is required. Periodical soil tests, soil rehabilitation measures, sound conservation policies, application of inorganic manure with right doses and right mixtures pay well at the end. If the soil has phosphate more than 40 PPM, K_20 more than 80 PPM, sulphur 30 PPM, organic matter more than 1 per cent with pH of 4.5 to 5.5, then the soil is considered to be nutritionally in good condition. Yearly application of NPU in soil is essential to compensate the loss of nutrient every year by harvesting of crop, leaching of soil etc. Calculation of application can be based, as follows (for mature tea): 1kg N_2 per 12 kg made tea, 1 kg phosphate per 50 kg made tea, 1 kg potassium per 10 kg made tea. Taking into account volatilization losses, leaching losses, (±) should be done as 60 per cent of the nutrient is lost and only 40 per cent is absorbed by the bush. By split application, nutrient absorption percentage increases.

Manuring of Young Tea on Age and Ground Coverage

Young tea manuring must be based on age and ground coverage. It can be based as follows: 1st year 30 kg N_2/ha, 2nd year 60 kg N_2/ha, 3rd year 80 kg N_2/ha, 4th year 100 kg N_2/ha and 5th year 120 kg N2/ha, it can be increased or decreased seeing the growth and coverage. Manure must have ratio as 2:1:3 N.P.U or 2:1:2. Application of Dolomite is equally important in party area, because here the pH is low. Due to leaching of Ca, Mg in waterlogged conditions, decomposition of organic matter is slow and the nitrogen remains locked up. After draining, decomposition of O, N is faster and nitrogen is used up in the process. Now a days sulphur application is of marked importance due to the limitation in the use of S.D.A. and S.S.P. However, application of sulphur improves drainage

Organic Matter Management

Organic matters are composed of decayed vegetation and animal residue. It is a reservoir of nitrogen and also contains phosphorus and sulphur. It increases water holding, exchange capacity of soil. Improvement of organic matter content in soil can be brought about by applying cattle manure @ 3-5 T/ha/yr or Neem cake @ 2-3 T/ha yr. Mulching with good mulching materials as, water hyacinth, Ageratums, Mimosa, etc. and planting of cover crops, as Napier, Guatemala, Mimosa, Lemongrass, retaining pruning litters an establishing good shade adds humus in soil. Two tonne/ha of organic matter is obtained by retaining pruning litter, 2-5 tonne/ha of organic matter is obtained from shade tree droppings, 5 tonne/ha from Lemongrash, 18 tonne from Guatemala, and 14 tonne/ha from Mimosa.

Soil Conservation

Loss of soil due to erosion, leaching etc. is high in hilly tea areas. A sound policy must be adopted to preserve the valuable top-soil, which is as follows: Minimum tillage practice, contours on slopes, strip weed control, infilling of vacancies. If not possible immediately, then to plant cover crops on the vacant patches, proper land levelling, establishing shade tree, reducing herbicidal load on soil, planting of shade trees on the base of the hillocks, will act a retaining wall. Having plenty of permanent/temporary shade trees along with sufficient green crops and cover crops in the tea gardens helps in protecting soil erosion and also supplying organic matters to the tea bushes.

Human Resource Management

Social and Personal Aspects of Tea Estate Executives–A Case Study

Introduction

Dibrugarh is one of the tea growing regions in Assam. It is surrounded by Naga hills on the south, Burma on east, China and Tibet on north and north Lakhimpur and Arunachal Pradesh on the west. As on June 1, 2005, there were about 390 tea estates in Dibrugarh covering an area of 69,030 hectares with an average annual production of 145 million kg. Average yield of Dibrugarh worked out to 2107 kg per hectare, average size of the estate being 177 hectares. Majority of tea bushes had already crossed the economic life (over 50 years). Based on data relating to area under different age group of bushes, 32 per cent of area contained bushes over fifty years. Average daily number of labour employed in Dibrugarh was estimated at 187,815 of which 90 per cent were field workers and remaining 10 per cent factory workers. Taking into account both field and factory average number of labour employed per hectare was 2.73 and productivity of labour (production per labour) 773 kg. Besides, tea industry in Dibrugarh gives indirect employment to a large number of people by way of ancillary and support services like fertilizer, tea bags, pesticides, roads, coal, electricity etc. Most interestingly, this industry engages more women than any organised industry due to nature of plucking job, which requires tenderness. Tea executives (managers) are the charge agents of the estates. They are solely responsible for overall growth and development of the estates and operating managerial functions in such a way as to achieve the goals of the estates. Their functios are numerous, complex and diverse. Maximum (field and factory) attention on utilization of energy (both human and non-human) and allocation of time (i.e. management of attention and time as well as utilization of energy) are generally considered the three 'S' for fulfillment of estate goals. Only reasonable, conscientious and intellectually sensitive persons can fulfil the vision, achieve mission and earn rewards from managerial career in the estates.

Methodology

Since the managers play an important role in managing the affairs of tea estates, a need was felt to know about the managers. Accordingly, a survey was conducted in tea estates of Dibrugarh for assessing personal, social and educational background of tea garden managers. The findings of such study may help in taking policy decisions while recruiting the executives. As many as 50 managers out of 390 gardens of Dibruagarh forming 13 per cent were selected on random basis through a pre-designed questionnaires which were canvassed during the field visits in the later part of 2005.

Personal and Family Back Ground

The owners and management of tea estates have firm conviction that leadership qualities are inherited. Garden managers are often recruited through personal contacts taking into consideration their family background, educational qualifications social status and economic conditions of families. However, over the years, a significant change has taken place in the recruitment of tea estates. The details are brought out in the following tables:-

Table 7.3: State of Origin of Managers

State of origin	No. of managers	Percentage
Assam	11	22
West Bengal	14	28
Uttaranchal	9	18
Rajasthan	7	14
Gujarat	8	16
Punjab	1	3
Total	**50**	**100**

Source: Field data

Table 7.4: Mother Tongue of Managers

State of origin	No. of manager	Percentage
Assamese	3	6
Bengali	20	41
Hindi	19	38
Gujarati	7	13
Punjabi	1	1
Total	**100**	**100.0**

Source: Field date

Nationality

All respondents of the study were Indian nationals. Only a few of them were U.K. citizens and directors of the companies owning tea gardens. None of the tea garden manager was non-Indian.

State of Origin and Mother Tongue

India is a vast country with diversified people having varied mother tongues and states of origin. It was, therefore, thought to establish if there was any regional predominance among managers in Dibrugarh. The managers were asked to name their states of origin and mother tongue. Data presented in Tables 7.3 and 7.4 exhibit the fact that managers having origin in Assam state and mother tongue as Assamese constituted 22 per cent and 6 per cent of total respondents respectively. Statewise classification showed that Bengalis accounted for the largest single group among managers. Mother tongue of the majority of the respondents was Bengali followed by Hindi. This is due to the fact that head office of these gardens are located either in Kolkata or Catchar valley. Bengali people dominated in Assam region.

Sex and Marital Status

Sex wise categorisation brought out the fact that all managers were male. It is believed by the top management that managing of the gardens is exclusively a man's job. All respondents were married.

Age

Age is a very important factor for managers. It helps in providing significant contribution to managerial qualities like dedication, devotion, diligence, determination, commitment, satisfaction, leadership style etc. Table 7.5 reveals that majority of the respondents were middle aged i.e. 41-50 years. The average age of tea garden manager was 46.5 years against all India average age of 40 years as per study conducted by Sagar C Jain in 1963. Young persons were not found suitable for the post of manager as all managers had to gather experience in the capacity of assistant managers for considerable years. Normally assistant managers are elevated to the post of tea garden managers.

Table 7.5: Age of Managers

Age-group (in years)	No. of Managers	Percentage to Total
31-35	6	12
36-40	8	16
41-45	21	42
46-50	12	24
51-55	2	4
56-60	1	2
Total	**50**	**100**

Source: Field data

India is a land of different religions. Caste, creed, community etc. are very important factors in the public life. Trade and commerce are also not free from this. Thus, it was considered necessary to examine the religion of managers. None of the selected managers was Muslim. One manager was Sikh, two were Christains and five Jains. Rest were Hindus, all of them belonging to higher caste. The details are shown below:

Table 7.6: Religion of Managers

Religion	No. of Managers	Percentage to Total
Hindu	42	84
Muslim	-	-
Christian	2	4
Jain	5	10
Sikh	1	2
Total	**50**	**100**

Source: Field data

Academic and Professional Qualifications of Manager

Education is of vital importance to human life. It is observed that high level of formal education is necessary to get entry into managerial position. Business now-a-days not only requires common sense but also specialised knowledge and technical skill. Thus managers of tea gardens in Dibrugarh were enquired about their academic and professional qualification. The findings regarding their educational qualifications are given below :-

Table 7.7: Academic Qualifications of Managers

Academic Qualification	No. of Managers	Percentage
School leaving	6	12
Graduate	33	66
Post-graduate	11	22
Total	**50**	**100**

Source: Field data

Table 7.8: Professional Qualifications of Managers

Professional Qualification	No. of Managers	Percentage
MBA, LLM Diploma in management	-	-
Trained in Tocklai	21	42
LLB	4	8
No formal professional qualification	25	50
Total	50	100

Source: Field data

Following observations are made based on data presented in Table 7.7 and 7.8:

- College is necessary to become a tea garden manager. About 89 per cent were graduate and above. Eleven of fifty respondents were holding post-graduate degree.
- Regarding professional qualification, it was noted that law and training course conducted at Tocklai experimental station were popular among the managers. About 42 per cent of total managers selected for case study were trained at Tocklai. This training offered the managers technical knowledge required in his job. Mostof the garden authorities had made training at Tocklai compulsory for their manager.
- None of the manager was MBA/LLM/diploma holder in management. About 50 per cent of them have no formal professional qualification. It is interesting to note that when all universities have been conducting courses on management, tea garden manager possessed formal qualification in management sciences. People concerned with tea industry and trade were of the opinion that practical experience was more useful than formal degree or qualification to serve as manager.

Social Status

Social recognition is an essential human need. In India, the question of one's prestige is more important than any other aspect of one's life. The social status of a manager, therefore, has the utmost impact on his managerial performance. As social status is difficult to measure by any scientific tool, it was decided to ask the manager about his feeling on the social status of his family and to verify the occupation of the father of the manager. Findings regarding the social status of managers are exhibited in the Tables 7.9 and 7.10.

The social status of a tea garden manager was considered excellent and good, according to the opinion of 12 per cent and 62 per cent respectively. About 6 per cent and 16 per cent of the total respondents shed light that their social status is 'not good' and 'bad'. Similarly, 14 per cent of total respondents that indicated are in different of the

Table 7.9: Social Status of Managers

Social status	No. of Managers	Percentage
Excellent	6	12
Good	31	62
Not so good	3	06
Bad	3	16
Indifferent	7	14
Total	**50**	**100**

Source : Field data

Table 7.10: Occupation of Father of Managers

Occupation of father	No. of Managers	Percentage
Businessman	28	56
Govt. servant	8	16
Army officers	3	06
Trade union leader	1	02
Tea company executive	10	20
Total	**50**	**100**

Source : Field data

social status. Most interetingly 28 managers (50 per cent) belong to business community while 8 managers further was government servents. About 10 managers have from Tea company executive and 3 are the sons of the Army Officers. The society appreciates a managerial position in a tea garden.

Conclusion

Data relating to social and personal background of tea garden managers of Dibrugarh (Assam) lead to the following conclusion:

- All managers were Indians and they were male

- Maximum number of managers (14 out of 50) hailed from West Bengal. Managers whose mother tongue formed the largest single group followed by Hindi speaking people.
- All of them were married. None was divorced or widower.
- Most of the managers were middle aged. Twently-one out 50 respondents were in the age group of 41-45 years.
- Most of the managers were Hindu (42 out to 50). No manager was Muslim. Three were Jains. One was Christian while one was a Sikh. None of the Hindu managers belonged to lower caste.
- Formal education is essential for managers. Eight-eight per cent of them were graduates while 11 out of 50 were post-graduate. No manager possessed formal qualification in management science. Four of them were law graduates, and 20 were trained at Tockali experimental station.
- Social status of the manager was good. Twelve and sixty-two per cent of them considered their social status as excellent and good, respectively.

Before closing, however, it may be mentioned that since the seventies of this century, industries in general have leaned too heavily on professional qualification of managers and professionalisation of management. The traditional pattern of selecting managers or the prospective executives according to their the family background has been given good-bye. In fact, there has occurred a sea change in the selection pattern of executive trainees/executives and in the compensation package. As such, it is felt that there is a need of making another study of the tea garden managers, keeping in view the spectrum of changes that have invaded the industries in general. This study conveyed a clear picture covering some important social and personal aspects of the tea garden managers engaged in Dibrugarh, Assam.

Crisis Management

The collapse of the Soviet Union that resulted in disappearance of the adjunct Eastern Bloc awakened the Indian tea industry and trade to new global realities. The recent years saw a new resurgence and aggressiveness with tea exports fanning out purposefully to high value hard currency areas. There has been a significant shift in the direction of Indian tea exports. Our exports so far were mostly in bulk form; now it has taken a direction towards value added form. The trade has, in a sense, experienced its own "perestroika". As a frame to this theme of resurgence, 1993 was *declared by the Government of India as the Year of India Tea, which aimed at consolidating and spreading the message of India tea across the globe. The tea industry too flagged off this year* with a tea convention, which attracted importers from all over the world and brought them in contact with Indian industry and trade. *The tea convention offered keen insights into the consumption patterns and preferences in the markets to which one caters. It focussed on the quality and price that were required for competitiveness in different markets.* The lesson learnt during the three-day convention would contribute to the formulation of appropriate strategies for our exports in the coming years. It is very encouraging to note that some tea companies have adopted fresh approaches by way of joint ventures and strategic alliances to take advantage of lucrative opportunities that lie in the international trading arena.

In tune with the process of liberalisation, the Tea (Regulation of Export Licensing) Order has been repealed. With the establishment of trade relations, new opportunities with countries like Israel, South Africa etc., were opened up. The internal market has become encouraging for the producers. Improved prices have been providing the much needed cash for ploughing back. There has been a change in the trend of consumption pattern. While growth in packet tea has been 6.5 per cent that of loose tea was 2.5 per cent. The withdrawal of excise duty on packets has in a big way contributed to this healthy trend.

Environment Management

Some of the importing countries, regarding minimum residual levels (MRL) of pesticides, have made the industry take up a campaign at grass-root level, to *teach and train the workers and management regarding use of certain pesticides. Sophisticated laboratories with state-of-the art-equipment were set up at Tocklai, UPASI and*

Palampur, each costing over half a crore of rupees, to check the residual levels. MRL has assumed particular relevance towards safeguarding tea exports to high value markets like EUC, Germany and Japan. Research also oriented itself towards discovering how tea drinking was *contributory element towards human health*. In this context, the Tea Research Association convened an international symposium in 1993, which examined the status of tea as a health beverage.

Productivity of Land and Labour

Today, the cost of tea is high; tea productivity per worker is about the lowest - tea workers produce only 730 kg per man-year! Land productivity per hectare is low. On an average, yield in North India that produces 73 per cent of the Indian tea and almost 100 per cent of the quality tea, is only 1610 kgs per hectare. Kenya produces over 2000 kg per hectare. Kenya produces tea at about Rs 30 per kg. In India, production cost of tea is nearer to Rs 50 per kg. So if Kenya retails tea @ Rs 50 per kg and India tea retails at Rs 80 to Rs 100 per kg, what explanation would one gives to the consumer, or what stand would one take before our Government against import of tea, say Kenya tea? After having accepted globalization in principle, which implies acceptance of products and services of good quality at relatively cheap prices, one will not be in a position and should not ask for protection.

Economic Axiom-Earnings of Workers to be Linked with Productivity

In the ultimate analysis, if one has to give a level field to ones' global competitor and still want to stay in business, one will have *to be an efficient producer*. The productivity of the worker and the *productivity of the land must improve substantially*. Talking about the productivity of the worker, quite often, one holds a view that with every new wage agreement, one must ask for increase in productivity. It is an economic axiom that earnings of workers should be productivity-linked but it is not an axiom that wage has to be linked with producitvity. Wage depends on other factors, the most basic of which is cost of living. Industry has no control over cost of living. One cannot de-link wages from the cost of living. One can, of course, use the argument of industry's capacity to pay. It is the duty of industry to pay fair wages to its workers while the duty of management of the industry is to see that human-productivity is improved to the extent that one *remains not only the producer of the best tea, but the producer of the most cost effective tea.*

Reappaisal of Protection Techniques with Cost Structure

To make the Indian worker more productive than his counterpart in other countries, one must consider productivity as a subject apart from wage agreement. This is an HRD function, which the industry needs for its own survival. The Indian tea industry must reappraise its production techniques, with particular reference to the cost structure. Labour cost constitutes nearly 90 per cent of the total cost; the aspect of worker productivity will have to emerge as a major component of a *visionary alliance between management and the worker*. On must not view productivity as a counter to *higher wage demand. One must consider productivity outside the forum of wage negotiations*. This is the only way by which one can lay the basis of a constructive exercise based on pragmatism and mutual trust and understanding. Deliberations on productivity will have to assume a broader canvas involving time and motion study of existing work practices in field and factory. *Value engineering studies will have to be made for re-designing equipment and implements*. But doing our homework worker productivity is not enough. After all, it is the manual worker who has to be productive. For this, training is required, but it is not enough. The worker must understand and appreciate why he on designing to be more productive. For this, motivating the worker is a prerequisite. In the past, the industry had higher wages paid. This has not led to established itself in a position where, the worker earned exactly the same amount as before but by working less hours!

Improvement of Worker Productivity, Land Productivity and Yield per Hectare

Together with worker-productivity, land-productivity and yield per hectare have to improve. In North-East India tea industry produces around 1600 kgs per hectare. Kenya produces 25 per cent more at

2000 kg. In India, we started planting tea nearly 150 years ago. Most of the tea land is exhausted, Seventy-five per cent of India's tea bushes are old and she has not much new land. Uprooted land does not have the same productivity as virgin land. Besides, uprooting and re-planing is an expensive exercise. If one has to keep one's plan target, so as not to starve either one's export or domestic market, one must go for extensive replanting and rejuvenation. Under ecology management, a certain universally accepted ratio of forest-land to other lands must be maintained. One cannot comment on these ratios, which have been evolved through years of research, experience and deliberations by experts who know their job. There are, however, huge areas of so-called forest, as they appear in government records but are areas that do not have any standing trees. Although the Governments is aware of this, it cannot part with these so-called forests, for maintaining the academic ratio. Rates of daily wages of tea plantation on labours for North and South India were given in Annexures 1-3.

Industry's Plea

Tea areas, because of the shade trees in West Bengal and the North East, can be classed as forests. In Kerala, they are converting potato and other land to tea and the findings of experts are that tea areas perform the same positive function as forest land so far as ecology and land erosion are concerned. Industry's plea is simple–tea *areas with shade are almost as good as forest and certainly much better than the degraded forests. As such degraded forests can be given to the industry for growing tea not only in the national interest but also in the ecological interest. And it is in this matter that the industry formed partnership with the Government to extend its wings and give effective support to the industry by allotting land–a big portion of which can be degraded forests. Pragmatism is called for, not legalism or bureaucratism*. Since these forests, on paper, cannot claim any standing trees, why not plant these areas with tea and shade tress! *Just classify shaded tea areas as forests and the ratio laid down for forest-land will be effectively maintained.* Just amend the definition of forest! Talking about the Government as an active partner, the first partnership contribution the industry seeks from the *Government is maintenance of law and order and rationalization of taxation*. The industry and Government have gone into a genuine partnership where it is in the interest of both parties to see that the industry keeps on growing and *generates increasingly more wealth, so that the Government can partake of it and get bigger amounts in coming years*. As a good partner, it is industry's duty to see *that both the Centre and the state earn increasingly more revenue from the tea industry*. The Government should achieve this by taking a smaller percentage of a big and growing cake, rather than a big percentage of a stagnating and slowly diminishing smaller cake. Hence, the necessity for a continuous growth of production through increased productivity of both land and labour and increased production with more land coming under tea.

Rationalisation of Taxes, Allotment of more Land and Maintenance of Law and Order

While the industry understands that the Government has certain basic fiscal needs that has to be and is willing to do its best, the Government also has to appreciate that if the industry is to prosper, taxes have to be more rationalized, more lands have to be allotted and law and order has to be maintained. However, with all the help and understanding from the Government, the industry will not be able to hold on its own in the new climate of free market economy and globalization, unless its productivity improves, most of which will have to come from the workers through industry's efforts. Demanding productivity from workers as a quid pro quo for increase in wages does not work. It is industry's responsibility to see that workers are trained and motivated to use this training in the overall interests of the workers, industry, state and the nation.

Involvement of Growing Relationship of Complete Faith and Dependence

"India is today the world's largest producer, consumer and exporter of tea, the only agricultural crop for which it holds this distinction." The industry also provides the statutory obligations under labour rules like housing, medical facilities etc., as also non-statutory items like provident fund, maternity benefit, gratuity–all these constitute a part of their wage bill. Against this backdrop one must think about the manpower involvement in tea. With the passage of time and more particularly now our thoughts should be more rational and pragmatic in approach. It is often seen that approaching a problem as a 'Leader' sometimes leads to disastrons results. It is therefore, imperative for one person solving the problem to reflect how he would have reacted to the consequences had the problems conceived. In other words, one should adopt a friendly approach for solving human related problems while dealing with welfare related issues. One must bear in mind the environmental and personal problems of the person, the community and the social pattern. Unless there is an involvement in growing relation of complete faith and dependence on the person, community and population as a whole., the success of leadership can never be achieved, be it social, educational, health, etc. This aspect of psychology is very vital, it eventually affects the potentialities of the property and affects the cost-benefit ratio. Progress takes place through science and technology on one hand, and social responsibility and the organisation, on the other. Unless this is understood, successful management skils cannot be imbibed. One may ask, what is managerial skill? The management skills can be broadly divided into the following areas:

a) Specialisation skill.
b) Systems and technical skills.
c) Human relation skills, and
d) Analysis, problem, decision-making and managerial skill

Decision Making and Human Relation

While the specialisation skills and technical skills are understood, the importance of decision-making and human relation needs a little elaboration. While running an estate, one is fully aware about the ultimate object of maintaing the estate viable even as the management is confronted with multifarious problems of the present days backdrops when the workers are apprehensive. On this, the management has to take a spot decision, if not responsibility, for the efficient management together with profitability. The legitimate rights of the workers as allowed by the law should be the last weapon to be utilized by then while the intelligent management should foresee an act in advance. The political climate in India has been changing very fast. The panters cannot remain in isolation. They are paid for to discharge their duties bearing in mind the highest production, lower cost, justice to the worker and none the less satisfying all other agencies. We should be quick to learn all these aspects while there is still time.

Employer and Employee Relationship

It is a fact that without active co-operation of the employees no industrial establishment can run smoothly and efficiently. One cannot afford to ignore employees in the present circumstances. During pre-Independence days, labour force was exploited to maximum extent for the benefit of the employers. But the era of exploitation ended with the emergence of independence. In the post-Independence era the Government has brought many legislations to protect the interests of the workers. If the laborers/employees feel that they are being deprived of benefits/concessions granted by various legislation and different industry-wise agreements, the situation might become explosive. It is the duty of the management to meet their obligation towards their employees. Once charter of demands/grievances are received from the employees, management should ensure to settle the genuine grievances by arranging meetings. In case of certain demands, which are not possible to meets immediately due to adverse situation of the managements the workers should be made to appreciate and realise the difficulty and allow sufficient time to the managements. All these issues should be sorted out across the table and the employees should not feel that the attitude of the management is apathetic towards them. Management on it's own also may arrange periodical meetings with the employees to discuss and decide the matters of mutual interest. Section 3 of the Industrial Disputes Act 1947 provides for formation of the "works committee" in the Industrial establishments. The purpose of forming works committee is to promote measures for securing and preserving amity and good relation between the employers and workmen. But it is a matter of regret that the workers' committees are not yet formed in our industry, perhaps, because of the negative attitude of the unions. However, it is learnt that the labour department of the West Bengal Government has advised for formation of the works committee.

Workers' Partenership In Industry

It is also necessary to persuade the workers to take keen interest in the progress of the enterprise in which they are engaged. They must be made to feel that the concern belongs as much to them as to the shareholders. Way back in 1920, Mahatma Gandhi propounded the idea of "*workers partnership in industry*" on the ground that the workers contributed labour while the shareholders contributed money. Both should have equal stake in the progress and prosperity of an industrial concern. In the peculiar condition in which our country is striving for rapid economic development, success will not be possible without securing the fullest possible cooperation of the workers. It is, however, added here that workers on their part should have a sense of responsibility and discharge their duty diligently and honestly to make the units in which they are engaged more and more meaningful. They should never adopt coercive and other illegal means for realisation of even their just demands and settle them only through prescribed means. This will help in maintaining industrial relations which is so vital for a labour intensive industry like tea.

Productivity of Tea Labour

The work in a tea garden is performed at the field and factory. The field work is related to cultivation and the factory work to production and dispatch for sale. No work-study has ever been *carried out in the case of the tea industry. The work schedule in the field and factory now being followed was perhaps introduced several decades back.* From the existing details, it seems that those schedules are neither scientifically based nor are they based on practical theories. They were formed and prescribed arbitrarily and are still in vogue, creating practical problems and difficulties to present day planters. Take the case of the task schedule of workers in the Dooars in respect of plucking and cold weather work etc. The trouble some days usually originate in the task of plucking by males and females. Details of labours wage settlement in Kerala, Karnataka and Tamil Nadu are given in Annexure 4.

Plucking Task Realistic and Rational

The plucking tasks, which have been fixed long back, are gradually becoming outdated. With scientific developments in the upkeep of tea bushes during the last two decades, the yield per bush has been increased considerably along with yield of green leaf per hectare. This naturally made it easier for the pluckers to collect more leaves in a round, resulting in much higher earnings and greater incentives for the pluckers. Any attempt to revise the task on the higher side has always been resented *by the trade unions. In the Dooars, there are many gardens where the task of plucking continues to be as low as* 15 kgs per day/worker (females 2 kg less) while the average worker plucks not less than 40/45 kgs in these gardens, during high season. This means that a worker plucks 15 kgs for his wage and the balance 25/30 kgs on extra leaf picked. It has unreasonably increased the production cost, which could have been reduced by raising the plucking task to a more rational and realistic level. This is not based on scientific principles and the matter, whenever raised in tripartite forums, was shelved by the government. Similar is the case with cold weather tasks like chilling, hoeing, pruning etc.

Lesser Task for Females

In all cases, the task for females was less than that of males, as the female wages were also less by a few paise than those of the males. With the enforcement of Equal Remuneration Act in 1976, the wages of female workers have been raised to the level of males but the lesser task remains. The unions strongly resisted the management's attempt to equalize the tasks of males and females in view of the equalization of wages. Since a large part of the workforce in tea garden comprise females, the management has been burdened with this extra loss. At the present moment, the tea industry is in the grip of a grave crisis. Amidst increasing costs of production every year the sale prices are reaching such a stage that it is doubtful whether any producer will be able to cover the cost of production this year. The question, therefore, arises whether our workforce has any positive role to play to save the industry from this crisis.

Role of Workforce

It is well known that labour productivity in the tea industry has continued to decline under the increasing pressure of labour agitations. The demand for higher wages was gained a new inpetus. There might be a need to raise the *living standard of workers, but higher wages cannot precede more efficient production*. In case of tea especially, the benefits of workers can only be sustained by increase in labour productivity in all departments. It is understood that *increasing productivity implies efficient utilization of available human, material and financial resources*. Regarding the human resources the industry feels that mental attitude to improve upon one's performance would entail maximum returns from the existing resources. What industry finds from available figures is very disheartening. In spite of management's efforts towards application of improved and scientific methods of tea farming during the last decade, labour productivity has remained stagnant, resulting in higher labour cost per unit. Neither the management nor the workers have ever given a thought to this problem and nothing positive has been done to develop consciousness among the workers about their duties and responsibilities in this regard. The gains of productivity depend on the increases in the levels of production and rises in prices of the industry's product relative to the general price level. If the price of the product falls or does not rise adequately or relative to the general price level, even a substantial increase in productivity of the industry will be unable to yield sufficient resources. This is the case with the tea industry today. Hence, neither productivity nor the price of tea is increasing adequately relative to the general price level. In both counts, it is facing a downward trent. Guidelines on wage issued by labour Liasion Commitee in Kerala, Karnataka and Tamil Nadu - (a) Employees Provident Fund Scheme 1952 and (b) Employees pension Scheme 1995 are displayed in Annexure 5.

Training to Newly-recruited Labour Force

Perhaps nothing has been thought and done for *imparting any sort of training to the workers in tea gardens on plucking, cultivation or manufacturing. This aspect can no longer be ignored and the impact on increasing productivity and ultimate reduction in production costs should be kept in mind.* The number of recruits from traditional labour families may decline gradually. For future recruits and the existing labour force, some sort of training in different spheres is imperative like plucking skills through practical demonstrations, application of fertilizers to minimise waste, art of tea-making in the factory and vegetative propagation and bush care.

Safety of Workers Under Insecticide Rules 1971

It is necessary that the provisions under the Insecticide Rules 1971 relating to safety of workers in using/spraying pesticides are complied with by the gardens in India.

Detailed Provisions in This Regard Are:

1) **Medical Examination** : Every worker is to be medically examined before employment and periodically thereafter. Any person showing symptoms of poisoning should immediately be examined and given treatment (Rule 37).
2) **First Aid Measures** : First aid should be given before the physician is called. The workers are also required to be educated regarding the effects of poisoning and how the first aid should be given (Rule 38).
3) **Protective Clothing** : Workers are to be adequately protected with the help of protective clothing and respiratory necessary devices. A complete suit of protective clothing shall consist of the following:
   a) Protective outer gunner/overhauls/hood
   b) Rubber gloves
   c) Dust proof goggles
   d) Boots
   e) Respiratory devices
4) Protective clothing should be made of materials to prevent or resist the penetration of insecticides. Materials should be washable (Rules 39 and 40).
5) **Stock of Antidotes** : Manufacturers, distributors and users are required to keep sufficient stock of first-aid tools, equipment, antidotes, injections and medicines to treat poisoning cases arising from inhalation, shin contamination, eye contamination and swallowing (Rule 41).
6) **Training Workers:** Manufacturers, distributors and users have

to arrange for suitable training of workers in observing safety precautions and handling of safety equipment provided to them.

Monitoring and Control of Processing Variables in Tea Manufacture

Production of tea from the tea plant originated as a culinary art more than a ago and remained so for many decades. Gradual increase in the popularity of the beverage and spread of tea plantations over many countries across the world resulted in a sustained development in the method of manufacture. Tea factories of today employ modern methods of biochemical engineering in the various steps of the production process. The statements at Table 7.11 provide information on the major *steps in tea manufacture, their objectives, the changes undergone by the leaf and other relevant aspects of the manufacturing process*. Rupture and distortion on of the leaf and loss of its water content are the main physical changes that take place when freshly plucked leaf is processed to manufacture black tea. They occur during the process of rolling, withering, drying and are accompanied by certain amount of change in chemical make-up of tea. But the main chemical transformation takes place in fermentation process. The nature and the extent of the physical and chemical changes of the leaf determine the ultimate quality of the product and its acceptability and market value. The processing variables, which influence these changes, can be measured with suitable instruments and in many instances can be controlled with the help of mechanical and electronic devices. The position in this regard now prevailing in most of the tea factories in India and the scope for improvement of the existing facilities are described in the paragraphs that follow.

Withering and Drying

The rate of removal of moisture in the withering and drying processes and the final moisture content at the end of the processes are determined by (a) temperature and relative humidity of the drying air, both at inlet and outlet; (b) air flow rate; (c) thickness of spread of the leaf; (d) period of withering and drying, and (e) uniformity of exposure of leaf to hot air.

Table 7.11: Bio-engineering of Manufacture of Black Tea.

Process Steps	Method	Purpose	Machinery and installation	Changes brought about
Withering	Partial dehydration of shoots (about 75 per cent moisture) to make them leathery for rolling, chemical changes etc.	Exposure to air under natural or controlled conditions	Withering lofts/drums/ tunnels/troughts / continuous withering machine	Lowering of moisture contents about 55 per cent; increase in caffeine, soluble sugars and amino acids; changes in proportion of organic acids and activity of leaf enzymes
Rolling	Rupture and distortion of tea shoots to allow mixing of enzymes and substrates	Mechanical bruising, tearing, cutting, breaking and twisting	Crank roller C.T.C. machine; Rotorvane; Triturator; Barbora leaf conditioner; continuous roller	Shoots cut and twisted; cellular constituents mixed; oxidative changes set in
Fermentation	Chemical changes of leaf constituents by enzymatic oxidation	Exposure to air under controlled temperature (about 30 degree C) and humidity	Fermentation floor/tray/troug h/drum m; continuous fermenter	Colour changes from green to coppery; polyphenol bodies oxides condensed
Drying	Stoppage of fermentation; dehydration to ensure keeping quality of product	Exposure to blast of hot air in a counter current drier (inlet: 80 to 100 degree c Exhaust: 50 to 55 degree C.)	Conventional tea drier; Tocklai continuous drier; Fluid bed drier	Moisture reduced to about 4 per cent. Product attains characteristic colour and appearance; some sugar is caramelized; polyphenols undergo epimerization

Source : Cha ki bat, November 1996

All the operating variables have to be properly regulated for obtaining a product having the desired characteristics and for economising on fuel costs. In the most widely used methods of withering, a bulk of tea leaves is spread over a withering trough and a mixture of heated air is blown through it. *Withering sections of many tea factories have as many as twenty or more of such troughs, and their operations have to be supervised and controlled until the leaves attain the desired degree of wither.* In the conventional type of tea drier, a blast of hot air enters at the bottom of drying chamber with mixtures of leaves spread on trays moving counter-currently to the flow of air. The hot air first meets the leaf that is almost dry and is leaving drier; the air passes through leaves of gradually increasing moisture content and is finally let out into the atmosphere.

Use of Ordinary Mercury Thermometens

Except for the use of ordinary mercury thermometers, virtually no other instrument is presently used *in the withering and drying sections of the factories for measurement of any of the large number of the operating variables*. The entire operation is thus left to the tea makers who have to adjust the conditions manually for the process to the processed smoothly. Not only that, determination of the end points of withering and drying are also left to the subjective assessment by individuals; moisture meters are rarely to be found in the withering and drawing sections of an average tea factories. *There seems to be justifiable reason why the situation should continue like this. Installation of digital thermometers with large display at suitable points in the withering and drying sections should not poss any problems.* Electronic instruments for measurement of many of operating variables such as pressure difference, and the so, forth could also be used with advantage for optimizing the processing conditions. It should also be possible to develop and use electronic devices for automatic control of some of the operations like maintenance of temperature of the heating air within the desired limits at the inlet and outlet ends.

Rolling

The design of the rolling machine and the conditions of the rolling *have direct bearing on the quality of the products, particularly for the leaf style, grade mix, bulk density and cup-age value of the tea produced as well as for the thickness of the liquor. A typical orthodox* roller consists of a circular table with bottoms fixed on the top, cylindrical box without a bottom and pressure cap. The box is loaded with withered tea-leaf and is made to move eccentrically over the table. The factors which affect the nature and the extent of rolling, and hence the degree of distortion and breakage of the leaf, are like (a) period of rolling,(b) design of the batten; and (c) cap pressure.

The bottens on the table and the cap pressure retard circulation of the leaf and consequently, the temperature of the leaf rises due to accumulation of frictional heat. Excessive heating can affect the quality of tea adversely. Rolling programme for each charge is, therefore, so adjusted that the leaf undergoes alternate spells of roll with and without pressure in a predetermined time sequence. *The other popular method of rolling makes use of the crushing, tearing and curling machine (CTC machine), which mainly consists of two engraved metal rollers running close together at two different speeds, usually 70 and 700 revolutions per minute.* The rollers work like a mangle and the leaf is cut, torn and rolled in the small gap between the surfaces of the two rollers. For satisfactory operation, the cutting teeth on the roller surfaces must be kept properly sharpened. The gap between the rollers should be carefully adjusted and uniform feed of leaf to machine should be ensured.

Basic Operations of Rolling Section Carried out Manaully

All the basic operations in the rolling section are at present carried out manually. It often becomes extremely difficult to supervise and handle with precision a fairly large number rollers that have to be used at the same time in a factory producing orthodox tea. The possibility of human errors in adhering to a precise time schedule for feeding of leaf, application of pressure and other operations cannot be avoided. Lack of coordination in the functioning of the rollers due to such errors can result in significant loss in the quality of product. Similar problems arise-although to a lesser extent in factories producing CTC tea, particularly in the matter of supervision and manipulation of the rate of feed of leaf to each of a number of machines in operation.

Suggestions for Using Electronic Devices for Automatic Monitoring

The possibility of using electronic devices for automatic monitoring and control of operations of orthodox rollers have been suggested from time to time by scientists and engineers interested in this field. Suggestions have been made for introduction of micro-process based control systems. One such system envisages the use of electronic sequential timer coupled with pressure gauge and motor drive for accurate and automatic operation of as many as twenty-four or more rollers in accordance with a pre-determined rolling programme. Likewise, it has been suggested that the common problem of overfeeding or underfeeding of CTC machines could be solved by the use of electronic devices that would continuously monitor and control the speed of the feed conveyors. Not much action seems to have been taken by the tea industry to follow up these suggestions. Certain other aspects of the rolling process for which automatic system would be useful, are the control of leaf temperature and adjustment of the gap between the pair of rollers in CTC machine.

Fermentation

The rate of chemical change of the constituents of the tea leaf during fermentation is determined by the temperature, humidity and the oxygen content of the ambient air. *The extent of change is dependent on the period of fermentation*. Instruments for monitoring the condition of the air in the fermenting room is at present very rarely used. *Even the period of fermentation is generally adjusted by noting the colour, feel and flavor of the leaf rather than on the bans on the objective measurements. Use of air conditioned space with provision of automatic control of oxygen content of air for the fermentation process to be processed at the desired level may not prove to be cost effective*. The installation of automatic records procced provide information of the various parameters that influence the process. The possibility of determining the end point with the help of automatic colour sensor would also merit-serious consideration. Over the decades, significant advance has been made in the development of machinery and equipment for manufacture of tea. What is lacking is the use of monitoring devices and control system for minimising the loss of quality in the end product caused by operator's error. Development and use of cost effective systems for performing the loss involved are expected to contribute significantly to overall improvement of the manufacturing process and the quality of tea produced.

Financial Needs of the Tea Industry for Sustainable Plantation Management

There is a general complaint in all industry circles about shortage of finance for development and expansion. It is also alleged that even when finance is available from the financial institution, the rate of interest and terms of repayment are prohibitive. The lack of generation of internal resources due to low profitability makes it imperative for the industrial units to look elsewhere for resources and, on the other hand, makes it difficult for them to avail of loan facilities. This dilemma is true for all industries to a greater or lesser extent and individual units in different industries have tried to solve the problem in their own way. Some of the ways adopted are acceptance of loans/deposits from shareholders and the public, issue of bonds as well as non-convertible and convertible debentures. Fresh issue of shares has, however, been conspicuous by its absence. The factors operating against issue of fresh shares are:

i) Low profitability which inhibits induction of additional shareholders as it would further reduce the rate of dividend per share.

ii) Obvious reluctance on the part of investors to invest in the shares of campanies with low profitability particularly because such shares, if at all issued, would under present circumstances, be offered only at a substantial premium which would make the investment all the more uneconomic.

It is, therefore, necessary to remedy the above situation in order to *attract fresh capital into industrials units seeking development and expansion and at the same time make it worthwhile for the industrial units/companies to invite fresh equity capital apart from loans, bonds, debentures, etc.* This can be achieved by a simple but novel device. At present, whenever fresh shares are issued, if at all, such shares command a premium based on the accumulated reserves of the company. The idea is that the new shareholders pay not only the per value or face value of the share but also make a contribution to the accumulated reserves so as to achieve two purposes:-

i) to keep the net worth per share unchanged; and

ii) to make the new shareholders equal partners in the profits and assets of the company, right from the inception of the company.

Joint Multi-stock Companies

What is required now is a departure from the *traditional conception of equity participation and to adopt a system under which fresh shares may be issued at par (without premium) to both existing shareholders and newcomers with the provision that these shares will not have any right to the accumulated reserves as on the date of issue of fresh shares*. The accumulated reserves will belong entirely *to the original shareholders. The newcomers may or may not enjoy the benefit of the reserves to the accumulated in future according to their desire*. In case, they desire to participate in future reserves, they will get dividend at more or less the same rate as the original shareholders. In case, however, they do not want to claim a share in the future reserves, they will get dividend at a higher rate.

Thus, there will be three categories of shareholders in addition to the original share-holders, viz.

a) new shareholders participating in past reserves as well as future reserves;

b) new shareholders not participating in past reserves but participating in future reserves; and

c) new shareholders not participating in either past reserves or future reserves.

Theoretically, there may be another category viz. new shareholders participating in past reserves but not participating in future reserves. However, it is not unlikely that new shareholders who would not like to participate in future reserves would like to participate in past reserves. Such persons would prefer to be shareholders of Category c, not participating in either past or future reserves

(a) Distribution of Dividents

Shares of Category paripassu will be issued at a premium and these shareholders will rank pair pass with the original share holders. Shares of categories (b) and (c) will be issued at face value. As for distribution of dividends, the procedure will be quite simple. *The total profit after taxation may in the first place be divided among the different categories of shareholders prorata to their net worth*. For category shareholders the total amount available will be distributed as dividend. For original shareholders as well as shareholders of categories (a) and (b) the total amounts available will be divided into dividends and reserves in such a way that they get a reasonable rate of dividend which may not be the same but the amount transferred to reserves per share must necessarily be the same. The calculations will be as follow:

Let, *total profit after tax be A and r be the percentage of A to T*. For share-holders of Group 1 i.e., category and group 2 i.e., category, the percentage will be r_1 and r_2 respectively as shown above representing both dividend and transfer to reserves. The dividends will be d_1 per cent and d_2 per cent, respectively such that $r1\text{-}d_1 = r_2\text{-}d_2$ = per cent transferred to reserve. For category (c) shareholders, however, dividend will be declared at the rate of r% and no amount will be transferred to reserves. Needless to say that for the above calculation, the equity capital on account of category (a) share-holders will be reckoned at par value and the amounts of premium on these shares will be reckoned as reserves.

What has been suggested above constitutes a new dynamic approach to financing of joint stock companies at different stages of development. Fresh issues at par may be made as and when necessary and as many times as may be necessary. Shares of different face values may also be issued at different times, if necessary. Accounting will also not be difficult. All that would be necessary is to split up the reserves to show the amounts of reserves for different periods synchronizing with the dates of issue of fresh shares. A bold new approach on the part of India industries seeking development and expansion but sufffering from shortage of funds is highly necessary on the above lines.

Financing New Patterns of the Tea Industry

The new financing pattern suggested above is suitable for all joint stock *companies and is particularly suitable for the tea industry, on both capital and revenue accounts*. The tea industry would, it is suggested, *do well to go in for raising fresh capital from the market on the above lines instead of depending solely on the financial institutions which are unlikely to provide all the funds that may be necessary*. Although the recent decision of the Government of India to allow a deduction of 20 per cent of the profits before tax from taxable income will make considerable amount available to the industry, it is apprehended that the industry may still not be able to meet all its financial requirements unless it decides to tap the capital market on the above lines. *In fact, the tea industry, which has already undergone a re-structuring of its shareholding and capital base in recent years in the progress of conversion of foreign companies into Indian companies under the Foreign Exchange Manaement Act, is ideally suited for injection of extra dynamism in its activities by taking steps to convert the tea companies into multi-stock companies on the lines indicated above*. Simultaneously, it should also resort to loans/deposits from the public as well as issue of bonds and debentures whenever necessary. The tea industry has so far been extremely conservative in these respects. Time has come when it should shed this conservative attitude and welcome new methods and techniques of raising finance. If necessary, the Companies Act may also be suitably revised to permit introduction of new financial innovations in the financing of the activities of joint stock companies on the above lines. In particular, specific provision may be made permitting formation of joint multi-stock companies and conversion of existing joint stock companies into joint multi-stock companies.

Strenghening Adoption of Bolder and Innovative Methods

Simultaneously, with the adoption of bolder and innovative methods of financing by the tea industry it is necessary that shareholders and the public are given sufficient incentives for investing in tea companies. The incentives that are immediately necessary are as follows :-

i) The entire expenditure for purchase of new shares of existing tea companies should be allowed as a deduction from the taxable income of the next year. This concession should be available only for purchase of fresh shares from the company and not for purchase of old shares from the market.

ii) For a period of at least 15 years, dividends received on fresh shares issued from a specified date onwards should be free from income-tax.

iii) Interest on debentures, bonds and deposits in tea companies made after a specified date should also be free from income-tax for a period of at least 15 years.

iv) Investment in tea companies, either for purchase of new shares or by way of deposits for a period of not less than three years, should qualify for exemption from capital gains tax when such purchase or deposit is made out of capital gains,

v) For deposits and/or investment in new shares, bonds, debentures of tea companies involving an amount up to Rs. 1 lakh in the name of any single depositor/investor, no enquiry about the source of the funds will be made.

The tea industry is very badly in need of resources for implementing the perspective plan up to 2015 while public sentiment for investment in the tea industry is for various historical reasons not at all favourable. The five old incentive package suggested above will help considerably in improving the credit worthiness of the tea industry. It would, therefore, be desirable for the tea industry to take up these suggestions with the government for its approval as expeditiously as possible.

Conclusion

Climate, land, water and biological resources form the basic prerequisites for tea cultivation in India. *Climate includes the factors of rainfall, temperature and humidity while land includes "topography", "aspect" and "soil". Biological resources include trees, shrubs and either natural wetlands and cultivated crops or the flora side and livestock*, wild animals and solid micro-organisms on the "fauna" side. All these natural factors contribute to the "property" value of an estate. Tea in North-East requires favourable climate, land and water regimes for successful results. *Ambient temperatures* required for raising tea in North-East range from 13^{0}C to 29^{0}C while

2000-5000 mm per annum could be the desired range of annual rainfall, provided it is properly distributed. The recommended soil pH levels are 4.5 to 5.5 for growing tea in North. While Darjeeling tea is raised on sedimentary soils, in Cachar, tea is raised on peat soils. *Topography also varies* in regard to tea cultivation in North. In Darjeeling, tea is raised along hill slopes while in Dooars, Terai and in Assam, tea is cultivated on level lands. While soil water run-offs is a major problem in Darjeeling, the problem in Dooars, Terai and in Assam is that of draining away excess water from soil through a system of channels and bunds. *Amongst biological resources, prominent ones are soil micro-organisms and natural flora such as shade trees and thickets provided by windbreaks. All these resources have a great significance to "sustainable" production of tea in estates.* Wind damage and hailstorms in Assam and parts of Bengal (during spring season) have been a significant factor in the destruction of tea plants. Natural wind-breaks are deemed to be good protection devices from these calamities. Similarly, shade trees such as Albizzia chinesis are considered to be a highly useful in preventing transpiration losses in extreme water-stress seasons. Cover crops in North Bengal and Assam, such as the Guatemala grass, act as natural nutrient additions to soils where replanting is resorted to. All these facilitating natural conditions are prerequisites for tea cultivation and for a good estate "property". Management practices in tea garden vary. However, where management practices, while not leaving aside the idea of optimizing harvest index, have been successful in conserving natural resources, this would be considered as a case of sustainable management practice with economic advantage.

References

1. Man and Development Journal, 2000-2002
2. Afro-Asion Journal, 1999-2001 Issues
3. IASSI Journal, Issues relating to tea, 2001-2004
4. Financing Agriculture, 1998-2004 Issues
5. Times Agriculture Journal, 2000-2003 Issues
6. Agriculture today, Varions Issues

7. Tea Board India Techno Economic Survey Reports (i) Darjeeling Tea Industry, (ii) Cahar Tea Industry (iii) Himanchal Pradesh Tea Industry, (iv) Tripura Industry (v) Nilgiris Tea Industry (vi) Coimbatore Tea Industry, (vii) Wynand Tea Industry (viii)

8. Diversification and Value Addition of Indian Tea, IASSI Journal.

9. Dailies-Economic Times, Business Lines, Eastern Mirron, North East Times, Financial Express.

10. Yojana, Kurkshetrya, India Today, Business World, Kishan World.

11. G.D. Banerjee Tea Plantation Industry in India - Structural Changes between 1850 and 1992, Law years Book Stall, Guwahati, 1996.

12. G.D. Banerjee and Srijeet Banerjee Darjeeling Tea Industry-The Golden Brew International Book Dustributing Comapany, Lucknow, 2007.

Chapter 8

Indian Tea Industry-Critical Eye

In the context of steep increase in cost of production and enmeshed in a net of heavy taxes, tea industry has to make earnest efforts to meet the demands of domestic consumption of low prices and also compete with other global tea producers to retain its share of the export market. To its better experience the tea industry had learned the hard way that it was not at all possible to depend on governmental policies which had led to downfall of tea. Such policies were primarily responsible for the erosion of India's dominant share of the export market all these years at one time not very long ago it was over 50 percent. Now it is barely 21 per cent. Added to this, the government thought of importing tea from other countries, this however, could not materialise due to strong protests from various tea associations. If Indian tea is not to go under, the industry should make effort to be self-reliant, otherwise, the fate which has all overtaken the jute, sugar and some other industries will affect tea also. There is a real threat to production if efforts are not made concertedly and consistently to increase the yield per hectare as expansion of the present area of cultivation can be ruled out. The industry must search all possible avenues for increasing exports. This is necessary if the dwindling foreign exchange reserves are to be built up. International contacts must be boosted up and for this, meets like the recent international convention on tea in the UK should be taken advantage of. Another world meet on tea was held in the United States. Tea is not so popular in the USA and in fact demand for it has been sliding down. But there is a vast potential market provided it is exploited properly. From all accounts, affluent America is in search of a healthy drink and the

Indian tea industry can play a great role to bring home to Americans the undoubted medicinal and health properties of tea. Such a campaign was undertaken in collaboration with the USA Tea Council. The international meet held in March 1991 took the initiative to act concertedly in furthering such campaign for the better of Indian tea particularly.

In view of this, there is urgent need to dwell upon the long pending issues of the industry. In this chapter an attempt has been made to discuss in brief the various critical issues of the tea industry which require special attention of the Government of India, tea association, Tea Board, Tea Trade Industry. The issues are being discoursed under different heads.

Innovation on Tea Bushes

It is an accepted fact that each asset has an estimated economic life in terms of its revenue yielding and service reandering capacity. Each asset is subject to wear, tear and waste due to normal use or consumption over a number of years. It becomes obsolete due to newer developments, and at a point of it time fails to command any value in market and turns to a scrap. This being the normal feature of an asset, economic enterprises are allowed under net income tax legislation of respective countries to set asides an estimated amount annually as "Depreciation"estimated annual diminution in value of the assets that spread over the asset's expected life of recovery of investment made. Although economic enterprises are currently allowed to make provision for depreciation on many assets. It is regrettable that tea producing units cannot make any such provision against their produced means of production-the principal property contributing to their revenue yielding capacity i.e., tea bushes. But there should not be two opinion that like other assets as plant and machinery, factory shed and buildings, mines etc., economic life of tea bushes is estimable, their productivity gradually diminishes with continuing consumption of tea leaves over a number of years. Hence at some times, replacement of tea bushes becomes imperative in order to hold the producing unit economically worthy.

In the spectrum of these facts, it is an obvious question as to why tea bushes shall not be treated as principal asset of tea producing units, why these units should not be allowed to make necessary financial provision by way of depreciation for recovery of investment on that. The governments of tea producing countries should review the connotation of 'asset', 'capital', 'investment' provision for depreciation' in real life perspective. It should be recognised that bushes ostensibly manifest all the facets of an asset and hence the producing units should be allowed to make reasonable provision of depreciation. This would essentially mean allowing the proprietor of tea bushes of open a channel for internal generation of funds, making the proprietor least dependent on borrowing and government assistance. As obvious, therefore, tea producing units would be self-reliant in matter of finance, fully responsive to the necessarity of extension planting and replacement planting which are pre-requisites to help the tea industry of a country to grow and prosper.

Organic Cultivation of Tea

Now is the time to ponder over seriously the necessity of introducing organic cultivation of tea which allows the plants to grow and mature as nature intended. Now is the time the companies in India engaged in tea growing and processing should take notice of the increasing sales of certified, organically grown black, green and harbal teas. Looking at the world tea market, it may be emphasised that not only Germany is insisting upon organic tea but it is selling profitably in other parts of Europe, Australia and Japan. The demand is likely to grow further since people all over the world, are becoming health and environment conscious. Enlightened countries now-a-days want that, in all circumstances, the ecological balance has to be maintained for the health of the present generation as well as the posterity. The World Health Organisation (WHO), social institutions registered in developed and developing countries are also campaigning massively for the maintenance of ecological balance. For imbalance growing continually is bound to cause colossal damage to our surrounding and health which in no way, can be recovered. Imperative is, therefore, to bid good-bye to the conventional growing methods of agricultural prudance which use chemical fertiliser, pesticides etc., and disrupt man-environment relation and natural growth of plant. Consumers are learning more about organic tea knowing that it has been cared for from beginning to end in a conscientious way. The soils were kept chemical-free, a farm plan developed to continually enrich the soil fertility. Tea bush nurtured in a way good for earth and workers and the leaves plucked and processed with documented care to ensure consumer of a contamination-free drink.

Consumer fee is that this cup of tea is the best way to support the cleaning up of the environment and to that the exposure of indigenous people to unneccssary chemicals. This feeling is sure to give them something extra which comes from participating in something larger than that of a cup of tea. It is indeed change towards a more gentle way of existing with nature and our fellow human beings. It is obvious that organic teas are making their way in wider markets. Now it is time that tea growing and processing companies in India should take a position to ride this wave into the future.

Violation of Pesticide Residual Limits

Not long past, Indian tea market in Russia received a serious jolt for supplying substandard tea to that country. Complaint regarding the quality of those supplies did not remain confined simply in the official files of the Russian Government but was brought to the floor of the domestic consumers cautioning them against the consumption of Indian tea. No matter who was the real culprit of the misdeed, it is true that the long-standing goodwill of Indian produce was severely damaged owning to that unscrupulous event. Indian tea, known for quality mark, acquired disreputation, no doubt. But before the stain could completely be removed another spot mark has surfaced very recently. It is disheartening to note that this time German has complained to the Tea Board against Darjeeling tea for violating German specification of pesticides residue limits. Recent complaints further include the produce of some other areas as Assam, Terai,

Dooars, etc. It is not a healthy sign, indeed, as far as export trade of tea is concerned. For, once a European country expresses extreme dissatisfaction against the supplies this may eventually turn as a cancerous growth among all the countries of the European Economic Community. And utter dissatisfaction, with cumulative effect, is likely to bring forth in them absolute aversion to Indian tea and a mood to lean heavily on other suppliers for necessary requirement. Obviously, the export trade will badly suffer. So will suffer Indian tea traders' endeavour in penetrating to new markets. The unavoidable effect is likely to be a glut of tea and the industry may eventually face depression for the causes created by the industry itself. So, it is time that tea producers and traders of the country make cautious approach to tea markets; they be more conscious to the tacit responsibilities that seller owes to the buyer in any transaction. For, just a stroke of insensible act on their part may vitiate the long-standing reputation of indent tea and the tradition that it has set. And once the country's image is lost in the world market it will take a pretty long time to regain. Obviously, the tea producers and traders, the Tea Board, brokers and the licensing authority have to act in a more responsible manner. Business ethics should in no way be sidetraked. It would be judicious to remember the old saying: Rome was not built in a day.

Now Quality Matters

It is of great concern to the tea industry in India that from on average of around 200 million kgs, India's exports have come down to an average of 165 million kgs for the last five years. If this trend continues the industry will heavily suffer in the price realisation front leading to a situation of unrecmunerative working. Sources indicate that the Tea Board and the industry have already taken up some promotional measures to boost up tea sales in the lost market. But the job does not appear easy. In the face of keen competition from Sri Lanka, Kenya, China, Indonesia, mere publicity and campaign, discussion at the meetings and statistical exercises will hardly enable the industry to increase sales and regain the premier position in world tea export.

For world buyers are increasingly taking to quality tea consumption from which there is no turning back to cheaper teas. Indian tea industry will have to comprehend this changing and emerging behaviour pattern of the consumer. Imperative is, therefore, to direct best effort to maintain quality production and quality export in bulk, in value-added form like tea packet, tea bags, tea caddies, etc. along with Brand promotion. It may be reiterated, higher segment of quality tea exports competition is less intense while that in lower segment is severe where price level matters most. India, no doubt, with track record of building up an image of quality tea producer and exporter, enjoys a favourable position in world tea market. But to hold the position more firm, regularity in supply and application of ethical business principles have to be ensured also. This will not only increase sales in the lost market but enable confident penetration into other potential areas ike South Africa, Israel, Pakistan, Ireland, etc. Eventually, industry's overwhelming dependence on one or a couple of buyers will be reduced.

Better Try To Stand on Their Own Instead of Taking a Crutch

News poured in that a host of growing establishments in Cachar, Tripura, and South India, producing plainer varieties of tea, are facing unfathomable financial crisis due to steep fall in tea prices resulting from loss of CIS countries, Iran and weak domestic demand. Reports further indicate the price of teas has sunk to such a low level at the auction centres in South India and North India that those establishments are unable to cover even the cost of production. And with a view to helping overcome this situation and survive, these establishments have urged the governments at the Centre and states, to grant adequate fiscal relief and provide for liberal financial assistance It has been stated that already a number of gardens in these areas are on the sick list and the list will definitely swell up if the governments fail to be generous. There is an alarming crisis indeed. And if no improvement in the situation occurs immediately not only those establishments and their work force but the entire socio-economic conditions in these regions will be affected. The Governments, as such, have obvious moral responsibility to rescue them from the death-trap. Contextually, however, some pertinent questions may be raised : For whose faults the said establishments have fallen in this distressed situation? For whose negligence some tea gardens have already been sick and a few more are likely to be sick in near future?

With regard to the causes of sickness of economic enterprises the observation of the Board for Industrial and Financial Reconstruction (BIFR), though not palatable, may be worth recalling in this regard. Faulty planning, improper utilisation of working capital, inefficient management, lack of vision and lethargy in developing new product have been cited as the responsible factors behind industrial sickness in general. At the very outset, therefore, it is imperative to ascertain if there are seeming signs of those maladies in the crippled tea growing establishments. Also it imperative is to find out if the ever undertook self-audit to locate where they stand and are heading to. Did they ever care to cure the ailment and grow healthy? Or, as is practised in India, the managements did simply wait for the opportune moment to pray for fiscal relief as well as long-term financial assistance. What is worth noting in this connection is that the tea industry in India is not passing through depressionary phase. Nor has it faced any sort of severe calamity so far. So, would it not be judicious to think twice if the government intends to be generous to individual establishments. For in a competitive economy opportunity cost is a decisive factor in making sacrifice. Individual establishments, therefore, should better try to stand and walk on their own instead of taking crutch.

The Uncertainty Ends

The last visit of Russian President Boris Yeltsin to India put full stop to the mundane talk of the tea industry. It was for disintegration of USSR and its fallout on India's tea which was the topic of deliberations for the tea trade and industry. A few years backs forum after forum and meet after meet, speakers 'visualised' a gloomy scenario for Indian tea. Some hardcore pressimists predicted a virtual decimation of the brew. Ministers sermonised the industry about the necessity of finding new markets, trade circles at large trembled at the very thought of entering the new markets amidst stiff competition from tea exporting giants like Sri Lanka. And as it is rightly said, 'necessity is the mother of invension', critical moments prompted the entrepreneurs to get out of the protectionist market arena with concentrated efforts to find green pastures elsewhere. The crisis proved a point well; it is dangerous to put all eggs in one basket. The crisis resulted in change of export pattern, with the emphasis now on hard currency buyers. The U.K. and Poland have become main targets, whilst business has now started up with Pakistan too.

The visit has proved we are needlessly pessimistic and get panicky even at slight hint. Not many visualised that things would change for better in Russia once the political uncertainties are over, the regenerated nation will engage in normal economic activity. Yes, it is well known, cut down to size politically and economically, it could no longer act like a world policeman and big brother for other proletarian regimes. Some experts had expected that Russia now would swing to the West and show no interest at all in India, the latter remaining like one more Latin American country at the doorstep of international financial bodies. Such pessimistic thinkings were proved wrong. To put the facts straight, Russia needs India's support not for geographical reasons alone but for others.

The visit is the aftermath of prolonged ground level talks between two countries at the official level with both sides gradually sensing that the year-long negotiations would not throw up a mutually acceptable formula on Rupee-Rouble exchange tangle and realising that it needed a political initiative to end the stalemate.

Lack of Planning Premises while Planning for Business

Although tea production increases over the year, the Quantum of exports hovered around less than 170 million kgs over the years.

Obviously the matter that matterns most in this context, why India's export stagnated over the years and who is accountable for. As usual the government has been blaming the exporters, who in tern, pass the buck to the overseas buyers. But in reality neither the government nor the exporter can shed the responsibility of causing a stagnant situation in tea export. For it is the individual and joint failure to make a correct assessment of the buyer economic condition, consumption pattern, etc. and diagnose the WHYs of emerging trend in the market. Probably, none of them at all takes care of planning premises while planning for the business. The necessity of forecasting with support data is either ignored or undermintered. Otherwise, acute shortage of fund compelling India's long standing trade partners as CIS, Poland, Iran to search for cheaper source of supply to meet their internal tea requirement, could be visualised earlier. In the same way, the far reaching impact of unethical business practice and that of violating the norms of pesticides residue limits could well be estimated beforehand. In fact it is not only the fund crunch of the *buyers but a combination of factors that dragged the country in the export 'Stagnation trap' in tea sector.*

But it was nobody's concern until very recently the question has come up on the floor; nor anybody realised the necessity of a cohesive approach to get escape from the trap. This is certainly indicative of our poor vision, business policy and the practice as well. Evidently, we failed to combat the unwanted situation, we stood imprepared in the face of unexpected events. So, where is the point of lamenting for the nonfulfilment of export target! It would be wise rather if all concerned with tea industry of the country imbibe in the lesson that business in the international market calls for sophisticated business approach coupled with adherence to business ethics. *Business is for those who care for business.*

Action Plan for Tea

The then Commerce Minister, Shri Arun Neheru directed the Tea Board to prepare an action plan for tea. The Public Accounts

Committee threw light on how the Tea Board could make a better effort for the development of tea industry. It is doubtful weather the Tea Board, as it is presently constituted, can ever frame and implement such plan. Instead of asking the Tea Board to prepare such plan, Government could have easily sized up the nature of the real challenges facing tea. An action plan announced by Government made available more land for tea and a target was set by the turn of 2000.

Close Interaction Between Tea Industry and Tea Research Centre.

It is often said that researchers and research institutions in India, of course, with the exception of IITs, mostly work on secondary data and on subjects purely theoretical which bear little or no relevance to the requirement of industrial users. Critics unhesitatingly indicate the absence of interaction between the said entities and, obviously, question is the meaningfulness of huge spending on research and development (R&D). In India, money spent on R&D is not small. In 1992, Rs. 4830 crores were spent on this account of which the Central Government's share was 80 per cent. And the government's spending on R&D took place through government research centres. CSIR complex and Tea Research Centres are a few of such institutions worth reckoning, well-equipped with manpower, scientific apparatus and research facilities. And as evident from the Annual Report these centres are deeply engrossed in studying and analysing scientifically the requirements of high tea yield, yield arresting factors and the ways and means to tackle the problem areas. Nevertheless, centres are continually experimenting the possibility of bringing in new areas under tea cultivation, Meghalaya, Orissa for instance. Since R&D entails heavy and regular expenditure with the expected result mostly remote, many economic organisation, even knowing fully the significance, cannot invest in this area. But organisations can obtain necessary assistance and able guidance from government research centres nowadays. What is needed in this regard uninterrupted communication and close interaction between the research institutions and economic organisation. This truth holds good to tea industry. It should take the expertise of Tea Research Centre continually in order to enhance competitiveness in the global market by holding the costline with increased yield and improving the quality of tea. Our presence in the international market is not commanding in any segment. We have high but not dominant share even in tea segment which is just 11.2 per cent. And over 30 producers are competing at the international market.

So, there is no point of becoming complacent just because the industry is able to meet the yearly export target. Rather it should be a matter of concern as to how the existing market can be held firmly in the event of growing competition. Surely in this matter R&D on tea cannot only provide a safe guard but lend help to flourish in the world market. Imperative need is therefore, the presence of mutual under standing and close interaction between tea industry and tea research.

Reminding the Commitment

Over the past few years, representatives of the tea industry frequently aired their discontentment for non-availability of sufficient financial incentives necessary for its healthy growth. And, indeed, the voice did not fall on deaf ear. The Government at the Centre and States has responded favourably to the industry's urge by making adequate provision of comforts through budgetary means. Quite some time has passed since the Ministry of Finance at the *Centre abolished excise duty both from bulk tea and packaged tea. Reduced further the corportate tax to 46 per cent, virtually scrapped the lock-in period of deposits. The State governments have also extended liberal contribution through* the withdrawal of entry tax, reduction of levy on green tea leaf, allowance for substantial deduction from agricultural income for funds invested for the development of plantations etc.

In the perspective of national economy, therefore, the industry owes an obvious responsibility to account for the utilisation of savings thus accruing to it since then. The industry is required to justify the receipt of concessions as this tantamounts to government investment in true sense. So, would it be unreasonable if the establishment in the industry are asked to give an account of their individual and collective effort taken so far for the healthy growth of the industry. Would it be unfair if the industry is asked to enlighten the country as to what it has done so far to increase man-productivity, land-productivity, production and plantation development to reduce cost of production, innovate non-conventional teas and to penetrate beyond the traditional boundaries. This is not only to remind the industry of its commitment but to make it conscious of the country's expectation interms of return. For investment, irrespective of nature and size, always entails a cost and some sacrifice which the society bears at the ultimate analysis. Evidently, perusal of investment return in vital in deciding whether to continue or discontinue the concessions allowed so far. Investment without reasonable return is absolutely unproductive meaning, national loss which cannot in any way be patronised. And investment opportunities are no less in the country at the moment. So it is time the tea industry should religiously remember its commitment.

Tea Board's Working Group Suggests Reduction in Import Duty

For some time there have been suggestions for reduction of import duty on tea. *Section 33AB of the IT Act already allows deduction from taxable income prior to apportionment in corporate tax and agricultural income tax and Section 80HHC allows such deduction from income tax after apportionment of taxable income.* However, it is felt that state governments will not be encouraged to reduce the incidence of agricultural tax further if they do not see an overall increase in the tax revenues from the tea industry. In such a situation, suitable steps need be taken to increase production, which will help the state governments to get larger revenues, thereby being encouraged to reduce the level of incidence.

The working group has also suggested that a uniform rate of sales tax be levied on sale of tea in consumer packs at the garden level to encourage tea producers to take active role in direct marketing.

As of now, some states now change 2 per cent against the general rate of 4 per cent. The suggestion now is to reduce it to 2 per cent uniformly for creating a favourable impact on the tea trade in non-tea producing states, which in turn would benefit consumers. It has further been suggested that the effective rate *of excise on instant tea be totally withdrawn instead of the stiff 25 per cent now to give a fillip to the sales of value-added teas.* Some suggestions have also been made on packaging *machineries and packaging materials.* The group felt that import of tea-bagging machine should be exempted fully from payment of import duties to encourage tea bag manufacturers to upgrade technologies and improve the level of quality packing. This in turn will induce higher exports of tea bags to meet the growing needs of consumers in importing countries. It may be mentioned here that in countries like UK, for instance, where consumption of tea in tea bags is very popular, the largest market share is held by overseas packeteers who buy their tea from Sri Lanka, Kenya and India. As of now, as much as 80 per cent of the market in *UK is controlled by tea bags.* The perception is that if quality products can be manufactured, then India can make a successful inroad into the tea bag market there. The working group has also submitted that the rate of import duty on tea processing and packaging material should also be reduced to at least 10 per cent from the existing level of 25 per cent. Government has already accepted some of suggestions and a few more are under consideration.

Multiplicity of Forms and Returns

Apart from the obligations common to all industrial enterprises such as income tax and other direct taxes, professional tax, sales taxes, customs and excise duties, there are about half a dozen Control Order under the Tea Act, and about 15 Acts on labour matters and an equal number of rules framed there under to be followed by the tea industry. Forms, returns or registers emanate from these Acts, Rules and Orders. Filling in such papers often requires specialised knowledge. Often a number of persons are required for the purpose and they may take substantial time too. There are, of course, some forms, registers or returns that are inevitable and inescapable. For example there, are Acts and Rules which relate to welfare of the workers of tea industry and their families, but the concerned records and returns may be rationalised and a comprehensive Act may be made and set of rules suitably framed to minimise the official work-load in tea estates and in the government departments. One is afraid by red tapism, by duplication of work the government has made out a case for compulsory computerisation. A centrally operated computer might timely feed various departments with required information with least disturbance to the industries. All said and done, apprehension persists. Government is a machinery. Computer too is, but its operation is in human hands. Human nature, as revealed in government, being what it is, one may draw a corollary to the Parkinson's Law stating that forms, registers and returns shall continue to multiply to cover up lethargy and lack of imagination in government officers!

Tea and Control

Situations may so arise in an industry, when some restrictions have been inflicted on it, to steer the activities of the industry towards a desired course. But in the dynamic and open economy the situations may often change when the regulatory measures cease to be effective. They may even be counter-productive. For due development of the tea industry, the Tea Act. 1953 was passed and some measures under it were taken. But now some of those measures are considered obstacles to further development in tea production and distribution. Accordingly, the industry's own men of consequence sat down to consider whether all those controls should be withdrawn, lock, stock and barrel. If not, which are to be retained and/or in what form. In such matters difference of opinion is quite possible. None the less, a consensus has now been reached. And on behalf of the industry the

Chairman of the apex body of the tea industry associations approached the government with a request to life forthwith at least some of the Control orders as they outgrew their utility particularly in the context of the government's policy of liberalisation and de-control.

The then Chairman Barooah, in his letter to Ministry of the Commerce, particularly mentioned five of the orders namely.

a) Tea (Distribution & Export) Control Order, 1957

b) Tea (Regulation of Export) Licensing Order, 1984

c) Tea (Marketing) Control Order, 1984

d) Tea (Warehouse Licensing) Order, 1989

e) Tea Waste (Control) Order, 1959.

Though he did not specifically state so it is known that even ordinarily most of these orders were not invoked for quite some time. In the few cases where these may still be relevant, the Tea Act the parent Act, in itself redundant, on certain aspects can very well take care of the situations. Multiplicity of orders and rules as such only create unnecessary confusion and should obviously be avoided. For example, the Tea (Marketing) Control Order, 1984 required the industry with certain exceptions to sell at least 75 per cent of their teas through Indian auctions. Now that producers are making their tea available in the market either through auctions or directly such restrictions are unnecessary. Government had adopted the policy of de control with a view to developing industry and making goods easily available to consumer. If in the process the middlemen suffer that is only to be regretted. Even so before the 1984 Order was issued, the brokers played an important role in tea marketing. They may do so again.

Similarly Tea (Regulation of Export) Licensing Order, 1984 requires the contracted prices to be registered with the Tea Board so that the importer is compelled to pay that price even if the auction prices fall after the registration. Such registration is unnecessary following the free convertibility of the Rupee. However, the industry is not against regulations if and where necessary in the interest of the industry itself. Maintenance of statistics in all aspects of production and marketing is one such requirement. The industry wants Section 10(K) of the Tea Act to be properly amended to include appropriate provisions in this regard.

Another matter : the Tea (Waste) Control Order, requires destruction or conversion of tea waste into compost in the presence of excise officials. With excise on tea the officials now plead lack of jurisdiction in the matter. Meanwhile stocks pile up causing health hazard and environment pollution. Consultative Committee of Plantation Associations has, therefore, rightly urged the Commerce Ministry to suspend with immediate effect Clause 4 of the order to allow the industry to take due action even before the order is formally rescinded. Appropriate actions should be taken forthwith. As in the case of controls in the past so in case of decontrols now it is the government policy at work. It need hardly be emphasised that an industry development require not merely quick decision but its expeditious execution as well.

Tea and Co-ordination

With little scope for increasing country's tea exports quantitatively, India looked for ways of stepping up unit value realisation. The more obvious method is to go in for volume addition more and more and it must be pushed vigorously. But there is another method, which is, if anything, more obvious little acted upon. This is to coordinate the efforts of major producing countries in export marketing and even in value addition. For reasons not quite clear, this question of collaboration has not been seriously taken up. The then Indian High Commissioner in Sri Lanka had been correctly quoted. He had said that this island neighbour was keen on the creation of facilities by Indian parties for processing raw materials available there with buy back arrangement with Sri Lanka parties. This would have helped

Colombo to better balance its trade with India. But an influential section of the tea industry opposed imports from the neighbouring country to South. There was, however, little opposition either here in this country or Sri Lanka for conducting their export marketing strategy rather than undercutting each other. But they ignored the advantages that could derive from cooperation. If they joined hands they could immediately increase world prices of tea. The point was they must jointly manage supply to international market side by side they had to work together to popularise this cheap beverage in western countries where promotion is costly. New Delhi, negotiated a strategy for joint marketing of tea with Colombo and Dhaka. The strategy aimed at joint ventures for blending and volue addition to make efforts of value added teas more profitable which is possible if only the major prodncers cooperated to manage supply.

Assam Psqyche and Tea Industry Need Pacification. A Healing Touch

For sometime the Government of Assam have been finding fault with the tea industry for not helping the State more for its socio-economic well being. Even the then Chief Minister himself had expressed his dissatisfaction at the celebration of ABITA, the Assam branch of the Indian Tea Association, pointing out that the sugar industry in Maharashtra had done so much for the rural areas there. A formal Press Release since issued by the Assam Government says *inter alia* : "The State Government has reminded time and again the dissatisfaction of all sections of the people over such attempts to ignore the State's larger interests finally culminating in the inclination of the Tata Tea Company to participate in the Haldia Petrochemicals of West Bengal with profits made out to Assam's tea without responding to Assam's industrial development which has been described by the people of Assam as a capitalistic exploitation design. The State Government has noticed more than one instance of large transfer of capital by Assam tea."

Non Traditional Tea Plantation Area Status For North Cachar

Tea Board declared the North Cachar hills district of Assam a " non-traditional area" for tea plantation.

Mr. M.K.Baruah, the then Chief Regional Executive of the Tea Board in Guwahati this disclosed in a seminar on tea. He said the concept of expansion of tea cultivation in non-traditional areas of the north-eastern region has gained ground. Many areas of high elevation, abundant rains and good soil in Arunachal Pradesh, Meghalaya, Manipur and Nagaland have already been identified. Of them, Arunachal Pradesh and Meghalaya have shown satisfactory progress. Meghalaya set up two nurseries in Umsing (Khasi Hills) and Rongram (Garo Hills). A scheme to encourage small growers by providing land and other support has already been introduced. The existing nurseries, in Arunachal Pradesh sat up with the assistance of Tea Board and private entrepreneurs showed bright prospect for tea production in India.

New Strategy To Boost Tea Export.

The Government prepared a strategy to increase the country's tea export to both rupee payment and general currency areas (GCA). Joint ventures for packaging and blending of teas on the lines of Tata Tea Ltd in the Commonwealth of Independent States (CIS) was encouraged. Besides Indian companies were told to participate in trade fairs and exhibitions in these states on a priority basis. In GCA, tieup arrangement was made with departmental stores as well as promotional campaigns through national airlines, brand promotion, besides more aggressive campaign through both print and electronic media. Visits by delegations to West Europe, West Asia and North Africa all major tea consuming countries were intensified. High level delegation visited some countries in this region in past two to three months.

Kerala Incentive to Tea Industry Sought by North-East India.

Leaders of tea industry in the country, Assam and West Bengal, approached their State governments to follow the example of Kerala which introduced an investment deposit scheme (IDS) under Agriculture Income Tax Act to encourage rejuvenation and modernisation of plantations. Under Kerala IDS, plantations were allowed a deduction of up to 20 percent from the previous year agricultural income. The amount so deducted was subject to the condition that if any withdrawal from the deposit was not utilised for the purpose for which it was sanctioned it should be treated as agricultural income of the year of withdrawal and assessed accordingly. The initiatives, according to Indian Tea Association, spoke of any Kerala Government's appreciation of the problems facing the plantation in securing additional land for fresh planting situation that reinforced the case for accepting replacement and rejuvenation within existing plantation. As this course for enhancing production and productivity implies medium term loss in crops, IDS, launched by Kerela a Goverment would serve to lower the effective overall rate of taxation on tea sector but also help in releasing additional internal funds for plough back. The overall, incidence of taxation on tea industry when compared with the burden on other industries, works out to 14 percent higher in Assam and 19 percent higher in West Bengal.

Tamil Nadu Plantation Extended

The Tea Board approved the proposal of the Tamil Nadu Tea Development Corporation for bringing an additional area of 3000 hectares under tea cultivation over a period of 1996-97. Out of this 2370 hectares were planted in Annamalai and the rest in Nilgiris.

Plantation Companies Plan to Market Packaged Tea

A number of companies owning tea plantation entered Rs. 2,000 crore packaged tea market soon. These companies were Haraison

Nalayalam Ltd. (HML), an RPG group company, and Premier Plantation, Ltd, a Poddar company, with its plantation in Kerala. Another company which entered the packaged tea market was Indiana Industries and it came out with a public issue for this purpose. Indian's tea unit in Kolkatta had a capacity to package 36 million kgs of tea. The project cost worked out to Rs 8.55 crore. The tea market is at present dominated by Brook Bond and its sister concern and Lipton and together they hold 60 per cent of the market. Premier plantation came out with a public issue to finance the acquistion of tea estates worked on lease. The Kerala-based company having its garden in the north of the state came with 36 lakh equity shares of Rs 10 each for cash at par. Premier tea processing plant could handle 20 lakh kgs per annum and plant and machinery in the processing plant was being modernised and upgraded. The company also acquired other business similar to its own. Indian used 29 sales depots and 1500 stockists to make it presence felt in the market.

Panel to Look into Tea Units

The Union Government reconstituted 30- member committee on tea industry with representatives from workers, planters, state and Central Governments to find out solutions to the problems faced by the industry. Sri P.A. Sanghma, the then union Minister of State for Labour, disclosed during his address in the 38th foundation day celebration of Assam Tea Plantation Provident Fund and Pension Scheme (ATPPF and PF) in Guwahati in September 1996. Sri Sangma regretted that only four to five percent of the gross domestic product (GDP) of the country is currently being spent on social security measures as against 20 percent in the developed countries. The ATPPF & PF Scheme launched in 1995 is the largest single industry social security scheme in Asia covering about 5 lakh laboures in 790 tea gardens in Assam with various schemes such as provident fund, penlion, life insurance and invalid pension. The scheme covered all tea gardens having an area of the 10 hectares and a labour force of 20.

Committee Mooted

The Commerce Ministry constituted a standing consultative committee on tea plantation in order to ensure better centre state coordination on matters relating to tea. The committee which is under the control of Commerce Ministry, includes representatives of State.

Centre and producer associations. It includes the Tea Board Chairman, and the State Secretaries of commerce and industry of tea producing states like Tripura, Tamil Nadu, Kerala, Assam, West Bengal etc. The committee could project the genuine grievances and needs of the industry towards persuading policy makers to cut across controversies and differences which often stem from attaching political considerations to economic problems.

Subsidy Scheme for Infilling

The tea industry submitted to the government a subsidy scheme to encourage infilling as a measure to increase production from land under cultivation. The industry opined that infilling of land gaps between the existing row of bushes could raise the crop size within three to five years. At present subsides are available for new plantation, rejuvenation and extension of existing plantation.

Teas and Ease in Nilgiris

After successful launch of Assam and Darjeeling lgos in Britain, tea gardens down South captured the imagination of British tea drinkers. The gardens of Nilgiri beckoned Englishmen not just for a cup of tea but an adventure-filled holiday of fun and floral. Thanks to Union Ministry of Tourism, the South Indian tea estates offered a round the year package holiday to British travellers beginning in the autumn. The idea, an original brain child of Ministry of Tourism, is not just aimed at exploiting the "Raj Nostalgia" of the average Englishman but also boosting exports of South Indian tea in Britain. A special advantage of introducing this kind of package tour was for travellers visiting the estates any time of the year. It also provides an opportunity of experiencing the entire process of tea making in the garden even as they sip their steaming cups of Nilgiris special. Yet the package not only offered visits to tea garden alone but also included charmed woods of Nilgiris and golfing at the famous course of Ooty, Wellington and Coorg. Under the package travellers from Britain were offered accommodation at the garden itself. The entire effort of the ministry aimed at promoting this concept in Britain. For this, a major media campaign assignment was given to Hindustan Thomson and Associate (HTA). Following the success of the South Indian package, similar promotional efforts were launched for the tea gardens of Assam, Darjeeling Manipur, Skkim etc.

Two Gardens Merge with Brooke Bond

Doom Dooma India and Tea Estate India Ltd. were merged with Brooke Bond India Ltd. (BBIL). All three companies were subsidiaries of the Unilever group. Unilever group had 74 percent stake each in Doom Dooma and Tea Estate as well as 40 percent in Broke Bond. After the merge Unilever Stake in Brooke Bond increased to 49.9 percent. Apart from enabling unilever to considerate its position in the tea industry, the merger gave Brooke Bond access to the huge cash surplus with the two companies. As a result BBIL restricted its borrowin. The merge ensured synergy as Brooke Bond was able to utilise 30 percent of production of the two plantation companies to blend the teas it produces. The merger turned the Brooke Bond into a bigger and healthier outfit which helped to have stable earnings and to compete in the market place in a more cost effective manner.

The Tea Traders Renew First Point Sales Tax demand

The tea trade requested the West Bengal Government over the years to replace the multi point Sale Tax (S.T.) with a first point tax. In a renewed effort to bring the State Government. round to their view, the Siliguri Tea Auction Committee (STAC) pointed out to the Commissioner of Commercial Taxes that all tea growing states in

South India are levying a first point ST. The STAC reiterated tea industry's argument that a first point ST will make collection more easy causing less harassment to trade than under the current multi-point levy. South Kerala has a first point ST of 5 percent and Karnataka and Tamil Nadu of six percent. Producers find a first point ST more acceptable than the multi-point tax even for packet tea and ex-garden sales simply because it means so much less paper work. Commercial tax officers have always resisted replacing the multi point tax with a first point levy on the ground that this will result in lower renewal. On the contrary, STAC feels that with about 300 producers and 10 brokers, collection will be assured and quick. It also claims that renewal will be more with fewer staff needed to collect it.

Tea Control Order Not To Be Relaxed

The Commerce Ministry ruled out the possibility of relaxing or repealing Tea (Marketing) Control Order promulgated in 1984. The order, which makes it mandatory for tea producers to sell 75 per cent of their total production through auction centres has been operating satisfactorily and no changes are necessary. The producers want the order scrapped, while the brokers and merchant-exporters prefer status quo. The ministry facilitated f.o.b. sale of Indian tea at the London auction.

Export Licensing Order Changed

The Government decision to repeal certain clauses of Tea of Regulation Export Licensing Order (TRELO) was overturned by the Tea Board. The Board decided that exporters wishing to use its logo accompanied with words like "Pure Indian Tea" should get their packets approved by it. The Commerce Ministry had recently dispensed with the necessity of the Board clearance. The 1984 order made it obligatory for exporters to have their packet approved by the Board in order to ensure packaging of international quality and checking under in voicing by exporters. The Board wants to ensure that its image is not sullied. It also desires to ascertain that those who use logos like Darjeeling Tea, Assam Tea and Niglgiris Tea actually export this item.

Concern At More To Curb Tea Board Activities

The Center moves to transfer some Tea Board development scheme to financial institutions created panic among some people. The Commerce Ministry proposed the Board to absent itself from the responsibility of executing some schem like 'A tea plantation finance loan scheme', 'A machinery and irrigation equipment hire purpose scheme' and 'A new tea unit financing scheme for non-traditional areas'. The brisk expansion of financing activity threw up the idea of single-window financing agency and in 1985 the Government brought in NABARD to finance the development of gardens in Darjeeling. The World Bank provided Rs. 43 core for the development of gardens in Darjeeling at the same time NABARD entered tea financing. A10-years scheme was drafted in this regard.

Economy-Ecology Sacks

The advent of paper packages in early 1990's at the auctions in Kolkata was a matter of pride. The lesser important producers like Bangladesh, Malawi, Sri Lanka, China have extensively introduced these sophisticated, hi-tech packages suitable for tea. It was with considerable enthusiasm that the industry graded B & A Sacks indigenous venture that also gave it the distinction of being the fifth or sixth manufacturer of paper packages suitable for tea in the world. Sri. Narendra Kumar, the then Chairman of CCPA, pointed out, plywood chests, that have traditionally packed teas, have been adding to deforestation of Assam. It is ecology, convenience and economy. The paper can withstand the normal rough manual handling in its stride. It would no be able to sharp 'Poeking'. More importantly, there would be no deterioration of quality of tea in package. Nor would sampling pose problems. Samples could be drawn from any portion of the package that is easily resealable with self-adhesive BOPP sealing tapes.

Assam State Electricity Board (ASEB) Starts Electrification of Labour Lines of Tea Gardens

The ASEB launched a scheme to electrify all labour lines in pursuance of the resolution of the State Standing Committee on Labour. According to the scheme, the supply of power to living quarters of the labourers improber and needed to be streamlined priority basis. The fund for the purpose was available from "Rural Electrification Corporation".

Tea Industry Wants Transit Insurance Policy Reviewed

The tea industry drew the Centre attention to the problem it faced while insuring the crop under the present Crop Insurance Policy which covered all risks right from the time of plucking the leaves to arrival of the processed tea at warehouses. Yet this policy was not realistic enough in the present context as it does not provide cover against pest attack and natural calamities such as drought and floods etc. Before the introduction of the policy, one had the choice to insure crops against hail storms, damage in storage and damage in transit separately.

Tea Industry's Status Elevated

The inter governmental group on tea accorded the status of an international commodity body by the Food and Agricultural Organization during the former's ninth conference held in Rome from October 7 to 10, 1991. The status allowed inter-governmental group to ask for financial assistance from common funds. This facilitated the groups' endeavour in promoting tea in hitherto untapped areas and allowed for research mainly into the health aspects often compared to other beverages and thereby lead to greater consumption and sale. The eight-member team led by Shri. P. K. Bora, the then Chairman of Tea Board had gone to the United Kingdom, Ireland and Poland to explore the possibilities of more export and to allay fears that India may fail to deliver the amount to tea required for international consumption, Shri P.K.Bora said Indian tea would be produced for export, changing the prevalent conservative "*residual approach*" *policy to a* "*production for export*". *The delegation got a great response from the authorities in the countries it visited, especially the U.K.*

Tea In Paper Sacks

The Bureau of Indian Standards (BIS) prepared and circulated a draft specification for finalisation of the use of multiwall paper sacks for tea packaging. The Tea Research Association (TRA) strongly recommended in favour of the paper sacks after carrying out extensive tests. Aluminium (Al) foil laminated inner-ply paper sack for bulk packaging of tea was introduced in the country at the Guwahati tea auction centre. The technology of the plant was provided by DRG Sacks of U.K. which first developed the Al-foil laminated inner-ply paper sack. All African countries, Sri Lanka, Indonesia, China and even Bangladesh have been using paper sacks now for packaging teas though it was somewhat new in India. The gaining of acceptance of paper sack in tea industry all over the world can be gauged from the fact that about 80 per cent of the total tea arriving in the U.K. at present is in the paper sacks. Other Western countries too are insistinghon paper sacks.

Inauguration of First Certificate Course in Tea Tasting

The Institute of Plantation Management organized a programme on "quality evaluation of tea through tasting skill". Neither most sophisticated technology nor most efficient systems can spell success on their own. It is the human resources. The competence and ability to perceive and act that has the pivotal role towards epitomising results. Suffice it to recall the words of wisdom of two great industrialists of 20th Century viz. Mr. Henry Ford-II of USA and doyen of Indian industry, late J.R.D. Tata, on the need for planned and on-going development of executive resource. Institute of Plantation Management in India (IPMI) has been entrusted the test of promoting knowledge and skill improvement of the persons already in employment or of those aspiring to take up career in plantation segment. It devises integrated programmes of training and instructions in the relevant agronomical, technical and management disciplines. The training does not remain confined to academic subjects or principles and practices of management but also includes enlarging of thinking and perceiving faculties of the individuals. The institute aims at broadening the intellectual and conceptual horizons of the trainers, besides building up their professional and managerial aptitude. The institute has emerged as a change agent and is instrumental in changing the outlook of this traditional segment by ushering in the scientific and productivity-oriented techniques and new management philosophy.

Planters Sign MoU with Hill Council

Darjeeling Planters' Association (DPA) signed a memorandum with the Gorkha Hill Council and nine other tea plantation workers' unions. Under the MoU which was in operation for three years till March 31, 1993, workers extended their cooperation in increasing the productivity of Darjeeling gardens. The unions rendered all necessary assistance to achieve optimum productivity and agreed to eight hours' duty in the tea gardens. The unions also recommended that owners exert their authority to ensure that all workers discharged their duties. To begin with the local body of the association interacted with all planters on a garden-wise basis for implementation of the MoU. The MoU created an awareness among the various trade unions in Darjeeling of the need to raise productivity.

Tea Board Scheme on Hire Purchase Equipment

In the interest of the tea industry the Tea Board had drawn up a scheme known a Tea Machinery and Irrigation Equipment Hire Purchase Scheme. The Board informed the apex industry association about persistent default in payment of Board's dues under that scheme. The Board requested the association of estate to persuade the defaulting members to clear the arrear amount at the earliest.

Consequent on the increase in the rate of interest on the government loan to Tea Board, the Board enhanced the rest of interest on the loans advanced under Tea Machinery and Irrigation Equipment Highre Purchase Scheme. Accordingly the existing rates were revised upwards.

Extension of Machinery Hire Purchase Scheme

The Board recommended the extension of benefits under Tea Machinery and Hire Purchase Scheme to tea estates that do not have processing capacity and were getting green leaf processed by other gardens within the same company or group. The extension benefited estates that did not avail the facility of the scheme because they did not have manufacturing capacity themselves. The Board received as many as 250 applications annually for loans under the schemes out of 13,000 tea estates in the country, only 1892 have factories where tea produced in other garden are processed. The scheme provides supply of tea machinery and irrigation equipment to tea factories and gardens on a deferred payment basis. The total value of equipment to any one tea estate or factory is Rs. 20 lakh, 14 lakh, Rs. 10 lakh each for each for machinery and irrigation equipment. The government enhanced the ceiling limit to Rs. 25 lakh from Rs.10 lakh at present.

New Exicse Forms for Applications For Registration

Pursuant to Finance Ministry notification No. 11/92, under new dispension of laws, the provision relating to licensing was replaced by the provision for registration of assessees accordingly. The new rule 174 (I) empowered the Central Board of Excise and Customs to specify the forms for "Application for registration and registration certificate". The Board drew up the forms for both purpose mentioned above and same are available at zonal collectorate.

Tea Board Survey of Tripura units

Tea Board conducted a techno-economic survey of tea industry in

Tripura which was a reappraisal of the earlier survey conducted in 1975. The survey recommended that Tea Board, State and the Central Government should take immediate steps to improve the present deteriorating conditions of the industry that earns much needed foreign exchange and employs 15000 workers in 6000 hectares of land.

Revised Norms For Consultancy Subsidy for New Units

Tea Board launched a subsidy to encourage setting up of new tea plantations on a commercial scale in non-traditional areas. The scheme provides for subsidizing the cost of preparing technically feasible and viable project reports as required under the New Tea Unit Finance Scheme of the Board. Since preparation of such projects requires considerable experience and expertise the entrepreneurs have been allowed to avail of the services of the approved consultants. The Board meets consultancy charge to the extent of 75 percent subject to a maximum of Rs 2 lakh for each of the project that has been found bankable and admitted for financing. New Tea Unit Finance Scheme (NTUFS) may retain the services of the consultants till such the loan is fully repaid. Keeping in view the desirability of retaining the services, the consultancy fees were disbursed in six instalments. First instalment is given at the rate of 25 percent of eligible amount after sanction of tea project by the Board under NTUFS. The balance sanctioned amount is be released in five equal annual instalment.

Participation In Fairs and Exhibitions in WANA Countries

Tea Board participated in the Damascus international fair since it was felt that Syria had a lot of scope of export of Indian teas, particularly packeted teas. Other events in WANA regions in which Tea Board participated during 1992-93 were Tehran international fair and Cairo international fair. Exporters sent their range of products well in advance for display/sale during these events.

Tea Board Opened Office at Moscow

The Board opened office at Moscow to recapture the markets of Commonwealth of Independent States [CIS]. The tea industry set up joint ventures of packaging and blending of tea on the lines of Tata Tea venture in Russia and other states of former Soviet Union. It entered into tie-ups with departmental stores and launched promotional campaigns through national airlines and more a aggressive campaign through both print and electronic media. Visits by delegations to West Europe, West Asia and North Africa, all major tea-consuming area was intensified. Two high level delegations visited some of the countries in these regions.

Darjeeling Tea Festival

Nevertheless, a large Indian consignment participated in the tea-cum-tourism festival co-sponsored by the departments of Tourism of the Centre and the state, the Darjeeling Gorkha Hill Council (D G H C) and Darjeeling Tea Planter's Association. These idea of having a festival where tourism would be promoted in the "Visit India Year" with tea as one of the highlights was first mooted in 1990 by the then Director General of Tourism Shir B.K. Goswami, who was also the former Chairman of Tea Board. The festival programme was a package which included items of interest for foreign tourist as well as the disceming tea imparters. A mock auction was billed and its proceeds were used for charitable purposes. An assorted fare of a football match was organized by the Sports Authority of India's sponsored by the Himalayan Mountaineering Institute.

Policy for Tea Export Oriented Units (EOUS)

Under the export-import policy for 1992-97, units undertaking to export their products may be set up under (EOU) or Export processing zone (EPZ) as out lined in Chapter-IX of Export-Import Policy, 1992-97. The Tea Board recommended the case of setting up of EOU Scheme by any unit with the proposal of importing tea by the said EOUs subject to compliance of the conditions like (i) export of tea blended with imported téa should be exported only in value added form, (ii) export of value added teas should be made only hard, currreny (iii) no sale of DTA Domestic Tariff Area by the said EOU1EPZ unit is to be permitted (iv) packets etc. containing imported tea should not be allowed to used marketing symbol of Tea Board (v) approval of such packets without marketing symbols should be obtained from Tea Board before export takes place. (vi) collector of Customs and Central Excise concerned should, provide bonding facilities for the factory premises including transit bond for the purpose of goods being taken from the port of importation to the factory prmises of 100 per cent EOU in question, (vii) monthly report of the import-export to be submitted to the Ministry of Commerce-J.C.C.I & E with a copy to Tea Board and (viii) to comply with all other export formalities of Tea Board and Govt. of India in this regard. Meanwhile market reactions indicated that export of tea in bulk form was short for 100 per cent EOUS.

Tourism Festival

With a view to attracting tourists to the state, the Assam Tourism Department in collaboration with certain tour operators and tea industry held a 'Tea Tourism Festival' from December 26, 1996. The department could not. however, make much of an impact because of the shortage of time and lack of publicity. Even though requirement of restricted area permits was removed from the state more than two years back to attract foreign tourists, the department did not have any figure that could indicate how much the state had benefited. According to state Forest officials, more than 2500 foreign tourist visited Kaziranga National Park.

Assam Tea Industry To Keep 20 Percent Profit to Fund State Projects

The tea industry in Assam set up 20 percent of its agricultural profit to build up a fund for special cell in the Assam Industrial Development Corporation (AIDC) or a separate body of investment in industrial and infrastructural projects in the state. This profit was entrusted to the Tea professional management which utilized the fund within seven years. The AIDC on new set up was responsible for identifying projects and taking investment decisions. The fund thus created was in the order of Rs 15 crore per year. The average annual profit of the tea industry in Assam during the last five years was Rs 120 crore 60 percent of total profit is considered as agricultural profit (Rs 72 crore) and 20 percent of this is Rs. 15 crore per annum. Shri H.P. Barooah, the then Chairman of Indian Tea Association outlined that tea industry in Assam is subject to heavy taxation in the form of 45 percent plus a surcharge of 15 percent as central corporation tax applicable on 40 percent of income and 75 percent as agricultural income tax on the remaining 60 percent of profit. Thus the cumulative tax burden on the industry is 65.70 percent as against 51.75 percent in case of other industry.

Assam Government Considered Tax Exemption for Tea Industry In The Lines of Kerala Scheme

Under the scheme the industry is allowed to set aside 20 percent of its profit for reinvestment in tea and development of tea industry within stipulated time. Shri Barooah stressed the need to 1) remove the Marketing Central Order 2) improve quality at the expense of quantity, 3) restore subsidies to boost tea plantation, 4) intensify marketing publicity, and 5) advocate more active participation by the industry in all trade fairs in West Asia.

Assam Tea Industry In Dire Straits

High production costs, government fiscal measures and land policy, acutre shortage of managerial manpower and deteriorating soil-climate environment are threatening the prospects of tea industry. The contributed initiation Central and State governments to mop up profit restricted the long-term growth of the industry as suggested by Chairman ABITA. Instead of sharply raising agricultural income tax, imposing price controls and various forms of cess, export restrictions and sale regulation, the government allow a proper scope for internal generation of funds to the turn of Rs 800 crore out of the total requirement of Rs. 1500 crore to achieve the targeted production in 2000 year.

The First World Tea Convention

The first ever world convention on tea in the United Kingdom was held in May 1990 to examine 'internationally the image of tea'. The convention discussed (1) how do the emerging conditions affect Britain's role and its significant impact on the supply and demand equation? (2) With the key role of producer countries' auctions what role the London auction would play which is the only international auction? (3) How will the European challenge of 1992 affect this British market? The UK market came under close scrutiny and financial services in relation to tea. The other areas of analytical study covered the role of brands within the tea markets pluse the question of generation of generic promotion. The role of catering tea in the UK received close attention as well as advertising and health. The convention emphasised the following aspects :- (a) Tea is a healthy (drink). Everyone has a degree of health consciousness. The consciousness is growing. (b) Tea is natural. It has no additive, artificial colouring or preservatives. (c) It is suitable for all occasion. It refreshes when we are hot warm when we are cold, relaxes when we are tired, calms when we are stressed and cuts across all barriers. (d) It is both economically important and environmentally acceptable. The convention encompassed all aspects of tea with promotions and public relations programmes aimed at the consumer.

Tripura Tea Industry In Doldrums

Lack of funds, bottleneck in transport, absentee landlordism, prevalence of indifferent and non-professional existence of managements and dearth of technical know-how are the main problems facing the tea industry in Tripura. As a result, the 53 tea gardens covering 6,481 hectares produce 531kgs of tea perhectare which is lower than national average. On an average, the state produces 3.5 million kgs annually which represents only 0.5 percent of the country's production. The state, has, however, the potential to increase yield to over 2,000 kgs per hectare. According to Techn-Economic Survey of Tripura is tea industry, growing of tea bushes from different stock, absence of appropriate tea husbandry, non-application of required inputs and inadequate replantation, inadequacy of processing machinery together with out-moded plant and machinery were common in the state. The cumulative affect of these factors was that the tea gardens were incapable of producing sufficient internal resources causing heavy indebtedness. Most of the units could not avail of the benefits of term finance for development activities.

Planters Failed to Match The Target Levels of Production

While addressing the 70th annual general meeting of Terai Indian Planters' Association at Matinga near Siliguri, the then West Bengal Minister for Food and Supplies, amended that the tea planters in the country had 'failed' to match the target level of production. With this trend the target of production of 1000 million kgs by could not be fulfilled. He also said since land was limited, emphasis should be laid on research so that more tea could be produced on available land . He appreciated that striking results had been achieved in the field of production and productivity of tea due to research efforts undertaken under the auspices of the two main tea research organisations.

Indian Tea Planters' Association (ITPA) Upset

The ITPA was upset following the withdrawal of investment deposit scheme and development allowance by the centre. The ITPA appraised then Union Commerce Minister, Shri Arun Nehru, that when plans were on to retain more funds for use in the industry the investment deposite schemes and development allowance were withdrawn. The ITPA said the industry found it difficult to mop up its own resources because of the existing differential and disparity with other industries in respect of tax burden by about 10 percent.

Centre Asks Assam government to Protect Tea Manage And Workers

The then Union Commerce Minister, Shri Arun Nehru, told Parliament that he had spoken to the then Assam Chief Minister to take steps for safeguarding the interest of tea garden owners and workers so that tea industry of Assam is allowed to grow unhampered.

Gujrat Invitation of Planters

Tea planters have been invited by Gujarat Government to explore possibilities of growing tea in South Gujrat. The State Government had promised to provide all possible assistance in this connection. The invitation came through the then State Food and Supplies Minister when he was addressing the second annual general meeting of All Indian Tea Traders' Association held in Ahmedabad. He asserted that the *Bulsar and Dang regions* of south Gujarat areas were very suitable for growing tea.

Tea cultivation in Uttar Pradesh

The Uttar Pradesh Government initiated Rs 24-crore scheme for tea cultivation in Chamoli, Pauri, Dehradun, Almora and Kausani (nonw in Uttaranchal). The scheme was financed through Jawahar Rozgar Yojna, Tea Board and the State Government efforts were made to farm Uttarkhand Tea Development Corporation and to set up a tea purchasing unit at Chamwat.

Two Cooperative Tea Factories in the Nilgiris District

At a cost of Rs. 5 crore, two more industrial cooperative tea factories were constructed in the Nilgiris district, announced the Tamil Nadu Rural Industries Minister. Then those factories were commissioned in 1995.

Modernisation of Hanuman Tea's project

It was learnt that the Hanuman Tea Co. Ltd initiated a scheme for packet tea project. The company entered the capital market with a right issue of four lakh equity shares of Rs 10 each at par.

Two New Brands From Esquire Tea

It was learnt that the Esquire Tea Plantation and Industries Ltd introduced in Maharashtra two new brand soft tea named 'Richmond' and 'Macmillan' with the intention of marketing them in rural areas. The company produced five new brands. The packaging unit is located at Daman.

Effect Of Increased Acidity Of The Soil

UPASI Tea Advisory Services reported that increases in acidic conditions of the soil increase the solubility of elements like, aluminium copper, iron, manganese, and zinc resulting in high concentration of these substances in the plants and causing serious injury to the plants. Also, large quantities of the macro nutrients like potash are leached to the lower depths due to ready solubility creating deficiency levels in the soil. It has further, been emphasized that extreme acid condition of the soil makes the bacterial activity slow is respect of nitrogen fixation and conversion of plant organic matter of humus.

Combined Use of Dicofol and Ethion

UPASI Tea Research Institute experimented the effect of combined application of Dicofol and Ethion at reduced dosage in tea. Five hundred ml each of the two acaricides were mixed and applied with hand operated knapsack sprayer in randomized block. The spray volume was Rs 400 ml per ha. The efficiency of this mixture stands as same to that of Ethion 50 EC or Dicolfoi 18.5 EC applied individually at the rate of 1000 ml per ha. Obviously, the residues of both the acaricides on tea could be kept low by mixing these chemicals at reduced dosage although controlling of mile, will, in no way, be affected.

Shipment of Indigenous Consumer Packs

Without any import content of teas, shipment of indigenous consumer packs from the country amounted to 107 million kgs annually during 1992-2005. Shipment of such consumer packs stood at merely 10 million kgs annually during 1907-2005. This indicated a remarkable growth in the export of indigenous consumer packs over the years.

Goodricke Group's Performance

Goodricke Group Limited was present in West Asia in the field of packaging and marketing of tea, reported Mr P.A.Leggatt the then chairman, at the company's 18th annual general meeting. Goodricke teas established a stronger position in the U.K., Germany and Japan. The crop harvested from the company's estates was 22.78 million kg annually during 1997-2002 compared to annual production of 20.15 million kg during 1992-1997. However it was informed that three of the group's gardens suffered substantial loss of crop due to hailstorms in the early part of 1999. A modern state of the art tea processing unit at Chulsi commenced operations during the year 1992. The unit replaced an 80-year-old factory which was gutted by a fire in early 1991 and had a capacity of 2 million kgs of made tea. The company emphasized on exports and this was reflected in the rise in foreign exchange earnings from Rs 10.87 crore to Rs 25.35 crore over the periods.

Peerless, Tata Tea for Barter with Russia

Tata Tea and the Peerless group separately negotiated with a Russian party for exporting a variety of goods not supported by technical credit. The basic idea was to formulate a barter arrangement under which goods were exported to Russia against items like potash and mineral resources from that country. Tea was totally absent or constituted just a small part of the export consignment by the Indian companies. However, the question emerged whether such barter agreements its the approval of the government. The immediate problem with this kind of trade was fixing the landed price of the imports. Earlier the International Monetory Fund had opposed such trading plans between developing countries. The Government simply took the initiative to bail out industries that had been trading with Russia. At the moment there was euphoria among the Indian tea companies after the Commerce Minister's promise to sanction technical credit for tea and coffee.

Tea Workers Threaten Strike

The coordination committee of tea plantation workers of West Bengal, at a meeting on April 10, 1994 launched an indefinite strike at tea gardens in Dooars, Terai and Darjeeling as the 25 point charter of demands submitted by the committee in July 1993 was not fulfilled. Meanwhile, the West Bengal Labour Minister held a meeting with the representative of tea planters' organizations and central trade unions working in tea plantation in West Bengal State Electricity Board at Siliguri to review the process under the electrification scheme in and around tea plantation worker accommodations in the tea estates of West Bengal.

Tea Planters Urged to Reinvest in West Bengal

At a meeting in Kolkata on 19th April, 1994, then the Minister for Commerce and Industry Govt. of West Bengal said that although the tea garden owners in the state had been earning huge profits they were not ploughing back even a portion of their income for the development of the sector. He said, the Government was willing to offer additional incentives and facilities to the tea garden owners if they reinvest part of their profit in the state.

Tea Leaves Remove Lead From Effluent

Scientists from the Harcourt Butler Technological Institute, Kanpur, reported in the Indian Journal of Environmental Health that chemically treated used tea leaves can serve as a viable, low cost absorbent to remove lead from aqueous solutions. The team also studies the adsorption capacity of various metal ions and concluded that tea leaves showed maximum adsorption with lead ions, followed by mercury cadmium nickel and copper ions.

Garden Demanding Darjeeling Logo

Sire tea gardens —Ambiok, Samabeong, Mission hill, Kumai of Kalimpong sub-division and simulbarie, Marionbarie of Kurseong sub-division members of the Darjeeling Planters' Association demanded the permission to use the Darjeeling logo. These gardens were denied the use of the logo when it was introduced by the industry and the Tea Board as a measure to ensure the quality of Darjeeling tea in the export market.

Tea Majors For Food Processing in Assam

Three major companies Williamson Magar, Tata Tea, the Assam tea mong several tea companies diversified into food processing deals with the Assam Industrial Development Corporation (AIDC) to set up 100 percent food processing joint venture EOUs in the state. The first of these projects were 300 million tonnes per year must room cultivation and processing unit with technology from the Netherlands at a cost of Rs 20 crore. The projects came up at Amin Nagar near Guwahati. The second project was banana processing plant located at Goalpara at a cost of Rs 4 crore with U.S. technology. The plant has a capacity of 4 million tonnes per year. In these projects AIDC and the private sector promoters had 50 percent stake each.

Tea in 'New Foundland'

Tea is 'gaining ground' in Laloo's land. The first tea garden in Bihar came up in Kishangunj district. The garden in run by Daftari tea estate private limited and employs about 500 workers. About eight lakh kg of tea is produced every year.

Target Set For Middle Course

To attain the ultimate objective of 1000 million kgs of tea production by 2000, phased production progress was outlined. The production target for 1998 was at 800 million kgs when domestic consumption and export demand were 640 million kgs, and 160 million kgs, respectively.

Packing Factory by Brooke Bond?

A tea blending and packing factory in Assam at cost of around Rs. 5 crore was set up by Brooke Bond India Limited. It was mentioned here, the premier tea company had no tea blending and packaging units in Assam. The company entered in this area as it was increasingly felt that such a set-up had immensely benefited the company in terms of strategical location advantage and also enabled it to further strengthen its presence in the valueadded tea sector, both in India and abroad. Brooke Bond had at its disposal tea produced by the three estates of Doom Dooma, all located in the state of Assam. Perhaps the company weighed its proposal in view of the fact that the state is in prominent position as a tea producer and Guwahati is a major auction centre.

For Mutual Benefit

After playing politics for a long period of time Sri Lanka at last realized the economic prominence of its next door giant neighbours and big brother, India. The India-Sri Lanka Joint Business Council (JBC) reached a broad agreement on joint promotion in the area of tea and tourism and greater exchange of information among the chambers of commerce and other such organization. The Sri Lanka delegation pointed out adverse balance of trade and urged for more purchase from their country. It pleaded for more Indian investment flow into Sri Lanka and more joint ventures. Anything from India was welcome to Sri Lanka except perhaps the 'IPKF'.

Tea For Farmer Czechoslovakia

Indian officials worked out details of a new trade agreement based on hard currency with Czechoslovakia republics, nearly eliminating barter trade with the East Europeans. The two arrangement, which were identical in language and intent, were initiated in the last week of November 1992 in Prague and Bratisiave, opening the way for a new commercial relationship. The former Czechoslovakia was the last East European country to end barter trade based on local currencies with India. Economic changes in both India and eastern Europe the old style of trading, nearly ended. Thus, the new agreements left the door open for barter. The Indian delegation ironed out ways to settle the balanced of rupees nearly 600 crore in favour of the Czechoslovakia which had accumulated under the previous trade regime. The fluctuating exchange rates added to the problem and the split of Czechoslovakia further complicated the issue. A "liquidation regime" was signed that allowed India to send goods to the two countries to settle the balance of rupees. The change over in the trading system had a negative impact in the initial stages on the amount of trade between the two sides. There was a transition period in the farmer east block nations before the policy changes came into effect. Governments in the region had balance between opening their economies to foreign investors and implementing the necessary laws to effect the changes. The new trade agreement helped the situation somewhat as the private sector plays a greater role.

Light For The Tea Labour Quarters

On Monday September 27,1993, the then Minister for labour, Government of West Bengal, informed that the employees and labourers of tea gardens in the Darjeeling and Dooars area were provided with the facility of electricity for their quarters, not available so far. This decision was taken at a meeting of the representatives of the tea garden owners, managements, trade unions, and the high officials of the State Electricity Board with the then Minister for Labour. Most of the managements of 262 tea gardens covering Darjeeling and Dooars implemented the electrification project. The State Electricity Board took the responsibility of giving electricity lines to the gardens. And the expenditure on connecting the lines with quarters, wiring etc was born by the tea garden owners. The State Electricity Board finished the job by December, 1993. Tea garden managements also extended a their whole hearted efforts in this matter.

Project Of Tea Cultivation in Meghalaya

The tea research station at Jarhat Assam had found from the soil tests that Meghhalaya can produce quality tea, comparing Darjeeling tea in flavour. Being convinced, the State Government had allotted several plots of land in Ri-Bhoi district for tea cultivation. The State Government had also constituted a permanent expert committee, with a farmer tea planter as its chairman.

Notable Improvement of GTAC

Guwahati Tea Auction Center (GTAC) in a span of 28 years, emerged as the world's largest etc. tea auction centre. From selling a mere 2.75 million kgs of tea in 1970, its annual sales at present exceed 195 million kgs. The total membership of the centre stood at about 950 comprising 600 tea estates, 285 buyers, 15 brokers and warehouse keepers. The GTAC primarily caters domestic market. With a view to participating in auctions actively, buyers from all over the country have set up offices here. The State Government is expected to earn over Rs. 15 crore from sales. Tax alone from the auction sales in the internal market. And the value of sales of from export is being estimated at Rs 150 crore annually.

Flood Relief by SVBITA

The Surma Valley Branch of India Tea Association arranged for adequate relief for the flood victims in Catcher and Hilakandi districts of Assam. Medicines worth Rs 30,000 were donated by Pathermara and Doyapara tea estates. Members of the Hilakandi circle distributed

1600 food packets to Indian Red Cross for distribution to flood victims.

Land Grabbing Protested in North Bengal

A tea nursery in Fumarika Tea Estate near Islampur in North Bengal was set on fire on March 5, 1995 for the second time. Jayshree Tea Company, owner of the nursery, had incurred a substantial loss due to rampage on that day. Thousands of tea bushes were uprooted, a nursery gutted and equipment was (generators and sheds), destroyed. The background to all this was the growing resentment over mushrooming of tea gardens in the area. Largely dependant on agriculture, people in the area said that agriculture produce per big ha in the area was quite high. And hence, large-scale encroachments upon agricultural land by tea gardens instigated the farmers to react adversely. They started filling up high drains laid for the purpose of irrigating tea gardens which was detrimental to farming because it caused the water level to go down. The Duncan Tea Estates got permission to start a tea garden projects in north Dinapur in 1991. The State Government later confirmed that others could also obtain no objection certificate by adhering to the guideline. It however specified that tribal land, land for deep tubewells and high-yielding agricultural land were avoided to obtain a certification. But tea companies flouted all guidelines, local residents alleged. There were different opinions as to the exact number of tea gardens in Islampur subdivision that did not possess no-objection certificate. But the gardens that had spring up enjoyed the advantage of irrigated water being situated in the Testa Command Area.

Industry To Improve yield

Addressing the 78th Annual General Meeting of Indian Tea Planter's Association, the then Minister of State incharge of municipal affairs Mr. Ashok Bhattacharjee, the chief guest, told the planters that the nation could not afford to leave the tea industry lose its importance not only as major provider of employment but also as a major foreign exchange eamer. In West Bengal, he said more than 2,00,000 workers earned their livelihood from the tea industry besides 7000 more were directly or indirectly employed in the activities, related to the tea industry. He pointed out that the industry so far paid little attention to research and development for improving yield from the plantation and bringing down prices. He advised the planters to direct maximum attention to this aspect of industrial activity.

West Bengal Budget, 1995-96

(1) Turnover Ta abolished, (2) Entry Tax abolished, (3) Rate of tax on inter-State dispatch of tea purchased from Siliguri and Calcutta auction centres will be uniform 2 per cent for the next year in place of the existing rates of 2 per cent and 3 per cent,(4) Sales Tax on jute goods reduced from 12 per cent to 4 per cent. (5) Reduction in Agricultural Income Tax not to effect tea. (6) 10 per cent surcharge on Sales Tax introduced, Rate of Sale Tax on fertilisers and pesticides reduced from 5 per cent to 4 per cent. (7) Basic Sale Tax rate on tea reduced from 7 percent to 4 percent. The comncessional rate of sale tax on tea brought down from 2 percent to 1 percent for re-sellers, and from 3 percent to 2 percent for manufacturers, with effect from May 1, 1995.

Consumer Choice of Tea

Consumers in the north India prefer leaf tea. South Indians prefer dust tea, as it gives a strong liquor. Dust tea is also used in the tea shops in Gujarat, Maharashtra and parts and Rajasthan. The growth in the market for branded packaged tea is much higher in the rural areas than that in the urban market. Available information indicated that the three major players in both rural and urban markets were (1) Brooke Bond (2) Lipton and (3) Tata Tea.

Elephant Menance in Tea Gardens

The forest development records revealed that since 1987, around 53 people, on an average, were killed by wild animals in the north Bengal forests. Most of the incidents occured however, in the tea gardens which are mostly situated in the remote parts of Jalpaiguri and Darjeeling districts, surrounded by dense forests and hilly rivers. Although many of these gardens had achieved glorious record for this performance, production and prices of tea, wild elephants, menace in the gardens caused high depredations. The elephants had not only killed workers and injured many but had also caused unaccountable loss of property, destroying in the pucca and kutcha labour quarters, the bushes and shade trees. The unabated destruction by wild elephants had caused a sense of insecurity and panic amongst the inhabitants of the gardens and the gardens' normal work was affected to a great extent. It was said " during the last 3 years", about 9 workers, including women and babies, were killed by wild elephants and about 50 pucca and over 200 kutcha labour quarters were razed to ground. Recently, on March 30,1995, as many as 5 labour houses were demolished by the pachyderms". Every year the gardens have to spend a huge amount to repair the damages caused by wild elephants and unless a concrete step from the Government is taken, it is "quite impossible to save the gardens from the depredation". Moreover, in view of the alarming situation the garden authority is seriously thinking to the extend any further plantation area though there was much scope for such extension due to surplus land available to the garden.

Energised Fences To Tackle Elephants

With repeated incidents of wild elephants and leopard entering tea gardens in the Jalpaiguri and the Malbazar area in recent times, the Forest Department of the government of Wet Bengal for the first time took the trouble in implementing measures to protect human habitation in the affected gardens. The State Forest and Environment Department installed energised tences around their labour colonies and commissioned solar lamps in the huts and paths 10 tea gardens in north Bengal. The Department subsequently took up other projects. Other gardens followed the footsteps.

Mujani Tea Estate To Reopens

Mujani Tea Estate, which was closed down on November, 6, 1994 by the management, reopened in the perspective of a bipartite agreement signed by the management and union a few days ago. The garden, which had 1600 persons on the roll of the labour register, was without electricity and drinking water since November 16, 1994 when the State Electricity Board had disconnected the garden's power line owing to default in clearing the pending power bill. Although none from the management's side was available to indicate the reasons for "suspending the work", the union leaders, however, said that the management told them of recurring loss incurred by the garden on the one hand and insecurity of officials perfected by the garden labour, on the other.

Proposal To Stop Plucking Withdrawn

In a press release, the Federation of All India Tea Traders' Association welcomed the decision taken at a meeting called by the Chairman, Tea Board on November 29, 1994, that the producing companies would not curtail production of tea in December. The release added that with the intervention of the Tea Board, all gardens made a genuine effort to maximise production of suitable teas as this was in the interests of Indian consumer. The Federation of All India Tea Traders' Association (FAITTA) hoped the production would not be artificially curtailed on the pretext of adverse weather and other factors which interfere with free market forces.

Tea Plantation Security Force Passed Out

Raised at a cost of Rs 2 crore almost entirely funded by the tea industry the Assam Tea Plantation Security Force was armed with 303 rifles and was specially trained to counter surprise attacks. To step up security in at least 100 tea gardens in Assam, which were identified as vulgerable to militant attacks, the newly formed Tea Plantation Security Force extended its security cover to more than 66 gardens from December, 1994.

Union Minister of State for Commerce On Tea

At the 101st Annual conference of United Planters' Association of Southern India (UPASI), the then chief guest, Mr, Krishan Kumar, the then Union Ministe for Non-conventional Sources of Energy and Minister of State for Agriculture said that as far as tea is concerned, our future lies in the improvement of productivity and quality, in the diversification of markets and value addition procedure. He added that several measure were taken by Agriculture Minister to improve productivity and enhance the research efforts in plantation crop including tea. A new tea area infilling subsidy scheme was approved for introduction production of tea by planting tea bushes.

DBITA's Book and Sports Grant Raised

Darjeeling Branch of Indian Tea Association's (DBITA's) scheme for awarding book grant to students from Jalpaiguri district securing the first ten positions in Higher Secondary Examination was raised form Rs 900 to Rs. 1200 for each candidate from the year 1994-95. The sports kit grants for 4 boys and 4 girls was also raised form Rs 1000 to 1200 at the same time. The said schemes were introduced in 1991.

Tata Tea in A Decade of Indianisation

Tata Tea Ltd, a 100 percent Indian-owned tea company, the largest in the world-under Tata management, completed more than two decade in 2003-04. Since Tata took over in 1983-1984 (1) the production of black tea went up from 137.8 million kgs to 163.1 million kgs (+ 34 percent) (2) the production of instant tea from 0.7 million kgs to 5.60 million kgs (+ 161 percent) (3) the production of packet tea from 4.1 million kgs to 15 million kgs (+270%). 4) the company pioneered the packaging of garden-fresh teas in polybags. And the market capitalisation went up from Rs 8 crore to Rs 3.200 crore. With a view to enhancing the welfare and well-being of large work force (58000 people) of the company and their families, contribution of the company, entirely voluntary, was in the following direction: (5) 63 hospitals and clinics; 1700 beds; 75 doctors and specialists; 130-bed general hospital at Munnar rated as that best Industrial Hospital in India; Rs 7 crore referral hospital recently commissioned in Assam. (6) 170 creches; 45 welfare officers 400 creche attendants, community health workers; 1100 under 5 children fed everyday; universal immunization of all under 5 children against communicable disease. (7) 110 schools; 280 teachers; vocational training centers to train for self-employment, educational centers for handicapped children. (8) Lab-to-land and community development programmes benefitting rural families in the vicinity of the company's via estates. Over the decade the shareholder funds increased from Rs 38 crore to Rs. 395 crore (10.2 times) largely by the accretion of undistributed profits. The dividend increased from Rs 4 crores to Rs. 45 crore (11.2 times). And market capitalisation increased from Rs. 8 crores to Rs. 2.2000 crore. For the seventh years in succession, however, Tata Tea achieved, during 2005-06, the highest income and the highest profit after tax. the company's performance, measured in terms of land key financial the parameter set it distinctly apart from other majors in the tea industry.

A comparison of the financial performance of the company with the average of eleven other majors in the tea industry reveals the following data.

Particulars	Tata Tea Ltd	Averaged of 11 other Majors
1. Profit after Taxes		
Percentage of paid up capital	186.8	75.1
% of Net worth	22.8	5.4
Percentage of capital employed	14.1	4.7
2. Dividend		
Percentage of equity capital	80.1	42.4
3. Retained earnings		
Percentage of equity capital	127.5	60.6

More Cups Per Kg Of Tea

Paramount academy of Technology (PAT) held its first workshop on CTC manufacture at Coimbatore in 1990. The workshop dealt with all aspects of CTC manufacturing and included practical demonstrations at CTC manufacturing units and tea estates. Shri Vijay Dudeja, the then chairman of PAT, pointed out that the CTC type of manufacture was introduced in India in the year 1931 which increased cuppage from 250 to 500 cups per kg of tea. He, however, regretted that despite the fact that many improvements in the CTC machine itself were made cups per kg of tea did not substantially increase. Mr Dudeja said that PAT had directed its energies in developing a process which would increase tea cuppage from the present 500 to 1000 per kg. The academy introduced a oneday seminar to the lovers of tea who enjoy a cup of tea every morning but know very little about their favourite beverage, tea growing, manufacture, types of tea and their speciality. This seminar was also of special interest to people indirectly connected with tea like bankers, governments, officials, tea machinery manufacturers and of course the tea consumers. It was for the first time that an institute exclusively involved in plantation crops was formed to promote research and development and to impart education on various department of plantation crops. The curriculum of that workshop included all aspects of CTC manufacture including its history, different styles, technical aspects like sharpening, different teeth profiles and a detailed analysis of connected processes of manufacture like withering, drying and fermentation. Shri Dudeja said that the next course by PAT was on "Tea Tasting;" the duration of which was two weeks followed by a general management course on "The art of negotiations." Mr Dudeja said that the plantation crops including tea were India's finest agro asset and an institute exclusively involved in all aspects of these crop was the need of the hour, Mr Dudeja added that the academy undertook to run refresher courses for personnel connected with the plantation industry and training of fresher in tea tasting, agricultural practices and manufacturing techniques. Simultaneously, the academy undertook research and development with the purpose of transferring technology to the growing regions. One of the major tasks undertaken was to develop environment friendly inputs for agriculture. The Paramount Academy of Technology sought assistance from well known universities abroad while drawing upon the work by Indian universities like the Assam Agricultural university and the Coimbator, Agricultural College, CSIR and others. The academy filled a vacuum that existed so far and contributed significantly to the growth of the plantation industry. The scientists and technicians of proven ability and excellence connected with the academy.

Contradictory Orders From Centre Over Cess

While the Union Minister for Commerce ordered that the Tea Board should collect the cess on tea, the Union Minister for Law viewed that the Tea Board was not legally authorised to collect the cess and only the Central Excise would do so. The Centre's decision in 1993 to abolish excise duty on tea, but to retain the cess was responsible for the creation of such a controversy. Following that decision the Central Excise Department, that used to collect cess on behalf of the Tea Board, withdrew from the responsibility. According to sources, the Tea Board had been asked to collect the cess themselves, but it get cleared from the Union Minister of Commerce of a scheme for recruitment of additional staff for collection of cess-submitted in July, 1993. The sources further add, the setting up of a new infrastructure for cess collection took long and posed serious problems as the Excise Department, which still collecting cess on behalf on the Board, would not do so after the current financial year 1994-95. Cess constituted the largest contribution to the annual budget of the Tea Board.

Withdrawal of Child Labour From Tea Estates

In view of worldwide concern voiced in respect of the Child labour in India, the general committee of the India Tea Association directed its members not to employ child either rather in the factory or in tea estates. It is expected that those already in the job will be automatically phased out within two to three years.

Tea Board's Planning To Raise Tea Yield

With a view to raising production of tea 1000 million kgs by 2000 A. D. from the current level, the Tea Board prepared a plan which included immediate and remote measures. Short-term measure as outlined in the plan comprised optimisation of inputs and improved cultural practices. Medium-term measures included in the plan were improvement of irrigation, drainage, rejuvenation, pruning and infilling while the long-term measures highlight such programmes as replanting and extension planting. The Tea Board hoped that implementation of this plant would enable the industry to achieve the targeted production.

India Blends To Promote Indian Tea Exports

"India blends", which was introduced in such countries as Russia, CIS, Egypt and Poland, was based on the idea of putting quality blend in teas of packets and marketing them at a competitive price backed by freight subsidy, sovereign guarantee, ECGC cover, warehousing, etc. Following a meeting of the task force on India Blend held on September 14, 1994, the exercise began with targeted volume of around 700 tonnes—500 tonnes from North India and 200 tonnes from South India. The brand name projected on international level was capable of competing with various Western brands already familiar to Russia and CIS countries. A reputed advertising agency was entrusted with the responsibility of selecting brand names and developing package designs for this purpose. It was further learnt that some members of the Marketing Task Force visited Russia to find out suitable agencies which received the shipments, arranged warehousing facilities and put into effect the ultimate distribution, apart from working out the details of the terms of payment. The Tea Board undertook the job of integration of the

"India Blend Project" into its overall promotional scheme for regaining lost markets.

India Joins Proposed Tea Producer Association

India joined the proposed "Tea Producer Association" that aimed at establishing a mechanism for meaningful interaction among the producing member countries on such matters as production, productivity and research, Following the meeting of the India-Sri Lanka working group, prepartory meeting of the proposed Association was had in 1995 at Colombo.

Tata Tea's R & D Activities Yielding Dividend

It was reported that the Research and Development activities of Tata Tea, comprising agronomic measures being applied to all of its South Indian gardens, had yielded average increase of tea from 2100 kgs per hector to 2700 kgs per hector. Company sources indicated similar experiments tried out in Sagmooea Rea Estate, Assam. It gave handsome dividend, the yield being 3028 kgs per hectare without any loss in quality. The package of economic measures, based on efficient management of carbohydrate dynamics of tea bush, was extended to other two tea estates Kellyden, Assam and Noweranuddy, North Bengal.

Hinduja, Ashok Leyland To Aid Indian Tea Exporters

The Hinduja and the Ashok Leyland companies relieved the Indian tea exporters to Iran, who had a difficult time owing to failure of that country's state trading organisation to honour the commitment to buy teas contracted. It was learnt that there two companies wanted to take 6.5 million kgs of tea at a commission of five percent. And surprisingly, the Union Commerce Minister forwarded their interest to the Tea Board in Kolkata. Industry circles felt to facilitate these companies to earn five percent commission amounting to $ 0.75 million, around Rs 2.5 crore in Indian currency, was not the mission of the then Union Commerce Minister and his men. It was something more significant and long term-to help the Hinduja emerge as the sole agent for the lucrative Iran market in the future.

CCPA Members To Increase Tea Wasters

At a recent meeting, members of the consultative committee of Planters' associations agreed to increase tea wastes with a view to improving the produce. Members further agreed not to reprocess or recycle teas during the new season commencing mid-March 1995. As a result of these measures, production of poor quality teas, jeopardised the industry's goodwill significantly. The CCPA took note of the fact that some small gardens, without declaring the quantum of tea wastes generated annually, supplied some of the wastes to instant tea makers. The committee asked member producers to abandon this practice.

Mundakoti Tea Estate Taken By Goenkas

Mundakoti tea estate in Darjeeling, owned by the Mittals of Amsing Tea Estate was taken over recently by the Goenkas of Wareen tea group. Darjeeling Plantations control four gardens in the hilly terrains of Darjeeling with a aggregate production of 9.5 lakh kilo. The new acquition added a further 5 lakh kgs taking the total production to around 1.50 million kgs annually. And thus the Goenkas became one of the five major tea groups which produced nearly 60 percent tea in Darjeeling. According to company sources, the Mudakoti tea estate has roughly 1600 acres under tea with an average yield of 650 kgs per acre. This yield was considered low compared to the four existing gardens under Darjeelign Plantation.

DBITA's Social Activites

Dooars Branch of India Tea Association handed over to the principal of Birpara College, a hall constructed at cost Rs. 1.54 lakh. The association donated Rs. 1.5 lakh to construct a few class rooms for the Sishubari High School, situated within the jurisdiction of Birpara-Madarihar Panchayat Samity, which were damaged by the flood in

July 1993.

ABITA's Social Activites

The Jorhat zone of ABITA donated 4 sewing machines and 14 accessories to the Jorhatamahila Samiti of Duliagaon, 3 kms from Jorhat. The association also donated a rest shed for the waiting passengers at Amguri town. The latest contribution of the ABITA was the construction of Lokopriya Omeo Kumar Das Julia School in the Sonitpur district, Assam, at a cost of Rs. 1.50 lakh.

Shifting of Plantation Institute from Kolkata to Bangalore

It was a disconcert news for the tea industry in general in eastern India and also the people of West Bengal to learn that the "Institute of Plantation Management in India", registered as a company in July, 1990 was shifted from Kolkata to Bangalore. The institute only one of its kind in India as well as abroad, was set up jointly by more than 15 companies (including Goodricke, Tata Tea, Warren Tea Williamson Magar, Duncan's Agro, Jokai etc. in a rented house in salt Take area, Kolkata, with the object of turning out duty qualified planters with latest technical expertise to meet the up-to-date requirements of the plantation industry. Training courses in tea tasting and plantation matters were also taken up. In January 1992 the institute approached the Salt Lake authority for a six-acre plot for carrying out plantation education. Where there was no response, the institute wrote to the Chief Minister of West Bengal directly to enlist his support for the institute's cause, adding that a strong lobby in New Delhi was very much active to set up the institute at Bangalore. Various other minister of the state were also approached, but with no effect. Ultimately, with the support of the then union commerce ministe, Mr P. Chidambaram, the so-allied southern lobby in New Delhi succeeded in sifting the matter with a grant of Rs. 1 crore from the union ministery, through the Coffee Board, for transfer of the Kolkata institute itself to Bangalore.

Cheers Mizoram

It seems something is brewing well for Mizoram in the days ahead. The state which harvests tea leaves four times a year chiefly from its plantations in Bitate and Ngopa, can well aspire to increase the rate to thirty with proper backup infrastructure power, modern pilot factories and good systems of communication. Mizoram's tea, despite poor processing and care, is of a quality that can hope to rival Darjeeling's with able assistance from the Tea Board, and the Tea Research Association of Darjeeling. In a Tea Board meeting held recently in Kolkata, it was pointed out that conducive climatic conditions, fertile soil, good hill incline and organic land regeneration provide solid reasons for Mizoram to be considered major tea producing state.

New system at Guwahati Auction

At the sales sub-committee meeting of the Guwahati Tea Auction Committee, held on 30 July 1992, it was decided that effective from sale No 36, orthodox tea sales at the Guwahati auctions would he held on Monday afternoons. This, would boost the sale of orthodox teas, replacing the present practice of sale after the C.T.C. tea sales. In addition, orthodox tea sales shall remain suspended every Friday three weeks prior to the day of sale to facilitate brokers distribute samples to prospective buyers for further export. Secondly reprints included a total, approximately 60,000 packages of dust tea sent in sale No 34 owing to the unsold lot of 30 per cent in sale No. 31. Since the market could not absorb this excess, the just out lots were reprinted in the succeeding sale No 35 a week later, leaving out 47,000 packages for the earlier sale. This was a result of increased dust offerings and persisted for some time to come.

Coffee planters Demand Debate

A move by the Centre to amend the Plantation Labour Act and the Minimum Wages Act met with stiff opposition from the Karnataka Planters' association. The then association chairman D. A. Umpathy

Gowda felt that a debate on the changes was necessary because coffee plantations in rural Karnataka, Kerala, and Tamil Nadu were already the victims of various taxes, and an unjustified consumer-price-index fixation system based upon high urban standards. Coffee plantations moreover, have to provide-several amenities proper to employed married persons unlike in other farms of industry. Unless the Government changes its mind, the chairman observed, the planters may have to look up to some other crop for their gains.

Multiwall Paper Sacks Open Up A New Era

In the good old days the planters depended on some established importing houses who used to bring in chests from the Scandinavian countries in the main and Sweden in particular. The tea circle then knew not only the Indian Tea Association (ITA), the main tea producers' organisation but also the Tea Chest and Plywood Traders Association (TCPTA). However, it did not take long for the Indian plywood tea chest industry to step in. Interestingly, one of the former presidents of the Plywood Manufacturer Association of India (PMA) is at the head of a top tea manufacturing company. However, slowly the industry was moving towards a problem because bulk packaging required softwood and that in turn felling of treas of certain species. In the early 60's, a U.N. Commission had suggested that wood-based industries should embark upon an *afforestation programme against the felling of tree*. It is doubtful whether any of those industries ever took the advice seriously. The Indian tea industry's need for tea chests is around 12 million sets per year which in turn calls for 1.2 lakh tonnes of timber and affects, as estimated by Mr. Narendra Kumar, the then Chairman of the Consultative Committee of Plantation Associations, about 6000 hectares of forest land. It is apprehended that deforestation at such scale will lead to ecological imbalance. Apart from this issue of environmental ecology there are compelling economic factors. The cost of plywood tea chests has been rising due to scarcity of wood. Those in the tea industry who can look ahead have been searching for alternative materials. For a time jute bags were also being experimented upon. The Tocklai Experimental Station has been on the look out for a quality of multiwall paper sacks.

The industry now has it from Mr. A.K. Das of Tockali that a type of multiwall paper sack been found suitable for the purpose and it can effectively replace plywood tea chest. Actually such sophisticated or hi-tech packages suitable for tea have long been in use is lesser tea producing countries like Malawi, Bangladesh, Sri Lanka and China. The Tockla sacks are made of extensible craft paper comprising five layers of paper to hold about 50 kgs of tea per sack. Knowing that the industry and trade at home and importers abroad must have to be satisfied about various aspects, the Tockla variety has been duly subjected to moisture test, tasters' evaluation, physical test and drop test. It was found that the comparative moisture content of teas stored for certain period of time in both plywood chests and paper sacks did not differ significantly. Tasters at Tockali, Kolkata and London could not also detect any difference between teas stored in the two types of countain. The Central Food Technology Research Institute, Mysore was reported to have undertaken physical as well as the drop tests. The former was carried cut to assess the performance of the sacks during transporting while the latter was to find out whether the sacks could withstand handling abuses.

To make the sacks acceptable to overseas buyers, note was reportedly taken of the quality requirements of U. K. and USA. As a matter of fact the tea associations of the two countries revised their specifications for the MPS used commercially for bulk packaging of tea. Then the industry have now looked forward to a new packaging era.

Consignment Tax In Assam

The state Government amended the tax laws in order to authorise tax officials to seize goods at checkgates so that cases of tax evation could be effectively dealt with. The Government considered levy of replacement tax to make good the loss of huge tax revenue due to transfer of tea, oil and plywood to other states. Assam, being a consuming State, should have logically opposed the levy of consignment tax. The industry supported the proposal in the hope that the State will get additional resources to the tune of Rs. 40 crore annually, if tea, petroleum produces and plywood are exempted from consignment tax, Assam will lose both ways and more advanced states will benefit at the cost of Assam. While the government's concern is appreciated, the case of the assessees, which include the tea industry, cannot be ignored. In terms of the Tea (Marketing) Control Order 1985, an amount of 75 per cent of tea is required to be put on sale at recognised auctions. Assam, producing over 60 per cent of the country's tea, cannot dispose of the entire production within the state and has to despatch a heavy quantity to the Kolkata auction. These will attract consignment tax. Therefore, it is not only that the cheapest beverage will cost more but its effect on export market will be more serious. India is facing a number of competitors in the world market and she will be easily priced out from the markets which seek cheaper varieties only. Consignment tax will attack tea industry and trade in another area. That is packet tea. Some tea manufacturers have arranged packeting of their produce in the gardens and have arranged for despatch of the same to distributors and stockists. They will suffer if such a tax is levied. Further, there are renowned blenders and packeters who operate on a centralised, all India basis. They have to distribute to different outlets in all the States. They would also be affected. All in all, though the Government's need for increased revenue is undeniable and a measure like the consignment tax can bring considerable revenue too, the industry and trade should not be so grievously wronged.

Storm Over a Tea Auction Centre

When an auction centre grows up, various factors contribute towards its development. Look at Cochin and Coonoor auctions. Quite old they are, coming up in 1947 and 1963 respectively but Madras as a city is much older than the two, yet a centre was not set up there. On the other had, Cochin and Coonoor, though minor ports then, were situated near the producing centres and that was the basic factor for formation of the auction centres there. Siliguri (1976) and Guwahati (1970) came up mostly on same consideration. Of course, unimaginative and some what repressive tax measures imposed by the West Bengal Government were other reasons for Siliguri to develop. Still other reasons were local patriotism or parochialism. London (1839) and Kolkata (1861) were a class apart. They developed because of historical reasons. Kolkata was the only transport centre nearest to the producing areas. London was the oldest and the largest receiving port. As the industry developed, the tea companies sought to create a sound commercial base in the country of origin. Therefore a market had to be developed locally and, as a first step, an auction centre camp up in Calcutta. Both internal distribution and external trade were beefed up. Calcutta as an auction centre grew by leaps and bounds. This was inevitable too.

A new auction centre was at Ahmedabad. Gujarat consumes a lot of tea. On that count, it has staked its claim for an auction centre. There were a number of practical problems affecting formation of an auction centre at Ahemdabad. First, All auction centres are located near the production centres and not near consuming centres. Secondly, even in normal condition, there will be a tremendous gap between production, offer and payment of 'prompt' and it will be found uneconomical in normal business practice too. Thirdly, some brokers and a few plantations cannot run the auction centre with 50-60 million kg of tea which Gujarat consumes. This has emboldened them but that is not enough. Fourthly, if the quantum of sales is transferred substantially, the Guwahati auction will be terribly affected and the services of about 3000 workers and employees as also the infrastructure there will be jeopardised. It means whether or not the Ahmedabad experiment will be a success, an existing and an established trade will be disturbed. Unemployment will loom large in front of people of an area where social and political unrest prevails.

Tea Industry Needs More Land

It is no longer a secret that if India is to maintain tis pre-eminent position in the world map of tea export and also keep the domestic market undisturbed, about 1100 million kgs of tea has to be produced by 2000. This is certainly a tall order. What then is to be done? What are the options or possibilities before the industry? More productivity? More land? The helpless condition of the Indian tea industry finds an echo in the words of the bewildered English poet.

Wandering Between To Worlds, One Dead And The Other Powerless To Be Born.

One choose more productivity; step up your R & D work. But a former chairman of the Tea Research Association himself had cautioned the industry: "We are already facing a *yield barrier* in the field." If this is not true of all gardens, it is at least true of a large number of them. May be all gardens shall have to face the same fate some day. After all, the Law of Diminishing Returns is based on observed facts. No wonder therefore that while infilling, replanting and better inputs are being resorted to, extension of land area wherever possible have also to be looked forward to.

The search for land started quite some time ago. The CCPA undertook survey some years back and finding some peripheral land available for extension planting, requested the State governments of Assam and West Bengal to make over the same to the organised sector of the industry. But the issue was not that simple. Problem is that different State governments had acquired some 'surplus land' under respective Land Ceiling Acts, portions of such land had been made over to landless people to settle, as a socioeconomic measure of the concerned government and portions to the Forest Departments. Land declared forest area under the Forest Conservation Act cannot, as per existing law, be handed over to the private sector. In this regard NABARD had suggested some time back and the Ramakrishnayya Committee also considered the feasibility of transfer of suitable forest lands to tea estates pointing to the similarity between plantations and forests in providing forest covers. NABARD had pointed out that one of the important purposes of afforestation was to provide tree canopy covers to avoid soil erosion as also to build up solid organic matter for better soil-water relations. The third purpose is to improve micro and macro-climate of the area to achieve proper ecological balance. Judged against these and other objectives of forestry, tea and coffee plantations fulfil these admirably. As a matter of fact, plantation crops provide double canopy effective ground cover against soil erosion due to the presence of shade trees which break the impact of rain drops at a high level and the bush canopy which provides 100 per cent ground coverage at proximate distance from soil.

The Pleasants And Unpleasants

Witness of many pleasant and unpleasant happenings, the year 2005 took farewell from the people. It is worth remembering that in the year only, Darjeeling tea estate had received the prestigious ISO Quality Assurance Certificate, in 2000 the first tea estate in the world to have earned this distinction. It is equally fascinating that produce of a Darjeeling garden was sold at a price highest ever any tea fetched in the world market, and the value-added tea received acclamation from new consumers. These are worthy events indeed, enough to add feather to the image of Indian teas overseas. But all was not well. The year could not keep the industry jovial and buoyant for long. Some unwelcome events frequently subjected individual units and the industry to serious perturbance, gloom and despair. Certainly it was matter of great concern that during the year the industry lost some of its friendly buyers, had to retreat from some markets and succumbed to export stagnation trap. The tea price, at the same time, fell to an unprecedented low level in the domestic market, and the militants at the North-east resumed killing and kidnapping of tea personnel extorting money with threat and coercion. These events, no doubt, have shacken the confidence of many tea units and disturbed the industry severely.

Does China Pose A Threat to Indian Tea Exports?

How misconceptions in history affect trade relations can be examplified by the tea trade between China and the United States of America. More than a century has passed away, it is yet hard to efface the impression that the tea consignment involved in the Boston Tea Party during the American War of Independence was not Indian tea at all but was of Chinese orgin. The mischief possibly occured because the consignment was sent by the British East India Company. What is more, since the historical tea party, tea imbibing was considered an anti-national act and Americans took to Coffee, more and more. The strange part of it is that when at a much china had thus stolen a March upon Sri Lanka.. A study by a University professor in India stated some time back that China and Kenya were forging ahead of India and Sri Lanka in the rate of progress of production, and consequently of export. Indian can be complacement at its own peril, he side, It has been said by another analyst that the average growth rate of Chinese export often can be put at 5.7 per cent in the last decade while the annual rate of increase in world tea trade had been to the tune of 1.5 per cent. Again, for a populous country like China domestic consumption of tea is quite considerable, unless production can be raised phenomenally. Exports cannot be increased. The Ministry of Agriculture in China is attempting to raise production by uprooting old bushes and improving upon agricultural techniques along with a programme of planting in new areas. Tea plantations in China cover one million hectares, one third of which is unable to provide good later date. Americans began to taste tea, again, it was the Chinese tea that they chose, though the Indian Black tea is by and large is better than the Chinese variety. Better quality Indian tea is priced higher but high price should not deter America. Some analysts state that China is back in the tea export trade in a big way. Already it ranks next only to India and Sri Lanka. China tea industry had thus high yields. On the contrary, one calls to mind that in 1984 when an Indian Tea Delegation visited China, it was given to under stand that tea is grown in 15 out of the 32 Provinces and that the tea area in China was of the order of 300,500 hectares. An average output per hectare, an American news report put it, at 630 kgs against the world average of 1020 kgs. According to the information gathered by the Indian Tea Delegation the average yield in the organised sector was about 1200 kg per hectare. Never the less, China has an edge in Green tea and special teas. According to the China Tea import and Export Corporation (CTIEC), in 2006 export of such teas recorded 80 per cent of world trade but in 2007 the market shre rose to 85 per cent. It is said that China's competitors in this field, Japan and Taiwean have been gradually withdrawing because of soaring domestic labour costs. This is situation where high-cost economy or an open economy is at a disadvantage competing against a totalitarian regime. India, as is well known, produces very little green tea. Black tea is her forte. As it is, her future in the world tea market is not all bleak.

Future of Sick Tea Gardens

The Exit Policy adopted by the Union Government supposedly under distress evoked mixed reactions in the tea industry which has sick estates in its fold. Sick industries were so long allowed to continue mainly because of compulsions of domestic politics; and now they are bidden good-bye reportedly because of IMF and IBRD compulsion. There have, however, been three factors limiting the full implementation of the policy: First, the exit policy will be acted upon only as the last alternative. Second, the retrenched worker will be offered a golden handshake; and third, if worker cooperatives take charge of the concerned units, all their past liabilities will be written off. The tea industry has been offered an additional facility in that the Government has asked the Tea Board to motivate owners of better-managed gardens to take over the weak or sick gardens and nurse them back to health. Of course, there is nothing unusual in this offer. Other industres were also asked to do the same long back. It did not work there and is not likely to succeed in tea industry either. For one thing, if the sick units can be taken over for good on terms of the better managed gardens, the latter might be interested. For another, the problems facing the sick units may be varied and not within the ambit of experience of the better units. Lastly, in the interest of many among the employees, some may have to be sacrificed. And this may not be to the liking of the unions or of the State Government concerned. It is because of this problem that the sick units had been allowed so long to stay on not in the interest of production, not for the economy at large. As hinted above, this is the problem that lies at the back of grim exit policy now adopted. It would have been practical to divide the gardens into two classes i.e. those which can be revived for fuller production and those which are beyond redemption. In this, it may not be much different from industries in general. And this is where the exit policy is relevant too. Considering that any addition by the sick industries might be a drop in the ocean for other industries, while the possible addition by such units in tea industry could be substantial, the tea industry stand on a slightly different footing too. Shri P.R., Dasmunshi, the then Commerce Minister, had asked at a specially convened meeting at New Delhi for preparation of a status report. The report indicated that about 145 units are weak or closed in West Bengal, Assam, Tripura and Tamil Nadu. The sick gardens cover about 32000 hectares of land and have potential for production of 48 million kg of tea.

Since 1989 when the idea of revitalising the weak and sick tea gardens was mooted at the New Delhi meeting and the report was asked to be prepared within a set time frame, the Tea Board sat unconcerned with the report in hand perhaps occasioning enunciation of new Parkinson's Law.

The Ramakrishnayya Committee reported that the major tea producing States in North India were not taking appropriate care and interestion the development of the tea industries. But some in South India took. As it is, one State Government in South India has reportedly taken even a World Bank loan for tea industry's development there . On the other hand, Assam and West Bangal, more particular the latter look to the industry not for the industry's well being but for its exploitation for filling the coffers of the Exchequer. The industry has been given no incentive. The Central and the State governments have been generally apathetic towards it. How can the sick and the weak estates be restored to health then?

Kerala Shows The Way

The issue is tea finance. More specifically how the tea industry can retain its resources, saving the same from the clutches of taxmen so that those resources could be ploughed back. Taxation of the tea industry in India has a peculiarity of its own. Since the historic U.P. case -*Commissioner of Sales Tax, Lucknow*-vs- *D. S. Bisht & others*- tea industry is looked upon both as an industrial and an agricultural pursuit. Not merely that, the agricultural part of the tea industry had been given a weightage of 60 per cent and the industrial part only the balance 40 per cent. Tea industry as an industry is taxed on this 40 per cent under the Income Tax Act at a uniform rate, one that is fix for all industries all over the country. On the other hand, agriculture being a State subject, the tea industry is subjected to tax on the 60 per cent content at rate varying in different States. But the rate of agricultural tax is nowhere below or even equal to the rate fixed for industries. As a results, tea industry is taxed usually at rate much heavier than that charged on other industries. States, however, wanted more not satisfied with what they constitutionally had, some state governments such as, Kerala, West Bengal and Assam sought to extend the agricultural content from 60 per cent to 100 per cent. Kerala and West Bengal passed laws and charged agricultural income tax on that basis. Actually both these States levied a tax not only exorbitant but also constitutionally arbitrary so much so that when the aggrieved tea producers sought a judicial review, courts of law, even the Supreme Court did not falter to strike down the tax. laws of both the States. Assam took a more reasonable path uring the

Sarcaria commission to so recommend as to increase the percentage suitably in order that the State's finances could look upon. Assam drew a blank. Possibly because at the time of its reporting, the Sarkaria Commission came to know that a case on the issue was being pursued at Supreme Court. West Bengal and Kerala had to retrace their steps. But West Bengal was unrepentant and continued with its persecution of the industry in another way resulting in further humiliation at the hands of the Supreme Court. Yet the governments appeared to be impervious to the deleterious effect of the taxes on the rate of the production which had either slowed down or become stagnant.

Credit goes to the new Kerala Government that of all the tea producing States, it has been the first and the only State to introduce a scheme for modernisation of plantation through what it named "Investment Deposit Scheme". In accordance with the scheme, under the Kerala Agricultural Income Tax Act, notified plantations are allowed a deduction upto 20 per cent from the agricultural income for the purpose of rejuvenation and modernisation. Kerala has now shown the way. If similar measures are also taken by Karnataka and Tamil Nadu in the South, and Assam and West Bengal in the North, the effective rate of taxation will be lowered and sufficient funds may be ploughed back for replantation and rejuvenation of the bushes. What the State Governments may lose immediately will be doubly returned in various ways through the development of the tea industry and its ancillaries.

Future of London As A Tea Centre

Tea has been a part and parcel of British life since it was first sold to public in London in 1687. And it remained as a monopoly trade item of East India compoany of Britain, almost throughout next hundred years. After shedding the monopolistic influence of East India Co on 20th November 1834 first free auction of tea in UK took place in Commercial Sales Rooms situated on the corner of Mincing Lane, and remained there till 1976. Tea producing estates and tea trading, blending, packing units were owned or significantly controlled by tea trade circle of London located in and around the city of London. Thus London grew to be the centre of the world Tea Trade and retained this position till the Second World War and for a short period after the war. After that, gradually at first and then rapidly, London tea scene underwent dramatic change, final shape of which has yet to come. Of late, it has been found that British corporate Giants are reluctant to continue their tea legacies in various parts of world, specially in India.

Recently controlling stake of The Assam Tea Co. Ltd., one of the very few remaining British-owned, London based, most coveted tea outfits, changed hands from Inchcapes to Mehtas of Bermuda at a consideration of US dollar of 30.4 million. Thus the British control of tea production and distribution is contracting sharply. Loss of these outfits is really a catastrophe to British tea interest. In view of the aforesaid facts, it would not be proper for anybody to think that London's prominence as global tea centre will reach its fag end soon, by ignoring truth. Because, UK-based tea blenders and packers still have a significant position in most tea consuming countries and their markets are destined to be expanded further with the changed political system in Eastern European Countries and Russia along with the emergence of unified European market, ask reality to come soon. Consequently, London will have greater role to play. It is still the only centre at which it is possible to purchase teas from widest variety of origins since it impart approximately 18 per cent of the world's total tea exports.

IS : 14000 Quality Management

It is all to good that people are gradually becoming conscious of environment pollution and ecological imbalance. A practical aspect of environmental pollution now relates to containg pollution. So much so that neither the governments nor the expert bodies can ignore any longer the complaints from the consumers. Answer to the problem has now been found in adoption of total quality management under ISO : 9000 which is an internationally accepted set of guidelines for quality systems. The Bureau of Indian Standards has issued corresponding specification published as IS : 14000:1988 which again states, among other, that "there is a world-wide trend towards more stringent customer expectations with regard to quality. Accompanying this trend has been a growing realisation that continual improvements in quality are often necessary to achieve and sustain good economic performance." "However, technical specification", the report adds, may not in themselves guarantee that a customer's requirements will be consistently met. There happens to be any deficiency in the specification or in the organisational system to design and produce the product or service." Nonetheless, the Bureau of Indian Standards has intimated the Tea Board of India of the situation. The Board, in turn, has also cautioned all tea industry associations that ISO : 9000 Quality Certification was going to be applied by EEC (European Economic Community) soon and tea, organic tea would be covered under it. In view of this fact it would be wise to scrutinise the quality system certification modalities at IS : 14000 series and impress upon their constituents the need for maintaining the specifications. The tea industry in India appears to be careful but taking a short-term view this leads to the complex question of ecological imbalance. For one thing, it involved continues use of wood which in turn means denudation of forests. The tea industry is under statutory obligation to provide the garden workers with fuel and as such felling of trees becomes inevitable. Besides soft wood trees have to be cut down to get logs for manufacture of packing boxes. On the other hand, a controversy still rages whether extension of fallow lands or lands with low-grade forestry can be turned into a greenery of tea plantation.

Change in Container System

There has been of late a change in the container system. Paper backed sacks are being used profusely replacing the wooden chests which were eminently reusable. Avoiding wastage they help in environmental protection. The pattern was therefore quite complex. By felling trees to get logs required for manufacture of plywood, one create an ecological imbalance, by using chests one helped environment. With sacks made with plastic, paper etc. one creates a problem for environment because these materials are neither reusable or recyclable. As a matter of fact, very stringent rules for recyling and packaging have recently been set down for trading with EC countries. Germany has masterminded the environment protection scheme which is being hotly debated within the Community itself. Properly known as the "Topfer Law" named after Klaus Topfer, Germany's environment minister, the scheme, stated briefly, requires waste collection to increase in stages until 80 per cent of packaging waste is collected by 1995. Of the waste that is collected, 90 per cent of glass and metal will have to be recycled, and 80 per cent of the plastic and paper. The British, French and Belgian governments have complained. *The Economist* informs use, that the law has played havoc with the economics of recycling in those countries also, among others. The situation may take an ugly turn. The Treaty of Rome allows a government to seek an exemption from a single-market law on environmental grounds, but only if it can show that the purpose of the law is not restraint of trade. The developing countries seeking market in Europe have to take up the issue in time.

Need For Training In Plantation Management

Are entrepreneurs born, and not made? For, it is a common experience that many successful businessmen of the past started form scratch: *sans* training, *sans* resources. The world has, of course, changed since then. Business has become so complicated now. It has left its linear path and it is extremely difficult now for the uninitiated to press forward. As with entrepreneurship, so with managers, professionalism has edged out hereditary captaincy in business. Even in professional management, the pattern has changed substantially. Now-a-days problems facing managers have become multi-dimensional requiring handling of various aspects of a given situation. May be they require different personalities to attend to them or approaches have to be different. Though there are some common basic traits in all management training, requirements of plantation is substantially different. This is not particularly because of the location of plantation being far from the madening crowd: an exile, as if from known urban environment of industries for the executives but because of unknown and complicated situation enveloping in the estates. This change in approach has been clearly brought out in a speech of a chairman of the Indian Tea Association.. "From his early years of isolation", he said, "The tea estate manager has necessarily emerged as a business-oriented multidiciplinary custodian of his large required at one end of the spectrum to be equally conversant with the latest agronomic methods as with modern factory operation at the other".

Though such appreciations of the working of managers is something commendable, it is too general in nature. In actual field of operation, Saonwalla's views are more relevant when he says that except for small gardens where the manager will have to carry the full burden of estate management, the industry will have to define a clear division of responsibility between the field and factory managers. Both are equally important and hence both these segments of management must be headed by competent and trained executives under centralised direction with long term corporate objectives.

Again, who can convince him to any other point of view when he expresses his firm conviction that the tea industry as a whole has failed to achieve its targets owing to serious lack of trained personel at all levels. One wonders the training of managing personal has become an issue today. The Indian tea industry which has behind it more than a hundred years' of experience, has failed to adopt a progressive and modern approach to the issue. The Ripes vanWinkel has woken up now to find himself surrounded by countries with modern perceptions. One would like to know how it could maintain its position as the largest producer and the largest exporter also.

Sometime back a few stalwarts of tea industry in North East India set up an Institute of Plantation Management in Kolkata. UPASI too mooted the idea of a course on the subject. This move was a sure step forward. This was really a need when the need for trained executives was so acute.

Only lately another move has been made but though it has government's blessing, some complications seem to have already developed. Regionalism in the matter would be a sad thing and unwarranted too. Rather, having the existing one at Kolkata with stress on tea plantation and the new one in South India serving other plantation industries would not be a bad idea. Actually, two institutes giving plantation management training are not too many. However, with good will and a desire to get through the training for managership is a must in any case, and it was taken up early too and it was permenently established at Bangalore.

What Cheer For Plantation Labour?

The Plantation Labour (Amendment) Bill, 1992, which has introduced in the Rajya Sabha some time back, is causing concern to the plantation industry, including the tea industry. The original legislation, was the Plantation Labour Act, 1951, which was last amended in 1988. And though the industries made several representations while it was being amended then, apparently no consideration had been given to those representations. The Lok Sabha is yet to consider the Bill. It is worthwhile therefore to point out that the Bill contains some proposals which while inimical to the interests of the plantation industries, particularly the tea industry, will not further the interests of labour either. To begin with, in defining "employees" the Amendment Bill has proposed to rope in Directors, Partners and the like. The intentions probably is to twist their arms for any default of their underlings. Since they are like 'absentee landlords' they may be held responsible only when the responsible local management cannot be identified for any grave default.

Secondly, in offering medical facilities there are already provisions for Garden hospitals and Group hospitals in the Act. That despite, an amendment seeks to provide for establishment of a Garden hospital within two years and a Group hospital within three years of registration of plantation. Such rigorous time-frame is unwarranted in view of the fact that the plantations are subject in these matters to rules framed by the State Governments. One need know also that the Sub-Committee on Amendments to the Plantation Labour Act, 1951 looked upon the huge expenditure on Group hospitals as unnecessary, if there existed appropriate arrangements for treatment of the patients. Even the Industrial Committee on Plantations approved of these decisions. Thirdly, provisions as to the safety have been blown to over-size by incorporating a separate chapter and new sections. While nobody will object to reasonable precautions being taken for health and safety of the workers, imaginary risks or hazards and protection there-from should not be provided for in law. Rather than the vague provision for periodical examination of workers exposed to insecticides as proposed, the existing arrangement of examination by the Medical Officer of the plantation once in every six months is quite reasonable and practical. It should be appreciated that the types of chemicals used by the tea industry, for example, are also used by the vast agricultural work force in the country for the unorganised sector. Yet no mentionable health hazard was heard from them. Moreover, the Tea Research Association has approved of the agricultural chemicals for control of weeds and pests. These have been found safe for consumers of tea and well tolerable for dermal and oral toxicity. Fourthly, where regulatory measures would have been enough, the proposal seeking blanket prohibition on employment of children is fought with problems for the workers family as well as for the plantation.

If enacted, the child worker will have to be retrenched and the family pattern of employment in a tea garden will have to be changed causing economic hardship for the family. A legacy of Industrial Revolution, the Western countries think of a child labour as hand and foot chained to a factory in a gingy/unhealthy atmosphere. Beware to Western thoughts, our legislators hardly appreciate that the children in plantation are actually employed in field operations in an open and healthy environment. Lastly, penalty clauses have been made unnecessarily harsh. It is strange that when unlike the old clolonial type management in estates, modern mangers on job are professionals, educated, humane and socially-conscious, such provision should be made. Moreover, one might like to know since 1951 when the Act first came into effect, how many cases are on record when the highest punishment had been awarded. Even so, harsh laws have never quite stopped contravention of law What then? What uplift do these provisions ensure of plantation labour? As it is let labour get what it should cut let not the industry suffer unnecessarily.

'Value added' Conventional Meet

It has become a fashion now-a-days to highlight in every available forum the need for getting extra land for tea cultivation; the disintegration of erstwhile USSR; thrust to be bestowed on value-added production of tea; and finally, the need to take R & D effort to the fields. Predictably these vital issues confronting the tea industry were thoroughly debated and discussed in the International Tea Convention, organised by the Consultative Committee of Plantation Associations (CCPA) to mark the 1993-Year of India Tea, as declared by the Union Commerce Ministry. The starting point of the year-long effort to promote the export of India Tea in the global market would be followed by advertisement blitz by the Tea Board, Indian. The convention which sought to foster global awareness of business opportunity, offered by Indian tea was well represented and moderately succeeded in spreading the objective for which it was organised. Remarkably, the much talked about subject of medicinal property of tea did not receive the kind of exposure was widely expected. There could be two possible reasons for this: the industry no longer consider it prudent to highlight the medicinal property of tea in commercial terms; secondly, the research efforts made in this regard by this country could not deserve focused attention in an international meet. The other reason could be that tea taster is not at all bothered about the laboured findings of researchers and in any case, his ardent love towards tea is beyond the supposed medicinal properties of the hot beverage. The then Commerce Minister, Sri Pranab Mukherjee, spoke with authority in the meet, as he had been well associated with the tea trade and industry in his previous terms as Finance Minister. He was well aware of the field and rightly pointed out in the meet that special emphasis should be made to transfer research work to the field. However, despite his spirited appeal, the meet could not establish convincingly that the plantation sector is a beneficiary of various research efforts undertaken for enhancing tea production by utilising the high yielding clones.

Yet, this problem is not limited to tea alone; it is utter lack of coordination between the research arena and fields which invite the criticism of eminent agricultural scientists. The Training and Visit (T&V) programme which is followed in case of food crops—could bring the research faculty in tea very close to the field. The country is yet to see the kind of co-ordinated effort of research faculty and farmers working hand-in-hand making the green revolution dream a reality in the India C. Subramanyam era of the late 60's. The plantations should realise that they could immensely benefit by utilising the research efforts made. The trade bodies have a definite positive role to play in this regard. After all it is in R&D efforts that the country's hopes are highly pinned.

Many speakers expressed concern that domestic consumption was going up without any corresponding increase of tea production. Of course the accusing fingers point to the uncontrollable population explosion. Can there be any solution others than to increase tea production manifold. The ongoing economic reforms package was widely welcomed by the meet which felt that it would immensely lead the country towards economic prosperity and for the tea industry, too, it argues well. The minister, too, appealed to the tea industry to utilise this opportunity for its betterment. The Indian tea has become competitive after devaluation of rupee. Strategically, India is excellently placed to yield to variety of demands of many foreign countries; that is bulk for blenders and packers, custom made consumer packs, tea bags for whole-sellers and retailers, speciality products like organic tea (the country has already thought for it) and processed item like instant tea. Many speakers expressed the apprehension that the image of Indian tea as premium product was no longer taken seriously in the international market and also about the progressive emergence of price-conscious consumers. While it is easier said than done to explore the possibility of finding new markets in view of USSR's disintegration, the fierce competition that could be expected from Sri Lank, Kenya even Indonesia was highlighted in the meet, However difficult it might be, the arduous task of finding out new markets is worth undertaking as the industry is seized of the hazards of relying largely on a single market on the basis of bilateral tradé agreements. There was consensus among the participants that the country should reorient its strategy towards value added products. There were spirited discussions on the export strategy. While many suggestions were offered by veterans of the trade, the need for strong branding attempts for the Indian tea was almost echoed by all. The then Tata Tea MD was more forthright when he asked whether it was possible to think of Sony without thinking of Japan and think of IBM, Coke and McDonalds without thinking of USA. Brand-oriented promotional activity for better export performance was highlighted by the then Goodricke MD, Mr. Bhasin, who was bold enough to say that acsiquition of sick companies in the West, which have already established brand image in the food processing industry should be considered along with the good-will for promoting Indian tea in value added form. His suggestion that tea should be given as a gift item on important occasions abroad by our countrymen reflected his unconventional way of thinking. It is our wrong approach of selling tea just like a commodity that costs the country enormously both in volume of sales and improved export performance, opined many. Though the meet could not stand out as in outstanding event, nevertheless it conveyed a message that the tea industry in the country was well aware of the problems it faced and it no longer brooded over the spilt milk—the disintegration of USSR. The meet visualised a better beginning for the brew, from the year 1993 onwards.

Jay Shree' Set Up A Tissue Culture Unit

At the recent 47th Annual General Meeting of Jay Shree Tea & Industries Ltd. (Under B.K. Birla Group) Mr. B.K. Birla, the then Chairman, announced that the company (obviously to diversify) was actively preparing to set up a tissue culture & horticulture export-oriented unit at Bangalore at an approximate cost of Rs. 15 crore, for which talks were going on with certain companies in Israel and Europe. Further, the company proposed to introduce a brand name, "Birla Tea', for all teas produced by it, especially for packaged teas, with confidence that a would establish itself in the market. Tea in polypacks would also be marketed soon. Finally, the chairman also pleaded for lowering of the present high level of agricultural income tax in West Bengal and Assam.

Goenka Shifts Sugar Project From Warren Tea

Report said that the Kolkata-based S.P. Goenka Group's plan for a sugar project was undergoing changes. The earlier decision to set up the sugar mill under Warren Tea has been sheived and the project will now be implemented by Kitply Industries, another group other company.

This is in keeping with the group's plan to consolidate all Agro-based business in kitply. Besides tea, all other businesses, especially those pertaining to plantation and forestry, will hence forth come under the Kitply umbrella. Waren Tea will continue to remain in tea and also pursue the group's effort to enter cement manufacturing.

Incidentally Warren Tea was perhaps the only tea company to have been given the clearance by the Finance Ministry to raise foreign funds through an Euro-issue.

Tata Tea To Increase Share in Asian Coffee

At a meeting of the Board of Directors, the Tata Tea Ltd. enhanced its stake in the Hyderbad-based Asian Coffee Ltd., from the present

9.5 per cent to a majority 64.5 per cent. The company further decided offered one ex-bonus equity share for every five shares of Asian Coffee in its bid to acquire the equity shares of the company. Tata Tea has, however, added that if, for any reason, it cannot acquire the additional shares, it will have the option of withdrawing the offer.

Company sources indicate, the terms and conditions of the offer, which are to be set out in the Letter of Intent, have to be cleared by the stock exchanges and Securities Exchange Board of India (SEBI). The issue will come out only on receiving the approval the said authorities.

Energy Conservation Schemes

The tea industry requires provision for constant supply of energy, It therefore approached the Industrial Development Bank of India which had prepared a number of conservation schemes to mention in particular, the Energy Audit Subsidy (EAS) Scheme and Equipment Finance for Energy Conservation (EFEC) Scheme. In a communication to Baratiya Cha Parishard, Dibrugarh IDBI explained the schemes.

Efficient use of energy is critical for our economic development. Energy conservation measures are cost effective, require relatively small investment and have short gestation as well as payback periods. Energy conservation is considered a quick and economical way to solve the problem of power shortage as also a means of conserving the country's finite sources of energy. Recognising the importance of energy conservation, several incentives and concessions have been provided to energy conservation projects by the Governments and the financial institutions in terms of concessiona/reliefs in income-tax, excise duties, customs duties, sales tax, subsidies, liberalisation of licences and loans at concessional terms.

It is in this context that IDBI has introduced two schemes, with a sharp focus on energy conservation objectives in industries. These schemes are (a) Energy Audit Subsidy (EAS) Scheme, and (b)

Equipment Finance for Energy Conservation (EFEC) Scheme. The schemes will be initially in operation for a period two years upto the end of the Seventh Five Year Plan. In the operation of the schemes, IDBI will have close interaction with the industry associations as well as National Productivity Council (NPC), Petroleum Conservation. Research Association (PCRA) and energy consultants.

Eligibility Criterion

Assistance under these schemes will be available for financing proposals for energy audit and/or energy conservation in financially sound industrial undertaking/companies which have been in operation for atleast five years. For the purpose of these schemes, energy conservation would include saving/reduction in consumption of energy per unit of output or improvement in efficiency of use of all forms of energy, including coal, petroleum and petroleum based fuels, natural gas and electricity. The saving/reduction in per unit consumption of energy would be assessed with regard to the standard datum level of consumption for the industry or in undertakings which have satisfactory house-keeping, operating and maintenance practices. The extent of conservation/saving/reduction in unit energy consumption would be assessed/verified by IDBI, if so considered necessary in consultation with NPC, PCRA or an approved energy consultancy organisation. Particulars of the two schemes under which assistance is available are as under.

Conclusion

With the bells ringing in churches,. horns blowing from ships and the jovial people welcoming the new calendar year 2008, we solemnly wish a very happy and prosperous new year for our patrons and for all those connected, in some way or other, with the tea industry of the country and overseas. Also we hope the new year be peaceful and tranquil to the tea gardens of the North-East region in the country that un-derwent severe torment due to rampant violence unleased by the militants last year. No denying the fact, the tempest that darkened the atmosphere, created a ful environment of fear and panic in industry circle had not only discouraged the ploughing back of profit but shattered almost all hope of fresh investment in the industry in this region though, of course, the situation has improved to a considerable extent. However, let gloom be an event of the past and the days ahead brisk and bright. Further it is hoped that the overall performance of tea industry this year be more gorgeous and glorious; production and export surpass the quantum fixed in this regard and the industry establish command in the global market as far as price and quality are concerned. But unless the Central Government and the Tea Board along with respective state governments jointly come forward with a package of incentive scheme and aggressive sales promotion programme, industry's own endeavour cannot be much effective and long-lasting.

Imperative is, therefore, introduction of further financial concessions for the highest producer and exporter of tea, highest price earner for the produce at the international market, besides providing for and creating Investment Allowance and Plantation Development Fund respectively as additional dose of stimuli to the tea industry. In fact, the necessity of such concerted effort to nourish the industry is indisputable. This may be vouched from the pre-budget appraisal of different industries of the country and, more particularly, in the spectrum of other industries' march, where the tea industry was, where it is now, and to what length it can move forward. Certainly, this industry deserves appreciation which is long overdue. Let the new year remove all disappointment; usher in an era of hopes; keep the tea industry brisk, buoyant and spirited in coming years also.

Chapter 9

Marketing Channel of Tea - The Pathway Movement

This chapter deals with marketing system of tea, modes of disposal of tea, seven marketing modes, primary marketing, development of auction centres, tea auction facilities, tea auction systems, advantage of auction sale, the Tandon Committee on Tea Marketing, ex-garden sales, mini-auction, auction for blended and packet teas. Besides, efforts have been made to devote critical analysis on new auction rules—Ahuja committee, 1981, marketing of Indian tea—domestic v/s exports, unrestricted import of tea to allow or not etc.

Marketing System of Tea

Tea is the most popular of all the beverages in the world. As the largest organized sector, tea is one of the oldest industries in India and holds a considerable potential for the economic development of the country. India has the largest area under tea and is also the largest producer, consumer and exporter of tea in the world. In 2005 India's production may be around 900 million kgs. which may account for about 29 per cent of world production. Tea exports from India has been projected at 205 millions kgs which may like to represent about 18 per cent of world export. In addition to contributing substantially to national and state ex-chequers directly and indirectly, it is the largest single export commodity earning foreign exchange.

Tea, being a perishable product, should be disposed of as quickly as possible. The economic viability of tea industry depends crucially on profitable disposal of its products. The marketing system of India tea deals with marketing channels and Government regulations on tea disposal. The marketing system of tea refers to the complex system of institutions and operations which intervenes between the producer of tea on one hand, and on the other hand ultimate consumer who drinks his cup of tea. Among the alternative means of disposal, the producer chooses the channel, which brings the best price to him within the purview of Governemnt regulations. The marketing channel in tea is the pathway of movement of teas through intermediaries from production in the garden to the hands of the ultimate consumers within or outside the country. The Das Committee in its study early in 1974 found that marketing of Indian tea was done by a two-stage process in which the first stage was the passage of Indian tea as a primary product via the various channels to (i) Indian blender packers, (ii) Indian loose tea wholesalers, (iii) U.K. importers, (iv) rupee country importers, and (v) non-rupee-non-U.K. importers overseas. In the domestic market, the second stage of tea marketing was a two -compartment affair, one of which was the marketing of packets in India by Indian blender packers and the other was the loose tea marketing system.

Modes of Disposal

Tea is marketed and made available to the consumers in two different forms viz. loose and packaged. Loose tea is not subjected to any further major processing after it is purchased at auction. It is sold to the consumer rather in the same condition or in blended form. It is generally not packed in convenient sizes before it is sold. In packet tea trade, on the other hand, tea undergoes further processing and different types of tea are blended and sold to the consumers in packets of conventional sizes. There are mainly three modes of disposal of tea viz. auction, ex-factory or ex-garden and forward contract. Among these the public auction system plays the most important role as Tea (Marketing) Control Order (1984) specifies that 75 per cent of the total output of tea estates should be sold through it. The inter linked modes of disposal of Indian tea are as follows : (a) Direct consignment to Landon auction, (b) Direct sale by forward contract to overseas buyers, (c) Consignment to Indian auctions, (d) Direct ex-factory sale to Indian buyers, (e) Direct sale by forward contract to Indian buyers, (e) Direct marketing (loose tea) in wholesale markets and. (g) Self-packeting and exports of packets overseas. Over and above, there are some sales of Indian packaged tea abroad and small scale attempts to sell packaged tea in home market by Indian producers.

The seven marketing modes are discussed below :

(a) Direct Consignment to London Auction

London auction is the oldest and pioneer of institutional marketing of tea in the world. Though over the years, the quantity of Indian tea sent directly for auction to London is coming down, still a good quantity of quality Indian tea is shipped directly to London for sale.

(b) Direct Sale by Forward Contract to Overseas Buyers

This practice was very common in the first quarter of the Twentieth century. Large buyers in the United Kingdom or the East negotiated forward for the purchase of the whole output of an estate, or for a part thereof, over a period of one year or more. The eventual disposal takes many forms. It might be shipped direct to the buyers for general trade distribution; it might be transported in varying quantities to different parts of the world, some of it might find its way to London auction; it might be retained at the port of shipment to be blended and possibly packeted there and reshipped to various consuming countries.

(c) Consignment to Indian Auctions

Most of the tea produced in India is sold through the seven auction centres situated in different parts of the country. Here tea is sold to the buyers through brokers, a middleman, who sells tea on behalf of the growers. The tea is sold to the highest bidder under the usual rules of sale governing such auction. The seven auction centers of the country are Guwahati, Kolkatta, Siliguri, Cochin, Coonoor, Coimbatore, and Amritsar.

(d) Direct Ex-factory Sale to Indian Buyer

Under this system, tea is old in the garden itself. This applies to sales from bought leaf factory. Tea produced in such factories is more regularly sold ex-factory to local collectors or dealers through whom it passes to merchants, who may sell it by auction or by private treaty or be shipped. Some estates located on the main road sell tea loose or in packets to retail buyers at the factory door, although the quantity is less. This gives a quick returns to the garden.

(e) Direct Sale by Forward Contract to Indian Buyers

Buyers and sellers make a contract even before tea is produced to sell it at a fixed price later on. The producer has to sell the teas to the buyers at the agreed price, irrespective of the price of tea later.

(f) Direct Marketing (Loose Tea) in Wholesale Markets

Growers sell their tea directly in wholesale outlet in the market.

(h) Self-packeting and Export of Packets Overseas

Tea is exported in packet form from the garden to different countries of the world in company's name.

Primary Marketing

Table 9.1 Primary Marketing of Tea

Details of Primary Marketing of Tea during 1980 to 2004 is given below.

Particular	1980		1990		1995		2004	
	Qty (1)	Pc (2)	Qty. (1)	Pc (2)	Qty. (1)	Pc (2)	Qty. (1)	Pc (2)
Indian Auction	306.96	53.89	482.25	66.95	428.36	56.66	464.70	52.79
London Auction	31.73	5.57	8.13	1.13	3.31	0.44	3.20	0.36
Singapore Auction	-	-	-	-	-	-	-	-
Total Auction	338.69	59.46	490.38	68.08	431.67	57.10	467.90	53.13
Export under forward contract	22.29	3.92	25.61	3.55	30.02	3.97	41.98	4.77
Ex-garden sale	208.56	36.62	204.35	28.37	294.33	38.93	370.32	42.10
Total sale	569.54	100.00	720.34	100.00	756.02	100.00	880.20	100.00

Source: Various issues of Tea Statistics, Tea Board, India, Tea Plantation Industry in India - Structural changes between 1950 and 1992 by Dr. G.D. Banerjee.

Note: Quantity in million kgs (1), Percentage to total sale (2).

The buyers at the other end of each of these channels are not distinct groups. There is considerable overlap and inter-mixture among them.

To describe this inter linkage, the buyers are categorized into several main types viz. (i) Indian packeteers, (ii) Indian (loose tea) wholesellers, (iii) rupee country buyers, (iv) U.K. importers/buyers, and (v) non-rupee overseas importers. Out of India's total production of 880.20 million kg in 2004, quantity sold through auction was 467.90 million kg (53.13 per cent), export under forward contract 41.98 million kg (4.77 per cent), and ex-garden sale 370.32 million kg representing 42.10 per cent.

Development of Auction Market in the World

The first organized sale of tea through auction took place at Mincing Lane in London. The East India Company sold its tea in India House, privately till 1838 but after it lost its monopoly of the Indian trade, all tea was sold in the commercial sale-room at Mincing Lane. For the first five years after 1834, tea sold at Mincing Lane was exclusively from China. On 10th January 1839, the first commercial consignment of Indian Tea was sold in the commercial sale-room by the East India Company, which was an event of great importance in the history of Indian Tea. As Sir Percival Griffiths in "The History of the Indian Tea Industry said. "The first importance of tea from the British territories in Assam consisting of eight chests, containing about 350 pounds, was put up by the East Indian Company in public sale in the commercial sale rooms, Mincing Lane, on the 10th January, 1839 and excited much curiosity". This was the first auction of Indian Tea. The first Indian Tea Auction Center was established in Calcutta on 27th December 1861. Calcutta Tea Broker's Association at first conducted the auction. Since 1947, auctions have been held in Calcutta under the auspices at the Calcutta Tea Traders Association (CTTA). There are 13 auction centers in the world at present out of which seven are in India. Table-9.2 shows the dates of establishment of the tea auction centers of India.

Auction market in Colombo started on 30th July 1883 for Sri Lanka tea. Chittagong Auction Center was established on 16th July 1949 to deal in teas of the then East Pakistan, (new Bangladesh). Nairobi auction market began sale on 7th November 1956 for the sale of African teas. Nairobi auction market has since moved to Mombasa on 14 July 1959. Before the war, Amsterdam was an important auction center for Indonesian tea. Sale ceased in that auction center in April 1940 but was resumed in January 1949 and then again suspended in July 1958. Auction sale was inaugurated in Antwerp in 1959 and later suspended in 1966. In 1960, auctions started in Hamburg but was suspended in 1965. These two auction centers handled Indonesian tea. Limbo acution market started operation in February 1970 and Djakarta auction on 11th December 1972. Thus, while London auction market is "cosmopolitan" in nature, other markets handle tea of the local producers.

Table 9.2 : Date of Establishment Tea Auction Centres in India

Sl. No.	Name of the auction center	Date of establishment
1	Amritsar	30th April, 1964
2	Calcutta (now Kolkatta)	27th December, 1861
3	Cochin	4th July, 1947
4	Coimbatore	22nd November, 1980
5	Coonoor	23rd March, 1963
6	Guwahati	25th September, 1970
7	Siliguri	26th October, 1976

Source- Tea Plantation Industry in India - Structural changes between 1850 and 1992 by Dr. G.D. Banerjee.

Tea Auction Facilities

Tea auction facilitates distribution of the largest quantities of the product in the shortest possible time, increases competition among buyers and sellers because of the concentration of the factors of supply and demand under one roof, improves grading and packing, offers advantages to the buyers in finding quickly the type and quantity he wants and extension of credit to buyers by financial institutions. The auction serves the buyers by enabling them to purchase tea of a much broader variety than they would otherwise be able to, moving from garden to garden individually. The consumer demands certain standardisation in tea blends. This ia an extremely delicate operation as the quality of tea manufacutred from day to day in different tea estater very greatly. To achieve this standardisations, the auctions allow the blenders to match teas from all over India with their blends. Buyers are afforded the widest choice to fulfil their particular requirements, be they for exports, whole sale, retail or blending, while the sellers are provided a platform for attracting the widest range of market through numerous buyers, both internal and domestic and foreign. No other commodity of such a varied quality can be disposed of in so short a time.

Tea Auction System

It has often been claimed that the tea auction system has withstood the test of time. The auctions have been found acceptable by both sellers and buyers and have the approval of the government as well. The auctions provide the producers a ready and reliable means of selling their produce. A now entrant, thanks to the auction system, does not have to necessarily worry about marketing his production. This is not the case with other products where marketing is an essential input. The tea industry has attracted many investors because one is in business straight away, without searching for markets. The producers receive the sale proceeds timely, 14 days after the sale, through a well established system of 'prompts'. The buyers have found the auctions beneficial as they can not only buy at a central point but can watch the operation of their competitors. They do not have to go from door to door for their requirements. Even for private transactions, auctions are the barometer. The brokers have been able to evolve an effective system whereby services are efficiently provided to both buyers and sellers. They have been providing market intelligence, manufacturing and agricultural advice to the producers and have regularly compiled useful data for the tea industry, including statistical information. However, despite its benefits, there appear to be some cracks in the system and now more and more. More and more producers are going in for direct marketing, by passing the auction system. This trend is likely to continue, as producers would like to exercise personal control over their production. The major buyers have supported the auction system in past. The former USSR bought the bulk of its quantity through auctions but the disintegration of the former Russia has brought in a change in the buying policies and purchase of the Russian Federation and CIS countries today are being done substantially through private sales. Similarly, other buyers, to secure quantities, are buying teas privately. In fact, the main supporters of Darjeeling tea have shown a clear preference for private sales during quality periods. The Tea Marketing Control Order of 1984 prescribes that the producers must sell 75 per cent of their production through seven recognized auction centers of India, Guwahati, Siliguri, Cochin, Coonoor, Coimbatore and Amritsar. This order, however, has no teelh and, in any case, may be withdrawn as India moves towards a free economy.

Advantage of Auction Sale

A tea auction center collects supplies of teas from a large number of go downs and canalizes them into many areas of high demand spread all over the world. As a mechanism of sale, the outstanding virtue of the auction is integrity the selling and buying are done publicly. The auction is economic gaps of money to the seller. As Goradia observes, the auction center is a meeting place, where up to 1000 gardens meet some 1000 buyers to trade 3000 to 5000 lots of tea every week, in the course of only 20 hours. The present system of selling tea in auctions through brokers, are selling samples to buyers and printing information catalogue originated in London. The same system, therefore, has been adopted in other tea auction centers also. The auction mechanism has some definite advantages: (i) The producer is assured of fair price on the prevailing market, (ii) assurance of continual flow of sale to the producers without fear of a buildup unsold stocks which may happen in case of other selling modes in times of recession (iii) no problem of bid collection as payment is automatically collected on the 14th day, (iv) the pushing nature of bidding in tea auction improves price and helps in maintaining a similar price level for comparable lots of tea, (v) free sampling, which costs less than 2 per cent, is a vehicle of sales promotion ideal for a commodity of such variety, (vi) as the auction takes place public the integrity of sale issimplicit to a producer regardless of his situation from the auction center or unfamiliarity with mechanics of trading.

Tandon Committee on Marketing

Thus, the system of tea auctions, which is more than a century old, has admirably stood the test of time. In spite of views occasionally expressed to the contrary, all committees and commissions set up in India and abroad have recommended the continuation of the auction system as the most efficient method of disposal of bulk commodity like tea. The last committee to examine the auction system in India was the Tandon Committee, which submitted its report in November 1978. After very careful examination of all aspects of the matter the committee confirmed the need to allow auctions to progress freely. The committee also recommended that efforts should be made to introduce in different auction centers useful practices followed in other auction centers and to achieve uniformity in rules in different auction centers as far as possible.

Ex-garden Sale

The Tea Board constituted a committee to examine the role of mini auction. The committee recommended that thus experiment should be watched alongwith the nodus operandi of the players and its impact on tea trade be examined to access the systemis advantages and disadvantages. The committee clearly envisaged the possibility of mini auction assuming bigger role in coming years. What is more remarkable is that the committee did not decry ex-garden sale and took a certain portion of teas produced being sold at ex-garden as a fait accompli and indispensable from the point of view of producers, particularly the weaker section. The need for ex-garden sale arose from the common wisdom of not putting all the eggs in the same basket, which inevitably reduce price. Moreover, having some volume of ex-garden sale is also important for maintaining a satisfactory cash flow position since in the sale through auctions it takes 3 to 6 months for the sellers to receive the sale proceeds. In this background the stipulation under the Tea Marketing Control Order, 1984 that 70 per cent of crop in 1984 and 75 per cent of crop in 1985 onwards should be sold through public auctions in India has been causing serious financial problems for the products apart from reducing the prices realized at auction. Stipulation of minimum of crop for sale through auctions in India was held good for two years ie, 1985 and 1986 but from 1987 onwards, the proportion started declining. This was due to considerable delay in sale through auctions, on the one hand, and reduction in prices as a result of too much tea being available at auctions, on the other. The existing auctions will also find it extremely difficult to handle the largely increased volume of tea smoothly and promptly unless their facilities are augmented. It is, therefore, proved that other methods of disposal of tea should be allowed to play prominent.

Mini Auction

Tata, which organized mini auction, filled the gap to some extent. It should be encouraged. Simultaneously, ex-garden sale, which in 1995 and 2004 accounted for 38.93 per cent and 42.04 per cent of total production, should be allowed to continue and, if necessary, to increase, depending on circumstances so that producers may receive the best possible prices for their produce and sale proceeds may also be received as early as possible, which is essential in view of their tight cash-flow position. The quantity sold through auction in 2004 constituted 53.13 per cent of total crop. Over the years, the sale through public auction in percentage terms started fluctuating and it may handle 45 per cent of the crop in immediate future and still lower proportion in the following years. As a result, a bigger role will be played by mini-auctions, London auctions, ex-garden sales as well as C and F export. Any dogmatic insistence on increasing sales through public auctions in India without considering the capacity of the auction centers on the one hand, and effects of such a policy on tea prices and financial position of tea producers, on the other, hand, will only create utter confusion in the tea industry and trade and an inevitable slump in tea prices. Mini auctions in particular have a big role to play as a method, which lies in between public auction and ex-garden sale. The Tea Board had drawn up a set of model rules to govern these mini-auctions so as to remove the scope for under invoicing and the evils associated with public auctions.

Auction for Blended and Packet Teas

There is need for other innovative approaches. Auctioning of blended teas and packet teas would be one such approach. It should cover not only teas blended and/or packeted by tea producers but also teas blended and/or packeted by buyers of loose tea. In fact, traders rather than producers may take the lead in organizing auctions of blended and packeted teas, which may be purchased by second stage traders for either domestic consumption or export. One immediate beneficial effect of this approach would be the elimination of the monopolistic hold in the matter of packet teas enjoyed by few packers with consequent reduction in prices it is ultimately consumers who have to pay exnorbitant prices for the teas purchased by them because of high profit margin enjoyed by traders at different levels of distribution channels and they do not get any relief even when auction prices nedecline. Table 9.3 indicates the percentage of offerings through auctions since 1910.

Table 9.3 Production and Sae of Tea during 1990 to 2004

(Note: Quantity in million kgs)

Year	Production	Sold through auctions	Per cent sold in auctions
1900	89.6	24.6	27.45
1910	119.6	34.5	28.85
1920	156.5	37.5	23.96
1930	177.4	42.0	23.67
1940	210.4	45.2	21.48
1950	275.5	113.6	41.23
1960	321.1	173.8	54.13
1970	418.5	241.3	57.66
1980	569.2	307.0	53.93
1985	656.2	505.3	77.00
1986	620.8	468.4	75.45
1987	674.3	472.5	70.07
1988	701.1	504.4	71.96
1989	684.1	477.4	69.78
1990	702.34	474.0	65.8
1991	754.2	501.2	66.45
1992	732.3	448.0	61.18
1993	760.8	441.7	58.06
1994	752.9	428.3	56.89
1995	756.9	428.4	56.66
1996	780.0	427.3	56.52
1997	810.6	442.2	56.99
1998	870.4	454.7	52.24
1999	825.9	460.5	55.7
2000	846.9	463.5	55.2
2001	853.9	460.15	53.8
2002	860.5	458.7	53.3
2003	870.5	461.5	53.0
2004	880.2	467.90	53.1

Source : Various issues of Tea Statistics

The Tea Market Control Order came into force with effect from 19th April 1984. It will be seen from the the data that quantity of offerings went up to 1991. It, however, showed a steady decline. With the ever-expanding middle class in India, packets and branded goods are becoming more and more popular. the number of producers of packet tea, the private sale of which is permitted under the Tea Marketing Control Order, has increased. The poly pouch with the "garden fresh" slogan is popularizing packet teas in India. The consumer packets, packed at the gardens, are sold directly and do not go through auctions. Improved communications have also helped in expanding the private sale market.

New Tea Auctions Rules—Ahuja Committee, 1985

The Tea (Marketing) Control Order, 1984 was promulgated by the Government of India in April 1984. This order made it obligatory for the organizers of public tea auctions and brokers to obtain a license from the Tea Board. Besides, all tea manufactures in India had to register themselves with Tea Board and sell 75 per cent of their annual production through the medium of public auction. The Chairman, Tea Board being the Licensing/Registering Authority was empowered to oversee the functioning of the tea auction centers and to issue directives whenever necessary to ensure that the public auction runs smoothly, efficiently and in the best interests of all concerned. The Tea Board, thus, became directly involved in the tea auction system. The public the auction system plays a vital role in the tea trade and industry. There are seven recognized auction centers in India at Kolkatta, Siliguri, Guwahati, Cochin Coonoor, Coimbatore and Amritsar. Out of the total Indian production of 886 million kg in 2004, 467.9 million kg of tea was sold through the auctions (details in Table 9.3). The tea auction committees at various centers have been reviewing the rules governing their respective auction centers from time to time and have been updating them in line with the changing times, conditions and need. Despite this, the Tea Board received grievances and requests from all sections of the trade to look into certain areas, which needed further improvement. The "Out lot" sales and distribution of free trade samples were the first amongst the issues raised with the Tea Board. In August 1985, by an administrative order, the Chairman, Tea Board formed a committee headed by S.S. Ahuja, the then Deputy Chairman, Tea Board, "to study the existing rules of all the public tea auction centers in India and to suggest changes where, necessar,y to bring improvement in the auction system". This committee on auction rules, also known as the "Ahuja Committee", submitted its final report and recommendations in the third week of April 1990. As its first task, the Committee identified eleven areas; (a) auction day, (b) catalogues, (c) prompt date, (d) broker's commission, (e) size of lots, (f) division of lots, (g) withdrawal of lots, (h) sale of out lets, (i) warehouse rent and insureance, (j) closing of catalogues, and (k) distribution of samples, for details examination. The Ahuja Committee submitted four interim reports and a final report, the recommendations of which were accepted by the Chairman, Tea Board. The main features of this report were as given below:

i. Auction Day— The Committee examined the possibility of conducting auctions at all the centers on the same day instead of separate days, as is the current practice, to avoid speculative tendencies, if any. The committee, however, recommended that the present system of holding auctions on different days at different places should continue as it was running satisfactorily. The auctions at each center have to be completed in two days and no more. For this, the auction committees have been asked to look into their infrastructure and make additional alternative auction rooms, if required. The brokers must be given fixed timings and must strictly adhere to them.

ii. Catalogue — The committee recommended that CTC leaf, orthodox leaf. Darjeeling leaf, green tea, all dusts and the supplemented teas be printed separately. This was because of sampling norms and proper maintenance of category-wise statistical data. The brokers have been asked to deliver samples, catalogues etc. strictly within the specified time limits so that the buyers are not inconvenienced.

iii. Prompt Date — The committee suggested no major change in the present system of payment of prompts at the various auction centers. The buyers and sellers prompt falls due on different days after the date of the sale at various centers. For example, in Coonor the buyers prompt is on the 12th day after the date of the sale and for the sellers it is the 13th day after the sale. In Siliguri, prompt is payable by the buyers on the 13th day which is paid to the sellers on the 14th day. In Calcutta, the buyer prompt is on the 14th day for leaf and 15th day for dust. Although there is no specification on sellers' prompt in Calcutta, the brokers disburse to the producers' prompt on the same day it is received from the buyers. The committee recommended that the payment of the prompt to the seller by the broker shall be the next working day immediately after the stipulated prompt date of the buyer. The committee has also recommended that the auction committee should not extend prompts unless the circumstances are exceptional.

iv. Brokerage — The sellers pay 1 per cent of the selling price to the brokers as commission. However, in South India, the brokerage is calculated on the selling price minus excise duty. Furthermore, buyers pay to the brokers, for various services rendered at the rate of Rs. 5 per 100 kg in Siliguri and Guwahati. In the South, there is no commission payable by the buyers to the brokers but there is a system of "lot money". Is this recommendation of 1985 yet to be implemented.

v. Size of Lots — In the North, tea estates (except Darjeeling) producing two lakh kg or more were to pack in lots not less than 30 packages during manufacturing periods between 1st July to 30th November. The only exceptions were to be BPS, small dusts and secondaries in the CTC category and tippy teas like BPS, Fannings, Dusts and Secondaries in the orthodox category.

vi. Division of Lots — In order to expedite the speed of sale in the North India auction centers, the committee recommended that brokers should not issue more than two contracts for 30 packages for under and more than three contracts for 31 packages and above. No buyer should get less than five packages in a division. However, for Darjeeling teas no change was recommended and, therefore, up to 15 chests one buyer, 16 to 30 chests two buyers and above 30 chests three buyers will continue.

vii. Withdrawal of Lots — In Calcutta, where auctions normally take place on Mondays and Tuesdays every week, sellers will have to give advance intimation to the brokers about withdrawal of any teas included in the catalogue for sale at the latest by 1.00 pm on

Wednesday of the week immediately proceding the week prior to the sale in question. This principle will apply to all other North Indian centers. In the South, this problem is not so visible and, therefore, no change was suggested.

viii. Sale lot Outlets— The Tea Board had earlier directed that teas remaining unsold in the auction room should not be sold as outlets. The auction committees have the option either to supplement the unsold teas in the following week's auction without re-sampling or reprinting them in subsequent auctions with fresh sampling. This practice is to continue. The quantity of Indian tea sold through different auction centers in India are presented below:-

Table 9.4: Dispoal of North and South Indian Tea Through Various Auctions During 1984 to 2004.

(Note: Quantity in million kgs)

Particular/year	1984	1887	1990	1993	1997	2004
Total production	639.9	674.3	720.3	760.8	810.6	880.2
Quantity sold through						
Kolkata	114.7	132.6	129.2	102.3	89.0	95.1
Siliguir	72.2	80.6	90.0	75.8	80.0	85.3
Guwahati	89.0	147.7	140.9	151.3	150.2	151.3
Amritsar	0.3	0.4	0.4	0.1	0.8	0.9
Total North Indian auction sale	276.2	361.3	360.5	329.5	320.1	332.6
Quantity sold through						
Cochin	64.0	52.3	52.3	52.0	56.1	58.5
Coonoor	23.0	27.4	36.9	41.0	44.8	57.3
Coimbator	27.5	31.5	24.3	19.0	21.2	16.3
Total South Indian auction sale	114.5	111.2	113.5	112.2	122.1	132.1
Total all India auction sale	390.7	472.5	474.0	441.7	442.2	467.9

Source : Same as Table 9.1

ix. Warehouse Rent and Insurance— In Siliguri and Guwahati, the sellers liability for rent and insurance is up to a specified time on the prompt date. There after the liability, passes on to the buyers. In Cochin, Coonoor and Coimbatore, the goods are at sellers' risk to the extent of sale price only until a specified time on the second working day after the prompt date. However, in Kolkatta the sellers bear additional 14 days' rent beyond the prompt date. The committee recommended that the system in Kolkatta, should be urgently reviewed so that the system prevalent in Siliguri and Guwahati finds acceptance in due course and progressively.

x. Closing Catalogue— The committee felt that the availability of teas for the domestic market, despite seasonality of tea production in the North, should be regular and adequate all through. Therefore, regular consultations were suggested to achieve this objective.

xi. Distribution of Samples— This has been a major area of debate and the committee's recommendations were elaborate. The committee felt that issuance of free trade samples to the trader could not be claimed as a matter of right. Free trade samples should be worked out and supplied in a manner that encourages genuine, regular and energetic buyers but at the same time discourages frivolous and/or casual buyers. The committee, therefore, specified qualification for small, medium and large buyers for each category of tea and for each auction center. The committee further recommended that over and above the minimum percentage purchase qualification, each buyer shall have to operate in at least 25 per cent of the sales held for the category concerned for the purchase year to be eligible for free trade samples in the immediate succeeding sampling year. The committee further dealt with matters like purchase of trade samples, restricted sampling of expensive teas, defined powers of the sampling committee and status of 'on account of concerned' teas.

Quantum of Samples— The brokers ensure delivery of proper quantum of samples to the buyers in order to streamline the system. Further, it was recommended that brokers, while sending trade samples, should clearly indicate in the challans the number of large, medium and small samples category-wise sent in a consignment with its total net weight. The quantity of purchase samples has been increased to 300 gm.

Bidding Rates — With a view to improving auctioning efficiency, the following scales of bidding should be introduced in Kolkatta, Siliguri and Guwahati :

Up to Rs 26.99	20 paise/kg
Rs.27.00 to 49.99	15 paise/kg
Rs 50.00 to 99.00	Re. 1 Per kg
Rs 100 & above	Rs 5 /kg

Claims for Shortages, Non-delivery, Damaged Teas : — The committee recommended that no claim for short weight be admissible unless the shortage exceeds 0.1 per cent of the declared weight per lot purchased by any buyer. The committee recommended that where lots purchased by the buyers were not to be found at the warehouse at all, either wholly or in part, a compensation amounting to 30 per cent of value of such teas be payable to the buyer.

Supervision:— The committee considered that way back in 1978, the P.L. Tandon committee strongly favoured the public auction of teas as the best means of bulk marketing and also desired that infrastureture of the Tea Board be strenghtened for the proper supervision and co-ordination of the public auction system. Owing to various financial and other aspects, this has possibly not been given effect to so far. Tea (Marketing) Control Order, 1984 issued by the government under the Tea Act, 1953, provides that 75 per cent of the tea production is to be routed through the public auctions, thereby clearly indicating the mind of the government of India in this respect. The committee, therefore, after carefully reviewing the situation, recommended that the Tea Board should devise ways and means of strengthening the infrastructure for proper supervision and co-ordination of the public auction system in North and South India to subserve the Government policy and the larger public interest.

The Ahuja committee comprised members, from all sections of the Indian tea trade and its recommendations were sent by the Chairman, tea board to the auction committees. The Tea Board accepted some of the recommendations made by the Ahuja Committee report and therefore it becomes a directive under the Tea (Marketing) Control Order 1984. The Auction Committees can, however, approach the authorities on specific issues with their problems and suggestions to ensure easier implementation of the Ahuja committee report. The report of the committee on auction rules is a major report on the auction system and is a valuable document produced after a great deal of effort and toil. It is a work of dedication and shows genuine interest in the working of the tea industry. The report will go a long way in further strengthening the bonds between the trinity of the tea trade, namely, buyers, sellers and brokers.

Tea Marketing Is No More A Fashionable Slogan

Signs of maturity were observed in the tea marketing scene, which was, perhaps, partly due to the effects of disintegration of the former USSR and partly to the economic liberalization move stoutly pursued by Dr. Manmohan Sign. Earlier, the glorious period of Indian tea marketing was restricted to production of teas on Indian soil to suit the needs of British blenders. Indian tea-sahibs were happy to satisfy the visiting agents, pack the produce in plywood chests and put them on to the holds of vessels sailing for London port. The estates were largely owned by the Britishers (at least the rich ones) and the accountants in London determined prices. It was a happy time, but, frankly, no marketing was involved. It merely served as commodity suppliers for big business. This situation continued for a long time through Independence. The first shock came from FERA. A great deal of hesitation regarding permissible share of foreign holdings, lack of decisions usually with Government of India, led to shifting of ownership of gardens. The British planters were losing interest an started developing an alternative source of supply for which Kenya was found to be suitable location. That is, however, another story.

With the loss of the London market, former USSR and East European countries appeared on the scene, strengthened by a long-term friendship treaty involving rupee trade agreement. Tea became an important item in this pact. Within a short time, the share of former USSR and East European countries surpassed 50 per cent of Indian export quantum. So, the need for exporting more than what India could conveniently do was not strong. However, an ambitious projection of 370 m. kg export by the turn of century, kept the tea industry busy all the while. The slogan of need for exporting more value added products like packet tea, tea bag and instant tea was heard from all corners. It was all for increasing the foreign exchange earnings. Some meek attempts were made to popularise Indian tea in foreign markets by way of subsising advertising expenditure of Indian exporters for their packs with the mention of Indian tea on it.

Foreign packers would also receive subsidy if they used a certain percentage of Indian tea in their blends and advertised that point. Funds for such activity was small and mechanism of payment quite complicated. As a result, real big tea marketers hardly cared for such schemes. But year after year some money, which appeared large in Indian context but chicken feed in the context of global operation, used to be dissipated. After the loss of USSR market when exports fell sharply, there was hardly any scope for toying with such experiments. Collaboration with global operators, attempts to establish brand image, realisings the need for consumer research, production of bio-tea and specialities etc. gave Indian tea industry a smart appearance. Convertibility of rupee as a part of liberalization plan provided necessary support for taking right steps. The devalued rupees had positively encouraged larger interest from general currency areas. Indian tea was found more competitive in the world markets. Breakdown of the buying system in CIS countries created such an impact in the international trade that the normal rules of demand and supply did not work. Export project called for substantial efforts in the field of marketing.

Collaborations Such as Tata-Telly, Meneil Magor Nestle are valid international tickets for global market destinations. Big contract by Iran did help to push up exports but such sales cannot be depended upon until demand for a particular brand arises from consumer level; going alone in the world market to establish a blend is a tough job. Big Indian business houses are glancing at tea for diversification like ITC who can use their overseas connections not only for bulk exports but marketing a brand as well. Internally, most of the big tea companies are vying for a better share of their brands at the consumer level. As a result, number of packs have appeared in the domestic market leading to a healthy competitions. A commendable step was taken by **Bombay Burmah group** by creating production facilities for **ecologically cultivated tea at singampatti on the southern tip of India.** There is a wide-open area in the speciality market, taping of which calls for marketing skill. This entails giving up the more fashionable and bureancreatic luxuries. It is encomaging to see that this view has been gaining credence, as is reflected in the growth of more mature marketing activities in the Indian teac sector.

Tea Market Trend

Tea is a tradition bound industry. The changing World order in the at three years, however, has left its own impact on tea. The coming down of the Berlin wall and the disintegration of the former USSR have led to many changes and opened up several opportunities for the tea world. The first, second and the third world are moving more and more towards freer economy, freer trade and freer investment. Consumerism has taken the front seat even in the developing and poor countries. Furthermore, the developed countries are moving towards healthier products and quality assuances. **Environment friendly bulk** packaging is being encouraged and to put pressure on the exporters, the disposal of "unfriendly" packaging material is being made the responsibility of the exporter. In addition, many new trends have emerged, particularly for Indian tea, some of which are discussed below.

Production

In 2005, the Indian production should reach 900 million kg, which will be second highest ever. Quality consciousness and the widening price concertina have put brakes on rapid growth of production. In 2005, if the weather is right, India should harvest a crop of 925 million kg. It is also clear that unless new areas are brought under tea cultivation, tea production will grow at a small rate of around 3 per cent per annum. Again, it is necessary to renovate tea areas, which are more than sixty years of age. A replanting programme of two per cent per annum will ensure a rotation over fifty years.

Domestic Market

India's per capita consumption of tea is amongst the lowest. Yet in volume terms India is the largest consumer. With the population having reached 100 crore, even if an Indian were to drink one extra cup a year, the additional requirement of tea for domestic consumption would be 2.55 million kg; if ten cups extra were to be drunk every day by every Indian, then the requirement would be 25.5 million kg. If one cup extra wre to be drunk every day by every Indian, the additional requirement would work out to 921 million kg per annum. India is indeed a very powerful market. Another important factor to note is that the Indians drink the very best of CTCs and are prepared to pay a premium for quality. Because of the strong domestic base, Indian tea prices are generally higher than the world prices. The superior quality of Indian tea and its vast variety has also helped in maintaining higher price levels.

Export

It has now become clear that the Government of India will not hinder in any way the exports of Indian tea. Procedures are begin simplified and restrictions have been eased or fully removed. The Government of India and the tea industry have been working towards improving per unit returns from exports and value added products have been gaining ground. While it is unlikely that the government will impose any restrictions on exports in the foreseeable future, the pressure from the domestic market will limit the quantum of India tea exports in the years to come. A strategy, therefore, has to be evolved so that even the export quantities remain around 200 million kg, the value will go on increasing. Barter deals and government-to-government buying appear to be thing of the past and trading in future, will be done in hard currency. The instrument of devaluation has its own limitations and with the move towards free-floating currencies in the major tea producing countries, the correct values would be established automatically. The former USSR is today an open market and although there is a preference for Indian teas in the Russian Federation and CIS countries, other producers, especially China, which has a vast common bordcr, may exploit the large potential of this market. The producer exporters are already playing a major role in certain importing countries and this trend is likely to spread further.

The Auction System

The major tea groups today are increasingly marketing their own teas either through domestic packers or direct exports. While the auctions will continue to be the barometer for price levels, more and more producers are likely to go in for direct marketing. The smaller producers, who have gone in for direct marketing through soft packs, may find the going rough unless they start putting in the essential marketing inputs like advertising etc. as well. Their present method of sale is virtually bulk-marketing through a third party. The quantity from these producers is likely to revert back to the auctions.

Import of Tea

From time to time, the idea of importing tea into India has been mooted. Importing cheap teas for domestic consumption will not solve the problem. Indians drink good quality tea and the imported varieties will not suit their taste. Furthermore, if 40 to 50 million kg of tea were to be imported, there would be a phenomenal price increase in the world markets. India has to be very careful so as not to upset the apple cart.

Promotion

As consumption of tea in certain developed countries is not increasing, the time has come to give a new "position" to tea. The world is today more health conscious than ever before and "healthfulness" could be the new slogan for tea. The "cheapness" slogan has to be discarded.

Quality

One way of increasing tea consumption in the world market is to ensure that the consumer is served good quality teas. Producers and importers of tea will have to make sure that sub-standard teas are neither produced nor imported. Universal acceptance of international standard ISO 3720 will help in lifting quality standards of all growths. India is, perhaps, the only country today, which strictly follows rigid quality standards.

Culture Products

All the tea bagging machines in India is busy fulfilling export-orders and some domestic needs. But the product of the future is instant tea. Time is not far when a "drinkable" pure instant tea, which is both hot and cold water soluble, will be on the shelves.

Bulk Packaging

While bulk packaging is still searching for an alternative to the tea chest, paper sacks are being used more and more. The real answer lies in convincing the tea importers to accept gunny bags, which are

Table 9.5: Country Wise Exports from India during 1947 to 2004

(in million kg)

Country / year	1947	1957	1967	1977	1987	1991	1997	2004
United Kingdom	127.2	135.4	117.2	74.3	22.4	22.5	25.4	25.0
% of export	66.3	68.0	53.8	32.4	11.09	11.09	12.7	12.1
Ireland	9.0	8.3	6.2	6.4	2.1	2.5	2.6	2.5
% of export	4.7	4.2	2.8	2.8	1.04	1.23	1.28	1.2
Netherlands	1.5	0.9	3.7	3.4	1.6	1.9	2.7	2.6
% of export	0.8	0.5	1.7	1.5	0.79	0.9	1.33	1.27
West Germany	Nil	1.9	2.2	5.8	4.7	4.7	6.9	6.6
% of export	Nil	0.9	1.0	2.5	2.33	2.3	3.40	3.2
Rest of W. Europe	0.6	0.1	0.5	0.9	0.5	0.6	0.8	0.8
% of export	0.3	0.05	0.2	0.4	0.2	0.3	0.4	0.4
Poland	Nil	Nil	1.8	5.3	10.7	11.9	14.0	14.7
% of export	Nil	Nil	0.8	2.8	5.3	5.9	6.9	7.1
Yugoslvia	Nil	Nil	0.5	4.7	1.4	0.2	0.3	0.4
% of export	Nil	Nil	0.2	2.0	0.7	0.1	0.15	0.17
Rest of East Europe	Nil	0.1	1.7	1.4	3.3	1.0	1.6	1.4
% of export	Nil	0.05	0.8	0.6	1.6	0.5	0.8	0.7
USSR	4.0	7.3	20.7	47.7	96.6	104.5	90.7	92.8
% of export	2.1	3.6	9.5	20.8	47.8	51.5	44.7	44.9
Afghanistan	Nil	Nil	5.7	8.6	3.6	1.6	0.8	1.2
% of export	Nil	Nil	2.6	3.7	1.8	0.8	0.4	0.6
Iran	3.9	5.6	1.8	6.6	18.9	14.8	11.7	12.8
% of export	2.0	2.8	1.1	2.9	9.4	7.3	5.8	6.2
Iraq	1.4	0.02	2.5	4.6	8.8	--	0.1	0.04
% of export	0.7	0.001	1.1	2.0	4.3	--	0.01	0.02
Persian Gulf Ports	4.4	2.6	3.0	6.2	7.0	5.2	6.8	7.02
% of export	2.3	1.3	1.4	2.7	3.5	2.6	3.35	3.4
Jordan	Nil	Nil	1.4	0.6	--	0.5	0.1	0.6
% of export	---	---	0.6	0.3	0.05	0.2	0.2	0.3
Rest of Middle East	0.6	0.3	0.05	0.07	0.3	--	0.2	0.2
% of export	0.3	0.1	0.02	0.03	0.1	--	0.1	0.1
Pakistan	Nil	Nil	Nil	4.6	0.6	0.3	0.4	0.4
% of export	--	--	--	2.0	0.3	0.15	0.2	0.2

Japan	Nil	Nil	0.3	0.8	1.4	2.0	1.9	2.3
% of export	--	--	0.1	0.3	0.3	1.0	0.9	1.1
Arab Rep. of Egypt	1.8	7.3	16.6	14.1	7.8	7.9	7.2	7.6
% of export	0.9	3.7	7.6	6.1	3.9	3.9	3.5	3.7
Sudan	0.7	2.0	10.0	13.6	0.1	--	0.1	0.1
% of export	0.4	1.0	4.6	5.7	0.05	--	0.05	0.06
Tunisia	Nil	Nil	3.8	1.2	1.0	1.7	1.5	1.9
% of export	--	--	1.7	0.5	0.5	0.8	0.7	0.9
Rest of Africa	Nil	Nil	--	0.4	3.7	7.0	9.8	9.5
% of export	--	--	--	0.2	1.8	3.4	4.8	4.6
Canada	8.2	7.7	3.9	2.5	0.8	0.6	0.1	0.15
% of export	4.3	3.9	1.8	1.1	0.4	0.3	0.05	0.07
USA	17.3	10.6	8.4	10.0	1.8	2.5	2.9	3.3
% of export	9.0	5.3	3.9	4.4	0.9	1.2	1.4	1.6
Australia	7.0	3.4	5.4	4.6	0.7	0.8	0.5	0.6
% of export	3.7	1.7	2.5	2.0	0.3	0.4	0.25	0.3
New Zealand	0.5	0.7	0.4	1.3	--	--	--	--
% of export	0.3	0.4	0.2	0.6	--	--	--	--
All other countries	3.6	5.0	0.1	0.5	4.3	8.1	13.4	11.95
% of export	1.9	2.5	0.05	0.2	2.1	4.0	6.63	5.81
Total	191.7	199.2	217.8	229.6	201.9	202.9	203.0	206.5

Sources : Same as Table 9.1

already popular in the domestic market. In the overall, the future prospects of tea appear to be bright and the tea industry in India is ready to face the challenges of the 21st century.

Marketing of Indian tea—Domestic Versus Export

Indian tea's popular slogan since Independence has been "World's" largest producer, consumer and exporter of tea". In 2004, however, Sri Lanka forged ahead and exported 290 million kg against Indian exports

of 204 million kg. In 1991 and 2003 too, Sri Lanka had exported more than India. Sri Lanka exports for these years were 212 million kg and 235 million kg respectively, against Indian exports of 203 million kg and 204 million kg. Another feature of Indian exports has been the sea change in its profile between 1947 and 2004. In 1947, U.K's share of Indian exports was 66 per cent and in 2004 it has declined to 12 per cent. On the other hand, the former Soviet Union, which bought no Indian teas till the 60's, became the major importer

Table 9.6: India's Share in World Exports During 1947-2004

Country/ Year	1947	1957	1967	1977	1987	1991	1997	1999	2004
India	191.7	199.2	217.8	229.6	201.9	202.9	203.0	204.2	199
% share	5.3.3	39.9	35.6	28.2	20.7	17.9	13.2	18.5	12.8
Sri Lanka	130.3	166.8	216.5	185.5	201.2	212.4	234.85	238.05	290.64
% share	36.3	33.4	35.4	22.7	20.6	18.8	21.24	21.52	18.87
Indonesia	3.9	38.8	26.6	51.3	90.4	109.6	103.9	102.5	98.57
% share	1.1	7.8	4.3	6.3	9.2	9.7	9.4	9.6	6.46
Bangladesh	N.A	4.5	Negligible	26.0	21.6	25.3	24.3	25.4	13.44
% share	Negligible	0.9	Negligible	3.2	2.2	2.2	2.4	2.3	0.87
Kenya	4.4	8.2	19.7	70.2	135.0	191.6	245.5	251.1	333.8
% share	1.2	1.6	3.2	8.6	13.8	16.9	22.2	22.7	21.66
Uganda	1.1	2.8	9.6	14.7	2.1	4.7	15.2	15.1	29.68
% share	0.3	0.6	1.6	1.8	0.2	0.4	1.4	1.4	1.93

Source : Same as Table 9.1

of Indian tea, accounting for 44.9 per cent of Indian tea exports in 1999.

Countries like Polad, Yugoslavia, Afgnaistan, Japan, Tunisia and even Germany bought no teas from India in 1947 but today are strong supporters of the Indian produce. Iraq, Iran, Gulf countries, ARE have been buying more but Canada, USA, Australia, New Zealand and the UK, have substantially reduced their purchase from Indian. In the 52 years period since 1947, African countries, particularly Kenya, have been giving stiff competition to Indian CTC teas and have gained popularity in the hard currency areas. Sri Lanka, on the other hand, a major producer of orthodox tea, has been stepping into the Indian orthodox exports and has taken the credit of catering to the entire expansion and demand in the orthodox segment. The only exception has been the former USSR which has supported Indian orthodox varieties strongly. Sri Lanka has been catering to the growing markets of ARE, Iran, USA and Pakistan. An encouraging

Table 9.7: Indian Consumption of Tea During 1947-2004

(in million kg)

Particulars/ Year	1947	1957	1967	1977	1987	1991	1997	2004
Consumption	98.5	112.9	180.7	302.0	446.0	520.0	635	720
Growth (% age)	---	14.6	60.1	67.1	47.6	16.6	22.1	13.5
Average annual rate of growth % age	---	1.46	6.01	6.7	4.76	4.1	2.8	2.7

Table 9.8: Indian Tea Consumption - as Percentage of Production

Particulars/Year	1947	1957	1967	1977	1987	1991	1997	2004
Consumption in m.kgs	98.5	112.9	180.7	302.0	446.0	520.0	635	720
Production in m kgs	254.8	310.0	384.8	556.3	674.3	741.7	81.7	880.2
% of production	38.7	36.3	47.0	54.3	66.0	70.1	76.9	82.6

Source : Same as Table 9.1

feature of Indian tea exports has been a rise in value added goods and instant tea. Packet exports in a 24-years span between 1981 and 2004 went up from 32 million kgs to 52 million kgs, thus showing and increase of 63 per cent. The instant tea export in the same 24-year period nearly doubled rising, from 0.78 million kg to 2.95 million kgs. Exports of value added teas have gone up in 19 years from 33.85 million kgs to 78.24 million kgs. In value terms, the earnings from packets increased from Rs 69.98 crore to Rs 836.65 crore; in the case of tea bags the earnings raised from Rs 3.26 crore to Rs 69.55 crore. The total value of Indian exports in 2004 was Rs 745.18 crore as against Rs 55.38 crores in 1947. India's share in world exports in shown in the table below:

Table 9.9: A State-wise Split of Estimated Consumption during 1991-2004

(Million kgs)

Particulars/Year	1991	1995	2004
Uttar Pradesh	44	50	65
Bihar	18	23	26
Maharastra	67	76	95
West Bengal	38	43	50
Andhra Pradesh	25	30	34
Madhya Pradesh	32	38	42
Tamil Nadu	21	23	26
Rajasthan	45	48	54
Gujarat	45	50	20
Orissa	10	12	42
Kerala	33	37	25
Assam	18	20	23

Punjab	40	45	53
Haryana	18	20	24
Jammu & Kashmir	10	15	22
Karnataka	26	30	37
Others	30	35	42
Total	520	595	720

Source : same as Table 9.1

In the domestic front also, the scene has changed. In 1947, Indian consumption was only 39 per cent of the production and in 1999 this figure reached 76 per cent. In the past, the equation was "Indian consumption equals production minus exports". In the eighties, this equation was reversed and on several occasions the governments had to restrict exports to conserve tea for the domestic market. The details of Indian consumption of tea in given below :-

The breakup of the Soviet Union has, therefore, had a strong impact on the Indian tea market. However, the exports have gained momentum over the years. Exports to Russia and other CIS members did not cross 45 million kg. Total Indian exports thus touched 206 million kg. Indian domestic market continues to grow at around 6 per cent per annum. In 1995, the domestic consumption was about 595 million kg. By 1999 this figure increased to 670 million kg. If export of 206 million kg is added to this figure, the production in 1999 was about 880 million kg. The CTC element of Indian consumption is over 94 per cent. In 2000, Indian requirement for CTC teas was around at 690 million kg, which went up to 705 million kg in 2001. State wise split of estimated consumption of tea is furnished below:-

New strategies will have to be evolved for the Russian Federation, CIS and Pakistan. Above all, exports will have to be given a clear priority over domestic need. While future supply and demand, on the overall, appears 'hand to-mouth' the future of speciality varieties, such as Darjeeling and Assam orthodox tea, would depend upon aggressive marketing.

Unrestricted Import of Tea: To Allow or Not

A proposal of Ministry of Commerce, Government of India, modified the export-import policy (1992-97) with a view to facilitating the EOU/EPZ to freely import teas for bulk re exports generating unfathomable dissatisfaction among many barons of the Indian tea industry. Tea imports were allowed with the rider that they should be used only for re-export with a 20 per cent value addition. But the imports were insignificant because the facility was limited to re-export of packaged teas, tea bags and instant tea. The Commerce Ministry sought the industry's view on allowing bulk re-export of tea blended with the imported product. Barons of the Indian Tea Association asserted: (i) having an exportable surplus, India does not need to import teas; (ii) if the imported low grade teas are blended with better stuff of the country to export as tea bags, packets, instant tea, its image would be damaged at the international market and exports would suffer in the long run; (iii) under the Exim policy (1997-2002) for tea were exporters were not allowed to sell any portion of the manufactured items in the domestic market. But the leaders of the Indian tea industry feared that once bulk teas, allowed to be imported, there would also be an option for unloading these teas in the domestic market. And a few larger business houses, facing stiff completion in the domestic market, would practically use the cheap imported product to reduce their prices in a bid to earn and maintain substantial profit and hold the domestic share; (iv) import of teas by India would raise international prices of teas while depressing domestic markets, a situation which would adversely affect the growth of tea industry that may eventually lead to recession. The aforesaid premises, as a corollary, led many barons of the industry to raise strong objection against the government's intention of further liberalise the Exim policy, which could open the floodgates for import of teas. They felt that the policy, if implemented, would not, in any way, help the growth of the country's tea industry. But, one should not be touchy and emotional while considering they policy of import. Rather, it imperative to visualize the necessity of imports in the perspective of reality and these is no denying the fact, that only such a study can help in commenting judiciously either in favour or against the policy.

Production Vis-a-Vis-Consumption

Whilst it is unlikely that the government would impose any restriction on exports in the foreseeable future, the pressure from the domestic market are likely to limit the quantum of Indian tea exports in the years to come. As stated earlier that with the country's population touch crossing the 100 crore mark, if every Indian drank one extra cup a year, the additional requirement of tea would be 2.55 million kg; again if ten cups extra were to be taken every day be every Indian, the additional requirement would be 921 million kg per annum. But how much can the industry with its present capacity if every produce at the maximum? It may be mentioned, that highest tea production was achieved in 1997 at 810 million kg. And it was high in 1998 with the crop amounting to 870 million kg, as indicated by Mr. A.K. Bothra, chairman, North Bengal branch of the India Tea Association at the 23rd annual general meeting of the association. And this achievement is, of course, due to maximum favour of all inputs, particulary the climatic condition. But he reiterated that the tea industry immediately requires more additional plantation area to meet the target of 1,000 million kg otherwise, tea production would grow at a small rate of around 3 per cent per annum. Nevertheless, it is necessary to renovate tea areas, which are more than sixty years of age. A replanting programme of 2 per cent per annum will ensure a rotation over 50 years. Obviously, the argument in favour of 'exportable surplus' needs to be reconsidered. It is a plain truth that if not today, tomorrow Indian will have to import sizeable quantity of tea ir or to curtail its export for the sake of domestic consumer. Otherwise, where is the guarantee that in the near future, domestic consumer. To otherwise, where is the guarantee that, in the near future, domestic consumers will not be strangulated with severe pressure of demand-pull inflation? Where is the guarantee that the industry will be able to maintain exportable surplus, as expected? These matters are, indeed, related with the industry's social obligation to two segments first, obligation to domestic consumers in terms of right price for the right product at the right time; second, obligation

Table 9.10: Export, production and per capital consumption of Tea in India.

Particulars/ Year	1950	1960	1970	1980	1992	1995	1997	1998	2004
Exports (m/kg)	181	193	200	224	190	167	203	205	206
Production (m/kg)	278	321	419	570	704	756	810	870	880
Population (million)	354	429	539	675	869	915	935	937	1005
Per capita (kg) consumption	1.27	0.29	0.39	0.57	0.61	0.93	0.74	0.79	0.95

Source : Same as Table 9.1

to the nation in terms of helping earn foreign exchange. Contextually, the observation of Mr Jimmy Hilditch may be referred to. In course of summing up the convention papers presented at the U.K. Tea Convention held in May, 1993.

The following table showed the future of India's exportable surplus of tea.

He observed: During the period India's "production has increased remarkably. So, too, has their population and the per capita consumption for the same period. With these statistic it is difficult to assess how India can feed internal demand and increase exports without increasing production".

Imports for Re-exports

There are countries like UK, USA, importing huge quantities high grade to re-export them in the value added form. It should not go unnoticed that international buyers are fast leaning towards packet tea, instant tea and tea bags. So, it is high time to catch them young. Indian tea barons should realise this fact. They should further appreciate that endeavour to re-export value added teas will help to find new markets and in contributing more foreign exchange to the national exchequer through non traditional way. This is likely to attract new investments also. This and two other significant matters should not go escaped our attention. First, India's overshelming dependence is on traditional buyers Russia and CIS, who were the principal buyers of Indian tea. Although, at the moment, India enjoys a comfortable position, the possibility of sellers in these markets should not be over-looked. The 'seller's market' at that time will be turned to 'buyer's market'. Second, China is preparing vigorously to exert its pressure in the international market. Tea is listed as one of the key export commodities. Due to overwhelming importance of hard currency earnings it was very likely that the China government provided all sorts of incentive to the tea industry. It is worth noting that between 1950 and 2004 total tea area in that country increased by more than seven from 155,000 hectares to 1,254,304 hectares. Output increased by more than three times over the same period from 41 m kg to 127 m kg. Export increase was for 10 times from 18 m kg. in 1950 to 185 m kg in 2004. Nevertheless, China has the greatest range of tea in different grades and varieties. China intends to be at the top of the list of tea traders in the world market. And there is no denying the fact, China may, at the earliest opportunity, penetrate in the Russian and CIS market. Keeping in view this possibility, the industry should right now find new markets, which may easily be possible by selling value-added teas.

Standard of Quality

Of course, the standard of quality matters much at any export trade. It may be recollected that only a few years back the quality of tea sold to Russia was so bad that million kg of tea were destroyed. Serious complaints were lodged with the Tea Board. Russian television cautioned the domestic consumers with the worlds: "Don't sip Indian tea". No doubt, industry's goodwill was severely damaged by this act of the exporters. The questions are obviously, who has to be blamed for this incident; what measures have been taken so far to prevent recurrence. The Tea Board, being the appropriate authority, should devise full-proof measures to ensure quality. Tea Board should (i) scrutinize every export order received; (ii) ensure the creditworthiness of the exporter; (iii) arrange intensive checking at the time of shipment; (iv) arrange random checking after unloading; (v) introduce mandatory use of the Tea Board's logo, subject to the fulfilment of stipulated conditions, for every export.

Conclusion

It is unlikely that with further liberalisation of imports, the domestic market will flooded with low-grade imported tea. For the Gresham's Law does not hold good in an open market. The law reacts in the opposite manner—good product drives away bad product. As far as India's domestic tea market is concerned, consumers here drink the best of CTCs. Not only that, they are prepared to pay a premium for quality. Because of the strong domestic demand, Indian tea prices are generally higher than the world prices. And it is to be noted further that in volume terms India is the largest consumer. Evidently, in the perspective of the country's consumer behaviour, it is doubtful that importers will be able to sell the low grade imported stuff to increase their profits and be able to exert dominant voice in the domestic market.

It was unwise to view that once India started buying of low priced tea, the price of its produce in the international market would have fallen. Some Asian sellers would have been benefited out of this transaction. From the viewpoint of open market economy, however, it is was felt that the aforesaid premise was not correct. In an open market mechanism only the appropriate substitute and its price plays a dominant role in determining the demand of the principal product and vice-versa. Since Indian importer intend to import only cheap varieties of teas, the price of Indian tea was likely to remain unaffected until new suppliers entered the market. And in this matter the only threat was likely to come from China—the Asian Dragon having a large variety and quantity of tea at its disposal.

In the light of the above study it was viewed that there was no point in getting jittery even though the Ministry of Commerce allowed free import of teas for re-export in bulk as well. The only necessity is to remain alert against the unscrupulous traders who may take the advantage of import liberalization policy of the Government of India just to further their own interest.

References

1. Bhatty, I. Z., Technological Change in Employment, A Study of References Plantation., The Mac-million Company of India Limited, 1978.

2. Banerjee, G.D., Structural Changes in Tea Plantation Industry of India, since 1956. PhD. thesis submitted in Jadavpur University, Kolkatta 1982.

3. Banerjee, G.D., Tea Industry in India Between 1830 to 1992— Structural Changes,, Published by Law Year's Book, 1994.

4. Banerjee G.D., Challenges Before Small Scale Industries, Published by Horizon Publishers and Distributors, Allahabad, Uttar Pradesh, 1997.

5. Karmakar, K.G. and Banerjee, G.D. Tea Industry - The Survey, 2005 NABARD, HO, Mumbai.

6. Banerjee, G.D. and Banerjee Srijeet, Darjeeling Tea- The Golden Brew, 2007, International Book Distributing Company, Lucknow.

7. Chowdhury, M. R., Oxford Book and Stationary Company, Calcutta, 1978.

8. Eden, T., Tea Third World, London.

9. Morission, R. D., Mcmorandum Relating to Tea Industry and Trends of the World, 1943.

10. Roy, Himanshu, Tea Prices Stabilisation, 1972.

11. Sarkar, G.K., The World Tea Economy, Calcutta, 1972.

12. Tea Board, India, Calcutta-Tea Statistics, Annual Reports, Techno-Economic Survey Reports etc.

13. Banerjee, G.D.. Tea Marketing A Review Indian Journal of Agricultural Marketing Mumbai, 2001, December (Annual Conference Issue)

14. Tea Marketing is no Longer a Fashionable Slogan, IASSI Journal, March 2000)

15. Banerjee G.D. and Banerjee Sarda, Sustainable Tea management IASSI Journal, January-March, 2004

16. Banerjee, G.D. and Banerjee Sarda, Tea Industry at the Cross Road, Yogana, Independence, Issue, 15 August, 2005

17. Banerjee, G.D. and Banerjee Sarda, Corporate Planning by Agricultural Development, Kurushkshetriya, March 2005 Issue Various articles published by G.D. Banerjee in Assam Review and Tea News, Chaa-ki- Bat, Financial Express, Economic Times, North-East Times.

18. Banerjee, G.D. and Banerjee Sarda, Chinese Pu'en Tea with Miraculous Functions, IASSI Journal, January-March, 2005.

19. Banerjee, G.D. Product Diversification and value Addition of Indian Tea, October-December 2006.

20. Banerjee, G.D. and Srijeet Banerjee, Darjeeling Tea - The Golden Brew, 2007.

21. Banerjee, G.D. and Banerjee Srijeet, Tea Plantation Industry - A Road Map Ahead, 2008

22. Banerjee, G.D. and Banerjee Srijeet, Export Potentials of Indian Tea, 2008.

23. Banerjee, G.D. and Banerjee Srijeet, Global Tea Trade - Dimensions and Dynamics, 2008.

Chapter 10

Thrust Areas of Tea Industry in India

It is common knowledge that plantation of *Camellia sinesis* in India was a British effort for consumption of its portion in their own country. The Britishers liked it mighy. In its praise, their poet sang of the "Cup that cheers but does not inebriate". Many others wrote also about it in many other ways. "Tea not only tickled the British palate but induced the nation of shopkeepers" to find new avenues for trade and commerce. In search of such an avenue, tea was pushed back to its country of origin. Old timers would remember how cups of hot tea used to be distributed in winter mornings by agents of tea companies. The service was free for the time being but not without motive. Before long, the imbibers became addicted to it so much so that even the poorest of them would try buy a cup of small earthern pot, as it was. The traders hoped, millions in India, rich or poor, buying it, that tea would erceate a substantial market in India. Thus, an essential exported oriented commodity got a home market too. Initially, apart from the poor people mentioned above, it was only the Britishers in India, who lived in style, and wealthy Indians who liked to imitate Englishmen, took to tea. Gradually the middle class people also adopted this tea culture. Today in most urban homes, hospitality starts with a cup of tea.

Tea industry in India has been growing since independence and it has been able to trade internationally the same volume undisturbed after meeting growing the demand in the country. The planters have played a remarkable role in the growth of the industry. By mere 33 percent increase in area under plantation since the year 1947, production has increased by 221 percent. This has been achieved by cultivation and large inputs of funds and management. Tea industry has successfully progressed and implemented massive development programmes which will increase the output of tea estates. However, to keep up with the development tempo, the industry requires substantial funds year after year so that more quantities can be made available for exports. Going by Recent escalation in cost of production due to sharp rise in prices of fertilisers, pesticides, fuel, transport, insecticides, vehicle, it was observed those percentage of cost increase will be highest in comparison to past years.

Recent announcement of export oriented policy is a welcome feature. As policy of higher target of export figure has to be attained and the remaining quantity is to be consumed in the domestic market. While doing this, one must ensure that this does not lead to spurt in internal prices. Moreover an increase in export volume beyond 220 million kgs will demand substantial increase in tea production for which availability of additional land for tea plantation remains the stumling block. However, the industry is not sitting idle and all out efforts are being made to maximise output. For increasing exports through value addition, a lot more is yet to be done. We have *increased value-added and not cost added exports. Value is added when 'Brand' is created and careation of 'Brand' is not an easy task.* No overseas marketer will part with its existing 'Brand' since it enjoys a substantial market value. Indian predominance with marketing ability and distribution network along with professional market can only do this job successfully. Nevertheless the industry, if approached, will assure these marketeers with supplies of the required quantities without any interruption. This is the first time that Commence Ministry *has publicly admitted that non-availability of additional land and higher tax rates are the main constraints faced by the tea industry in its development.* The industry appealed to Commerce and Finance ministies for making essential amendments in Section 33AB of the Income Tax Act so that development funds were available to the industry without any waiting period.

The TRA's invention of high yielding clone producing yields around 7,000 kgs per hectare benefited the industry. It has also established a full-fledged Bio-tech laboratory at Tocklai and perfected the technique of tissue culture at the Lab stage. Tissue culture plants are now grown in natural conditions. This has a lot of positive impact on the tea industry and will make available millions of plants in excellent health for propagation in tea gardens. The TRA is collaborating with the national laboratories with a view to enhancing the photosynthetic capacity of the tea leaf and. The process would make the bushes more productive. All these projects made significant contributions to the functioning of tea industry. Here attempt has been made to deliberate on the critical thrust areas of tea industry. These areas are being debarted by the scholars planters, policy makers', producers, trades and others involved in tea industry. Some of these are given below:

Prics Determine Costs Rather Than The Other Way Round

The future lies in exports, since the domestic market will not grow much faster than population. And to open up access to foreign markets, a price correction was indispensable. Attempts to rig domestic prices would be self defeating; not only would they shunt the industry out of the international market but they also reduce growth of domestic demand., Hence the industry must adopt a new regime in which prices determine cost rather than the other way round. The industry is full of absentee land-lords who took profits but reinvested little. That was the right thing to do when State and Central taxes were high. Output was growing and worst teas were found. Even there is no buyer to purchase the tea estates. The industry has to invest in replanting, improved curbing, better packaging and stricker marketing. Those planters who can invest must retain tea estates and those were cannot must sell out. New investment will make the difference between selling poor teas at a loss and quality teas at a profit.

Changes Sought in Child Labour A ct

With a view to abolish child labour especially in plantation on areas, the Bengal /Word Bank asked the centre to amend sections 24 and 27 of the Child Labour (Prohibition and Regantation Act), 1986 which states that employers only needs a "fitness certificate" from a medical practitioner to employ a child. Section 24 of the Plantation Labour Act, 1951, which prohibited employment of children below 12 years was delected by an amendment in 1986. The amended Child Labour Act prohibit the employment of child labour According to official estimates there are at least 8, 300 children employed in 275 gardens in the state of West Bengal on a regular basis. A much larger number is employed during the "flush" or the plucking season. According to Labour Department study, child labour is employed due to cheap availability, non-availability of local labour especially in plucking season, and availment of subsidised ration offered to the plantation workers.

Assam Company Targets West Asia for Packet Tea

The Assam Company Ltd. (ACL) sells packet tea in Lebanon and Jordan with tie-up arrangement with a company at Muscat, a maker of detergents and bisuits-having a wide distribution network in the Gulf and West Asian markets. It started business in Saudi Arabia, Oman, Qatar, the united Arab Emirates and Bahrain. The ACL is yet to enter markets like USA and Japan. The cost of entering such markets are too high and market is too small.

A Pleasant Surprise for Tea Industry

Addressing the Annual General Meeting of the Tea Association of India in Kolkata Mrs. Jayati Chandra the than Chairperson, Tea Board supported along with the then Minister of Commerce granting concession to the industry under Section 88 of Income Tax Act. The industry received a pleasant surprise in the budget, 1995.

Destruction of Tea Wastes

The Control Board of Excise and Customs understands that tea waste has been piling up and has assumed critical dimension due to unwillingness of excise authorities to supervise destruction of tea waste or its conversion to compost in view of the abolition of Central Excise duty on tea. The matter has been examined by the Board and it has been decided that since the collection of cess on tea continues with the Central Excise Department, the Central Excise officers may continue the supervision of destruction of tea and issue certificates of destruction of tea waste. The existing version of para (d) of the Commodity Manual relating to tea is accordingly amended.

Brooke Bonds' Entry into SSI area

The Government sought details of of Brooke Bond Lipton Ltd. plans to enter into ice cream business. The manufacture of the item was reserved for the small scale sector. Similar notices were also served on the state owned Mother Dairy and some other companies planning to manufacture and sell ice-cream in the guise of "frozen deserts". Brooke Bond entered into an agreement with certain sections of the Kwality group to manufacture and market ice-cream. The agreement between these two companies and KIC Food and Yankee Doodle violated the reservation policy. The Government sought more details about the agreement from Brooke Bond Lipton and Kwuality. Some of the SSI ice-cream companies are in fact big units-masquerading as small units. All important manufacturing units were inspected by joint teams of the department of Small Scale industries and the Ministry of Food Processing Industries to find out all the facts.

Under the current policy, large companies, both Indian and foreign, are permitted to enter SSI areas only if they undertake to export 75 percent of total value of production. The companies will have to obtain a licence under the provisions of the Industries CD-development and Regulation Act, 1951.

New Tea Projects New Mumbai

After the successful commissioning of its state-of-the art tea processing unit at Chulsa, Good ricke Group Ltd (GGL) launched two new project—instant tea plant and export-oriented packet tea unit—near Mumbai. G.G.L., which owns 17 tea estates mainly in the Dooars, requires to make a fresh investment of about Rs. 20 crore or so in these new projects for value addition to its tea. This apart, the management wants to continue the ongoing modemisation of the tea factories and expansion of computerisation at all operational levels. Commenting on immediate prospect. Mr P.A Leggatt, the then Chairman of G.C.L. said that the proposed instant tea project and the plant started commercial production in July 1995. The capacity of the plant was 6 lakh kgs of instant tea powder of both the cold and hot water soluble variety. The new packaging and tea bagging unit (near Mumbai) which produces packets and tea bags for export were operationalised. Both these projects not only added value to teas but ensure higher profit margins in the coming years. As for marketing of teas, the then G.G.L. Chairman made a significant observation. Due to the increase in world production it was not longer remunerative to pursue export perse. The majority of consumers were not connoisseurs of high quality flavour teas but would opt far average cut of tea as long as it was not two inconventint to prepae or look too long to brew. This was precisely why G.G.L. was going for value-added teas for which there was ready international market.

Tea Industry Bengal and Agricultural 1-T

The tea industry in Bengal production has witnessed stagnation of during the last ten years. The industry, therefore, requested the State Government to lower agricultural income tax to more reasonable levels to promote long term growth. The West Bengal Government brought down tax rates from 82 to 70 per cent in 1993-94 Budget. It is yet to make upon its mind on the industry's request. Restructuring of tax rates in 1991 led to an increase to 83 percent on the highest slab. The government reduced rates to 70 per cent in 1994 and an allowance on investment was permitted. However, this rate is still the highest in the country. The allowance remains on paper. Among tea-growing states, agricultural income tax rates are 60 per cent in Assam and 65 per cent in the southern states of Karnataka, Kerala and Tamil Nadu. The West Bengal Government imposes tax on Rs. 60 of every Rs 100 of income and the Centre on the remaining Rs 40. The States 70 per cent rate of tax means a burden of Rs 42 while the centre's 46 per cent rate imposes a burden of Rs. 18.40. The total tax on every Rs 100 of income is thus Rs 60.40. In contrast, other industries are subjected to an income tax of Rs 46 on every Rs 100 of income. This makes the tea industry's tax burden 14 per cent higher. The industry also pleaded for an amendment to the Bengal Agricultural Income Tax Act. 1994, to permit an allowance on investment. Bengal's Finance Act of 1994 entitles an assessee to a deduction of 20 per cent of his agricultural income if the amount is utilised within the previous year for specific purposes. The industry's stance is that post tax profitability to tea companies being low and cost of a green field project being high a company requires accumulation of a certain amount of capital over a period of time as the promoter's contribution to a project.

The proposed amendment allowed the company a deduction on deposits made with either the West Bengal Industrial Development Corporation or the West Bengal Finance Corporation. As for the notification for the industrial development scheme, the tea industry is in favour of a provision for investments both within and outside the tea plantation sector. The industry has also raised the issue of making donations for worthwhile causes. Even the West Bengal Government sought donations from the tea estates. The industry wanted that such expenditure be deducted from tax calculations. Tamil Nadu and Kerala allowed such expenditures to be deducted in computing taxable agricultural income. The other important Plea in the memorandum submitted by the tea indensity to the Govenment is with regard to merger to healthy and sick companies. The term Industry wants the Agricultural Income Tax Act 1994 to be amended to allow carry forward and of accumulated losses in certain cases of amalgamation.

Tea Production and Trade in India

The gradual decline in total production of orthodox teas in India is largely due to the curtailment in export to CIS countryside. The largest scale diversion to CTC manufacture is a direct result of the decline in demand for orthodox teas. One must, however, ensure that the shift from manufacture of orthodox teas does not result in a reduction in supply of this export-oriented product. On the export front, sharp decline in share of exports to CIS countries, Iran etc. resulted in fall of exports coming to the Calcutta Auctionsl. Total sales of all teas on an average amounted to 94.6 million kilograms. While there was a marginal increase in sale of CTC and Darjeeling leaf teas, sale of orthodox leaf teas dropped by about 7 million kilograms, on an average. On the price front the average price realised for leaf teas during the last five years was Rs. 50.94 per kilogram and Rs. 45.23 per kilogram for dust teas. However there was a decline in an average price per kilogram in all the auction centres in India. Such a sharp drop in prices has spelt untold misery for the producers, fluctuating price hurt the buyers, destabilise export markets and brokers suffer as they get a fixed percentage on the sale price the Calcutta Tea Traders Association (CTTA) is concerned about the sale of teas through the auction system and a suggestion has been put forward by certain section to repeal the Tea Marketing Control Order 1984. One is of the opinion that the auction system is the best method for disposal of a bulk commodity like tea. It is the auction system which ensures that tea is available in adequate quantities and at reasonable price throughout the year. It is, *therefore necessary to sustain the auction system both for the export market as well as for catering to the domestic market. However, the Government of West Bengal has exempted teas entering Kolkata from the purview of entry tax. This exemption will act as an incentive to producer to route larger quantities of teas through the Calcutta Auctions.*

Simplification and Rationalisation of Sales Tax

The Association has made several representation to the Government of West Bengal for simplification and rationalisation of the sales tax law applicable to teas sold in the Calcutta Auction. Teas sold in West Bengal are subjected to multipoint sales tax at varying rates resulting in cumbersome paper-work and delays in completion of sales tax assessments. It is suggested that a flat rate of sale tax of the 2% on all internal sales by brokers at the Calcutta Auctions will result in higher revenue generation and also make it attractive for buyers to purchase tea at this centre. It is hoped that the State Government will favourably consider our suggestion for interest of the tea trade and industry at Kolkata.

The CTTA's main function is to administer the Kolkata Auctions and sales were held as per schedule during the last year. This is due to close co-operation amongst buyers and sellers of teas and the continuing support of its member, CTTA is to run the Calcutta Auction in more efficient manner in the years to come. The fortunes of the Calcutta Auctions are closely linked to the demand for Indian tea abroad. Kolkata has traditionally catered to the export market and the constituents of CTTA comprise not only most of the leading exporters of Indian tea but also firms with vast experience in the domestic market. The CTTA has been assisting the Commerce Ministry and the Tea Board in their efforts to promote Indian teas in overseas countries.

Pesticide Residue in Tea

Pesticide residue in tea has become a burning problem. Individual estates do not have the infrastructure to test pesticide residues. It is becoming vitally necessary for both Government and Tea Board to set up laboratories to ensure that no teas which have pesticide residues over prescribed limits are exported or sold in the domestic market. Several merchant exporters who are members of CTTA are of the opinion that testing laboratories should be set up in Kolkata and Cochin as most exports are routed through these centres. While it is the fact that nome of the tea associations have the infrastructure to test tea samples as well as consignments of tea, the Tea Bboard may wish to undertake the job on a commercial basis. This would require scientific personnel and inspection officials for pre-shipment inspection of each consignment of tea. The various associations would agree to actively participate in the proposed commercial venture. The Tea Board may therefore consider preparing a project report for setting up testing laboratories for the benefit of the tea trade and industry.

Safe gaurd the Interest of Exporters-Buyers

While liberalisation must continue and controls must dismantled, it is necessary to safeguard the interests of exporters-buyers by preventing shipment of substandard teas, whether the tea is in packets or in the loose form, in the greater interest of the country's exports. The genuine exporters would not be averse to some inspection to ensure that the proper tea is being exported. It has been reported that packets of established exporters are being duplicated by third parties. Some of these duplicate packets were found to contain substandard teas thereby tarnishing the image of the established exporters. The Tea Board may, therefore, consider steps to protect the interests of established exporters by way of according approval to packet teas for exports and ensuring that such approvals are given within 24 hours of the application. In India, tea as a beverage is facing increasing competition from variety of soft drinks. It is, a general opintion that urgent innovative steps are required to counter the challenge of other beverages. It is felt that a strong domestic market will play a positive role in case of inadequate export levels.

Adequate Space in Warehousing

Warehousing is an integral part of the auction system and it is the responsibility of the CTTA to ensure adequate availability of warehousing space throughout the year. Owing to certain legal hurdles, the CCTA is not in a position to augment the warehousing area on a permanent basis. This has resulted in shortage of warehousing space during the peak period as the warehouses registered with CTTA are utilised by most producers for auction as well as private sale and shipment of teas. Tea Board is, therefore, expected to allow the CTTA to independently augment the warehousing space during the peak period till such time the CTTA is in a position to process the applications for registration of warehousing space on a permanent basis.

Major Areas Indian Tea Industry

The target of 1000 million kgs was not achieved in the year 2000 but it may be achieved in the year 2005, not that the industry did not want but it was not feasible to increase production upto 200 million kgs in two years (1998-1999). Increase of 200 million kgs in 5 years may be realistic and the industry must ensure to achieve this. Indian tea has a large domestic market which annually consumes around 80 per cent of the country tea production and is growing at the rate 3 per cent annually. It is interesting to note that whereas Jammu and Kashmir has the highest per capita consumption of 1594 gms. followed by 1525 gms in Punjab, 1222 gms in Gujrat, 1100 gms in Kerala and 1000 gms in Maharashtra, it is as low as 232 grams in Bihar, 276 gms in Orissa, 366 gms in Tamil Nadu and 376 gms in Uttar Pradesh. In West Bengal it is 464 gms. per capita. Average per capita consumption in the country is 643 gms. There is good scope for increasing the consumption of tea in the rural areas of our country particularly in the low consuming states. Tea is not only a cheap refreshing drink but it is established as a health drink and that is why it is becoming a favourite drink in rural India also.

Tea Exports

Tea exports have been hovering around less than 200 million kgs during the last 10 years and could not reach at least 220 million kgs in 2000. Side by side, the industry should give greater stress on value addition by making more exports in tea packets and tea bags. Efforts should be made to introduce flavoured teas also. Brand promotion is seriously needed to bring forth the supreme quality of our teas abroad and thus create loyal consumers. India has assiduously built up an image of quality tea producer and exporter in the highly competitive world market. Eventually, it is our quality which will sustain our market share and reputation. An important aspect of export activity is the introduction of 'India Blend' under the brand name 'Nargis' for promotion in Russia and other CIS countries, and European countries. This will certainly improve our export position in these world markets.

Tea Prices

The average unit price realisation in the domestic auction centres in the last five years had no doubt made gains but was still below the 2000 level. Increase in production costs due to annual growth in inflationary trends fully mollified price improvement and there were no real gains to the tea industry. The lowering profit margins lead to lower earnings and high tax rates that take away a large chunk, thus leaving very little finances for plough-back into the development programmes. A fair price realisation to the tea producers is a must in view of the large scale technical requirements for developments.

Land for Extension

In order to achieve a faster production rate in future, additional lands are need for extension purposes. The surplus ceiling lands lying unused within the tea plantation are still vested with the State Governments. The West Bengal Government has changed its old land policy by leasing out such vested lands to tea estates. But grant of NOC for seeing up of new tea estates in north Bengal in still being delayed. The Assam Government still continues to hold large tracts of such surplus lands vested with it but its land policy of 1979 does not permit handing over to the corporate sector. A change in this policy would enable the corporate sector to put such lands under tea cultivation within a short time. Then there are lands on the periphery and nearby which can be easily brought under tea by the existing tea plantations. Another source of additional land is the existence of degraded forest lands which is of no use of anyone and lying sterile. It is vital that the Union Government re-examinits policy vis-a-vis degraded forest lands for tea cultivation since such a move could serve the dual purpose of quick afforestation at no cost of the Goverment. and simultaneously augment production of tea.

Tea Board Assistance

Substantial increase in the rates of loan finances and subsidies in the Tea Board's developmental schemes have considerably brightened the rapid growth in production. These new rates of assistance from Tea Board should encourage even those who had not been attracted to develop their tea estates further. In view of the very limited land availability for tea extension purpose, uprooting and replanting would have to be raised to at least be 1 per cent per annum from the existing level of ½ per cent per annum. The new rate subsidy on replantation would be able to considerably compensate the revenue loss by uprooting. Similarly, handsome increases in the rates of assistance and subsidies for infilling and interplanting would meet the growing requirement of the industry.

World Bank Assistance

The tea plantation Industry has been informed of the proposals for obtaining World Bank Assistance for faster growth in tea production over the next Five Year Plan period beginning from April, 1997. While welcoming the proposal, the industry has suggested that:

(1) rate of interest be not more than 7 to 8 per cent;

(2) Tea Board Finance and Subsidy Schemes should not be disturbed;

(3) Tea Board should be the nodal agency for implementing the scheme;

(4) the tea industry be a part of the negotiating team with the World Bank. Presently the Industry suffers from unsteady flow of development loans as recently NABARD has suddenly stopped

refinance facility on all development loans till further notice. The industry must be assured of release of vested surplus lands and degraded forest lands for extension purposes. Other measures like replantation, infilling and interplanting, rejuvenation pruning, irrigation and drainage etc. would play a major part under this plan for World Bank Assistance.

Incentive u/s 80 HHC

Section 80HHC of the I.T. Act, 1961 allows full deduction in respect of profits earned out of exports. The intention of the section is to provide incentive for more exports. While all industries, including Tea Merchant/Exporters derive full benefit under this section, the Income Tax authorities allow deduction against only 40 per cent of the total income to the Tea Producer/Exporter. This is so because 40 per cent of the income of the producers is taxed under central income tax and the balance 60 per cent under state agricultural income Tax. The Association would once again appeal to the Finance Ministry for amending the provision under Section 80HHC as to allow the same benefit to the tea industry as is being allowed to all other industries.

State Agricultural Income Tax Rates

No doubt the State Governments of Assam and West Bengal did reduce the agricultural income tax rates in the past, the present rates of 60 per cent and 70 per cent, respectively, continue to be the highest incidence of tax on tea as compared to all other industries. An agricultural commodity like tea, which is prone to all the vagaries of nature and price fluctuation, continues to bear this heavy tax burden thereby causing difficulty in internal resource generation. In order to do justice to the tea industry in the matter of taxation, An appeal was made to the State Government of Assam, West Bengal and Tripura to bring their agricultural income tax rates at par with the corporate tax rates. This tax incidence on the Indian tea industry is the highest amongst all tea producing countries.

Tea—A Health Drink

Arising from the growing global consciousness on health vis-a-vis food products a unique opportunity exists to stimulate tea consumption on the basis of its health benefit. There is now emerging scientific information that tea actually possesses beneficial aspects with regard to human health. Among the established benefits are fluid balance in body, zero calorie content, protective effects in heart disease and stroke, in combating cancer, possessing some anti—viral and antibacterial effects etc.

Export Incentive—Fiscal relief

Tea producer-exporter is being allowed the tax benefit under Section 80HHC of the Income Tax Act only to the extent of 40 per cent of its profits from tea exports whereas the tea merchant-exporters are reaping full deduction benefit for income tax purpose like all other commodity exporters. The tea plantation industry has been pointing out to the faulty explanation under Notification No:600. dated 25th May, 1991 of the C.B.D.T. for limiting the extent of tax benefit to 40 per cent of the profits from tea exports but nothing seems to be happening for long. Deduction under Section 80HHC in respect of export profit must be allowed from the composite income of a tea producer-exporter in computing business income. As Assam tea is the main constituent in tea exports, full tax benefit has been allowed under Section 80HHC to the tea producer-expecters. It is exputed that other tea growing States will extend their support in this direction.

Import of Tea

To allow import of tea into India has been a demand of a multi-national in spite of the Government's denial on this issue. Tea producers strongly feel that there is no necessity of importing teas because there is neither a shortage nor there is any deficiency in quality. Opening up of imports would only lead to flooding of poor quality teas which would adversely affect consumers and drain scarce foreign exchange reserves.

Growth of Domestic Market

Indian tea is fortunate to have a large domestic market which is growing at the rate of 3 per cent to 4 per cent annually, but the annual per capita consumption of tea is only about 650 gms. This needs to grow in the coming years. A strong domestic market is essential for the health of industry. It is therefore proposed to develop it by making better quality teas, better distribution in the rural areas and small affordable packets.

The Tea (Marketing) Control Order, 1984

The Tea (Marketing) Control Order has now become completely redundant in our liberalised economy in the context of free marketing. There should not be any compulsion for putting 75 per cent bulk teas in auction and it should be left to the choice of a producer how to sell his teas. The tea producers should market tea as a consumer product, not as a commodity.

Land for Extension in Assam

As the tea industry has already launched tea development on a large scale to achieve a target of 1000 million kgs by 2000 A.D. need for large area of additional lands for extension of tea areas has become very pressing and urgent. Large areas of surplus lands suitable for tea growing are still vested with the State Governments. With the change in its land policy towards setting up of new tea estates the West Bengal Government leased out such vested lands for the tea development purpose. The sanctioning of NOC for setting up of new tea estates in north Bengal got momentum. The Assam Government still has large tracts of such surplus lands vested with it which are suitable for tea cultivation. One is aware of the Assam Land Policy 1979. The Government's concern was to help the educated unemployed by setting up small tea gardens on such lands which the tea industry greatly appreciated. Still the progress in this direction has not been encouraging which is rather a set-back to the tea development in Assam. The tea industry in the Corporate Sector has both financial and technical expertise to bring about rapid development in the growth on such lands. The State Government may sympathetically consider giving back such lands to the original tea estates or allowing the tea corporate sector for allotment of such lands. This development in tea would have a cascading effect on overall economy of the State in general and of the rural area in particular. It would generate additional employment of one labour in each new acre coming under tea cultivation in the rural area of Assam.

Agricultural Income Tax

Due to the extremely high rates of the agricultural income tax on tea income the total tax incidence on tea income has been highest among all commodities. Even though tea being an agricultural commodity suffering all the buffeting of uncertain weather and market conditions, it has continued to bear the heaviest tax burden on its meagre income leaving small amounts from internal generation for development. Tea plantation industry is grateful to the Assam Government for bringing down the agricultural income tax rate from 75 per cent to 60 per cent thereby providing relief to the industry. But the tax incidence still continues to be pretty heavy as compared to all other industries. In order to bring equity with all other industries and enable it a level playing field in this area. It is therefore appealed to the State Government to bring the agricultural income tax rate at par with the corporate tax rate. Such a relief would make the industry competitive in the international market. Tax incidence on teas in India is the highest amongst all tea producing countries.

Depreciation on Tea Bushes

Unlike other industries there is no depreciation available on the tea industry's major asset, the tea bush and, therefore, one of the major sources of internal generation of funds is closed to it. It is for this reason that extension planting has not been upto the desired level. Other industries are able to recover their investment of capital nature of plant and machinery by as much as 80 per cent within 4 years and almost 100 per cent in 7 years even though such plant and machinery have an economic life of over 40 years. But the tea Industry is denied this facility. At current costs, the capital expenditure on tea plantation is Rs. 1.25 lacs per hectare. Around 100 million kg of the additional production of 242 million kgs over next 6 years would have to come from extending area under tea. It is strongly suggested that the tea bushes—the tea industry's major asset—should be equated with them. And the cost of extension planting and replacement planting should be treated as capital expenditure, and thus be allowed the normal depreciation under the Income Tax Act.

NABARD —Direct Financing

In today's liberalised economy, not only India but in almost all the tea producing/exporting countries (including China and Vietnam) cutting costs while maintaining quality has become the basic objective. The interest cost to long-term borrowers for development is now among the most important factors. Since the NABARD's development loans are refinanced through banks, this process adds to cost of borrowing. Our need for large-scale development in tea to make it competitive, makes it imperative that this financing is done directly by NABARD which will bring the interest cost to 11 per cent per annum. It is hoped that the Union Government and NABARD would consider this suggestion in all seriousness and urgency.

Role of Tea Board

Tea Board has been playing a very important role in the development of our tea industry which is quite commendtable. In view of rapidly escalating extension costs the current rates of finances and subsidies under various schemes of Tea Board now fall short of requirement. The unit cost of planting has already been revised to Rs.96000 per hectare w.e.f. October, 1993 by NABARD subsequently it was again revised. The Board has also now revised its rate of development finance to this level. Replanting/replacement, have been less than 1 per cent p.a. against the annual requirement of 2 per cent of area under tea. This subsidy rate also was revised upwards based on the current planting cost. So were the subsidy rates on infilling and rejuvenation.,

Infrastructure

Presently Assam's essential infrastructure like roads, bridges, telecommunications etc. are in a poor shape. This is causing serious impediments in the States economic growth and creating doubts in the minds of otherwise keen large-scale and medium-scale investors. Being located over wide-spread areas of Assam, the tea plantations depend solely on telecommunication for contacting the outside world and commercial centres and roads and bridges for to and from movements of goods as inputs and marketing of teas over long distances. But all these facilities, being in a poor shapes, have been causing considerable problems. Infrastructure gets further set back by serious recurring floods. Situation is quite the same in north Bengal where all its tea plantations are located. The State and Central Governments must pay attention to alleviation these serious infrastructure deficiencies. Rapid economic development calls for quick improvement in the country's total infrastructure.

Labour Productivity

Labour costs are escalating steadily without any matching labour productivity improvement making us in-competitive in the international market. In this situation it is the interest of both the tea industry and the tea working population to come to a realistic understanding under which the labour are required to improve there productivity level. In order to meet the competition abroad and to keep the domestic supplieds at a reasonable price to the common man, need for improvement in labour productivity in now a must and the labour wages and benefits must be linked to productivity also. Serious thought should be given for rationalisation of staff and labour on the basis of scientific study.

Panel Wants Subsidy For Tea Raised

The standing committee of the Commerce Ministry has sought an increase in subsidy for replantation of tea to keep pace with the growing demand. It warns that exports may be hit if the government fails to act soon. The committee emphasised the need to expand cultivation to Arunachal Pradesh, Mizoram, Nagaland and Manipur which have the "climate and soil conducive" for the purpose. "It is the only viable option" its report said, adding that the annual growth of tea consumption during the last four decades *was 4.9 per cent against the population growth rate of 2.1 per cent*—an indication that per capita tea consumption is increasing steadily. Referring to export potential of Indian tea, it said that in 1981 about 43 per cent of tea production was available for exports which declined to about 17 per cent in 2005. According to the report, the tea industry employs over a million persons and an additional one million are indirectly employed in ancillkary occupations. Therefore, to boost tea production, it is necessary to revise subsidy for replantation as most tea bushes in the country's estates are "over 50 years old and yields are no longer at their best." In 2005 tea production was 880 million kgs from 512000 hectares.

As regards expansion of tea cultivation, the report said the Kangra valley in Himachal Pradesh, with a 150-year tradition of tea cultivation," offers an excellent opportunity" to increase yields. While 1,158 tea gardens are spread over 1,857 hectares there, the per hectare yield is 464 kgs against the national average of 1,761 kgs per hectare. To bridge the gap of demand and supply the committee said it was "*worth examining' the proposal for importing tea to meet domestic demand and for value added re-exports. This was necessary, it said, in view of the time lag of minimum of ten years for new estates to produce tea.* The committee noted that the tea industry had not been doing well on the export front in the recent years. In the 1980s and the earlier years of 1990s, the industry "*failed to achieve the level of performance" of 1981 when it exported 241 million kg of tea*. While there were occasional upswings in the exports, it has been "*a downhill journey thereafter*". On the export front, it suggested that greater efforts and vigorous propaganda were needed to boost Indian tea sales in the CIS countries. It noted that Russia was "*tilting*" *towards third country imports of cheaper tea from Sri Lanka*. However, it pointed out that despite shortfall in the targeted offtake, the 1993-94 off take by Russia was higher compared to the previous year. "But the slight increase gave no solace to Indian experts as it was insignificant compared to pre 1990 offstake."

Tea exporters incurred the wrath of German importers on two fronts—on deployment of *child labour below* 14 years of age in the plantations and secondly on the higher lėvel of chemical *residue than the maximum residue level (MRL)* permitted by German law. Deployment of child labour does not pose a "serious problem" as their percentage is estimated to be between 1 and 1.5. The committee recommended that the Commerce Ministry should consider amending the Plantation Labour Act, 1951 with a view to "*impose ban*" *on deployment of child labour in tea plantation.*

As regards presence of MRL, the committee noted with satisfaction from media reports that the *German Tea council has come forward to help out the Indian exporters in retrieving an impaired image of Indian tea. For getting better global price, the standing committee suggested India entering into a "marketing pact" with its major rival Sri Lanka, and getting away with bargain prices. "Such an agreement could fetch food returns for both producers"*, it said. It noted that the Sri Lankan tea industry has much more at stake when global prices get depressed since it has no domestic market to fall back upon. Perhaps a beginning was made in 1992 when a few Indian companies "teamed up" with Sri Lankan businessmen to offer their expertise to 22 Sir Lankan tea companies accounting for more than 85 per cent of that country's production. The standing committee noted that production of tea apart, not much attention was paid to the promotion campaign abroad in respect of Indian tea.

Indian tea : VAT's the Solution

The Government of India appointed a high powered committee to look into the problems faced by the Indian tea industry. The committee, under the chairmanship of the then Union Commerce Secretary, Mr Tejendra Khanna, examined all aspects connected with the development of this industry. These inter alia included costs and profits of the industry and the overall economic policy affecting production and exports. One of the problems of the committee was to examine declining export potential of this industry, Although, traditionally Indian tea has been one of the major exporters, over the years, it share in exports has declined. In fact, the Indian tea faces stiff competition from China whose black tea is making considerable inroads into CIS countries and from the Kenyan and Sri Lankan teas which are attempting to replace Indian tea. The disturbing export prospects for the Indian tea is partly attributed to stagnant consumption of tea in developed countries and partly to inelastic supply and low productivity of the industry.

Revamping the Tea Industry : The second important problem of the committee was of revamping the tea industry. It called for serious efforts. The Eighth Plan accorded high priority to the scientific management of tea gardens, replanting of old and uneconomic tea bushes by high yielding plants, reduction in regional disparity in tea productivity, extension of tea cultivation in traditional and non traditional areas through encouragement of various farming systems and popularising of the Indian teas in the global market. While recognising the importance of all these aspects mentioned in the plan document, the most important aspect was to revamp the overall tax policy. This had to be tuned to give a boost to this industry.

The tax policy related to direct as well as indirect taxes. Here the issues related to indirect taxes required more elaboration only. The most important aspect of indirect taxes related to tea industry is the archaic nature of sales taxes. The tea industry is adversely affected by the comparatively heavy sales tax burden. Although the sales tax is said to be a single-point tax, in effect, it s a multipoint tax levied at a various stages.

Variations in tax rates at the auction centres : First, the tax is levied at the time of auction often at various auction centres. The rates of tax vary from one state to another affecting diversion of the trade from one state to another. Whereas the rate of tax on auction in West Bengal is 4 per cent, Assam it is only 2 per cent and in the southern states of Kerala and Tamil Nadu, the rate is 6.25 and 5.5 per cent, respectively. The variations in tax rates at the auction centres affect the economic activity of the sellers as well as purchasers. To illustrate the economic effect of tax on auction let us take the case of Guwahati auction centre, which was established in 1970. When this centre started functioning there was no tax being levied on auction of tea there. Even today the tax rate is the lowest in the country. As a result it has evolved as one of the world's largest CTC tea auction centres and is now the second largest tea auction centre in the world with 867 members auctioning tea valued at Rs 555 crore in 1989. Secondly, tax is levied after auction on the inter-state sale if tea moves to another state for blending and packaging. On such transactions instead of a state sales tax, a Central sales tax is levied at the rate of 4 per cent. Thirdly, the tax is levied once again at the time of sale by the first registered dealer such as Lipton, Brooke Bond, Tata Tea, etc. This tax varies from 2 to 13 per cent in different states. Although, majority of states (15) levy sales tax at the rates ranging between 6 and 8 per cent, two states have low rates of 2 to 4 per cent and six states levy rates between 10 and 13 per cent. Finally, there is a surcharge as well as additional sales tax on the basic sales tax in some of the states.

Incidence of Tax - Cascading and Pyramiding Effects : The combined incidence of all these taxes on the tea industry is pretty high, which is hidden in the price of the commodity. Also, the total burden of the tax is much as compared to the levels prevailing in other countries exporting tea. Above all, the burden of tax is heterogenous, varies from one state to another, leads to pyramiding, and cascading effects and thus causes adverse economic effects on the auction activities in the state and exports of tea abroad. Although, theoritically there is no tax when tea is exported, yet the tax levied at the earlier stages (viz., at the time of auction or at the stage of inter state transactions) does cause adverse effects the price of tea. The effects are two fold: cascading effect and pyramiding effect. Cascading refers to inclusion in the final sale price of taxes paid at initial or intermediate stages of production (as well as of taxes levied on these taxes at later stages in the production process. Pyramiding, on the other hand, refers to the fact that, if sellers onset their sale price at a fixed gross margin (mark-up-system) over costs, then if those taxes include a tax element the absolute size of the mark-up profit will be correspondingly larger. Thus, with cascading the final sale price of the commodity increases by an amount larger than indicated by taxes; with pyramiding,. the final price paid by consumer may be still higher, but the additional revenue (from the increased absolute margin collected in the comtax cost price) flows not to the Government but to the seller. The present taxes and duties of tea in India is presented in Annexure 6.

Fiscal Reforms : With the above adverse economic effects of the existing sales taxes the most important fiscal reform for the country is to switch over to a system of value added tax (VAT) to replace the existing sales taxes. This is the need of the hour. It would be extremely useful to take the tea industry out of woods as the main technical achievement if value added tax form of sales taxation is precisely eliminate the cascading effect. It would therefore remove the deficiencies of the existing tax system and would consequently encourage exporter. Since VAT would not leave any trace of tax for transactions entering into exports, the industry would offer Indian tea at competitive prices in the world through reduction in costs, elimination of cascading and removal of pyramiding of taxes.

In last two decades more than 30 countries of the world have switched over to this tax. If Indian tea has to compete with Kenya where VAT is in force Indian tea industry has to do away with the existing taxes causing cascading and pyramiding effect. To sum up the argument, the existing sales taxes are levied at various points and affect the ultimate price of Indian tea. It, therefore, leaves it behind when facing competition with other teas of the world. It is, therefore, necessary to introduce VAT on tea. The modus operandi of introduction of VAT as well as its administration, is neither difficult more does it require major administrative reshuffle. Also it is not at all necessary for a state to switch over completely to a system of VAT. Tea could be singled out for this purpose. The states of Karnataka and Andhra Pradesh have already adopted this tax for liquor. Without making much efforts, therefore, VAT must be introduced to help Indian tea.

Acurtain Raiser Finding

A scientific prediction on market position in 2004 and a look at certain developments, both positive and negative, that would determine the course of events globally is given below :

1 Crop shortfall: Global 135-140 million In Sri Lanka around 30 per cent with some permanent damage and slow recovery on plantations consequent to extensive damage and inconsistent weather.

  The wiping out of the production surplus carried over from 2002 in 2003. It means that most packers and user countries' reserves would be very thin.

  North Indian Winter: January to April; Political turmoil in Kenya and damage to tea in Africa and Sri Lanka could have a negative impact on production in 2004.

2. Currencies: Recovery of Sterling, drop in value of the Rupee.
3. Duties and Taxes: The abolishing of export duty in Sri Lanka and the removal of import duty in Germany.
4. Low stocks and low tea inventories held by most packers in importing countries due to restricted supply, cost of finance and uncertainties resulting from the recession.
5. Re-appearance of the CIS and East Block buying through intermediaries.

6. Removal of Advalorem Sales Tax will encourage manufacture of quality tea as there is no taxation on high price teas.
7. Market-oriented management in Sri Lanka; consequently. plantations will be able to respond and meet specific requirements.
8. Russia and Argentina bilateral agreement will absorb a large volume of (10,000 mt till early 2004) low quality teas.
9. The possibility of some key North African and Middle Eastern markets opening buying offices in Colombo.
10. The commencement of the EEC common market would open up opportunities for established tea trading houses in Europe to expand into new markets.
11. The availability of larger volume of better quality CTC tea which would give the local exporters the confidence to go out and secure larger orders which could be fullfilled from this volume.
12. The improvement of Syrian quality standards and the gradual opening up of the Iranian market.

In contrast, the negative factors are as follows :-

1. Inconsistent weather pattern affecting quality and yields. Damage to tea caused by the extreme and protracted drought.
2. Carry forward losses from 2003 affecting cash flows and consequent cut back of essential inputs to plantations.
3. Reduced buying by CIS and East Block in India in particular, making available a range of teas from India on the World Market.
4. Ability of some producer countries in particular to serve key tender markets due to cost advantage.
5. Increased preference for CTC teas in Pakistan, eg market share of Kenya has increased from 44 per cent in 1985 to 65 per cent in 2001. Similar pattern developing in Eygpt.
6. Turkish, Georgian and Vietnam teas appear on the world market.
7. High cost of finance in Colombo, which is considerably higher than most other key producer countries. eg Sri Lanka 19 per cent. India 14 per cent, Indonesia under 10 per cent (subsidised) with ability to give extended credit.

In conclusion when comparing the pros and cons, one could conclude that the industry which took, a severe beating in 2003 will see some recovery in 2003 particularly from a producer point of view. The expected increases in price would be most welcome to the producers who had incurred heavy losses in 2002 due to sharp drop in production and relatively low prices that prevailed. This would be subject to the curtailment of the already inflated cost of production which is considered to be amongst the highest of most producer countries.

Tea Convention, New Delhi : January 21-23, 1993

The deliberations at the Tea Convention 1993 were all solemn and serious. In the convention some interesting statements were made; some of these are listed below; call them the 'quotable quotes' of the convention.

A buyer from Pakistan stated, "Pakistani tea consumers have the palates of princes but pockets of paupers."

A speaker taking a cue from hand stitched garments which command a premium as opposed to machine stitched, posed a question, "Why can't we promote Indian teas as hand-picked, hand made and hand-packed."

- Quipped a delegated, "Add to it, for the hen-packed!"
- Taking of the difficulties of exporting teas to Pakistan, a producer stated, "I tried and tried to sell to Pakistan directly but finally got the order via Indonesia".
- "One kg of tea could buy a barrel of crude oil some time back, today you need 15 kg of tea to buy a barrel of crude."
- A speaker's suggestion of importing cheap teas into India for domestic consumption was rejected by one and all. It angered many and a delegate, visibly upset, called the proposal 'INSANE'.
- There was no answer to the question as to why a blender sells its branded packets in UAE without the company logo.

- "Tea is a renewable resource. When we export tea we export sunshine, water and human energy-all renewable. Tea exports are not like some other exports which cost the country heavily as resources are depleted." The Chairman of a session posed a question, "We shall export Yes. But let us ask the Government export for what? 40 percent of export earnings go towards payment of debi Import of fertilizers is fine as it increase our food production. But why import petroleum products which are not environmentally friendly. Exports must also help the economic freedom of the country."
- There was a mention of the 'Global Village' that the world is becoming today. A foreign delegate commented, "In tea we think global but act local."
- "In Germany, since 1947, there was a tax of DM 4.15 per kg on imports of tea. This has been removed in 1993." This should help in improving the consumption of tea Germany."
- A producer has decided to ask for Rs. 100/- per kg more for his offerings.

"Pure Darjeeling tea means 100 per cent Darjeeling tea in Germany. But in other European countries a blend of 60 per cent Darjeeling and the rest from other growths gets the Darjeeling label. These blends, when they come into Germany, cause problems. Labelling is important and should define the grades correctly."

The Commerce Ministry sources stated that the anomaly is being removed.

- "In Germany a panel of tasters protects quality today and not chemical analysts. This is through a recent Government legislation."
- "Exports to EEC countries will have to take bulk packing material like the tea chests. Packing waste management is the responsibility of the exporter."
- "Value addition really means branding, otherwise it is commodity trading".

"With affluence comes 'choice." Therefore, the 'marketing of choice' is the slogan in the developed countries".

"Zimbabwe has some areas producing 4000 kg per hectare. By 2000 AD, 800 million kg can be added to the world production—higher than the current production of India."

"Tea—The World's Natural Drink"

"New innovative products are the only answer to brand loyalty in the West for Indian value added exports".

"Indian products are technically right but not consumer-oranted."

"We in India seem to be drinking teas through our eyes and not through out palate."

"A buyer buys where it is easy to buy. In India there is the nonsense of registration which does not make buying easy."

"The average Japaneses believes that tea by and large grows in England, a little bit in Japan and the rest in Malaysia"

"Coffee, Tea and Cocoo are the three hot drinks—the market for all three is declining. The clod beverages are gaining".

"We Ministers do not buy or own tea. Every one brings up tea, so each morning the taste of tea is different."

"At the various international tea stalls, it is the pretty well turned out Sri Lankan lady with ago looking pack of Lanka tea who attracts and not India tea."

"Every one has to be a high quality but low cost producer."

Taking Tea

There were not many surprises in the 1993-94 Budget, but it certainly ensured the determination of the Goverment. to pursue the policy of economic liberalisation and globalisation of Indian market. In the process of doing so the Goverment exercised caution to fight out adversaries by way of providing for food subsidy, fertiliser subsidy, rural reconstruction, social welfare for backward community restructuring of rural banks etc. Nevertheless, there were divergent comments from various quarters to suit respective, political, economic interests like (progressive) 'growth-oriented', Investment friendly; poetic budget, etc. On the other side 'IMF dictated; 'Dunkel budget 'antiopor', 'pro-foreigner' etc.' Although, there was not any special mention about tea industry except continuance of exemption of excise duty, substantial reduction of corporate tax, in addition to saving on excise duty, provided for additional funds and incentive for investment in tea industry for increasing productivity and opening up new areas for tea cultivation. That was imperative keeping in view continuous growth in internal market and need for higher exports. In order to meet this demand both vertical and horizontal growth is called for.

Although the record of performance at all India level on account of yield per hectare is fairly impressive, there is scope for further substantial improvement. In 1971 all India yield rate was 1175 kgs. per ha while in 2005 it was around 1739 kgs per ha. Average of North Eastern Indian figures however compare lowered at 1175 kgs per ha. and 1630 kg per ha respectively.

Average yield per hectare

Year	All India	North East India
1951	909	939
1961	1066	1064
1971	1271	1175
1980	1461	1416
1990	1730	1631
1995	1771	1679
2000	1679	1639
2002	1739	1630

In order to achieve a moderate target of 1100 million kg. production by the 2015 AD, it is essential to invest in tea gardens for raising productivity in North India sector. In spite of a glorious past, it's falling behind South Indian average of 2004 kgs per ha (2004 fig). It is true that tea companies were scared to invest in spite of high profitability due to terrorist activities during the past several years in Assam and border states. Grim stories of abduction, extortion and murder of tea executives were regular newspaper headlines. When the Special Tea Protection Force was about the join duty after completion of training, ghastly killing of.

Increasing productivity of tea and opening up new areas for tea cultivation is a national issue which calls for large investment.

The basics for capital input has been cleared in this Budget. But it is unfortunate that politics, as usual, has been allowed to enter into this business. ITA is a resourceful and respectable organisation. It is time to act more aggressively for a national cause, which may need pulling strings from strategic corners of the corridors of power. Special Tea Protection Force must be enlarged and activised. It must be ensured that the Force does not become a tool of political game. Promises have been made to make new land available for tea cultivation. Strong Pursuasion is necessary to bring it into reality. West Bengal Goverment has proposed a heavy 'Salami' of the order of Rs. 30,000 per hectare which seems unreasonably high. It is a good sign that agricultural income tax has been reduced to 60 per cent in Assam and West Bengal too has followed the track. These matters must be settled to the satisfaction of all. Time is crucial Tea industry prepared itself for a future working on the present. The Budget admitted a huge fiscal deficit and a large budgetry deficit but it had many good points and certainly created a climate of investment. Tea companies took full advantage of it and dealt with the situation in wtih a firm hand. There was one important area in the tea taxation system which was not touched in the Budget. MODVAT has been applied to two important industries such as capital goods and petroleum products which will be undoubtedly very helpful. But in tea industry, heterogenous application of tax makes it very complicated and raises cost at the ultimate-end-product level. Sales tax at Guwahati auction centre is 20 per cent whereas at Kalkata it is 4 per cent, in Kerala it is 6.25 per cent and in Tamil Nadu 5.6 per cent. There variations effect the economic activity adversely. Then if the tea moves to another state for blending and packing it attracts a Central Sales Tax @ 4 per cent. Thirdly, it is again taxed at the time of sales by the first registered dealer which varies widely from 2 per cent to 13 per cent. Finally, there is a surcharge on all these taxes in some states. The total impact of all these taxes, which is hidden in the cost, is substantial. It has a piramyding as well as cascading effect on Indian tea in the global market. The only way to correct it was application of value-added tax system. Although the Budge had gone, but time for it has not yet gone. A high-powered committee was set up to look into the problem of Indian tea industry headed by the Commerce Secretary. This problem must be carefully presented to the committee so that a favourable decision is taken. ITA, TAI and UPASI should take it up seriously.

Rs 500 Crore for Tea Welfare

The Assam Govt. has decided to economic prepare a package for tea community witha Rs 500 crore. Cheif Minister Tarun Gogoi Govt. of Assam has entrusted three Congress tea organisations to prepare the package to be palced before the Centre for funding. The congress tea cell chairman, Bhagirat Karan, said Gogoi would take up the matter with Prime Minister Manmohan Singh who is a Congress MP representing Assam in Rajya Sabha. Sources said Singh has already agreed in principle to spare the amount in the next fiscal.

The package will lay stress on improvement in four key areas, including drinking water, healthcare, education and self employment. Besides the tea cell, the Assam Chah Mazdoor Sangha (ACMS)and the legislature forum of the Indian Congress (Intus) are engaged in preparation of the package. The three organisations played a key role to keep the congress's tea vote bank intact during the January panchayat elections held against the backdrop of a slew of anti congresss agitation and call for boycott of elections by the Assam Tea Tribes Students' Association and other tea bodies.

Karan said : "We are now giving finishing touches to the package. It will be submitted to the chief minister soon." Prasising Gogoi for according top priority to the welfare of the tea community, Karan said the chief minister has assured that he would take up the matter with the Centre to ensure funding of the package. Once sanctioned by the Centre, the tea tribes welfare department will implement the package under "active supervision" of the three tea organisations that have recently pressured Gogoi to raise the budgetary allocation for the department by Rs 7 crore from Rs 30 crore.

The package demands the setting up of five "group hospitals" covering the tea and Ex-Tea Tribe population in the state. Each of these hospitals would cater to the need of a cluster of two to three contiguous districts, Karan said. Under the package, funds will be used to set up public health centres in tea garden areas with a population of more than 10,000 and upgrade educational infrastructure in tea estates.

The package aims to mitigate the drinking water probelm in the tea gardens through installation of adequate numbers of tubewells and hand pumps. Addressing the problem of unemployment among youths of the tea community would be another important component of the package, Karan said. Many educated unemployed were taking up arms because of lack of job opportunities, he said.

Grants-in-aid would be provided to the educated unempolyed to encourage them to start their own ventures, including piggeries and dairy farming, he said.

Conclusion

If India is not to miss the boom in the international tea market and forgo valuable foreign exchange, it has to increase the output of this beverage rather fast. Rising consumption demand at home must not stand in the way of maintaining the exportable surplus at its present level, let alone developing it. This is no doubt easier said than done. The demand for tea is outstripping supply, not only because of the natural increase in population but also because ever newer layers of people are taking to the drinking of this cheap beverage. This is as true of tea as of sugar or for that matter any other article of mass consumption. Keeping this in view, the Elevanth Plan Set on output target for tea at 1000 million kgs and export target of 300 million kg, both targets are, in one sense, ambitious. True, there is not enough surplus land to bring under tea cultivation. Equally true, productivity is not easy to raise quickly. The state governments in tea-growing areas are dragging their feet in making available to tea estates adjoining lands. Even degraded forest land may not be readily available. The environment and forest ministries tend to hold a rather extreme view. Thus it is difficult to increase tea production. If the wide gap between the per hectare yield of different tea estates in the same agro-climatic zone could have been minimised the Elevanth Plan target was not difficult to attain or even to surpass. In any case, a multipronged strategy was adopted by the Union Government. In this context a special committee was set up to exptore the possibility of converting about 50,000 hectares of coffee land in South India into tea and rubber plantations. The home demand for coffeee has been stagnating around 60,000 tonnes and the export potential has been more or less tapped. Diversion of some coffee land to tea and rubber plantation did not adversely affect coffee interests. It helped increase tea and rubber production. Tea fetched more foreign exchange due to increase in shipments. And a rise in rubber production reduced its imports, saving foreign exchange. Narrow interests of any group must not be allowed to obstruct diversion of excess coffee land to tea and rubber cultivation.

Further, the various issue of tea industry were deliberated in various Annual General Meetings of different tea associations and these were compiled and given in the Annexures 8-12.

Chapter 11

Role of Research Bodies for Sustainable Development of Tea Industry

Back drop

Once, the then Prime Minister late Pundit Jawaharlal Nehru invited Professor P.M.S. Blackef and Professor A.V. Hill to advise him on the national science laboratories he was about to set up. One day, Dr. Shanti Swarup Bhatnagar, the then CSIR chief, was showing Professor Hill round the national physical laboratory. Professor Hill reportedly said with half a smile, "Yes, *a grand building indeed. But where are the researchers*? Our Cavendish laboratory was started in a hut". A hut is not essential for successful work or an edifice. Yet if a country can afford a neat building instead of a hut to house a research institute there should be nothing against it. The question is to choose between essentials and non-essentials. We have failed there. We have failed to keep many of our brilliant research workers content and offer them necessary infrastructure and other facilities. Thus, what we need is the selection of priorities and judicious distribution of finance over them. But first of all adequate finance is required. Take the tea industry. The only organisation that carries on research on tea in North East India is the [Tea Research Association] (TRA) complex with headquarters at Tocklai in Assam. Though said to be the biggest tea experimentation centre in the world, its purse is lean. For a long time it is being financed partly by the Council of Scientific and Industrial Research (CSIR) in spite of it having a membership of about 800 planters. Currently it faces a resources crunch, a serious one because the *CSIR refused to oblige it any longer.* Only the intervention of the then Union Minister of State for Commerce, Mr.

P.R. Das Munshi, took it out of the woods not that the CSIR was at fault. Itself short of funds, the CSIR argued that tea should come under agricultural research and not industrial research.

It is estimated that the overall R&D spending on the farm sector has been 0.17 per cent of GNP., which means about Rs 600 crore, but the amount going to tea has been a paltry one. the need for stepping up investment in research and development in the tea industry was assessed in a national conference. This was essential, said and the government also realised the importance of R&D *in this important industry and a R&D scheme with a corpus of Rs 10 crore was constituted.* Though the government belatedly woke up to the need for research in tea industry, the scheme subsequently earned the confidence of the industry. It is an open secret that tea units have become member of Tea Research Association, but some tea estates have been callous to research. Firstly, one of the reasons may be that tea cultivation had reached a plateau and not much could be achieved from the existing estates. Another reason may be the feeling among a large number of planters that growing more tea was government's headache so that more foreign exchange could be earned. In that case, result of any useful research would be brought to their knowledge. This view got support from a publicised comment made in good faith by a Commerce Ministry official. He said that whether or not a planter could afford TRA *membership the fruit of research should go to him so that the industry developed.* A third reason appears to have developed from a sort of disenchantment. The planters know the *tea industry is heavily taxed. The more they produce and earn, the higher will be the rate of agricultural tax on them, sometimes a prohibitory one. So why take all the trouble?* Strangely enough, these problems are peculiar to North East India. In the South, the UPASI tea research centre does not appear to have faced some of these problems. No wonder the planters there have contributed their quota to the research fund as the businessmen and tea planters in the North are also aware that investment is necessary before a return is expected. If they can be convinced that research is necessary for the good of the industry they would surely not fall back.

Direction of R&D in Tea

Between 1965 and 2005, the area under tea India increased from 3.4 lakh hectares to 5.5 lakh hectares and the production rose from 366 million kgs to 900 million kgs. For a 56 per cent increase in area the production increased by 146 per cent. This increase in production and productivity was possible because of the R&D activities of the Tea Research Association (TRA) and United Planters Association of South India (UPASI). In North India, in 2005, the average yield of TRA member gardens was 40 per cent more than that of non-member gardens. By 2006, the yield of member-garden became almost 90 percent more than the yield of non-members. The tenth plan envisaged a production of 1000 million kgs at the end of the plan period in 2007. This represented an annual growth rate of about 4.5 per cent during the nineties, which was achievable. Out of this, less than 1 per cent as expected, came from increase in area; the balance 3.5 per cent came from better productivity resulting from the R&D efforts of the North and South. In the eighties, TRA member gardens which received R&D support from Tocklai showed a productivity growth of 2.98 per cent against an overall growth of 1.72 per cent in Assam. In West Bengal, during the same period, TRA member gardens' productivity was 2.72 per cent per year against an overall West Bengal figure of 1.78 per cent. Today, in the North, the yield in a replanted area in four years after planting is 2,200 kgs per hectare or more than the average yield of the whole of North India, i.e. a hectare worth of tea plants on ground for four years only is matching the productivity of the whole tea area in the North with over hundred year heritage! *This is due to thanks to the technological innovations in the management of young tea developed by TRA.*

Technological Innovations of Tea Research Association (TRA)

The TRA has already made technological and manaement innovatios in developmnt of young tea plans, some of this are presented below:

- Apart from releasing its own clones (40so far) and biclonal seeds (15) TRA has assisted its member gardens to develop *70 clones of their own.*

- *New pruning and skiffing techniques* not only increased production manifold, but also affected more equitable distribution of crop throughout the season. This reduced the peak load in factories and made it possible to make better teas. Studies on plant nutrients enabled optimization of application rates and better utilization of inputs: Techniques and technologies for integrated control of all major pests, diseases and weeds enabled the tea estates to be free from pest, diseases and weeds and thus maximised production. New approach to water management located water logging even on 5000 ft. high hills of Darjeeling and new techniques and technologies to get rid of the excess water both in hills and plains resulted in phenomenal increase in yields in hitherto uneconomical estates.
- In the field of tea machinery, TRA has developed and *commercialised McTears rotor vane, Continuous tea drier, Barbora leaf conditioner, Boruah continuous tea roller*, Tocklai tea breaker and a Continuous withering and a Continues fermenting machine.
- A method of production of instant tea from green leaf has been successfully scaled up to pilot level and the technology has been sold through Tea Board. Tea based food colours have been produced in the laboratory to replace those produced synthetically.
- Work has been done on *alternative packaging materials*, like multi-walled paper sacks and synthetic lining materials for chests to replace aluminium foils.
- *Effective extension services* through twelve advisory centres in Assam valley, Cachar, Dooars, Darjeeling and Tripura have enabled the member gardens to take full advantage of the fruits of research. Regular training courses in field management, manufacturing, drainage, tea economics, both for managerial and supervisory staff, are fulfilling the task of human resource development for the industry, both for traditional and non-traditional tea areas. Such training are being supplemented by publication of the tea encyclopedia and by magazines and handouts like Two & A Bud, Annual Scientific Reports, advisory bulletins, advisory leaflets and special bulletins.

- *Economic evalution of the Tocklai* recommendations are being continuously done to ascertain cost benefit equation of such recommendations; time and motion studies are being done to identify measures for improvement of productivity.
- *A 32-bit computer* has been set up at Tocklai for electronic data processing of all research results since 1911, for quick references as well as for creation of a Technical Data Bank for multiple uses.

Fruits of R & D Activities

The fruits of the R&D activities have enabled the industry to cater to the ever-increasing home consumption and contain the exports, at least quantum wise, if not share-of-the-market wise. The industry has been able to maintain a steady annual production growth of nearly 4 per cent and at the same time produce the highest quality of tea in the world. All this is due to the excellent work done at Tockali. Tockali has, however, now arrived at a stage where yields have already reached a plateau and development of processing equipment has been limited to improvisation of the mechanical devices of the equipment and machinery, working principles of which have been known for the last four decades. In the meantime, with the increasing per capita consumption in this country, combined with growth of population, our home requirement has been increasing by almost 20 million kgs a year. We have also, in the last few years, lost our prominent position as the biggest exporter of tea in the world market and our share of the market came down from 45 per cent to 13 per cent in 2005. The government understandably, is concerned about it and wants to ensure that we maintain our predominant position as an exporter. These two factors, growing home requirement plus the necessity of maintaining our export at least at 28 per cent, are responsible for computing the targeted production of 1000 million kgs by 2006 AD. This represented a compound growth of 4 per cent per year, which we have achieved in the past. But, it is no longer going to be easy to maintain this growth rate because, as things stand today, most of the additional production will have to come from the existing area and will have to be processed in the outdated factories and machinery, which are in use today. *We are already facing a 'Yield Barrier' in the field; in the factory we have reached the level of saturation in the use of conventional mechanical devices. So, a completely innovative and state of art approach has be strengthment.* So long, our plant breeding work has been purely a selection job-not a creative one. But to break the yield barrier, to produce planting materials in terms of both quality and yield, we have now to turn to biotechnology. and we are successful to contain extent the TRA has developed drought resistant, disease resistant plants that need minimum of fertilizer and are capable of producing 7000 to 10000 kgs per hectare. This objective was achieved only through *use of genetic engineering techniques such as protoplast fusion, recombinant DNA, polyploidy somaclonal and mutation breeding. The aim is to exploit the genetic diversity available in tea.* Such plants produced by genetic engineering will be multiplied in the Tissue Culture Laboratory for propagation in a short time.

Tissue Cultue Laboratory

The Tissue Culture Laboratory has been organized and work is in progress. Initiation of the callus of the tea plant was made in the basal medium from various sections of the plant. Through modification of the medium, induction of massive callus, differentiation and regeneration were attempted. *Collaborative arrangements with the Biotechnology Division of Bhabha Atomic Center were made to take advantage of the latest techniques and facilities available there.* There are large gaps in one's knowledge with regard to nutrient uptake of the tea plant. The line of work, therefore, confined to the study of the uptake and metabolism of the different nutrients and their identification as limiting factors in crop productivity through the use of radio-tracer technique. For this purpose, a Radio Tracer Laboratory was set up. The necessary clearance from the Bhabha Atomic Research Center was received and the N-15 analysers are already functioning were intiatiation of fundamental streties.

Initiation of Fundamental Studies

Fundamental studies on *sink-sources relationship with special reference to the use of growth promoters and growth suppressors have also been initiated and some valuable clues on the metabolic processes of the tea plant have also been obtained.* So far as tea processing is concerned, the entire thinking and approach needs a fresh look. An innovative approach is required to streamline and will be a continous process both in concept and in designing of the processing equipment. Basic research is absolutely essential in the understanding of biochemical reactions and enzymology involved in tea quality related to withering, fermenting and synthesis of volatiles in processing of tea. Findings on these are to be taken into account while developing tea-processing technology, which will be continuous, automated, energy efficient, less space consuming and computer controlled; i.e. latest in technology. What we have now is antiquated. Thus, the thrust of TRA's R&D is only in one direction and that is sophistication of our percepts and concept so that an altogether new horizon is broken in the very basics of our understanding in tea processing and productivity. To attain this, there are two primary prerequisites.:

- The first is to provide a sense of direction. For this we need a National Committee for tea research, which will lay down the guidelines of R&D work to be done and undertake co-ordination among the different tea research organisations as well as other research bodies in the country. The National Committee for Tea Research was formed and committee for assisted by a "think tank" consisting of the best scientists and technologists of the country drawn from various scientific institutes together with persons of eminence and vision in the field of production, marketing and administration.
- The second *is the resources.* To do all this work in R&D, TRA needs funds. The government should contribute adequately, if not generously.

The tea industry not only earns quite a sizeable amount in foreign exchange of but is a contributes to the exchequer every year. This, is an industry that directly or indirectly, employs 3 million people; creates jobs in rural areas, employs women at least to the tune of 60 per cent of its workforce and generates one employment for an investment of Rs 20,000. Yet, this sector on an average, recieves about Rs 3 crore for research and development as against a total expenditure of Rs 3400 crores - just about .09 per cent.

	Nature of the project	Rs in lakh
1)	Biotechnology	89.18
2)	Development of tea machinery & tea processing equipment	90.43
3)	Water management	134.98
4)	Field technology, production and protection	234.73
5)	Substation & soil testing laboratories	214.95
	Total	764.27

TRA's Proposals to Tea Board

Accordingly, TRA had proposed to the Tea Board a few projects, which the Tea Board approved. These were:

Source: TRA's Annual Report

Subsequently, it was given to understand that there had been certain cuts and, out of the projects only the ones on biotechnology, tea machinery and soil analysis, at a total cost of Rs 394.56 lakh had been accepted and a formal approval was received. The association, therefore, set up four soil-testing laboratories with its own resources with the expectation that expenditure would be reimbursed. However, later, to TRA's disappointment, it was advised that there had been a drastic cut in the allocation and that only the project on Biotechnology had been approved to the extent of Rs 41.80 lakh, and the association would have to find the funds to the extent of Rs 48 lakh within the estimated cost during the Seventh Plan. But that is the past. *Let one think of the future! Let one hear what the government proposes to do to make up for the lost opportunity.*

Government's Proposal for the Lost Opportunity

It is, however, not the government alone that one should depend on for funds. The industry also must bear its share. The industry's contribution so far has been rather low compared to its turnover. The all-India, all industries average expenditure on R&D is 0.63 per cent of the turnover. Certain industries and units spend as much as 2 per cent to 4 per cent only. In tea industry it is less than 0.3 per cent.

The smaller units in North India are being asked to pay just about 0.1 per cent only. All sections of the industry, however, must contribute their bit. The smaller sections may contribute proportionately less in case they are less prosperous. But contribute they must. There must be involvement of every sector of the industry. To this end, the Tea Act should be amended as recommended in the status paper of National Committee for Tea Reasearch so that unless a tea estate is a member of one of the R&D stations, it just cannot be registered with the Tea Board and excise authorities and hence cannot function as a commercial entity. Fortified with the formation of National Committee for Tea Research, and arrangement of adequate funds from the government and the industry, the TRA can undertake their research and development in full-scale as recommended in the CSIR review committee report and the status paper, by recruiting the best scientific talents of the country and by setting up the moist modern laboratory complex and equipping it with the latest scientific instruments.

Tea Research Association (TRA)

The Tea Research Association (TRA), a unique corporate research body in India, incorporates both public and private resources to *promote sustainable development of tea research in North East India. TRA*, which was formed in 1964, has its tradition in the great and magnificent R&D work in tea that has been conducted at Tocklai experimental station for nearly a century. The contribution of Tocklai in increasing all aspects of tea productivity is too well known and well acclaimed in the international arena of research. Tea Research Association was formed basically with the objective of broadening the scope of Tocklai's activities and bringing the results of its R&D efforts to all tea estates. The R&D activities of tea research association has been funded by (i) *subscriptions from the member estates, (ii) grants from the Council of Scientific and Industrial Research (CSIR) and (iii) the Tea Board*. The tea industry is deeply committed to Tocklai and its research. This is evident from the fact that in the last 30 years the contributions from tea industry to TRA have more than doubled. Tea industry has also supported a special research fund *for hi-tech research in Tocklai and recently this has been augmented by special grants on biotechnology and tea machinery by the Tea Board as well*. The major resource of TRA thus comes from the tea industry. It is of interest that The total fund diverted to tea R&D constitutes about 0.30 per cent of the total turnover of the tea industry as against national industry-wise average of 0.63 per cent. The cost of research on tea in thus significantly less than that of other industries. Even with this resource limitation Tocklai has and continues to contribute significantly towards the growth and improvement of tea industry. TRA, which has completed 41 years of its services to tea industry, got momentum in increasing the overall productivity of tea and making future project strategies.

Research Policies at Tocklai

Applied research at Tocklai aims basically at *addressing field and factory issues of tea productivity*. These issues are given to the working scientists by a feedback system through the field advisory officers. The advisory officers of TRA visit tea estates, collect samples relating to the issues that the estates face and pass them on to Tocklai for evolving appropriate technologies for their solutions. This system has worked extremely well and Tocklai indeed is one of the few organizations in the world where a good and effective liaison has been established between the scientists and the clients who are the users of Tocklai's R&D findings. To cater to the requirements of basic research connected with tea, the following directions have been identified.

Genetic Approach To Plant Improvement: To bring quantum leap in tea yields, TRA greatly emphasised the application of *biotechnology and its integration with conventional methods of tea breeding* to evolve tea cultivators that utilised more sunlight and optimised nutrients so that each plant produced more shoots per unit area. With this objective in view, special techniques for tissue cultured tea, which ultimately helped in production of more planting materials, and bio-engineered plants, with high attributes for yield and quality, were developed. This was done in addition to conventional work like production of highly productive seed and clonal varieties. Tocklai developed an ideal plant type that helped in improving more yield per unit area by partitioning more of photosynthesis towards the production of pluckable shoots. This genetic approach brought about a significant change in the current concept of tea breeding in terms of higher productivity and quality.

Soil fertility microbiology : Improving soil fertility is a key area of research at Tocklai. It has been established that unless soil fertility and biological characteristics of the soil are maintained at their optima, the tea varieties may not be as productive as they are supposed to be. Great stress has, therefore, been given to soil research, particularly in identifying the physical, chemical and biological attributes of soil that are of consequences in the growth of tea. Tocklai quantified the essential elements in the soil that are needed to sustain tea *throughout the entire period of its growth*. Thus, properties of soils that permit concentration of these elements at the root surfaces and inter-cellular spaces for effective operation of the root vis-a-vis cell absorption mechanism were identified.

Nutrition : *Optimum nutrition is essential for productivity. Tocklai developed operation schedules for application of need-based fertilizer for higher productivity*. However, great stress has been given not only towards application of nitrogen, but also on their effective utilization by tea plants. It is known that tea utilizes less than 25 per cent of the nitrogen applied to the fields; the challenge before the Tocklai scientists is to find out how to make tea plants use more of nitrogen so that its use becomes more cost-effective. TRA established that an inter play of soil and biological factors determines the nutritional need of tea. Therefore, the role of organics assumed additional importance in understanding the nutritional needs of tea. By using radio isotopes, Tocklai worked out the limits of plant's responses to applied nutrients, and ways to overcome them. A related approach was evolved to find out the enzyme system within the plants that regulated nutritional needs of the plant. A third approach was to study the soil microbes to find out their roles in nutrient uptake by tea plants. The selected strains of soil organism helped better utilization of some of the nutrients if they are applied in relatively lesser quantities.

Overcoming limiting factors : Water : The TRA recognizes that even if better plants are produced by genetic or conventional means, their yield potential cannot be fully exploited unless the effects of limiting factors that interfere with productivity are minimized or totally eliminated. Even some of the existing tea varieties respond well if the limiting factors are removed. Excess or lack of water in some seasons, for example, can severely interfere with the growth and productivity of tea unless the water requirement of tea are maintained at the optimum. The TRA has, therefore, given great stress on integrated water management to enable tea plants to remain physiologically active throughout the season to produce more yield of quality. Tocklai emphasised that there is no generalised formula to overcome water stress in plants, but by taking consideration of the environmental and soil factors, it is possible to develop working models to replenish or remove water under diverse growing situations. What is, however, needed is to develop creative solutions that take cognizance of local situations as problems of water management are highly area-specific.

Pathogens & weeds : The changes in agricultural practices over the years have had their repercussions on pests, and pathogens of tea. The increased abundance of these organisms very often does not allow the utilization of full yield potential of tea and they also interfere with the physiological functioning of tea leaves. The net result is that even plant with good yield potential fails to come up to the expected standard. Tocklai has been pioneer in developing strategies to effectively deal with the vast spectrum of tea pests, pathogens and weeds with appropriate pesticides. Tocklai has also pioneered the rational use of pesticides so that they do not interfere with tea environment in any way and also do not leave any residues in made tea. These achievements notwithstanding, Tocklai realises that pesticides at a certain point may start giving diminishing returns. Therefore, currently stress is being given on the use of biocides and biological control agents for effective and lasting control of pests and pathogens.

Tea processing : The TRA's contribution in the area of machinery development is well known. It developed processing equipment that automates the entire system of tea processing without in anyway affecting the quality. A corollary to this approach is the development of devices to monitor each step of tea manufacturing by biosensors.

Integrated management of energy is another area where pioneering work was done at Tocklai. This apart, up-scaling of existing machinery and development of machines that consume less energy have also been undertaken.

Flavour : The TRA emphasizes that tea productivity must integrate both quality and quantity. The bio-chemists at Tocklai identified the biochemical basis of tea quality, particularly flavour, and the way it is built up during different phases of manufacturing. Using the most modern equipment, the volatile flavouring constituents of tea were identified, and based on the proportion of different volatile compounds, a flavour index of tea was also developed. Further research was conducted on get an insight of the dynamic mechanism within the cells that regulate tea flavour. This aspect of research is of paramount importance for Indian tea as it is known over the world for its quality.

Future Thrust

Tea research appreciates that to achieve a major break through in tea research, it is essential that an era of modern research begins at Tocklai. With this objective in view, TRA is actively co-operating with Tea Board and other agencies. It has raised a corpus, which is utilized for carrying on basic research on different aspects of tea productivity and flavour. Biotechnology is one such area where a good deal of resource is being diverted. Biotechnological approach ultimately integrates production and processing dynamics of tea so that a unified concept on tea productivity emerges. This concept extended in developing new plant types with attributes of higher productivity and quality. The TRA also recognises that to conduct research of a high order, a conducive ambience to research is also essential. To this end TRA drew up a blue print for setting up an ultramodern laboratory complex at Tocklai. The complex has most modern equipment. It provides all necessary back-up services and infrastructural facilities to ensure the scientists the best equipment and resources to meet the challenges ahead of them. Indeed, the Tocklai scientists are fully aware of these challenges and have accepted them in a truly scientific spirit. An international conference on R&D in tea, for example, admitted that Tocklai continues to pioneer tea research in the world today.

Tea Research Body set up

Tea Research Association formally came into being in January 1964 after a meeting of the founder members on December 30, 1963. India Tea Association Tocklai experimental station administered the new research body. Mr S.P. Sinha presided over the inaugual meeting and preferred to see Tocklai become a research station for the entire tea industry. For this he proposed the formation of Tea Research Association open to all but utilising the resources of Tocklai and of other stations in North East India. " To achieve this," Mr Sinha said, "It would be necessary for the Indian Tea Association that to agree to lease its Tocklai station and ancillary buildings to the proposed Tea Research Association as well as all its scientific staff'. It was further made clear to the Indian Tea Association that the government would not permit the new body to grant to the staff any higher scales of pay and amenities than those enjoyed by comparable officer in other government research stations. Where higher salaries were paid by the Indian Tea Association to existing staff, the association would be responsible for meeting the difference between the Indian Tea Association (ITA) salaries and those paid to scientists of similar status in other research stations falling under the general supervision of the Council of Scientific and Industrial Research (CSIR). Accordingly, the Indian Tea Association had agreed, to lease the whole of its scientific station and the machineries and equipment therein to the Tea Research Association on a nominal rent of Rs 1,001.

Agreement between the Council and the ITA : The agreement was reached between the council and the ITA on the special financial liabilities, which the association had to continue to shoulder as long as the staff concerned remained in service. The article of association and the rules thereunder was drafted and came up for acceptance later on during this meeting. The annual subscription payable by members varied according to the size of membership, but on figures based on 1962, the cost of Tea Research Association to its members was approximately Rs.30 lakh per year of which 50 per cent was borne by the government. So far membership acreage was 385, 586 acres (156,041 hectare) which represented a subscription of Rs 3.89 per acre (Rs. 9.61 per hectare). It was hoped that once the association was under way, many more tea companies would come forwarded and join. As yet membership only represented 51 per cent of the total acreage in North-East India; of non-Indian Tea Association gardens only 14 per cent of the acreage had so far applied to join the association. But the government and the Tea Board wished that all should join.

Expansion of Research : About the development of scientific research work in India, the industry did not take long to realise that science would play a major role in the growing and manufacture of tea, and as early as 1900, the Indian Tea association appointed its first scientific officer, Dr. Mann. He had his research headquarters in the museum in Calcutta, although much of his work was done in the tea districts. The move to Tocklai was made in 1911. It was from these small beginnings that the Tocklai experimental station was set up and over the years research in the tea industry has expanded steadily. Tocklai (1963-64) employed 21 officers and approximately 800 junior staff and labourers.

Work at Tocklai

The work at Tocklai was covered by ten different branches, which were kept separate for the administration of their research and advisory programmes. Otherwise, they worked together as an integral whole. These included four branches, which were basically related to research, four were experimental and two were advisory. The four research branches were the physio-chemical branch, the Botany branch, the plant pathology branch and the bio-chemistry branch, which conducted research respectively on the environment in which tea was grown; on the tea bush, on its pests and diseases and on made tea. The basically experimental branch comprised the agricultural branch, engineering development branch, tea tasting branch and the statistical branch. The function of the agricultural branch was to develop improved cultural methods, often based on research in other branches, and to test them out under field conditions while the function of the engineering development branch was to do the same for methods of manufacture. An important adjunct to the agricultural branch was the Borbhette experimental garden, which covered 40 hectares, where practical field experiments were carried out. Simultaneously, the engineering development branch had a well-equipped workshop and a pilot factory in which new machines were fabricated and tested and amongst other things it invented the famous McTear Rotor vane.

The function of the tea tasting unit was to ensure that no new cultural or manufacturing practice adversely affected quality and to confirm whenever quality was improved; besides tracing and correcting faults in manufacture, which could lead to loss of quality. As fundamental knowledge accumulated, it became necessary to test out the research findings and to disseminate the results of research and practical experiments to tea growers. For this purpose, there were advisory branches at Tocklai and Nagrakata in West Bengal. The former had offices stationed at Tocklai itself, on the north bank of the Brahmaputra. Advisory officers provided garden managers with advice on all aspects of tea culture and assisted in conducting the experiments required to test out Tocklai findings under local conditions. That was the organization for which one should owe the Indian Tea Association a measure of gratitude for making Tocklai, which had become the largest research station in the world entirely dedicated to tea.

Hope for Future

Concluding his speech, Mr Sinha said the Tea Research Association had a great future before it. Today, everybody was aware of the urgent necessity of producing more tea and of increasing India's foreign exchange earnings. The Tea Research Association could do much to assist in this matter by helping the industry to improve the quality and yield of tea. Already during the last 55 years, (i.e., from 1950 to 2005) the average yield in North-India has increased from approximately 939 kgs of made tea per hectare to 1700 kgs per hectare i.e., about twice that amount and much of the credit for this must go to past research and experiments at Tocklai. He was confident that even more could be done in the future and that the engineering department at Tocklai could help further in developing a continuous manufacturing system by which tea would pass continuously from one phase of manufacture to the next. Work on various machines to achieve this end was already well advanced at Tocklai and the new continuous dryer was commercially available during 1964. All these matters were of vital importance if India was to continue to compete successfully with tea produced in other countries such as East Africa, Ceylon and Indonesia.

TRA—CSIR Round Table Conference

A TRA and CSIR round table conference was held in the latter half of December 1990 at hotel Taj Bengal in Kolkata. Among those who spoke were, Mr. A.P. Mitra, the then director general of Council of Scientific and Industrial Research (CSIR) and Mr. Vinay K. Goenka, the then chairman of the Tea Research Association (TRA), which organized the conference. The then CSIR chairman said that his organization's laboratory facilities and the services of scientists would be made available for tea research. He stressed that increased attention on the question of improving machinery and plantation techniques was required to be paid in order to enhance tea output substantially. More expansion of the area under plantation would not alone do, he added. It was felt that it should be possible to produce 1,000 million kgs of tea annually by the year 2,005. The conference was attended by the directors of several CSIR laboratories. Mr Vinay K. Goenka said that the tea industry in India needed substantial science and technology support since production had not been growing as fast as it should have. Referring to Indian tea in the international market, Shri Goenka pointed out that one of the disquieting features with regard to production of tea in India was that it still is weather dependent to a large extent and actual production of tea had always fallen short of the target in production. Can India through greater inputs of R&D, give more stability to the projected growth? India has one of the largest bases in science and technology in the world and is much better placed in this regard compared to majority of tea producing countries. So if India cannot achieve this goal who can?

Steady increase in Foreign exchange earnings : For about three decades, the volume of exports of tea remained in the vicinity of 200 million kgs as the policy of the Government of India has been to allow exports only after meeting the internal demand of tea. In other words, the increase in production on year-to-year basis was retained by ever-increasing rate of domestic consumption. As a result, countries like China, Sri Lanka and Kenya forged ahead in the international market and our share in the world market declined sharply. There has been a steady increase in the foreign exchange earnings due to increase in unit value realization though volume of exports has been static. A special feature of the tea exports is that the industry consumes negligible amount of foreign exchange in terms of raw materials of components. There is, therefore, a tremendous need to pool our resources and imbue the tea industry with greater confidence through the support of science and technology. The round table conference focused attention on some of the thrust areas in agriculture and engineering.

Thrust Area in Agriculture : A manger's emphasis is towards development of tea cultivars with attributes of high yield and quality, not otherwise possible to achieve by conventional means. Towards these objectives a special effort was made to study the somatic embryogenesis as a first step towards mass propagation of elite clones. Production of haploid plant by arther, ovary and pollen cultures was taken up for developing a pure diploid homozygous-line of tea plants. These plants, in turn, were used as progenitors in evolving plants with high productive potentials. Emphasis was also given to study the basic genetics of tea so that hybridization for quality and yield of a high order were reality.

- In search of higher productivity, a physiological approach was taken up to find ways and means to reduce the high respiratory losses by tea. In effect, this helped in increasing the photosynthesis by tea plants which ultimately reflected in higher productivity. However, attention was paid to increase the low harvest index of tea genetically and by chemical means.
- To increase the productivity of existing tea, special research was done to overcome the constraints towards productivity. Thus, research on bio-control of major pests and management of tea plantation in particular was carried out both in the field and laboratories. The other area of research thrust involved management of water, particularly location of outfalls and identification of potential drought and waterlogged areas by

using remote sensing and aerial photography. The principal object of these studies was to achieve major break through in tea productivity within a short period of time.

Thrust Areas in Engineering : Since tea productivity cannot be considered in isolation of quality, a major research endeavour of TRA was to devise tea machinery on the basis of enzymatic reactions during different phases of tea processing. A major breakthrough had already been achieved in identifying the important flavour components of tea and their role in the development of aroma complex of tea in different areas.

In the area of machinery development, stress was given to make the tea processing a continuous operation – the ultimate objective was to make the whole system automatic. Current R&D activities involved monitoring the level optimization of tea during different phases of manufacturing like withering, rolling and drying. Attention was paid to the development of a moisture-detecting device to accurately read the moisture content of tea-leaf at different points of manufacturing.

An adjunct R&D effort was towards conservation of use of energy in tea factories. The then methods of tea manufacturing required about 0.4 to 0.5 KWH of electric energy and 1.2 kg to 1.6 kg of coal or 0.4 to 0.7 liter of TD oil to manufacture 1 kg of black tea. Research was conducted to reduce the use of energy while not compromising with the functional efficiency of different tea machines. There is every reason to hope that conservation of heat energy in the driers is possible by improving the combustion and the drying efficiency; and by reducing the loss through the chimney, drier exhaust and conduction. This apart, other possibilities of energy conservation were also being explored.

Along with developing the new tea processing techniques, considerable attention is being paid to identify chemical compounds of pharmacological importance in tea. There is evidence that some of the tea pigments and chemical can be used to alleviate chronic diseases like blood pressure, heart ailment and even cancer. Tea leaves also have compounds that are of high nutritional values. By integrating these two aspects, tea can be propagated as a health drink for the populace at large.

Tocklai's Significant Contribution – Development of Tea Growing and Processing

The pioneering research carried out at Tocklai has been contributing significantly towards the development of tea growing and processing. During the last decade alone, per hectare yield of tea in North East India increased by 25 per cent primarily because of the R&D activities at Tocklai and effective transfer of the results of research to the planting community. This helped the industry to cater to the ever- increasing home consumption and maintained the level of export for earning valuable foreign exchange. The industry was able to maintain a steady annual production growth rate of nearly 2.5 per cent and at the same time, produce the highest quality of tea in the world. Tocklai experimental station commonly known as "Tocklai" has been serving the tea industry, especially in north east India, for nearly eight decades and has become synonymous with the research on tea in the country. The contribution of this oldest and largest tea research institute in world has benefited not only tea planters in India but also the tea industry all over the world. For the greater interest of the industry, the Tea Research Association (TRA) was formed in 1964 to take over the management of Tocklai experimental station and other outstations. The present budget of the Association is of the order of Rs. 5 crore out of which 50 per cent of the recurring and 33 per cent of non-recurring expenditure incurred as per government norms and is paid by the Government of India as grant in aid. Since inception, the TRA has been receiving such grants from the CSIR and the Tea Board. The various research projects of TRA are carried out in Tocklai in its seven research departments— Botany, soil & water management, agronomy, plant protection, engineering & manufacturing technology, Biochemistry, statistics and agricultural economics. The region's specific research and technology transfer are done through a substation at Nagrakata in Dooar (West Bengal) and six other branches at Darjeeling, Terai (West Bengal), Cacher, North Bank, Upper Assam (Assam) and Agartala (Tripura). The advisory department with its extension network throughout the tea districts basically deals with the transfer of technology at field levels. TRA publishes a six-monthly journal Two and A Bud, a reference book, the tea encyclopedia, and annual scientific report, papers, memorandum, wall charts quarterly bulletin and advisory leaflets, and occasional bulletins. All members get a copy of these publications. The continued services of TRA vis-a-vis Tocklai to the tea industry through research and development specially during the last few years are mentioned in the following paragraphs area-wise.

Planting Materials : Tocklai was the first in the world to evolve the vegetative propagation method for tea. Breeding for high yielding, drought tolearant, high quality tea cultivars has been an ongoing effort. As stabel certain Tocklai has so far released 40 clones and 15 bi-clonally seed stocks of its own and through garden selection scheme 108 other clones have been recommended to suit the need of different agro-climatic regions.

Two more clones, TV-29 and TV-30 are now ready for release. A germplasm bank has been established and a new species of tea named Camelia irrawadinsis has been described. Some of the Tocklai-released clones have already crossed over 5000 kgs/ha made tea mark in quite a few commercial plots. In the endeavour for still better planting material, tissue culture technique is being adopted and re-germination of plantlets from various plant tissues has been achieved successfully.

Plant Physiology : Studies have shown that tea leaf becomes fully efficient once its grows over half its normal size; it retains its peak photosynthetic ability for about six months before it is shed at about 18 months. Drought-affected leaf recovers it photosynthetic ability much faster while water logged ones do not do so for a long time after the cessation of waterlogging. About two-thirds of the dry matter produced by the bush is lost in respiration and only about 10 per cent is harvested. Photosynthesis is impaired at temperature above 30°C and hence shade is highly essential. A study of the direction of movement of photosynthesis in tea bush using radio-active carbon source has shown that a strong base exists of determining pruning time, as re-growth of bushes following pruning was found to be related to the starch reserve in the roots prior to pruning. Diurnal change in dry matter accumulation has indicated a gain of 10 per cent if plucking is deferred till noon. The relationship in periodicity of growth of root, shoot and seed has been determined. Seasonal dormancy is related to short day-length and low temperature, which can be broken by gibberellic acid by neutralizing the effect of growth promoters like triacontanol to give increased in yield during plucking season. Growth retardants have been used with success to promote frame formation in young tea. Standardization of grafting has been made and it has been found that the stock influences only the vigour of the scion and not quality.

Plant Nutrition : Application of urea and ammonium sulphate at the same rate of nitrogen per hectare yields similar results. About 40 per cent of the nitrogen is lost through leaching and 10-20 per cent in gaseous form; the gaseous loss is higher with urea. In plots receiving continuous doses of nitrogen for over 50 years, it has been found that high dose of N caused increase in accumulation of thiamine, an amide, in the roots' nutrient absorbing system and soil microbial spectrum also underwent an adverse change. Balancing N with P and K improved the situation. Very high dose of N alone did not boost the yield though correspondingly some other research institutes reported high yield increase. However, positive response was possible in young tea with high dose of N in the range of 180 to 200 kgs/ha (depending on the varietal difference of the tea plants) when balanced with adequate potash and phosphate. Tocklai, therefore, advised its members to desist from using very high doses of N, and beyond 135 kgs/ha is advised only in specific situations. Potash response was found to be universal and related to time, level of application and soil potash status. Application of phosphate caused an increase in aluminium phosphate content of the soil. Missouri rock phosphate can replace the costly super phosphate fully in mature tea and by fifty per cent in mixture for young tea. Mycorrival fungi are being isolated to help enhance the phosphate uptake in young plants.

Increase in white root portions helps increase the root action exchange capacity. Response of various types of tea to captions is more or less specific. Soil pH can be brought to desired level through amendments by application of pyrites or dolomite as the situation demands. Deficiency symptoms for important macro and micro elements like N, K, Mg, Zn are identified and corrective measures are made available. Foliar application of Zn is more effective than soil application. Zinc sulphate is the cheapest of the zinc sources.

Agricultural Practices : A plant population of 14 to 18 bush per 10 sq. m is considered to be healthy health. Leaving an extra leaf in un-pruned tea increases yield. Mulching helps conservation of moisture, suppresses weeds, induces feeder root proliferation and adds to the organic content of the soil purning litters act as mulch. Cultivation helps aeration and stops localized waterlogging.

Plant Protection : Economic control measures for the commonest pests and diseases of tea, shade tree and green crop used in North East India have been developed. This has become possible through studies over the decades on the life history of all important pests and diseases, which are influenced by season, temperature, rainfall, soil or cultural operations like pruning, plucking, manuring, shade, drainage, cultivation, etc. Further, the study helped identifications of the vulnerable stage when chemical control becomes most effective. For the first 30 years, efforts on chemical control were confined to recipes of home made pesticides. But following the pesticides boom in the 1950s about 400 pesticides received from all over the world were tested for biological efficiency and the ones effective under our conditions were recommended after checking on their phytotoxicity, taint and harmful residues. In addition, large varieties of spraying equipment were tested and the suitable ones were recommended with all relevant information on when, how and where to use the. Biological control of some pests like aphids and scale insects their application on in thousand per hectare has been found to be optimum, a higher population showed adverse effects after 4---5 years. Planting procedures have been standardised. Need for rehabilitation in uprooted areas has been documented. A new method for bringing up young tea was developed, which has the dual advantage of higher early production and sustained later productivity. Growth retardants have been successfully used to suppress heavy rain flush without loss of crop and labour management during rush plucking season. Introduction of longer pruning cycles helped uniform crop distribution. Standard plucking developed by Tocklai is more advantageous than black plucking. Soil fumigation has done the dual job of controlling primary root diseases and shortening the rehabilitation period in some situations. Survey on pests diseases led to the discovery of many species and genera of fungi and insects. A quick and efficient method for enmatode extraction and another for blister blight control dicots have received recognition.

Weed Control : Introduction of chemicals for weed control helped in arresting the menacing spread of Miamian in the nineteen sixties. Since then a wide range of herbicides have been tested against both dicots and monocots and a cost effective spraying schedule is now available to deal with all types of weeds in North East India. Pre-emergent autumn application of weedicides is more cost efficient and equally effective as application in growing season. Developing a solubilization technique has reduced cost of application of expensive weedicides like glyphsate. Long-term continuous spray leads to a shift in weed population indicating the necessity for changing herbicides. Characteristic damage symptoms produced on tea through inadvertent application have also been identified.

Water management : Drainage and irrigation led to higher productivity in tea in waterlogged and drought-prone areas, respectively. Retaining water table at 90 cm below ground level has been found to be significantly superior to shallower or deeper water tables. In areas with high water table caused by lack of suitable outfall, pump drainage or re-allocation of the main outlet drain solved the problem. Subsurface drains at 1.2 m depth was superior to surface drains 75 cm deep. It has been found that 20 per cent of rain goes as run-off and 80 per cent contributes to the water table problem once the soil has been saturated with early showers. Studies on run-off co-efficient, rainfall data, slope of the land, soil texture, presence of seepage etc. have been made to formulate the drainage system, its depth and spacing, suitable for a particular area. The areas provided with improved drainage system, have recorded on an average about 25 per cent increase in yield as compared to the conventional drainage in waterlogged areas. Irrigation requirements for each sub-district have been estimated through a study of rain in relation to crop and these estimates are now being verified under field conditions. Experiments have shown that in young tea, drip irrigation is more effective than sprinkler irrigation.

Shade : Tocklai has established that a light even canopy of shade is essential for tea plantations of North East India with the exception of the high elevations of Darjeeling. Shade trees cut off the high isolation detrimental to photosynthesis. Shade reduces tea leaf temperature and thereby saves the leaf from sun scorch or physiological death and ensures photosynthesis during high temperature regime. It also reduces incidence of pests and diseases like mites, red rust and Porla. It helps increase in leaf area accumulation of dry weight. It has buffering effect and prevents high fluctuation in soil temperature; on a moderate estimate, it adds organic matter by way of leaf fall to the tune of 80 kgs/ha.

Tea Machinery : In Tocklai's effort to make tea manufacture a cost-effective continuous process, the following machines have been invented; some of them have been used extensively all over the world. The machines are (1) McTear Rotor Vane, (2) Withering Tunnel, (3) Continuous Tea Tray Dryer, (4) Continuous Fermenting Machine, (5) Marlboro Leaf Conditioner, (6) Boruah Continuous Roller, (7) Tocklai Tea Breaker, (8) Storage system for, continuous Withering Machine and (9) Continuous Withering Machine, a modified version of the fermenting machine.

Tea manufacture : For better utilization of biochemical processes in tea manufacture, the components of the tea shoot, their nature and transformation during withering, rolling, fermentation and drying are identified. That the chemical withering is necessary to make good tea has been established. During rolling and specially during fermentation the oxidation of catching gives rise to TF and TR; the former contributes towards brightness, and quality while the latter towards strength and body of the liquor. The role of chlorophyll in appearance, trapezoid compounds like linalool in flavor effect, of pectin on fermentation, and of sugar on polyphone biosynthesis have also been established. Defect in manufacture can be identified by organoleptic tests. A floor level fermentation test has been developed to provide "chemical index" for assessing degree of fermentation. Categorisation of Tocklai released clone vis-a-vis their compatibility in relation to its strength flavor and self- drinking characters have improved clonal tea blending.

Packaging Material : In view of the growing shortage of conventional packaging materials for tea and to keep up with the modern packaging method to suit the requirements of buyers all over the world, Tocklai has been experimenting on available alternative packaging materials. To mitigate the shortage of aluminium foil for use as tea chest lining, three alternative lining materials were tested and finally approved by Indian standard institute, The Bureau of Indian Standards. Multi-walled paper sack is another promising pack.

Experimental Methodologies : Statistical inferences are drawn for a perennial crop like tea by very long time-scale field experiments. The first scientific estimate of loss of crop in tea due to pests and diseases was done and methodology was developed to carry out such estimates economically and efficiently in future. A mathematical model has been developed for evaluation and enunciation of biochemical parameters responsible for briskness, brightness, strength, colour, quality and valuation of tea made through CTC and orthodox methods of manufacture. Methodologies have been worked out to improve the efficiency of comparison of experimental treatments and reduction in the cost of experiments for long-term trials.

Economic Studies : Economic evaluation of Tocklai's recommendations on control of re-dust, red spider, weeds, various pruning cycles, plant density and assessment of Tocklai clones and seeds have been done. Estate development projects, rejuvenation and replanting have also been evaluated under commercial conditions. Another major breakthrough has been the motion and time study, which led to the identification of measures for improvement of productivity of tea labor. Energy balancesheet of the work involved in plucking a tea shoot has indicated areas for reducing fatigue and increaseing the productivity of estate workers.

Institute of Plantation Management, Bangalore

Plantation sector plays an important strategic role in Indian context. It is labor-intensive and export oriented. Passing through the romantic and scientific era, it has entered a new phase, namely liberalization and globalization. This phase has thrown new challenges and problems for a modern day plantation manager who has to compete and deal with new realities. Plantation manager has to extend his/her vision from the ground level to global scene. In view of the new changes the need to sustain and improve this sector's strategic tip was identified as a critical need. To fulfil this need an institutional mechanism was considered appropriate. Ministry of Commerce foresaw this need and took initiatives in this direction leading to establishment of Indian Institute of Plantation Management, (IIPM) Bangalore.

Considerable thought on the part of the government and the enlightened leaders forming the plantation sector had gone into conceptualizing the idea of this institution. Initiative came from the Ministry of Commerce, Government of India, in early 1990s. A working group was set up comprising members from the government and industry to deliberate on the various aspects for setting up the institute. A steering committee set up by the Ministry of Commerce gave the initial thrust that was needed for establishment of this institution. Institute evolved around an innovative reach-out model of institutions to meet the management training needs of the sector as a whole.

Premise of IIPM

IPM is based on the premise that competitive edge of a sector can be strengthened through people. Hence, a continuing effort is needed to constantly update the management skills. Continuing efforts are also needed to prepare a new generation of enlightened leadership. Vision of IIPM is to contribute to this efforts. IIPM is not just another institute of management. As a unique sectoral school of management it has distinctiveness. This distinctiveness comes from the sectoral requirements. Plantation sector in India has a geographical spread as well as a distinctive ownership spread. It has presence of both the corporate as well as owner-managed organization. In case of owner-managed organizations, building up the managerial capacities of next generation assumes a special significance. These requirements add to the distinctiveness of the institute. Application of known management skill and techniques to agro-based industry functioning in a highly competitive environment is a major concern of Indian

Institute of Plantation Management. The plantation sector is unique in view of 'flattened hierarchies' with plantation manager operating far away in the remote areas. Being labor intensive, the people-factor is critical to its success. Plantation manager has to be down to earth and at the same time be prepared to face the ever-changing world of global competition. Indian Institute of Plantation Management acts as an intellectual resource center in this endeavour.

Reach-out Model: Uniqueness of IIPM

IIPM is unique because it has designed itself during its inital stage of development around a new innovative reach out model. This model reverses the traditional concept of education as one-way traffic. Under the rech out approach institute reaches out its client system through on-site training and education. On-site education becomes a learning experience for the educator as well as it reduces the theory and practice gap. Further institution reaches to the place where it is required. This tends to correct the ivory tower bias of the academicians. In case of plantation sector the reach out model is an appropriate one as the numbers involved is very large and geographical spread as wide. While interaction with a select group is organised at the central facility, interactions with larger numbers are responsible only through reach out concept. Reach-out model is aptly suited to the requirements of the plantation sector and is also an innovation in management education.

Mission and broad objectives of IIPM

Mission Statement: IIPM is committed to the cause of sharpening strategic tip of the plantation sector by continuous improvement in management methods through management training and education. As a sectoral school of management, it has designed its activities and programmes around the concept of plantation management.

Foundational Principles : IIPM is an exclusive, sectoral school of management. It is based on five foundational concepts or principles that define its scope of activities. The five basic principles have been identified, keeping in view the think-tank requirements as well as the management education needs of the owner- planters and the plantation managers. The foundational concepts are as follows:

- Strategic think ahead forum;
- Creation of elightened leadership;
- Continuing development of the best plantation managers;
- Action based research; and
- Intellectual self-reliance and enhancement of intellectual capital.

The institute's educational paradigm is centred around the creation of future enlightened leadership for the plantation sector.

The institute's training paradigm is centred around the concept of the BEST plantation manager (B = Behavioural, E = Economic, S = Strategic, T = Technical). The training programmes are designed keeping in view these four dimensions to make them relevant and useful to the participants.

The institute's research paradigm is defined by action-based research. The approach to research makes the research meaningful and useful to the practitioners. Action based research also allows practitioners to contribute to the development of experience-based knowledge.

The institute acts as a strategic think ahead forum by providing intellectual support. For this purpose it brings together academicians and practitioners for strategic scenario mappings.

Broad Objectives : The board objectives are given below :-

- To impart continuing management education to professional managers and owner-managers in the plantation sector and associated agro-business enterprises, with a view to bring to them latest techniques and ideas in management.
- To train young professionals/young entrants and estate inheritors for entry-level managerial positions in the plantation sector.
- To conduct policy research for policy making at the government and institutional levels.
- To conduct the research in policy, strategic, managerial and implementation problems of the plantation sector, in order to improve the management of plantations, as well as to augment the existing body of knowledge in plantation management.
- To act as an information and intellectual resource centre and

act as think-tank for policy, strategic and operational issues for various segments of the plantation sector and the associated agro-business enterprises.

- To serve plantation sector and the associated agro-business enterprises by undertaking management consultancy services on strategic and operational aspects of managing plantation enterprises.
- Training the small growers in better management of their plantations.

Scope in Institute's Activities : The institute explores the possibility of undertaking of the activities as enumernted below :

- To fulfil its role as a think-tank and intellectual support resource. The institute conducts interactive brainstorming workshops and seminars on themes of importance and relevance for the plantation sector.
- Institute conducts short-term executive programmes (STEPs) for the professional managers and owner managers. These programmes are designed to provide new techniques for effective handling of managerial and operational issues.
- Institute undertakes action-based research with a view to field test the ideas and concepts developed at the institute.
- Through its writers' forum, the institute encourages the practitioners to contribute towards development of the experience-based knowledge for enhancing the intellectual capital.
- The plantation information network of the institute aims at strengthening the database in the plantation sector at the national and international levels.
- To meet the future managerial talent requirements, institute would in due course consider initiating a longer duration programme for the new entrants and estate inheritors.
- Institute undertakes consultancy assignments in policy, strategic, implementation and operational issues of relevance to the plantation sector.
- Institute participates in inter-institutional programmes for exchange of scholars. In collaboration with other leading

institutions it also offers facilities for the post-doctoral work.

Foundation Stone Laying Ceremony

A significant milestone in the growth of the Institute was achieved during the year 1998-99. Foundation stone laying ceremony of the institute was held on 14th May 1998 at 12.30 p.m. at IIPM project site in Bangalore University campus.

The then Hon'ble Minister of Commerce, Mr Ramakrishna Hegde, laid the foundation stone of the institute. The then Hon'ble Chief Minister of Karnataka, Mr J.H. Patel was the chief guest of this function and laid the foundation stone for the academic complex. The Commerce secretary, Mr P.P.Prabhu, laid the foundation stone for the hostel complex. An additional secretary, Mrs. Rathi Vinay Jha, and several distinguished invitees from the plantation sector, also graced the function.

Micro Propagation of Tea: Achievements and Future Prospects

The production and the productivity of our tea lands are on the decline because most area under tea is cultivated with seedling tea obtained from plants that are 75 years old with low yield potential. A significant result of this old plantation is a low plant population density and hence a poor productivity potential. Replanting or consolidating these areas by infilling with high yielding quality clones help in mitigating this problem to a large extent. But slow progress of the replanting and infilling programmes, apart from the high investment involved, is attributed to the non-availability of suitable clonal materials in sufficient amounts. The traditional method of vegetative propagation by single node cuttings, though very useful, is slow and has not been able to meet the ever-increasing demand for clonal plants. Industry's experience in Sri Lanka is that using this system the industry is unable to meet the demand for plants for long established clones produced in recent years. In the case of any new clones that may be introduced, it may take well over 10 years before mother bushes are established on a scale large enough to supply the needs of the industry. Developing a viable micro propagation system for tea helps to alleviate this problem, for it. A large number of plants of existing clones of desirble traits within a short period of time are produced. Thus any new clone produced by selection or breeding is multiplied quickly for large-scale planting. This helps in enhancing tea production by increasing the productivity of tea lands, with uniform product of high quality, thereby making the industry more viable. This technique of rapid large-scale clonal propagation has been adopted for a wide range of plants. Production on a commercial scale was first accomplished with orchids and soon afterwards with an ever-increasing number of ornamental foliage plants and flowering plants. Over the years this technique has been developed for a number of fruit and woody ornamentals, trees and some speciality crops and commercial production of many of these crops are well underway. However, in the genus Camellia, the propagation by tissue culture techniques has had only a limited success and still less in the case of tea. Camellia(Sinosis [CL). O. Kuntze] saneness, the queen of Camellias.

WUC .T (1976) and WUC .T Hear et al. (1981) were able to obtain a limited number of plants from cotyledon callus. Koto, M. (1982, 1985, 1986) obtained embroys and also regenerated plants from slices of cotyledons from Camellia sinosis and C. japonica and was also successful in obtaining few plantlets from stem callus. The possibility of regeneration of shoots and growth of buds and callus nodal, from nodal explants have been reported by Phukan and Mitra (1984). Growth of buds and callus formation on explanted organs of tea was reported by Sarwar (1985). Nakamure (1988) produced rooted plants from shoot tips and maxillary buds and induced adventitious embryos on cotyledon callus, but could not obtain proliferation of the shoots grown in culture. Work carried out at the tea research institute of Sr Lanka showed that tea can be propagated successfully using tissue culture techniques. Arulpragasam and Latiff (1986) developed a method for the proliferation of shoot tips in culture. Seniviratne et al. (1988) successfully rooted plants to field conditions. Arulpragasam etc. (1988) developed a system for successfully regenerating plants from cotyledon callus cultures, which were also acclimatised to field condition. The progess achieved so far in the sucessful regeneatrion of plants form existing moistens, de novo formation of organ primordial from callus utilising the stops of ex-plant establishment, propagate multiplication, plant regeneration, acclimatisation and planting out in field plot was reviewed by Arulpragasam (1988).

Current Research

The present work relates to the successful development of an efficient and reproducible method for the commercial production of tea clones using tissue culture techniques. The term "clone" is used here in its classical meaning to denote a group of uniform individuals that have originated from a single plant and have been reproduced only vegetatively, in contrast to its recent usage to denote a plant developed from as single cell.

Ex-plant : Soft-wooded nodal segments with maxillary buds, collected from mother bushes of clones TRI 2025 and TRI 3017, pruned 4 months previously, were used as ex-plants. Ascorbic acid was used as a vitamin as well as an anti-oxidant. The cultures were incubated in a growth room at 22-24°C under a light intensity of 2000 Lux from fluorescent lamps with a 16h photoperiod. After about four weeks in culture the maxillary bud of the nodal ex-plants began to grow out and by the eighth week produced about 2-3 maxillary buds.

Prevention of Contamination and Browning : The nodal segments, 1.5-2.0 cm in length, were dipped in 95 per cent ethanol for 45 second, trimmed to 1.0-1.5 cm length and swirled in 2.0 per cent mercuric chloride for 20 minutes followed by three rinds in sterile distilled water. Before sterilization, the ex-plants were kept immersed in a 1.5 per cent solution of polyvinyl pyrolidone for 30 minutes. This procedure prevented browning and reduced contamination to a great extent.

Establishment : The sterilized nodal segments were ex-planted in a solid medium consisting of MS inorganic salts at half strength and the organics. The details are given in the following table:

Proliferation : At this stage the ex-plants were transferred to a solid proliferation medium which had the same composition as the establishment medium except that the inorganic salts were used in

Table 11.1: Composition of Media used for Establishments of Nodal Ex-plants

Component	Concentration (mg 1.1)
Major elements	1/2 Ms*
Minor elements	1/2MS*
Myo-inositol	100
Thiamine- HCl	0.4
Ascorbic acid	2.0
IBA	0.1
BAP	2.0
Sucrose	30,000
Agar	8,000

* Murashisge and Skoog (1962) mineral salts
Source-Assam Revised and Tea news, Angust, 1995

full strength and the concentration of BAP was increased to 2.5 mgl and the concentration of IBA reduced to 0.01 mgl. The increased BAP concentration enhanced shoot growth and proliferation while the tendency to form callus at the cut end was reduced appreciably at the lower auxin concentration. The maxillary buds produced on the nodal ex-plants developed into shoots 10-15 mm in length within six weeks in the proliferation medium. These were dissected out and transferred to fresh proliferation media. Larger leaves were trimmed during the transfers. This process of dissecting out and transferring was carried out every six weeks. By repeating this procedure every six weeks it was possible to obtain about 610 plantlets within a period of one year from a single nodal ex-plant. This technique was found to be very efficient, reliable and reproducible. Using this process we were able to obtain about 32,000 plantlets within a period of one year, starting with 50 nodal ex-plants. The plantlets thus obtained in culture can be rooted in vitro (Seniviratne et al, 1988) or in soil directly and gradually acclimatised to green house and field conditions. Experiments on rooting of plantlets on a large scale are in progress and the results so far are promising.

Discussion

Once the protocol for the large scale rooting of plantlets produced in culture is perfected it would be only a matter of time for this procedure to be used for the commercial production of tea plants. This would help in meeting the increasing demand for good quality, high yeilding clones for the re-planting and infilling programme of the tea producing countries. This procedure will not only be the final step necessary to multiply the existent vegetative plants of known characteristics, but can be used to rapidly multiply and selected clone for field evaluation. The commercially cultivated seedling tea is extremely heterogenous and consists of hybrids of various combinations. It is unfortunate that this vast wealth of genetic material is being lost gradually due to re-planting with a few selected clones. Germplasm preservation is therefore one of our urgent needs. Institute has already established an in vitro germplasm bank at Talawakelle. However, this requires a large land which could otherwise be used profitably. In vitro cultures of individual genotypes would occupy only a very small space, and hence micro-propagation techniques could be used for maintaining a large collection of the desired genotypes. This technique would also help in facilitate exchange of genetic material between countries. Embryo culture has been successfully accomplished at the TRI (Arulpragasam, 1998). This method could be used to ensure the survival of many "difficult" crosses in our breeding programme with clones of known characteristics.

Recombinant Variety

Another culture, which has not been successfully carried out in tea, is a proven method for stabilizing the recombinant variety and the useful traits of the F_1 hybrid plants. Plants developed by this method can be rapidly multiplied by tissue culture techniques.

Production of Disease, Drught and Other Stress Tolerant Plants

One of the most exciting prospects is the production of disease, drought and other stress tolerant plants. A method for the culture of callus derived from cotyledons and the regeneration of plants from these callus cultures has been worked out (Arulpragasam, 1998).

Cotyledon callus culture lends itself to long-term culture, a feature, which could be used in the selection for strees and disease tolerance. Further, some clonal variants produced in callus culture could be used for the production of new lines.

Propagation of Clones from Commercial Production

The rapid propagation of elite tea clones is now feasible using tissue culture techniques and this can be used for the commercial production of millions of plants annually for re-planting low-yielding seedling tea. This would give better prospects for this export-oriented commodity in countries like Sri Lanka, which depend on tea as a major foreign exchange earner. Mass clonal propagation of tea could have a positive impact on the economy of countries with large tea growing areas.

For crop improvement in the agricultural sector, micro-propagation is the final tool necessary to rapidly multiply any new variety or clone whether it is produced by the conventional methods of selection or by breeding or by the more sophisticated methods of genetic engineering, protoplast fusion or gene transfer.

Micro-propagation by Somatic Embryo-genesis

When compared to micro-propagation by maxillary enhancement, somatic embryo-genesis can yield a larger number of plantlets at a time. But it is necessary to assess the field performance of somatic plants for their uniformity and possible variation. This could be done easily in the case of tea, as the final product is the vegetative part, unlike other where yield is related to fruiting and evaluation may require a number of years. If the frequency of variation is low enough and acceptable, then propagation by somatic embryo-genesis leads to lower operating costs. The potential of this method should, therefore, be investigated.

Application of Tissue Culture Techniques in different levels of conflexity

The value of tissue culture techniques is that they can be applied at different levels of complexity. Each country should design its programme in a way so as to take maximum advantage of the technology according to its needs and specific situation. Otherwise there is a danger of the developing countries becoming more technologically dependent on technologically advanced countries. Co- operation at the sub-regional, regional and international level of the tea producing countries will help to stimulate research, to train experts, to disseminate specialised knowledge and promote contracts between them.

Conclusion

There is an urgent need in tea producing countries to increase the availability of good quality and high yielding clones. This could be achieved by developing a viable micro propagation system for these elite clones. But, so far, the micro propagation of tea has had only a limited amount of success. The successful development of an efficient and reproducible method for the commercial production of tea clones using tissue culture techniques is of paramount importance today. Repeated proliferation of maxillary buds in vitro was obtained by auxiliary enhancement, by which process it is possible to obtain 30,000-35,000 plantlets within a period of one year, starting with 50 nodal explants. Prospects of extending this technique to other exiting fields such as germplasm preservation, development of disease and stress tolerant plants and production of new lines are emerging.

Selection criteria for Drought Tolerance in Tea

Abstract : Various physiological and bio-chemical criteria were evaluated for drought tolerance in tea under conditions of soil moisture stress. Water potential, stomata diffusion resistance, relative turgidity, water saturation deficit, transpiration rate and pro-line and epicuticular wax contents, were found to be correlated, with drought tolerance. Hence these parameters may be used as selection criteria for drought tolerance in tea selection and breeding programmes.

Introduction : Screening cultivars that withstand severe soil moisture deficits is an important facet in the overall crop improvement programme. The severity of the effect of water stress depends mainly on the plant type, and drought tolerance is the ability of a plant to perform satisfactorily under such conditions. Plants circumvent the ill effects of drought through a number of physiological and biochemical mechanisms. These mechanisms are basically responsible for maintaining relatively higher plant water status under conditions of severe soil moisture deficits. Tocklai released cultivars have been classified into categories (tolerant and susceptible) based on their degree of drought tolerance (Berea and Bezbaruah, 1970). Hence an attempt was made to correlate some of the physiological and biochemical parameters with the degree of tolerance.

Materials and Methods : Water potential was measured with a pressure chamber instrument Stomata diffusion resistance and rate of transpiration were measured with L1-16000 steady state pro-meter. Relative turgidity (RT) was determined after Weatherly (1950) and water saturation deficit (WSD) was estimated from its simple relationship with RT (Barrs. 1968).

Free pro-line and epicuticular wax contents in leaf samples were estimated following the standard methods of Bates et.al (1973) and Silva Fernandez et al (1964) respectively.

Clones TV1, TV14, TV16, TV18 and TV20 as drought tolerant and TV2, TV3, TV4, TV5, TV6, TV13, & TV15 as drought susceptible were used.

All the experiments were conducted under identical conditions of soil moisture deficits. Under laboratory conditions, drought was imposed by withholding irrigation till most of the plants exhibited wilting symptoms in the leaves.

Results and Discussion on Water Potential and Leaf Water Content

Water potential was measured in the 3rd leaf from top of the apical bud. It was observed that drought tolerant clones consistently exhibited higher water potential than susceptible ones. Water potential reflects the build-up of plant water status, which could be observed in the difference of leaf water content. Details are out lined below:

Stomata Diffusion Resistance and Transpiration rate : It is known that soil moisture stress increases stomata diffusion resistance and simultaneously decreases transpiration rate. However, the increase and decrease in stomata diffusion resistance and

Table 11.2: Effects of Soil Moisture Deficits On Water Potential and Leaf Water Content in Two Categories of Clones.

Category	Clones	Water Potential (bars)	Leaf water content (mg/cm)
Drought	TV1	16.27	18.40
Tolerant	TV16	17.00	20.33
	TV17	16.80	20.46
	TV18	17.27	
Mean	16.84	19.73	
Drought	TV2	19.27	17.64
Susceptible	TV3	20.73	16.75
	TV4	20.20	17.45
	TV6	19.27	
Mean	19.87	17.28	

Source : The Assam Review and Tea News, August 1995

transpiration rate respectively was more in drought tolerant than in susceptible clones (Table 11.4). These two interrelated physiological processes help in building up of plant water status. The difference in value of these parameters between the two categories is a contributing factor for drought tolerance.

Relative Turgidity and Water Saturation Deficit : Plant water status can also be reflected through measurement of relative turgidity and water saturation deficit. In this study, tolerant clones exhibited higher relative turgidity and lower water saturation deficit than susceptible ones (Table 11.4). TV1 exhibited highest relative turgidity and the lowest water saturation deficityl, whereas, the reverse was the case in TV3.

Higher quantity of pro-line and epicuticular wax was found in the leaves of tolerant clones than suscepitble ones (Table 11.5).

Other than pro-line and leaf wax content, the parameters mentioned above are in some way or the other connected with the plant water status. Hence among them, a good trend of relationship was

Table 11.3 Effect of Soil Moisture Stress on Stomata Diffusion Resistance (RS) and Transpiration Rate (TR) in Two Categories of Clones.

Category	Clones	RS (Sec cm)	TR (ug cm.S)
Drought	TV1	24.43	1.68
Tolerant	TV17	21.83	1.85
	TV18	19.88	2.30
	TV20	24.10	1.92
Mean		22.56	1.94
Drought	TV2	19.11	3.70
Susceptible	TV3	18.63	2.81
	TV5	17.08	2.80
	TV15	17.08	2.58
Mean		17.98	2.97

Source - The Assam Review and Tea News, August 1995.

Table 11.4 Effect of Soil Moisture Stress on Relative Turgidity (RT) and Water Saturation Deficit (WSD) in Two Categories of Clones.

Category	Clones	RT (per cent)	WSD (per cent)
Drought	TV1	72.29	27.71
Tolerant	TV17	68.86	31.14
	TV18	68.79	31.21
	TV20	71.60	28.40
Mean		70.38	29.62
Drought	TV3	57.54	42.46
Susceptible	TV4	67.67	32.33
	TV13	59.71	40.29
	TV15	65.55	34.45
Mean		62.62	37.38

Source- TRA's Field Trial, The Assam Review & Tea News, November 1994

observed. Increased stomata diffusion resistance exhibited by drought tolerant clones infers that the stomata respond more quickly to drought. This reduced the transpiration rate and thereby helped in building up of plant water status. This enhanced plant water status could be reflected through higher water potential, leaf water content, relative turgidity and lower water saturation deficit.

Deposition of epicuticular wax may be correlated with reduction in transpiration rate and increase in stomata resistance. The role of pro-line in drought tolerance may be in the manipulation of osmotic adjustment.

Table 11.5 Effect of Soil Moisture Deficits on Pro-line and Wax Content in Leaves.

Category	Clones	Pro-line (ug/g)	Wax (ug/cm)
Drought	TV1	316.66	119.78
Tolerant	TV17	320.83	132.70
Mean		318.75	126.24
Drought	TV3	268.83	95.20
Susceptible	TV13	296.67	105.87
Mean		282.75	100.54

Source - The Assam Review & Tea News, November 1994

Conclusion

Drought tolerance in tea could be assessed through some physiological and bio-chemical parameters under moisture stress conditions.

- It could be correlated with high water potential, stomata diffusion resistance, relative turgidity, pro-line and cuticular wax content and lower transportation rate and water saturation deficit in tea.
- The plant water relationship parameters exhibited quicker and better response to soil moisture deficits than pro-line and cuticular wax.
- These parameters may be used as selection criteria for drought tolerance in selection and breeding programmes of tea.

Role of Tea Research Institute of United Planters' Association of Southern India (UPASI)

The Tea Research Institute has six divisions namely Botany, Plant Physiology, Soil Chemistry, Entomology, Plant Pathology and Tea Technology which are involved in tea research. The research findings are disseminated to planting districts through six advising centres. In the Annamalis the advisory service is redered by Research Institute, thus catering to the needs of entire tea industry in South India. The research highlights and major activities are enumerated below:

- Mechanisation of crop harvesting is one of the priority areas of research. It was found that plucking average could be substantially increased by the use of Kawasaki motorised harvester. The annual plucking average of the single man operated machine was 182 m, kg, whereas for two-men operated machine, it was 295 kgs, integrated with hand plucking. It was found that Folar 52.5 FW post emergent herbicide at the rate of 2.100 kgs a/ha gave control over weeds for a longer duration. In another study 'Triclopyr' at the rate of 1.00 litre along with Glphosate formulation at 1.75 litres in 450 litres of water/ha gave control over weeds occurring in tea fields.
- The changing pattern of carbohydrate reserves was studied in relation to pruning. Carbohydrate levels in the roots sharply declined following pruning up to 45 days and then slowly began to increase. The reduction in carbohydrate resource in the roots from the time of pruning to two leaf stage was about 5 per cent.
- A protocol for the production of high frequency somatic embryos using immature cotyledons of UPASI-9, UPASI-10 and CR-6017 is being standardised. Plantlets were derived from cotyledonary explants of UPASI-9, and UPASI-10 through somatic embryos and after hardening these were planted in Vandiperiyar and Valparai to assess their field performance. Protoplast isolation from embryogenic calli from immature cotyledons of TRI-2024 was tried. The protocol for viable protoplast isolation was standardised and further work in this line is in progress.
- The work on role of enzymes in tea processing was continued. Addition of biopectinase in orthodox manufacturing led to an

improvement in TF, TR and TLC. In another study, the addition of bioprotease resulted in the development of rosy aroma and aromatic compounds in general were found higher. Polyphenol oxidase (PPO) was extracted from Agaricus bisporus and purified and added during CTC manufacturing. It was found that TF, BI, CI and certain VFC group II compounds increased due to this treatment.

- Foliar application of magnesium sulphate at the rate of 15 kg/ha combined with 10 kg zinc sulphate along with 500 ppm of manganese and 100 ppm of boron significantly increased the yield over control. Soil application of 60 kg S, applied as sulphate of ammonia, was found at par with that of Green Plus (organic manure) and iron pyrite. In Nilgiris, the highest yield in Assam seedling was obtained at 350 kg N/ha.
- The experiment on drip irrigation in Nilgiris in UPASI-9 indicated that the effect of 2 mm water applied once in three days was comparable to that of 2 mm water applied daily and they were found significantly superior to 4 mm and 6 mm water applied at three days' interval and control.
- The work on integrated pest management continued. In the laboratory, cent per cent mortality of adult shot hole borer beetles was achieved within 5 to 7 days when *Beauveria bassiana* suspensions were applied at 10^7 and 10^8 spores/ml. The research on sex pheromones of *Helopelitis theivora* indicated the presence of 21 volatile compounds released by unmated females.
- A combination of chlorpyrifos and cypermethrin gave satisfactory control of tea mosquito bug and similarly, for the mid cycle control of shot hole borer a combination of profenofos and cypermethrin was found useful. A new acaricide fenpropathrin was found effective against red spider mites, while application of fenpyroimate gave good control over purple mites.
- The work on pesticide residues was continued. Studies on deltamethrin showed that its residue levels in black tea on 7th day ranged between 0.03 and 0.18 when applied @ 180 ml/ha and varied between 0.14 and 0.19 ppm when applied @ 200 ml/ha during wet season, respectively. In the case of dicofol the

level of residues was 1.18 and 6.69 ppm on 14th day when it was applied @ 1000 ml/ha in dry and wet season, respectively. During 1999, a pesticide residue survey of Nilgiris teas was conducted and residues of endosulfan, quinalphos and chlorpyrifos were not detected while 90 per cent of the samples had residues of ethion and dicofol, but all were below the MRL prescribed by European Union (EU).

- For blister blight control, a new triazole, Tebuconzaole (Folicur 250 EW) was found effective at the rate of 200 ml/ha applied at 7 day's interval. Research on biofertilisers was continued. Seven isolates of Azospirillum and three isolates of phosphobacteria were isolated from the soils of Annamalais. The population level of phosphobacteria was higher in treatments where the biopreparation was given alone or in combination with lower dosage of rock phosphate.
- The optimum fermentation time and theaflavin level were found influenced by humdification and supply of fresh air in drum type fermenters. Work was carried out for developing a preparation of liquid tea concentrate and chilled tea beverage with natural tea flavour. A carbonated tea beverage with artificial flavour has also been attempted and standardization of the methodology is in progress.
- The advisory officers made more than 1130 visits to estates and conducted more than 60 training programmes for the field staff and executives of member estates. Area Scientific Conferences were organized in Meppadi, Gudalur, Valparai, Coonoor, Munnar, Chikmagalur and Vandiperiyar. Training programmes on Hazard Analysis and Critical Control Programme (HACCP) were organised for the executives of member estates of Valparai, Coonoor and Vandiperiyar with the help of Tea Board and the Bureau of Indian Standards.
- The eighth Joint Area Scientific Symposium (JASS VIII) was jointly conducted by the Central Travancore Planters' Association and UPASI Scientific Department at Vandiperiyar on 23rd and 24th April 1999. The traveling symposium included field visits and presentation of papers on topics, such as mechanisation of pruning, new planting, soil and water conservation, weed

control, ecology and control of thrips, tea mosqutio bug, shot hole borer, shear harvesting, shredding of tea prunings, soil of Central Traveancore and replanting.

The UPASI-106th Annual Conference

The UPASI in its 106th annual conference held on Coonoon on 21st September 1999 suggested a separate set-up to study the implication of WTO on plantation sector in order to work out a strategy to meet the challange. It called for diversification of the export markets for South Indian tea and said that it was with this objective that an international tea convention was organised by UPASI in Cochin in September 1999. It also called for rationalisation of agricultural income taxation rate structure and incentives and facilities, including exemption of export profits. Another issue touched upon by it was the re-orientation of the land policies of the State Government to make them conducive to the expansion of plantations. The conference also suggested extending the definition of plantations to crops like cashew, peper, nutmeg, cloves, cinnamon and even oil palm and exempting these crops from land ceiling. Mr. Jacob Thomas reiterated the plantation industry's commitment to the welfare of the workers and their families in the areas of housing, health care, education, family welfare, child care and community development. Mr D.P. Bagchi, the then Principal Advisor (Agriculture), planning commissioner and secretary to the Government of India highlighted the importance and economic significance of the plantations, especially in South India. He stated that in order to survive in the coming years, there cannot be other way than being competitive and world class. He said that reform process was irreversible and the state Governments had also to fall in line sooner or later. He agreed that producers-exporters of plantation commodities should also get the benefit of tax exemption from export profits. A recommendation was made by Planning Commission to the Commerce Ministry to consider holding a national level meeting to go into the taxation issues relating to the plantation sector, especially agricultural income tax.

ICAR projects : UPASI Krishi Vigyan Kendra (KVK).

Need based production and practical oriented training programme and rural research and development activities are organised by UPASI Krishi Vigyan Kendra under the sponsorship of Indian Council of Agricultural Research (ICAR) and Tea Board.

Training : Eighty-two On Campus and eighty-seven Off Campus training programmes on various subjects like tea cultivation, coffee cultivation, horticulture, agricultural engineering, home science, woolen knitting and bee keeping have been organised for the benefit of Nilgiris farming community, rural youth, extension functionaries and estate personnel. Over 4837 beneficiaries were trained during the year, bringing the total number to 65,689 since inception.

Field Days/Seminars : The following seminars/workshops were conducted :

- A workshop on cultivation and marketing of medicinal aromatic and culinary herbs was conducted on 27-28 April, 1999. About 250 farmers participated in the programme.
- A workshop on spices cultivation was conducted on 12 August, 1999 and 60 farmers were benefited.
- A workshop on mechanisation in tea was organised at Kotagiri on 2 August, 1999 and at Gudalur on 22 November' 1999. About 255 farmers were benefited.
- Entrepreneur Development programme on sources of finance and marketing was organised for ex-trainees on 23 and 24 August, 1999 and 54 ex-trainees participated in the programme.
- A workshop on the use of Computer in tea factories was held on 15th November' 1999 and 22 personnel from various (INDCO) and Boughtleaf factories in Nilgiris participated.
- In collaboration with District Industries Centre (DIC) Udhagamandalam a farmer meet was organised at UPASI-KVK on 14 December' 1999 and 175 persons attended the Programme.
- Women in Agriculture Day was celebrated at UPASI-KVK on 31 December' 1999. About one hundred women participated.
- A Seminar on Recent Development in Tea Manufacture was organised on 31 January, 2000. About 141 personnel fromvarious Indco and Boughtleaf factories participated.

- A district level farmer meet was organised on 7 March 2000. 264 farmers attended this programme.

Publications : The following publications were broughtout:

1. Factory Manual
2. Mechanisation in Tea
3. Higher level pruning and higher yield
4. Foliar application of nutrients to increase the productivity in tea
5. Nutritional management for high productivity in tea
6. Four issues of KVK News, a technical institutional newsletter of UPASI-KVK (quarterly)

Frontline Demonstration

Tea : Foliar application of nutrient on tea has been taken for frontline demonstration in Thummanatty village. The total area selected for demonstration is 10 acres. Land is owned by growers, the farmers holding size ranged between 30 per cent and 100 per cent Manganese, Boric, Magnesium and Planofix spray was given twice during the month of September and October 1999. Diammonium Phosphate spray was carried out during the month of November. Urea, Muriate of Potash and Green miracle spray was given thrice from January to March 1999 at an interval of one month. The yield recorded in the control plot is 5000 kgs of green leaf per annum. The yield recorded in demonstration plot is 7000 kgs of green leaf per annum. The increase is 2000 kg of green leaf/per annum.

Vegetables : UPASI-KVK in collaboration with Central Potato Research Station, ICAR Muthorai, Ooty, Horticulture Research Station, Ooty, took up projects of potato, cauliflower and fresh Bean.

On-farm testing

Role of Raw Material on Tea Quality : is defined below :-

Raw material with 50 per cent coarse leaf

Raw material with 25 per cent coarse leaf

Raw material with 15 per cent coarse leaf

The experiment shows that raw material with 50 per cent coarse leaf produced very poor quality, low bulk density and higher electrical power consumption. Raw material with 25 per cent coarse leaf treatment is producing low quality, low bulk density and higher power consumption. Raw material with 15 per cent coarse leaf produce good quality with high bulk density and less power consumption.

Tea Processing Unit - Imparting Practical Training

Imparting practical training on tea manufacturing to the Boughtleaf and Indco personnel is the major objective of the unit. The following areas were given importance in the training programme.

- Importance on quality raw material.
- Temperature maintenance at different stages of tea manufacturing.
- R.C. mixing.
- Factory house keeping.
- Machinery maintenance.

During the year, five programmes were conducted for Indco, Boughtleaf factories, unemployed youths, estate executive/staff. In all 70 participants attended the programmes. During 1999-2000, the factory had produced 25621 kg made tea and the average price realisation was Rs 64.68 per kg. The highest sale price achieved during the year was Rs 76.24 per Kg. of tea.

Instructional Farm : The Instructional Farm is being used for on-farm research, training-cum-demonstration activities and production and supply of planting materials for small growers of Nilgiris. Over 1.60 lakh of high yielding clonal plants, 3,000 Silver Oak shade tree samples were raised and supplied to small growers. During the current financial year (1999-2000) 1,38,631 kg of green leaf has been harvested. The average yield per hectare is 3,535kg of made tea (or) 13,863 kg of green leaf per ha.

Tea Board Small Growers Development Projects

Under the Tea Board project, training for small tea growers, demonstration plots and crop diversification scheme were continued for the development of small tea growers.

Training for Small Tea Growers : As many as 38 On-campus and 44 Off-campus training programmes were conducted during the year for the benefit of 2,554 Small tea growers and practising farmers. Special programmes on quality plucking, foliar application of nutrients and fertiliser management were also conducted at various villages in Nilgiris on regular basis. The training programmes on rejuvenation pruning, infilling and replanting/new planting were organised for the benefit of the growers who have applied for Tea Board subsidy.

Demonstration Plots : Frequent visits were undertaken to Demonstration Plots laid out in different villages and demonstrations on various cultural operations like Pruning, Plucking, Manuring, Foliar application of nutrients, Shade regulation and Plant protection measures such as Pest, Disease and Weed control were carried out. Over 48 demonstrations were organised during the period under report [1999-2000] and 473 small farmers participated in the demonstrations.

Crop Diversification Scheme: Under the Crop Diversification Scheme, 3,15,788 clonal tea plants and 7,107 Silver Oak seedlings were supplied to the Small tea growers and SC/ST farmers. Necessary advice on soil conservation, lining, contour planting and post planting care, were given. Over one hundred visits were made to the project villages during the period under report for implementation of the programme.

Field Advisory Visits : The scientists of the Kendra undertook totally 270 field advisory visits to the small tea growers and suitable advice on the various agricultural practices and remedial measures. A detailed technical report was sent to the individual tea farmers subsequent to the field visit.

Other Activities

Certificate Course on Tea Husbandry and Tea Technology : A three month intensive programme on tea husbandry and tea technology was conducted 1st March 2000, and 16 trainees had undergone this programme. An extension training in the theory and practice on crop production, plant protection, post-harvest technology and middle-level management aspects connected with tea plantations had been imparted during this programme. Use of computer for inventory management and certain field practice management was also incorporated in the course syllabi to make the course more meaningful and practical oriented.

Project on Integrated Watershed Management : UPASI-KVK took up an integrated participatory watershed management project in the Thuneri watershed in Nilgiris district under the Hill Area Development Programme, which consists of three micro watershed namely Thummanatty, Kenthorai and Kothumudi. The integration of all line-departments and the participation of the village communities in the planning, resource mobilisation, implementation, monitoring and evaluation is the main focus of this project. Village meetings were conducted in each of the villages within watershed area in order to make people aware of the proposed watershed project. The [Participatory Rural Approach] PRA was conducted in 11 villages along with the line departments. The data were analysed with the villages and came out with a detailed watershed management plan.

Women Cell activities : The Kendra has formed nine self help groups for women in adopted villages. The women are regularly trained on plantation crops, horticulture and home science aspects. They are motivated to save monthly and use the amount saved through micro credit system among the members. The groups are in operation for six months and they could save over Rs. 90,000 which is utilised for meeting immediate needs of the members. Necessary steps are being taken to link the groups with banks in order to avail the credit facilities from banks under NABARD Finance scheme for self help group for women.

Two workshops on the entrepreneur development were organised for women involving the resource persons from District Rural Development Agency (DRDA), District Industries Centre (DIC), Tamil Nadu Housing Development Corporation (TAHDCO), Tamil Nadu Corporation for the Development of Women and Khadi and Village Industries on 23rd and 24th August and 14 December 1999, in which 64 women trainees participated.

Thummanatty Experiment to Develop Strategies for Improving Quality and Better Price Realisation

The Thummanatty members at the Farm Science Club, which is an agricultural forum, took initiative in conducting the experiment. The experiment was carried out between 9th and 15th November 1999. The green leaf harvested at Thummanatty village were brought to the UPASI-Demonstration Mini Tea Factory and processed. The farmers adopted the green leaf standard as recommended by the UPASI.

The graded tea was sent to M/s. Contemporary Target Co. Ltd., Coonoor for marketing through Coonoor tea auction. The Thummanatty tea was catalogued as "UPASI-Thummanatty clonal tea" and sold in sale No. 47. The Thummanatty clonal tea fetched the highest price among the Boughtleaf and Indco tea factories. The leaf grade sold at the maximum price of Rs. 74 per kg. and dust grade sold at the maximum price of Rs. 70 per kg. Significantly, the price difference was Rs. 15 when compared to the medium quality factories which fetched an average price of Rs. 55. As per the Paramount Tea Marketing News, it is gratifying to note that the UPASI-Thummanatty clonal tea of small sector fetched the top price next to Parajulie, Swarnajulie, and Mayura teas. Based on the average price realisation the green leaf price per kg. is fixed at Rs. 13.40 when the average green leaf price in the small growers sector in that region was Rs 9.00. Further experiments are being made in the different regions of the district in order to create an awareness among the small grows on the quality upgradation.

The National Tea Research Foundation (NTRF) Projects on "Pacha Taints, Role of Enzymes in Tea Processing and Development of a Protocol for efficient Somacional Variation" are being continued while projects on Pesticides Residue in Tea, Soil Test crop response on rationalisation of nitrogen and potassium manuring and Forecasting of Blister blight have been concluded. The VIII Plan projects on Strengthening of laboratory Analytical Facilities and Maximisation of Tea Productivity and Miniature Manufacturing Unit" were continued under IX Plan Projects on "Physiological and Biochemical Basis of Clonal Selection, Collection and Evalnation of Germ Plasm, studies on improving quality of South Indian Black Tea and exploration of bio-fertilision in tea for increased productivity and soil health are being continued, under the financial assistance of Tea Board, a new birnding for Quality Control Laboratory and Advisory Centre was constructed at Coonoor and it was inaugurated by Mr. S.S. Ahuja, the then chairman of Tea Board.

Role of Tea Board in Conducting Tea Research

Providing support to scientific research on tea and allied areas are the major functions of the Tea Board as defined in the Tea Act. With the change the requirement in the recent years particulrly in production and poroauctivity and quality, efforts were concentrated towards higher production and also quality through scientific research. The thrust areas have thus been identified and new research programmes have been started in Ninth Plan. The activities of tea research are the covered in a network from apex body i.e. Tea Board with its research station at Darjeeling Tea Research Centre (DTRC), Tea Research Association in the North East, UPASI-TRI in South India and various institutes in different corners of the country. There was shift in oinentation and development of new programmes of research in different fields as conducted by various institutes to avoid duplication of fundamental research. In fact the information of one institute was shared to launch advance programme in other institutes in the same field. Tea Board had overseen all such programmes of research from its apex committees and participated in the scientific advisory committee meetings of the premiem Tea Research Institutes. Already there was coordinated effort to interact in different areas in the meetings of NTRF where project details were scrutinised at regular intervals and institutes like TRA, UPASI and eminent scientists in the fields participated in such useful proceedings. Tea Boared accordingly suggested new scheme to give financial support for the benefit of the tea industry.

The Quality Conciseness

The quality consciousness has gained momentum, both nationally and internationally. Development of standards and refining methods of testing were constantly undertaken at various forums. Upgradation of quality of tea, mainly in South India, was a major effort of the board by launching special research schemes to look afresh into the gamut of various determining factors. Financial support was accordingly given in this area. At the international level, the requirement of quality had undergone change and accordingly the board had to document various requirements on quality under the World Trade Organisation (WTO) regime.Technical committees under the codex were preparing documents on technical aspects and the board had to really participate and support various activities of committees to harmonise standards at par with international requirements. The board had to change the areas of financial support like quality consciousness, standards, awareness programme on the international developments, finding new areas of production innovation and so on.

Abstract of Research Programmes

Grant in Aid

Major financial support towards grant-in-aid was given to Tea Research Associantion and UPASI-TRI for their ongoing research activities. The financial requirements of both the institutes have increased in the recent years since the equipments, chemicals and also manpower have started costing too high to get financial support from their internal resources. The board considered the requirement and reviewed the position. It is expected that the effect of new funding pattern on account of grant-in-aid to TRA will be revised soon along with new financial support to TRA.

Darjeeling Tea Research Centre (DTRC)

Although much could not be done at this centre due to non-creation of scientific posts, the Government has taken up the matter positively, hinting at engagement of six number of grade-A scientists on contractual basis. If this is materialised, the scientists will be recruited in different specialised fields who can undertake experiments for the benefit of the Darjeeling tea gardens. The areas like flavour chemistry on Darjeeling tea, plant protection aspects, physiological and agronomical requirements, developing high yielding clonal materials for Darjeeling hills will receive a boost. The ongoing activities of the research centre were going on as usual.

Sponsored Programmes

Tea Board is looking after various sponsored programmes of research on which specific grants were sanctioned. There were a number of such activities which immensely benfited the tea industry. Such schemes were always specialised in nature and were not covered by various research institutes through their ongoing programmes of research. The board had advanced either cent per cent or given partial grant as support to various host institutes once the programmes were identified and launched by them.

i. Network Programmes on Bio-technology : The Department of Bio-technology, Government of India, has initially launched a DNA finger printing programme with Bose Institute, Kolkata. The board had given partial financial support and also hosted initial works at its DTRC, Kurseong. The Department Bio-technology (DBT), subsequently constituted a high level Task Force to identify areas of concern through which tea industry can be benefited by introducing bio-technological tools. Accordingly, institutes like Coucil for Social and industrial Research (CSIR), Palampur, GB Pant Institute, Almora, Delhi University, ICAR, Bose Institute, Kolkata, TRA, UPASI-TRI had formally collaborated and identified programmes of works at different institutes. The total project cost may be around Rs. 5 crore on which the board is to provide 25 per cent financial support to DBT for the network of bio-technology in tea.

ii. Himachal Pradesh is Revamping its Tea Industry : For this an elaborate programmes have been drawn identifying 6000 hectares of land to cover new plantation. Technological support to the existing, as well as to new areas, is essentially required. Accordingly, the board has recasted the existing scheme of Himachal Pradesh Krishi Viswa Vidyalaya (HPKVV), Palampur on which R&D findings were generated. The programmes were revamped for which the university was working to change the requirement of research.

iii. On the Health Benefit Aspect of Tea: Specific programmes were launched by TRA at the Indian Institute of Chemical Biology (IICB), Jadavpur. The board had given financial support to procure capital items of equipments under the programme along with some recurring cost on chemicals, etc. New areas had been identified for experimentation and demographic studies on the effect of black tea to prevent dental caries, diabetes, anti-tumorous effects, etc. were carried out. Results were in the positive direction.

iv. Mechanisation in Tea: It has gained momentum with the increased shortage of labour in various areas. Himachal Pradesh is acutely suffering from shortage of labour. To find alternatives, mechanisation had been introduced in tea plucking, pruning through innovative research by CSIR Complex, Palampur. The board had given capital support in mechanisation, procuring various mechanical equipments which were suitably modified and commercially developed for the tea industry.

v. Technical man-power : This is essentially required for the development of the tea industry in the North East, particularly in the states of Nagaland, Tripura, Manipur, Arunachal Pradesh and Meghalaya. Various state governments have approached for financial support to train man-power deputed by them at TRA for short term training programmes. The board had given financial support to run these programmes.

vi. Seminars, Conferences and Meetings : A number of seminars, brain storming sessions were organised by the board to develop innovative ideas on product development, quality aspects of tea, flavour chemistry of Darjeeling tea, packaging aspects, environmental requirements and phytosanitary certifications. The board had given financial support to all these activities.

vii. International Organisation for Standardization (ISO) Meetings : Tea Board arranged to host the Tea Sub-Committee meeting of the International Organization for Standardisation in November 1999, in which scientists' delegation from tea producing and importing nations participated. The deliberations for 4 days were successful to review the international standards on quality of tea, packaging of value-added items, residue, environment, etc.

viii. Hazard Analysis on Critical Control Point (HACCP) : Tea Board organised ten 1-day awareness programme-cum-trainings on ISO-9000 and HACCP amongst the tea industry in India. HACCP certification in the free trade environment will promote export of tea as per requirement of World Trade Organisation (WTO). This new package was adopted by the board for the production of tea in India and accordingly, a scheme was also launched for giving financial support to the tea gardens.

Plan Schemes

During the 3rd year of the 9th Plan, eight Research Schemes, four each at UPASI and TRA, were implemented. All these programmes were ongoing activities in various fields like bio-technology, pesticide residue, heavy metals in tea, bio-chemical aspects on quality and in quality upgradation of tea. During 9th Plan, both capital and recurring components were given by the board unlike previous Plan Schemes.

Brief of each of the Schemes under 9th Plan are given below.

i. United Planters' Association of Southern India - Tea Research Institute - UPASI-TRI (4 Schemes)

a. Collection Evaluation, Documentation and Conservation of Tea Germplasm, the Development of Genotype and Cultivars with High Yield and Quality : Although the scheme was launched during 1997-98, real work started in the second year after the capital equipments were procured. All germplasm in tea were collected and catalogued systematically for developing elite genotypes. Chemical characterisation along with finger printing were also progressing satisfactorily. Long term experiments were also laid out on nutrition, shade, and for bio-technological works.

b. Studies on Improving Quality of South Indian Black Tea: Field level quality control laboratories were established under the 9th Plan Project, particularly at the advisory centres so that entire South India was covered, to facilitate works. Procurement of capital items of equipments had been done and testing works were progressing.

c. Physiological and Bio-chemical Basis of Clonal Selection in Tea for Quality, High Yield and Drought Tolerance : Attempt was made to link physiological aspects of tea plant to identify important attributes so that duration of traditional clonal selection programmes could be reduced. This fundamental work, although complicated, may boost in future, tea breeding works.

d. Exploration of Bio-fertilisers in Tea for Increased Productivity and Soil Health : Bio-fertilisers in the acid soil of tea, particularly in the hills, is an important aspect for future. Strains developed by ICAR were experimented in different locations in South India along with local microflora. Capital items were purchased and also the laboratory set-up was ready for further experimentation.

ii. Tea Research Association (TRA) (4 Schemes)

a. Collection, Conservation and Evaluation of Tea Germplasm: This project has started to collect and conserve all tea germplasms and started finger printing works along with allozyme studies. The field level works were undertaken and also chemical works were progressing.

b. Management of Bush Architecture for Increasing the Productivity of Tea : To increase the productivity of tea by modulating suitable bush frame and also the pruning cycle, field level experiments were laid in different tea districts in North East India. Capital items were purchased.

c. Studies of Heavy Metals : Studies in heavy metals in tea project were progressing very well. Procurement of equipment were done and large scale tea samples were collected for analysing various metal contents in tea.

d. Studies on the Metabolism of Polyphenolic Constituents of Black Tea : TRA launched this project at Indian Institute of Chemical Biology, Jadavpur, which is capable of handling such fundamental studies on polyphenolic compounds. The analysis works were progressing on total polyphenols, TF,TR, in line with the objectives.

Technical Support

Technical support to the tea industry from the Board has ever increased in the free trade environment. Self-certification on the product for standard quality is the common requirement under all agreements of WTO. Accordingly, tea importing nations are depending on the trust of the tea exporters and producers in respect of quality of tea and packaging substances. Institutions like ISO, EEC, USEPA/FDA/ Japan Tea Association, German Tea Council were all entrusting importance on the self-certification of the imported product as per their requirement of quality.

The stipulations in all **standards in the developed nations have been upgraded,** based on their self-certification requirements. The tea industry was informed by the board regularly about the requirements of quality in various countries which were not uniformly formulated. In the recent years, the requirement on the quality of tea in Russia and the Netherlands have changed to environmental aspects like metals, myco-toxins. The requirements of packaging has also changed in the European countries. Exporters are now required to specify the content of packaging materials and also to stipulate its end use, printing on the package regarding bio-degradability. Similarly, environmental considerations in the developed nations have come up as a major issue in the recent years. Tea as well as packaging substances are covered under such regulations.

The European countries have adopted **common directives on the phytosanitary aspects,** including packaging waste, pesticide residue. The standards, as formulated by them, were well defined and the requirements were also stringent compared to other quality zones. Germany is having separate stipulation on this aspect; tea exporters were often faced with constraints to satisfy such regulations and the board had to advocate with scientific data, on case-to-case basis.

Pesticide residue stipulations in the EEC were differing from FDA, Russia and Japan Tea Association. The stringent stipulations on various pesticides, particularly in case of Germany, sometimes created embargo. However, if the same product was meant for export to other destinations, where these stipulations were not required, the teas were smoothly exported. These issues were taken up with Indo-EEC Forums for redressal.

Harmonisation of pesticide residue standards globally was an attempt under ISO as well as Codex Residue Committee. Tea Board participated in deliberations at the national level to support harmonisation programme under Codex for adopting common standards on residue. The issue for liberal standards considering tea as a brew was also put forward.

Phytosanitary Certification is a new development as required under EEC guidelines. Countries like Russia, the Netherlands are insisting for such Phytosanitary Certification at the time of importing tea. Since it is not clear on the criteria of such certification, the exporters were guided by Tea Board to get clarifications on the importers' requirements and in some cases, the Central Plant Protection Department came to rescue.

Organic tea is a new dimension to the tea industry. During the year, concerted efforts were made to standardise the national level Accreditation and Certification Programmes. Tea Board participated in several deliberations of the National Committee and drafted regulations along with the guidelines on package and practices of Organic as well as Bio-dynamic teas. These are now ready for notification.

Quality Control and Self-Certification of tea is a major issue. Tea Board launched several schemes in this direction to establish quality control laboratories for the benefit of the tea industry in North-East and South India. The board had also launched HACCP self-certification, quality control programmes. The tea producers as well as the tea packegers had taken the advantage of the scheme by participating in the programmes for acquiring HACCP and ISO 9000 Certification. The board had extended financial support for acquiring such certification.

(ISO) Standards, although voluntary in nature, majority of the tea producing and the tea exporting countries are honouring its stipulations. The board organised ISO Tea Sub-Committee Meeting in India during November 1999 and took advantage to focus India's stand on the quality of tea and packaging sub-stances. Specific issues like iron contamination in tea, identifying substance characteristics in tea, were specifically included in the ISO activities for future. Green tea standards, which were predominantly based on Chinese type and grades, were modified to specifics on Indian green teas in respect of catechins.

The standards of quality of wood panel, jute packaging substances, craft paper were reviewed. Bureau of Indian Standards (BIS) invited views of the board on these specific issues and accordingly these were sorted out. The Prevention of Food Adulteration Act (PFA) also reviewed a number of issues of the Shadow Committees on Residue, CCFIX residue and the board passed on its comments to these international meetings accordingly.

A new issue came up during the year in respect of **genetic manipulation in tea.** Although the requirement, was at its preliminary stage at the international level, some nations like the Netherlands, Canada had started imposing such certification. Tea Board interacted with the Committees of Codex on Genetic Manipulation and also with the concerned countries which were insisting for such certification. Tea Board had started issuing such certification for the sake of export of tea.

Domestic marketing of tea has also faced constraints in view of residue and metallic contamination in tea particularly in the Western sector. Focus was mainly on the lead and iron content in tea. The board had to intervene in a number of cases and fixed guidelines on tea production to control metallic contamination. Also, the board had launched advanced research programmes on these lines. All these issues were also taken up with PFA and with the concerned consumer forums.

The board was also involved in the activities of **Task Force on packaging, electronics in tea** and accordingly put forward the requirements of tea industry to specialised bodies. The industry is now using several electronic gadgets for automation in the factory.

Survey on the environmental issues, packaging substances, metal contents, factory conditions were taken up by the board in specific ways with various concerned laboratories like IIPO, Central Food Laboratories and also quality testing laboratories in the private sector. The requirements of the tea consumer in the domestic front were cared for, in view of taking up of such specialised programmes.

The board was also involved in the committees like Council of Management of Tea Research Association and its various committees, IIP and committees of UPASI. Since the board was giving major funds to these institutions, their activities were constantly looked after and reviewed from time to time. The increased responsibility had been vested on the board in respect of tea research in India for which token grants were also given to support various activities, in addition to major grant-in-aid from the board. The tea industry is also spending massively in the small grower sectors. **Soil Suitability Certificate became a major issue.** A number of soil laboratories all over India were recognised for such soil testing and all such reports were considered before any registration was granted to an organisation as a new Planter of Tea. Technological support to these small growers were also taken up particularly in the North Bengal and in the North East separately. In case of South India, small growers was attached to UPASI for technological feedback. The board was extending financial support to these specific programmes.

National Tea Research Foundation (NTRF)

National Tea Research Foundation (NTRF) is constituent body under the Societies Act and also recognised by the DSIR and Income Tax authorities for the purpose of exemption of income tax. NTRF has completed about 10 projects so far at various host institutes, results of which were given to the tea industry in South and North East India. Ten more research projects are in progress at the moment and more schemes are in the process of adoption and launching. The financial outlay of all these research schemes, so far undertaken by NTRF, had exceeded Rs. 5 crores.

The findings of some of the projects were widely accepted in the tea industry like disease control, new planting material, pesticide residue protocols, manufacturing of tea and so on. NTRF also had taken up new schemes recently on the health benefit aspect of tea. A number of institutes derived financial benefits to launch new research schemes on these aspects particularly to use tea as preventive dose and curative medicine. NTRF also organised various seminars and brain Strorming sessions to identify newer areas of scientific research like project diversification. New fields were opened by NTRF like publication of tea research newsletter periodically and cataloguing of research scientists along with subjects. NTRF has also started to function as apex body of tea research for dissemination of scientific information to tea research scientists in various specialised disciplines. More programmes are underway for taking up as its future programme of work.

The Expenditure statement for the year 1999-2000 under research is given below:-

Table 11.6 : Expenditure statement by NTRF during 1999-2000 under Research

Name of the Scheme	Actual expenditure
A.	
1. Grant aid in Assam Agricultural University, rorhat.	0.90
2. Scheme on improvement of tea culture in the hilly areas of Himachal Pradesh.	3.50
3. Contribution to UPASI scientific department for organising 'Advisory Service and project on chemistry of tea'.	8.00
4. Grant-in-aid to TRA, on account of sharing of expenditure of Tea Research Association, TA/DA to members for participating in the meeting of National Committee on Tea Research and other concerned expenditure.	250.00
5. Darjeeling Tea Research Centre, Kurseong (DTRC)	6.60
6. Short Training course for Non-Traditional /Traditional/Backward areas in North East India.	
7. Workshops/Seminars/Conferences relating to ongoing schemes and other projects and DTRC, Kurseong/Awards	1.35
8. Promotion of mechanisation in tea leaf plucking and other field operations in tea gardens in Kangra, Himachal Pradesh	4.92
9. Project on epidemiological and clinical studies on black tea (IICB).	2.00
Total A	**277.27**
B.	
1. UPASI-TRI collection, evaluation, documentation and conservation of tea germplasm, the development of genotype and cultivars with high yield and quality-UPASI	8.85
2. Studies on improving quality of south India Black Tea-UPASI	11.75

Name of the Scheme	Actual expenditure
3. Physiological and bio-chemical basis of clonal selection in tea for quality, high yield & drought tolerance-UPASI	20.00
4. Exploration of bio-fertilizers in tea for increased productivity and soil health-UPASI.	20.00
5. Revitalisation of tea research in Darjeeling hills, DTRC, Krseong.	
6. Management of bush architecture for increasing the productivity of tea	0.16
7. Studies on heavy metals: Part-1 Heavy metals in Tea, Part-2 Heavy metals in Tea soils	4.56
8. Studies on the metabolism of polyphenoli constituents of black tea	12.28.
9. Indian Institute of packaging	1.00
Total B	**87.27**
Total of A+B	**364.54**

A decade and half of NTRF-1988 to 2003

NTRF registered on 7 June 1985 as an Association started functioning at the premises of the Tea Board in 1989. It is an independent interactive functional body, funded by Indian Tea Industry and National Bank for Agriculture and Rural Development (NABARD). In liaise with the Tea Board India, NTRF Supports innovative research on all aspects of tea on the basis on non-conventional approaches, other than traditional research carried out by two prime tea research institute-TRA, Tockkai for North and TRI-UPAS, has South Indian Tea industries respectively particularly areas covering plant physiology plant protection and pesticide management to meet global standard, quality improvement and Human health aspects of tea.

Creation of Corpus Fund

In the first national conference on Tea Productivity and Development, held in Kolkata in August 22, 1987, the then Hon'ble Minister of Finance and Commerce Government of India, Mr. N.D. Tewari announced that a compos found of 10 crore to be created for the promotion of research in the field of tea production and productivity.

The Ministry of Commerce in their letter declare September 11, 1987, addressed to the Chairman, Tea Board requested for necessary action of noise Rs. 5 crore as R & D contribution for tea industry for confirm fund. A matching contribution would also available from NABARD to create the Corpus Fund.

In a meeting convened by the main chairman, Tea an Board September 27, 2987 of the leading the planters and representatives of the two premises institutes, Tea Research Association (TRA) and Tea Research Institute United Planters' Association on Southern India (TRI-UPASI) unanimously agreed for raising funds of Rs. 5 crore of which Rs. 4 crore and 9 crore with be contributed by North India and South India tea industry. The funds collected world be suitable invested, interest's income assuming there is will only be used for the purpose of carrying and research of different facts of tea. A small committee consisting of Chairman. Consultative commiittee of Plantation Association (CCPA); representatives from TRA and UPASI was contributed to advise chairman Tea Board on issues connected was raising of funds. TRA raises the bills for contribution to the NTRF in March, 1988 @ 8 paise per kg. of grade tea for the year 1985, subjects a maximum of Rs 4000 to all tea estate in North India. Similarty TRI-UPASI raised bills for such contribution to all tea estates in South India. Income tax exemption on the contribution by the tea companies to the campus fund was granted by the government U/S 35 (i) (ii).

Genesis for forming the NTRF

In pursuance of the decision taken in the meeting held in December 22, 1987, in the office of the Managing Director NABARD, Mumbai, two Committiees namely Administrative and Technical Committees was contributed in December 30, 1987. The Administrative Committee (AC) will decide (1) subject to government instructions from time to time the pattern of investment of the compus funds keeping review the object or maximising returns and best interest of the tea remember in the country and (ii) all matters pertaining to deposits investment patterns and withdrawal which will be required from time to time. The committee shall have the power to invite exports to the meeting, workout proper investments patterns and monitors the fund utilisation. The Technical Committees will finalise appropriate procedure for inviting resemble scheme from appropriate agencies to consider and (iii) prove research scheme for implementation and funding from the corpus by inviting export as and when needed. Both the committees should meet at least once in a quarter. On finalisation of "Memorandum and by Laws with the approval of Tea Board, NABARD, Industry and Ministry of Commerce, NTRF was registered in June 7, 1988 under the West Bengal Societies Act XXVI of 1961.

The management of affairs of the NTRF was vested to the governing Body or Seven Members comprising of the Tea Board Chairman as President, there representatives NABARD, the chairman CCPA, the chairman TRA and the president UPASI.

Activities

Research and Development Activities of NTRF

NTRF operates in liasion with Tea Board India for supporting innovative research on all aspects of tea from cultivation on to consumption to human health effects of tea. Benefits accused out of the investments of conpus Fund are provided for worthwhile high quality research.

The main emiteria for research support are as follows:

- The project must be innovatives, not routine and must identify the areas where research could be fruitful for Indian the industry at large and have some social values.
- The project must have some practical implication internus of enhancing growth, productivity, processing, and towards establishing health and other financial aspects of Indian Tea.
- Research in disciplines such as genetics, plant development, molecular biology, enzymology, bio-technology, flavour chemistry, production engineering, medicine attributes of tea besides tea economics and management from the core of fund support.
- Research institutions recognised by DSIR, Ministry of Science and Technology, Govt., of India, as eminent national Institutes and those posses back research infrastructure of laboratory and scientists, can submit projects to NTRF for financial grants in

identified areas related to tea.

(ii) Other than research projects

The activity of NTRF besides funding research project include.

- Collection of data from NTRF projects of develop protocol from recommendation for enhancing productivity, quality and human health aspects of tea.
- Collection of research findings pertaining to improvements of quality and yield of tea and their commercialisation.
- Publication of research reports review, Quarterly News Bulletin, Annual Scientific Report in which research data generated under NTRF funded projects at different institution are documented.
- Organising Seminar and work shop including publication & of their proceedings.
- Internacting with producers and research institutions to identify research problems relevant to the activities.

Trends of research Support from NTRF

NTRF within the period of first 15 years did approve and sponsors a large number of research and development projects to various host institutions covering various areas. Detail is are given in table 6.6.

Table 11.7 Area Wise Projects Taken up, Institution Involved and Grants Approved since inception upto March, 31, 2003 by NTRF

Area of Research & Development	Projects Taken up	Host Institution involved (No.)	Total & D grant approve d (Rs. in Lakh)	Percent age to Total (7)	Percent age to Total (4)
1. Plant physiology, Breeding & Development	4	UPAcSI-TRF (2),. TRA (1), IHBT (1)	83.68	13.41	8.87
2. Soil Nutrition and Water Management	4	UPASI-TRF (2), AAU, Jorhat, Assam (2)	65.59	10.51	8.87

4. Quality Improvement	5	UPASI-TRF (2), TRACD, IHBT (2)	86.48	14.18	11.11
5. Work Study : Ergonomics	1	AAU, Jorhat, Assam (1)	4.64	0.75	2.22
6. Human Health benefits	16	C.U. (3), HCB (2), ITRC (2), Presidency College, Kolkata, (2), Bose Institute (1), CNCI, Kolkata (3), VIMS, Kolkata (2),	4140.53	22.52	35.56
7. Product Direnfication	1	J.U. (1), Tata Memorial Centre, Mumbai (1)	20.45	3.28	2,22
8. Promotion	2	RRL, Jorhat Assam (1) CCPA (2)	6.40	1.02	4.44
Total	45	18	623.96	100.00	100.00

Note-AAV-Assam Agricultural University, BCKV-Pridhan Chandra Krishi Viswavidynlay, RRL-Regional Research Laboratory, Jorhat

1 HBT -Institute Tuxicology Research Centre, Lucknow

1 TRC-Vivekananda Institute of Medical Sciences, Ram Krishna Seva Pratishan, Kolkata, IICB- Indian Institute of Chemical Biology CCPA-Consultative Committee of Plantation Association, Ju-Jadavpur University

Source- A decade and half of 1988-2003 National Tea Research Foundation (NTRF) C/o Tea Board India, Kolkata, June 2004

Institutional Interface

For the first time in the history of research in India. NRRF inducted Agricultural Universities, other universities, National Laboratories in India with specialised still and hightoned research by providing research specific grants. These the spectrum of research support by NTRF is not restricted to the two classical tea & research centres in India, TRA Tocklai in North and UPASI-TRF in South India but to other research institutes of excellences and universities as well. As many as 18 organization and 45 projects were supported by NRRF out of 18 organisations. There are 2 tea research body, 9 national laboratory and 7 university colleges, out of a total of 45 projects, 15 projects were supported by tea research bodies, 18 National laboratory and 12 universities/college.

Further are outline has been made to

Name of the institutions, number of projects solely funded by NTRF and number of projects completed upto 31 March 2003 of those institute and also the amount of monetary of rant releases so far to each one of those are presented in table 11.8

Table 11.8 Projects Approved Completed and Grant Released on 31 March 2003 by NTRF.

Institution	No. of projects approved	No. of project completed	Grant amount
1. UPASI-TRF/Valapari, Coimbatore	10	6	189.06
2. TRA, Jorhat	5	4	10.58
3. IHBT, Palampur Himanchal Pradesh	4	4	84.86
4. University of Kolkata	4	1	54.85
5. ITRC, Lucknow	2	1	12.68
6. VIMS, RKMSP, Kolkata	2	1	4.88
7. Bose Institute, Kolkata	1	1	6.35
8. AAU, Jorhat, Assam	3	1	18.46
9. IICB, Jadavpur, Kolkata	2		40.67
10. Visva Bharati, Santininetan	1		2.80
11. Presidency College, Kolkata	1		8.07

12. North Bengal University, Siliguri, WB	1	1	3.67
13. CNCI, Kolkata	3	-	5.39
14. Jadavpur University, Kolkata	1	-	2.00
15. RBL, Jorhat, Assam	1	-	2.00
16. BC.KV, Nadia, West Bengal	1	1	4.25
17. Tata memorial Centre, Mumbai	1	-	5.06
18. CCPA, Kolkata	2	2	6.40
Total	45	23	525.93

Contribution Tea Industry organised conference/seminar for promotion of Indian Tea

I. Break up of amount released upto 31.03.2003

(a) towards completed projects (33) Rs. 407.03 lakh

(b) towards on going projects (22) Rs. 118.94 lakh.

II. Approved balance amount due for ongoing projects Rs. 97.99 lakh

Source: A decade and half of National Tea Research Foundation (NTRF)

NTRF, C/o Tea Board, India, Kolkata 70001, June 2004

The vast data lease generation from its a perspective of resember results from various completed projects will not doubt provide the core materials for developing practical recommendations for Indian Tea Industry. The gains accrued from each projects and their benefits to Tea Industry not over emphasised.

National Tea Research Foundation - Governing Body Mealing

15th meeting of the Governing Body of the National Tea Research Foundation was held on 4th December, 1997 at the Tea Board's Office in Kolkata and was chaired by Mr S. S. Ahuja, Chairman, Tea Board. Mr S. Patra, Assistant Secretary, attended this meeting on behalf of the Association. The meeting inter alia observed the following issues.

1. NTRF would launch a priced Tea Research journal of international standard and would seek assistance of Indian Institute of Chemical Biology in this regard.
2. NTRF would incorporate eminent scientists/personalities in its governing body and spread its activities to various parts in the country.
3. Internet linkage for NTRF.
4. Two eminent persons would be selected to monitor South and North Indian tea projects under NTRF. Names of Dr Akarim (ex-UPASI) and Dr D N Barroah (ex-TRA) were mentioned in this connection.

Indian Institute of Plantation Management

During the period under review, Bangalore University leased out five acres of its land in Jana Bherathi campus of the Indian Institute of Plantation Management for establishing its offices. The IIPM, in turn, would have to support the University academically in related subjects like Botany, Sericulture and Management besides maintaining roads and other infrastructure onthe campus. IIPM was also granted Rs. 5 crore by the Union Commerce Ministry to construct the first phase of essential infrastructure on the 5-acre land granted by the Bangalore University. The Institute was also granted income tax exemption under section 80 (a).

The 8th and 9th meetings of the Board of Governors of the Institute were held during this reporting period. Besides these, the IIPM in collaboration with Tea Board also organised several Training Programmes in West Bengal and Assam also at the ITA office in Kolkata.

Assam Agricultural University

Assam Agricultural University at Jorhat requested the CCPA to arrange for practical garden training for its students studying BSc (Agriculture), Tea Husbandry and Technology streams. At the request of the CCPA the Association arranged for this training in its member gardens as per its share of allocation.

North Bengal University

During the period under review, North Bengal University approached the CCPA to arrange for practical garden training for its students purcuing Post-Graduate Diploma in Tea Management as in the previous year. The Association, at CCPA's request, advised its member gardens to provide the usual facilities to the students selected for this training.

References:

1. Annual Scientific Report 2004-05, NTRF, Kolkata, West Bengal
2. Salient Research Outcome of the completed projects funded by NTRF, August 2003
3. A decade and Half of NTRF (1988-2003), June 2004, Kolkata, West Bengal
4. Tea Research A New Perspective, Proceedings of forests workshop of NTRF, 30 April 2005, West Bengal
5. NTRF, News Bulletin, Various issues, Kolkata, West Bengal
6. Annual Scientic Report, Various years, Tea Research Association, Tocklai Experiment Station, Jorhat, Assam
7. Annual Report, Various yeas, TRA, Jorhat
8. Annual Report, various Issues, consultative Committee of Plantation Association (CCPA), Kolkata
9. Annual Report, Various Issues, UPASI.
10. Annual Report, Various Issues, Tea Board, India, Kolkata
11. Annual Report, Various Issues, Indian Tea Planters Association, Kolkata
12. Annual Report, Various Issues, Indian Tea Association, Kolkata
13. Banerjee, G.D., Structural changes of Tea Plantation Industry in India since 1956. Ph.D Thesis submitted to Jadavpur University, 1982
14. Banerjee, G.D., Tea Plantation Industry in India between 1965 and 1992- Structural Changes (1966), Law years, Book Stall, Gowahati.
15. Banerjee, G .D., Primary Marketing of India, Tea Indian Journal of Agricultural Marketing, Annual Conference Issue, December 2000
16. Banerjee, G.D., Tea Marketing is not longer fashionable Slogan,

IASSI, Journal, April-June 2001

17. Banerjee, G.D., & Banerjee Sarda Sustainable Tea Plantation Management, IASSI Journal January-March, 2004
18. Banerjee, G.D and Sarda Banerjee, Tea Industry of the Cross roads, Independence Issue, 2005
19. Banerjee, G.D., History of Darjeeling Tea Industry, Assam Review and Tea News, December 1999, Vol. 888, No. 10
20. Banerjee, G.D...... Development Issue of Tea Industry, Assam Review and Tea News, February 2000, Vol. 88, No-12
21. Banerjee G.D., Development Issue of Tea Industry March 2000, Vol. 89, No-1
22. Karmakar K.G. and Banerjee G.D. The Survey of Tea Industry in India, Occasional paper, National Bank for Agriculture for Rural Development. Development of Economic Analysis and Research (DEAR), Ho. Muradabad, September 2005
23. Banerjee G.D., Market Research in Tea Consumption, Chai Ki Bat, Bharatiya Chai Parishad, Kolkata August 1989, Vol. 34, No-8 (Part-1)
24. Banerjee G.D. Market Research in Tea Consumption, Bharatiya Cha Parishad, Kolkata, October 1989, Vol 34, No11 (Part -II).
25. Banerjee, G.D., Biotechnology for Indian Farmers Financing Agriculture, Finance Corporation, July-September, 2001
26. Banerjee, G.D., All Hands in Deck. Times Agriculture, Journal October, 2002
27. Banerjee G.D., Economics of Organic Farming, Agriculture Today, October 2005
28. Banerjee G.D., Eco labelling of Agriculture Products -Challenge of 21 Century, Agriculture Today, December 2005.
29. Banerjee G.D. and Banerjee Srijeet, Tea Plantation Industry - A Road Map Ahead, 2008.
30. Banerjee G.D. and Banerjee Srijeet, Global Tea Trade- Dimension and Dynamics, 2008.
31. Banerjee G.D. and Banerjee Srijeet - Export Potentials of Indian Tea.

32. Banerjee G.D. Organic Farming - A Glance, Suvikalpa, Nabcon, Nabard, Mumbai.

33. Banerjee G.D. Agricultural Marketing Infrastructure in Nagaland, Nab Law, Nabard, Mumbai.

34. Banerjee G.D. and Sarda Banerjee, Product Diversification and Value addition in Tea, IASSI Journal January-March 2005.

35. Banerjee G.D. Agro-Processing Sectors - Challenges and opportunities October-December 2006.

36. Baneerjee, G.D. and Baneeji Srijeet Tea Industry A Road Map Ahead, Abhijeet Publication, New Delhi, 2007.

37. Baneerjee, G.D. and Baneeji Srijeet Global Tea Trade Dimensions and Dynamics, Abhijeet Publication, New Delhi, 2007.

38. Baneerjee, G.D. and Baneeji Srijeet Export Potenticals of Indian Tea, Abhijeet Publication, New Delhi, 2007.

Chapter 12

Sustainable Development of Tea Industry in International Perspective – Areas of Concern

It is observed from the earlier chapters that issues of tea industry have been discussed taking into consideration its development/ growth, promotion, production/productivity, extension/replacement/ new planting/diversification of exports, primary marketing (Indian auction, London auction, exfactory sale, exgarden sale, forward contract etc), labour, wage and employment, government taxes and levei etc. All these were mainly concentrated with reference to India. The readers may perhaps desire to know what are the issues of the tea industry in its various facets with referance to other producing countrie. In this context, efforts have been made to collect information/ news, write-ups from various journals, news letters of different tea assciations, Tea Board, national dailies and the gists/focusses made by the authors through their articles published in reputed national and International journals. All these have been compiled and presented in this chapter.

German Importers Appreciated Corrective Measures by Tea Growers

German tea importers were satisfied with the corrective measures adopted by Indian tea growers to control application of pesticides and phasing out of child labour. This allays fears of tea exporters to Germany being seriously affected if the Government had failed to conform to German standards. The then Chairman of Indian Tea Association Mr. S.K. Bhasin recalled that Indian exporters earned the wrath of German importers on two fronts. The issue of deployment of child labour below 14 years was objected to by the Germans. The second issue was the highest level of chemical residue than the MRL stipulated under German law. ITA advised planters to phase out child labour and control use of pesticides.

Exports of Tea to Poland

Under the Indo-Polish Trade Agreement a provision for export of tea to Poland in non-convertible Indian rupee was made with effect from 10th April 1992 in addition to earlier provision. The provision fixed for tea was like (i) black tea- North India- Rs 370 million and South India Rs 130 million and (ii) value-added tea Rs 100 million. It was clarified that the provisions referred to above pertained to only those exports which were paid for non-convertible Indian rupees.

Liquid Market Grows in Japan

There has been a remarkable growth in demand for liquid tea in Japan, reports Trade Scope. In fact to day more than half of the total volume of leaf tea consumption comprises raw tea used in making liquid tea. Even though black tea has a long history as canned beverage, the amount of tea consumed in this form used to be very small indeed. However, the advent of automatic vending machines brought with it a boom in canned coffee which could also be consumed in winter. This was followed by a fad for "Oolong tea". The volume of liquid tea consumption has also increased in the restaurants and fast food outlets to save labour have resulted in introduction of liquid tea products. The developments can also be seen in other establishment such as tea rooms and hotels.

Recently, the expansion of the liquid tea market has showed signs of slows down. As with 'Ooolong' tea, then represents a temporary slump after a period of rapid growth, after which a second growth phase can be expected. It is widely held in the industry that market for liquid tea will increase to a level similar to that for 'olong tea'.

No more CTC for Russia

The then USSR tea representative in Kolkata was aggrieved with the notice from the Union Commerce Ministry restricting it from lifting CTC tea from Indian autions. The Soviet officials who handled the tea trade felt it is a kind of infringment on our right to lift 135 million kgs of "all varieties of teas" as was determined by trade protocol for 1990 signed by the Government of India and the USSR. The prohibitory notice was issued on October 11, 1990 and the Soviets withdrew from CTC purchase from October 22, 1990. However, since they had already procured 115 million kgs of all varieties, the import was not very major. Moreover, according to Soviet office they were free to buy other tea grades. In fact, they are "buying then but lent at dearer prices". The industry sources believed the move was prompted by the heed to bring down tea prices. The Russians started buying again from January, 1991.

International Tea Seminar in Bangladesh

The Bangladesh Tea Board convened an international seminar on tea in Dhaka, Bangladesh on 10 and 11 December, 1990. The seminar discussed tea production, management and research, improved yield and quality, research towards higher production of tea, micro propagation and integrated pest management, how tea plantation harmonised environment, integrated water management, tea financing, packaging and improvement of quality of tea. tea marketing and tea as beverage in 21st century. Scholars and tea technologists of international repute at home and abroad presented their papers in the seminar.

Common Tea Market in SARRC Proposed

The government pitched for a common tea market among SAARC countries with arrangement for collective marketing in international markets. While Sri Lanka and Bangladesh mooted this concept, the

Indian Government sounded the domestic tea industry on the matter. This line of thinking prompted by the bleak prospects for the Indian tea industry which fell short of the Eight Plan target of 100 million kgs. One view is that most bushes in the country are 50 years or more old with little virgin land for new extension on the gardens. The economics of planting in non-traditional areas is yet to be undertaken while small growers have their limitations. Then there is a fear of an imbalance between demand and supply in due course. The other view is that the industry had done little to break through.

For an Indian Market in Germany

Germany is not an important market for Indian tea, at first sight. It imported annually 6000 tonnes. German tea drinkers are the most quality concious in entire Europe. They look down on tea bags and donot hesitate to import the choicest Darjeeling teas by air. Indian tea exporters, however, have a fight on the their hands. If Indian teas are to recover the ground lost over the years in the EC, not only to Sri Lanka but also to Kenya, Malawi and Indonesia are to be explored. What is more the trend is towards teas in other EC markets. At the same time, the market for packaged tea continues to dominate in EC, EC companies, especially the UK-based multinationals.

CIS Was Offered Credit to Buy Tea

The Union Commerce Ministry chalked out a two-pronged strategy to retain the single largest market for plantation companies in the commonwealth of Independent State. Unveiling the plan at the opening of the UPASI conference the then Deputy Minister for Commerce Salman Khurshid, stated that lurred the CIS states with new line of credit and offer of counter-trade. The then Defence Minister Mr. Sharad Pawar, returned from the CIS with the impression that counter trade was an effective way of retaining the markets for Indian commodities in the erstwile Soviet Union, said Khurshid.

Tata Tea in Russian Tie-up

In a major globalisation effort, Tata Tea Ltd (TTL)—a blue chip company in the Tata group—sat up an Indo-Russian joint venture to boost exports of Indian teas and other agro products. The joint venture was named Tata Krasnodar Industrial Ltd (TKIL) in which TTL with its associates and Krasnodar Tea Company were equal partners, each holding 50 percent of TKIL equity TKIL acquired the ownership of a tea blending and packageing plant at from Krasnodar Tea Company as part of the agreement. Immediately after the take over of the plant, TTL secured an initial order for the supply of 3 million kg of black tea worth Rs 16 crore. The tea was used in the packaging plant at Sochi. The packet-tea was sold under the brand name "Tata Krasnodar" and carried the inscription "An Indo-Russia Star Product".

Speciality Tea Explored Market in UK

The successful launch of the Darjeeling logo in 1987 and the Assam logo by the Tea Board made consumers increasingly aware of the specialy tea. They would not mind sippling quality tea on week day but speciality tea is must for weekends, holidays and occasions. Large funds were being spent by the UK Tea Council and leading blenders for promoting Indian tea in the quality market segment. "Logos have certainly helped to authenticate the origins of the varieties being sold by millions of sterlings spent on advertising and marketing also play "crucial role".

Steady tea supply to UK

India assured Britain that it could provide an uninterrupted supply of a wide range of tea to it in conformity with the requirement of a quality conscious market. A high level delegation led by Tea Board of India was on a visit to Britain. It held a serious of meetings with the UK Tea Association and the Tea Council of Britain with a view to exchanging Ideas. The talk assumed special importance in view of the inter-governmental meeting of the Food and Agricultural Organisation in Rome where tea plantation and its trade got prominace discusion. According to Mr. P.K. Bora the then Chairman of Tea Board the talks with the UK Tea Association were very fruitful. The Association is the parent body of British tea traders and importers. Indian tea exports now stand poised for a sharp growth with pronounced policy shift from a wither to conservative " residual" approach to "production" approach. Perfectly matching blend specifications and offering world class packaging for self placement in retail counters the world over, Indian tea is praised for greater thrust in discerning markets. A wide array of Indian teas are now packed in tea bags to suit the life style of tea drinkers on the move. India growing base in instant tea has closely followed the world trend owards "convenience" tea.

Japan Black Tea Market Growing

Japanese market is turning to black tea, away from the familiar olong and traditional green teas. Recently a tea auction in Darjeeling recorded a highest ever price of and Rs 2000 per pound and the buyer was Japanese. The total tea consumption in Japan is 120,000 million tonnes a year. Out of this black tea accounts for less than 15 per cent. It is pushing its way into the green tea market especially in tea bags. Unlike the CIS or Iran, Japan is economically sound. Therefore, under the present circumstances, Indian black tea producers and exporters should grab this opportunity to enter the Japanese market. Tea Board sent signals to black tea merchants to pay special attention to promoting black tea in Japan in the light of tough competition and their miniscule share in the market. Promoting tea in Japan requires considerable marketing might and financial muscle. Since independence, industry lacks adequate marketing infrastructure in Japan. Marketing Indian products is done there in collaboration with Japanese breweries and soft drink companies taking advantage of their vast distribution network. The leading breweries in Japan developed links with major Indian tea companies like Good rich, Harrison Malayam, Brooke Bond Lipton India Ltd. Mcleod Russel and Duncan Agro Industries.

New Packaging Regulations in Germany

All exporters of tea to Germany faced the problems of German legislation and organically produced teas to all EC countries arising out of EC legislation. The objective of the German legislation was to stem the tide of packaging waste which threatened to engulf not only Germany but all Western Europe. It applied to all merchantdise and not just tea, whether imported or domestically produced. Under the German legislation, all packaging materials must be environment friendly and must be returned to the manufacturer and distributor for recycling. This phase of ruling became law in Germany in January 1993 when shops were obliged to take back all packaging. The standard, foil-lined plywood tea chests used for leaf grade were out—unless Indian exporters were prepared to take them back. German tea helped exporters to develop chest which collapsed after use, for easy re-shipment to India. Average cost of disposing of tea trade chest was between DM 40 and DM 50 depending on the location of the importing firm. The extra cost passed on to consumer. A recent—survey carried out by trade chain concluded that 98 percent of the "packaging around packaging" was superfluous and eliminated 80 percent of it. A leading German daily news paper claimed that 50,000 tonnes of packaging annually fell into this category, "Superfluous". The German legislation, which covered packaging for retail tea market, also since April 1993, inspired EC to adopt similar legislation for EC as a whole. The EC legislation on organically produced teas, in fact, covered all agricultural products and food stuff. It was designed to protect consumers and applied to both domestic production and imports. It was fully implemented throughout 12-nation EC, from July 23 of this year.

Indo- CIS Trade in Tea

The Commerce Ministry produced ECGC cover for tea industry to enable it to overcome credit problems and boost exports to Russia. The ministry and industry believed that such a cover was necessary as only limited quantities were purchased by Russia in repayment of the rouble debt that India owed to the former Soviet Union. The need was recognised and a delegation led by Government of India on the Tea Board sorted out the problems in the way of exports to that country. At a meeting with Commerce Ministry officials in New Delhi, most tea exporters felt that debt repayment arrangement with Russia need to be 'firmed' up. They also expressed themselves against making available tea supplies to Russia in the escrow account due to the fear that it covered "over-invoicing' and diversion of dollars to other account units. Further escrow account was getting "discounted" in Russia and there was also problem of opening letter of oil credit against escrrow account. Unless steps were taken to prevent over-invoicing coupled with a firm tie-up with Russian bank export escrow account would not take off. No Russian buyer came forward to buy tea from India against hard currency due to shortage of dollars.

How To Ensure Minimum Residual Level (MRL) checks

The Tea Board expressed its inability to comply with demand of the German Tea Association (GTA) that the Board either regulate the pesticide residue level or share the cost of analysis of Indian tea. The Tea Board move followed the enforcement of quality control regulations in the German and the European Community (EC) markets. The issue also triggered fears among the industry that tea consignment could be rejected on a large scale by the markets. The Board advised the GTA that does not have the infrastructure to check and license only those export consignments which conformed to the German quality control regulations. The Board assured the importing countries that every efforts were made to monitor and check pesticides residue level in Indian tea. The EC set separate deadlines for eradicating different chemicals. The date was January 1, 1998. The Board's meeting on December 28, 1997 at Munnar in Kerala took up research programmes in collaboration with the trade in German and EC markets which enforced stringent yardsticks on pesticide residual levels. The meeting also requested the Tea Research Association, the Council of Scientific and Industrial Research in

Palampur and United Planters' Association of South India to set up laboratories. Even chemicals which are not used in India have been mentioned in the check lists brought out by inporters. Most of the residue was in the tea leaf and not in liquor which is consumed. But importers insist on quality checks on leaf. At the Board meeting, industry representative felt that immediate steps were taken to generate data on residues of Dicofol, Ethion, Chloropyriphes and Teradifan (which is banned in India). The Board however was silent on the German Tea Association's demand for sharing the cost of analysis which was DM 400 per analysis. The Board launched a campaign to convince importers that only a small fraction of residue is dissolved in liquor when tea is brewed in hot water.

It wanted the Tea Research Association to generate data on chemical MRLs (minimum residual levels) in dried tea as well as the tea left over after brewing to convince the importers.

Will India Import Tea

The Union Commerce Ministry allowed import of tea from any source if the importing Indian company undertakes to re-export the commodity. Announcing this, the then Union Minister of State for Commerce, Mr. A. Sreecharan, said, "There is no bar on import of tea if the importer gives an undertaking to re-export the entire quantum after adding value." In an informal chat with reporters, he said the Union Government allowed hundred per cent export-oriented units to import tea for blending and re-export. One such unit came up at Falta export processing zone and another came up near Pune. The two EOUs were being set up by Hindustan Lever and Alpha Exports. These two companies were allowed to source their supply from any country. According to Mr. Ardhanareswaran, special secretary, who was with the minister, the ministry did not object if tea was imported for value addition ending in re-export. He said countries like Sri Lanka, Mauritius and Bangladesh evinced interest in supplying tea to Indian companies if they opted for re-export as stipulated by the Commerce Ministry. He said "the emphasis is on value addition to earn as much foreign exchange as possible".

Tea in some European Countries

Most of the countries in Europe prefer coffee to tea, of course, except the United Kingdom where 54 million people drink 70,000 tonnes of tea against 1.53,000 tonnes of tea consumed by 350 million Europeans per annum. After UK the Federal Republic of Germany (FRG) is the second largest consumer of tea, the consumption amounts to 16,000 tonnes annually. The country imports high quality tea, specially of Darjeeling. Intake of tea in France registered a conspicuous rise from 8, 439 tonnes in 1984 to 25, 952 tonnes in 2007 of Prospect for the Netherlands also looked bright as revealed by the tea consumption figures of the country from 9,229 tonnes in 1984 to 1,80,852 tonnes in 2007. It was noted that FRG, France and the Netherlands together accounted for 55 per cent of the total European tea consumption. Tea is not a traditional plant in Europe. From Asia it was taken there by the European merchants. It was the Dutch and Potugese who first brought tea to Europe and, not as many people think the British. The Portugese pioneered the trade routes with the Eastern world and the Dutch first brought tea to Europe in 1610.

Descidence over Russian buying

Tea exporters were reportedly divided over the issue of including tea in the basket of commodities to repay India's outstanding rupee dues to Russia. The producer-exporters were clearly opposed to large quantities of tea being included in the annual repayment of India's rupee loan. At a meeting convened by the Union Commerce Ministry to discuss Indian trade with Russia funds worth Rs. 500-600 crore was allotted to Russia to purchase indian tea in 1993. The producer-exporters said this would put India back to the days when the Industry and trade became totally dependent on the Russian rupee trade (the Russians buying about 60 per cent of Indian exports) to hold the price and the market share in export, Russia's forced withdrawal from the auction in 1992 compelled the Indian tea industry to live up to the glabal competition from other producers for foreign exchange. India did not do badly either. Despite the poor crop India exported about 180 million kg with the Russian federation importing Rs 40 million worth of tea. Their question now is: Shall we chase volume export as we were doing all these years, or shall we chase hard currency as we learn- to-do last year aided by the full convertibility on trade account. That advantage was lost when the Russian purchase was received with the backing of Rs. 500 crore. Tea prices reached heights where the hard currency buyers did not find Indian tea competitive. Some of the tea producer-exporters feared that Russia would buy the best Indian tea under the loan repayment programme and sell it in Europe for dollars. The Government should not allow anything that will threaten Indian export in an area of growth. However, producers who are not exporters welcomed the return of the Russians. They were demanding that the Russians should be allowed to buy more than Rs 600 crore worth of tea. They knew the tea prices would soar if the Russians start buying. Though differing on some points, the merchant exporters badly agreed with the producers. They said the Russians could buy more as Indian production was around 740 million kgs in 1993. They could mop up a part of the extra production. The non-exporting producers said that home market should be able to bear the higher price in case of a large Russian mop-up because tea price has always risen at a lower rate than other commodities. India is the largest CTC maker. Most producers wanted the Russian to buy more CTC saying that with more cuppage this worked out to be cheaper for them compared with orthodox. With large purchase the CTC price would then jump and so will the companies profits.

Trade Protocol Between India and the Russian Federation

The Tea Board disclosed that a trade protocol had been signed between the Government of India and the Government of the Russian Federation for the calendar year 1992. As per the said protocol, the provision for export of tea from India to Russian Federation for the calendar year 1992 was 60 million kgs on rupee payment basis at the exchange rate prevailing in India between the designated currency and Indian rupee on the date of payment based on the policy of the Reserve Bank of India. Import and export of goods from each other outside the ambit of this trade protocol was permitted on the basis of counter-trade, commodity exchange, barter, buy-back operation but through payment in freely convertible currency or any internationally recognised form of business cooperation subject to compliance of laws and regulations of the two countries. The trade agreement signed between India and the Russian Federation of February 22, 1992 provided for import of 120 million rupees worth of Indian tea for the latter. The quantity may vary between 50 million kgs and 60 million kgs. There was no indication as yet as to how the quantity will be apportioned between CTC and orthodox. India had already signed two more agreements for tea, one with Uzbekistan which, was to buy three million kgs and the other with Kazakhistan which was to import to million kgs, while the deal with the Russian Federation the largest in the Commonwealth on Independent States (CAS), removed a great deal of uncertainty surrounding exports of tea to the erst while Soviet Union. Industry and trade circles hoped that much of the remaining uncertainties would disappear when Indian and the ukrine, the second largest state in CIS, were able to reach an agreement. If all the deals struck with the member states of CIS took care of about 100 million kgs, the tea industry and trade assured of stable market conditions. At the moment, the deals covered between 55 million kgs and 65 million kgs. Significantly, although the agreement with the Russian Federation was signed on February 22, 1992, trade circles viewed that buyers on behalf of it participated in the auctions only by the third week of March 1993. This was because they sorted out other issues including the crucial one of payment against exports made last year. As it is known, on instructions from the appropriate quarters in the erst while Soviet Union, the designated buyers had stayed away from auctions for almost nine weeks. The crstwhile Soviet Union was the largest importer of Indian tea for the past several years and the quantity it had been buying rose progressively from 120 million kgs to 135 million kgs in recent years. It had also emerged a major importer of CTC tea.

Managing Companies's Tea Culture in Sri Lanka

The management of Sri Lanka's 449 state-owned plantations, which was taken over by 22 managing companies in the private sector, introduced new approach in different facets of tea plantation culture. A new plucking system was introduced where-by three leaves and a bud were plucked, as a matter of policy during rush crops. To ensure omission of non-essential chemicals and inclusion of essential for the replacement of plant nutrients and sustainability, fertiliser mixtures were changed to conform to demand of the soil at different fields. In addition, foliar spray on an intensive scale was applied to promote flushing of green leaf. Long-standing pruning practices were changed drastically. The cut-across prune culture in the low country replaced the hard prune carried out in the mid and high-grown areas, thus saving the frames of branches developed over many years. Shade practice followed earlier was discarded and the South Indian pattern of bee villeas was adopted. Production, as a result, shot up by 48% over the previous years just in 18 months.

Coffee And Tea In The New Europe

Sponsored by Tea & Coffee Trade Journal, an exhibition and symposium on tea and coffee was held in Vienna, Austria between September 20 and 22, 1994. The symposium on tea featured raw materials, product manufacturing-trends in technology, marketing, specially market, new designs for retail shops, brand imagery, blending flavours, herbal, organic. The exhibitors included major tea packers, tea importers, manufacturers of tea packaging equipment, tea bag and paper markers.

Green Tea Sales Hip in Japan

According to a report of World Coffee and Tea, the sale of green tea which was caused to fall by the consumption of Western-style teas,

Kocha again picked up in Japan. The regaining position in the market was said to be the outcome of selling tea in cans. And the sales growth followed the same trend as that of Chinese oolong tea, it was observed. The sales forecast of canned green teas for the next few years indicate a rise between 50 to 60 per cent annually.

Fall in Chinas Black Tea Exports

It was reported that a considerable quantity of China production of low-grown black tea was being converted into the production of green and jasmine teas. This trend was attributed to higher profits being contributed by these teas from domestic sales to China's increasingly affluent and huge population compared to exports to the world market at relatively low and depressed prices.

Tea in UK

UK Tea Council reported tea accounted for, 43 per cent of all the beverages the Britishers consumed during the last five years. In the hot drinks sector, tea's share is 62 per cent. Instant tea contributes only 2.2 per cent of all brewed tea for the past few years. "Speciality tea"—a blend of teas that have been especially prepared for consumption at a certain time of day—is becoming more popular. The loose-leaf share of tea remained steady at 13 per cent for the past few years. The use of tea bags, however, accounted for 84 per cent. The average cost of a brewed cup in UK is only 2 pence (around 3 US cents) including milk which accounts for half of this cost. Adding the cost of sugar, which is only 30 per cent of the breved tea, the cost per week on an average is 47 pence (61 US cents) per week for tea.

Incentive to Sri Lankan Tea Producers

Steps taken in 1992 and 1993 to liberalise the economy are significant. With effect from 21st December, 1992 the Sri Lanka Government abolished all taxes on tea. The ad valoram sales tax on teas sold at Colombo auction as well as the export duty on teas were done away with. As a result, tea producers get the assistance of about Rs. 3.00 per kg in the form of reduction in production cost, observed Forbes and Walker. Further, the abolition of the ad valorem sales tax provided an impetus to the producers in directing their attention to the production of quality teas and thus making the tea more attractive to international buyers.

Sri Lanka Consider Long- Term Management Agreement

At the centenary celebrations of the Colombo Tea Trader Association, the then President D.B. Wijatung, said that the Sri Lanka Government considered long-term extension of its agreement with private companies for the management of state plantations. In 1992, the Government had entrusted the management of the loss-making state plantations to 22 private companies for a period of 5 years. According to the President, the Government made long-term agreements, with a view to infusing fresh thinking and new blood into the tea industry of Sri Lanka.

Privatisation of Lankan Tea industry

Sri Lanka Government's policy of gradual privatisation of the tea industry in the country was watched with sympathy and interest. Apparently the question of higher productivity induced the government to take the decision. Currently a controversy is raging at various levels in India also about privatisation of the PSUs. The protagonists of privatisation argue that with a view to making profits, private enterprises increase efficiency and productivity. The detractors argue that the Nehruvian model of State-sponsored enterprises was most suited for the forward looking but presently a backward economy, like India's. The Government is changing that policy under, as they say, World Bank and International Monetary Fund compulsions. In Sri Lanka, the issue had been studied in detail with special reference to conditions in tea industry there. According to the report of the study, privatisation is urgently needed by the industry for any further development. The efficiency of the private enterprise in Sri Lankan tea industry will be appreciated by the cryptic comment that last year's crop excess was shared between the private and the state sector of the tea industry in the proportion of 65 per cent and 35 per cent, respectively. According to the Development Plan drawn up by the Tea Board there, the entire tea industry in Sri Lanka is dependent to a very large extent on the private sector today than ever before for further stability. In 2006, private sector's contribution was about 200 million kgs. towards the total of 360 million kgs. On the other hand, the targets for the state sector could not be achieved and had actually fallen short of expectation through marginally. By 2007 private sector's contribution is expected to rise through higher productivity, through the adoption of replanting, infilling and other recommended agricultural practices.

What should interest India in the matter is not just the common pursuit of privatisation. In addition there are a number of facets to the issue to see and consider. The first point of contact between Sri Lanka and India on this issue is the joint tea export effort. Much of the credit for this new initiative reportedly goes to the late Ranjan Wijeratne who held the portfolios of Plantation Development and Defence before his death. The minister lobbied successfully for privatisation and for joint India-Sri Lanka foray in export market. It is also reported that the Union Commerce Ministry in India is already seized of the problem. There is yet another aspect. In the massive privatisation programme, participation by foreign companies, was also mooted. A large number of foreign companies including some important Indian companies made a bid. Chances of Indian managements replacing Lankan management had however aroused protest in Sri Lanka with the Chamber of Commerce and the tea brokers warning the Government that handing over management to Indians would be dangerous. In an editorial one newspaper said: "The implications of handing over vast tracts of land yielding "green gold" to Indian plantation companies will be apparent even to political neophytes." It asked, "While the Indian investment guaranteed by Sri Lankan law is *per se* welcome, would not investment in very sensitive regions of the country at this particular point of time in fact be a negative catalyst in strengthening ties between the two countries?" The feeling needed to be assuaged. And Rupa Karunatillake, the then Minister of Plantation Industries made a public statement that "the government was only privatising management, and not selling the estates". Whether or not, there be a joint Indo-Ceylon export effort or an Indian company is allowed to run a private sector tea estate, future of privatisation of industries in Sri Lanka should be carefully noted by the industry and the Government here in India where an almost similar bid is on.

Tea Exports to Egypt Require Certificate of Origin

The Ministry of Economy and Foreign Trade in Egypt is learnt to have issued a directive revising the decree No. 619 of 1998, which made the Certificate of Origin mandatory for all imports into Egypt. As per the directive, exports of tea to Egypt should indicate the country of origin only on the invoice, which should be certified by the Egyptian Embassy/Trade Office in the supplying country free of charge. The new regulation allows manufacturers to ship tea to Egypt either from the country of production or their branches and distribution centers in other countries. It is reported that the new decree has come into effect from November 7, 1999.

Sri Lanka Tea Exports

On the basis of quantity bought by the major importers of Sri Lanka teas for the period from January to December 2006, the CIS still remains as the single largest importer although year to year figures show a marginal decline. Other notable declines have been from Turkey, U AR and Jordan. On the other hand, the U AE continues to rank as the second large importer of Sri Lanka tea and has shown a growth rate of around 16.6 per cent compared to the same period last year. Other significant gains in imports have been from Tunisia, Syria, Iran, UK, Saudi Arabia and Germany. However, the notable feature of Sri Lanka tea exports for the period January to December

2006 was (i) marginal decline in tea exdports, (ii)"fall in value added tea exports, and (iii) short fall of Imported Ire-exported tea.

London Paper Blackens Indian Tea Industry

The Sunday Mirror of London recently published a report alleging the use of child labour in Indian tea plantation. The paper claimed its reporters visited tea estates in Assam and found evidence of child labour in the plantations. The newspaper report has named England-based George Williamson Ltd. as one of the users of child labour in the plantations under its Indian subsidiary controlled by Mr. B M Khaitan. However, George Williamson has categorically denied the allegations made in the report.

Duties and Taxes

Duties and taxes on tea in different producing countries (other than India) like Bangladesh, Indonesia, Kenya, Uganda, Tanzania, Malawai, Russian Federation, Mozambique, Mauritius, Taiwan, Japan Argantina etc are presented in Annexure 7.

World's Largest Tea Party

With a view to setting a record and finding place in the Guinness Book of Records, Hong Kong threw the world's largest tea party on the last Saturday of November, 1999 which was attended by 4,950 guests to brew pale green Chinese tea. Thousands of Hong Kongers gathered in small groups with colleagues, friends or family to sit cross-legged around tea pots and thimble cups on mats spread across a fair ground by the harbour. The Teaism Alliance Hong Kong, a charity organization founded by tea expert Yip Wai-Man, put together the events and auditor Price Waterhouse authenticated the number of participants.

US Tea Association Celebrating Centenary

The USA Tea Association is now more than one hundred year old. Born as the Tea Association of New York on January 5, 1899; it was rechristened as the Tea Association of the USA in 1912.

Training Workshops in Kenya

Mr. Surajit Ghose, Engineering Consultant, had just returned from Kenya having successfully conducted fifteen (15) days' of Training Workshops, between 7.12.1999 and 23.12.1999 "On The Theories & Practices of Maintenance Engineering and Management in Tea Factories" at all the twelve zones of the Kenya Tea Development Authority (KTDA) covering all their forty-five (45) tea factories. The Training Workshop was requested for by Mis KTDA to be organized by Mis Vikram Forging & Allied Industries Ltd., Kolkata the most leading developer and manufacturer of Tea Processing Machineries & Equipment since several decades in the world and a leading supplier of tea machines and spares in Kenya. The participants were all the Technicians and the Management personnel of each of the factories. The course materials for the Training package covered the following areas and 'were mainly prepared from the book "Guide to Maintenance Engineering & Management Practices in Tea" written by Mr. S Ghose.

General	Tea Processing M/Cs	Management
1. Machines	1. Withering Trough	1. Maintenance Management
2. Lubrication	2. Rotorvane	2. Energy Management
3. Bearings	3. CTC	
4. Drives	4. CTC Roller Sharpening	
	5. Fermenting M/c	
	6. Drier M/c	

A one day Training Workshop was also conducted at the Changwi Tea Factory of Mis Gteorge Williamson, Kenya, for the Technicians and Management personnel of four of their tea factories at the Kericho area.

First World Tea Festival In Russia

The First World Tea Festival which was organized in Moscow continued upto May 2003. Mr Vladimir Vo1kov, the Festival's Director ofInternational Programme said: "We believe that a global event connected with tea and the cultural tradition of various nations will draw worldwide attention to the cultural, historical, health-improving, aesthetic and economic value of tea". A number of tea related events were arranged. Pavillions for main tea producing and consuming countries, namely China, Japan, India, Sri Lanka, Kenya, England, Russia were set up.

Pakistan Trade Delegation In Sri Lanka

Sometime in the first week of October, 2002 a trade delegation led by the then Pakistan's Minister of Commerce, Industries and Production, Mr. Abdul Razak Dawood, visited Sri Lanka to finalise the Free Trade Agreement (FT A) between the two countries. The Pakistani Minister visited the country earlier for bilateral trade discussion when the two countries signed the framework agreement of free trade. Pakistan is the second large trading partner of Sri Lanka in the SAARC region. The Sri Lanka Government expects to increase exports to Pakistan and thereby to reduce its existing trade deficit. The agreement includes the free movement of goods between the two countries through the elimination of tariffs.

Publicity of Indian Tea In Russia

In a bid to regain the lost market in Russia, the Tea Board of India publicized Indian Tea through TV channels and popular dailies of that country. The campaign programme, at a cost of RS.6 crore, started on October 24, 2002. India's export to Russia has sharply declined in the last couple of years due to Russia's leaning on Sri Lanka. This situation has prompted India to launch massive campaign.

Iran Temporarily Bans Tea Import

Iran imposed ban on tea import to support the country's tea producers. Nemat Yavarzadeh, who heads the tea producers' association in northern Iran, said the embargo was meant to boost production of local producers and to help disposing of stock of tea. In the past also Iran imposed temporary ban on tea import as locally produced tea was lying unsold and cornered by the imported teas. However, the embargo could not alleviate the sufferings of the local producers, as smuggling of tea in the country was rampant. Iran produces around half of its domestic annual consumption leveling 100 million kgs of tea. Iran has gradually relaxed state control over tea trading in recent years as part of reforms to liberalise the industry.

Tea Becoming Favourite Beverage in China

Liu Qinjin, a prominent Chinese expert on tea and Professor with the Food Science Institute of South-West China Agricultural University, said that tea drinks are poised to become the new favourite type of beverage in China, and will compete with the dominant carbonated drinks in taking the lion's share of beverage market. Over the past few years, the growth of tea drinks market has exceeded 300 per cent, making it the third favourite beverage in the country, after carbonated drinks and bottled drinking water, The consumption of tea as a drink is developing fast in China.

Tetley to Sell Private Label to US Company

The Tetley group sold its private label tea business in the US to Harris Tea, an American company, for a consideration of $ 15 million. The proceeds of the sale were used to bring down Tata Tea's (Great Britain) debt-equity ratio, which stood at 1.8: 1. Tetley has firnled up distribution arrangements in Pakistan and Bangladesh. Though the global tea market was under pressure, during the 10-month period ended December 2001, Tetley's sale raised to 3 per cent. In the UK, though the tea market has grown by less than 1 per cent, Tetley has managed to increase its market share to 25 per cent, higher by 4 per cent over the last year. Its closest competitor in the UK, PG Tipps, has 23.5 per cent share of the market. Tetley has a 41 per cent share of the Canadian tea market, 11 per cent share of the US market and 16.2 per cent share of the Australian tea market.

ISO 9002 for Glasgow Estate

Glasgow Estate (selling mark Agra Ouvah), Sri Lanka, after pursuing Quality Management Systems Programme, has received the ISO 9002 certification from the Bureau Yeritas Quality International (BYQI). The certification from BYQI qualified Glasgow Tea Processing Centre to be included in the Department of Trade and Industry - Q.A. Register in London, which is the foremost Directory of Companies both in the UK and abroad. This inclusion allowed for Glasgow teas to be available throughout the world as a product which is processed to the highest possible quality standards of a "Food Factory". Establishing quality circles involving the active participation of staff along with the repair and replacement of machinery and upgrading of the factory brought about a tremendous change in the productivity and hygienic conditions of the factory. Glasgow estate is a property of Agrapatana Plantations Ltd for whom the Managing Agent is Lankan Tea and Rubber Plantations (Pvt) Ltd.

Tea in Italy Gaining Popularity

Attempts to grow tea in Italy go back almost two centuries to 1810 when some English residents tried to grow the herb in Sicily. There were further attempts in 1973 and 1981, but it is only recently that tea plants have actually managed to grow and survive in Italian soil. The quality of tea now being produced in Italy is far better than even before. One of the novelties is the production ofa black tea named "Te delle Tre Tigri" (Tea of the three tigers). This tea has a delicate and slightly aromatic flavour, judged by connoisseurs as really excellent. Its flavour is somewhere between Indian Darjeeling and Chinese Keemum.

Tea is becoming more and more popular in Italy. Italians tend to prefer light tea drunk with or without lemon, either hot or cold in the summer. All year round, supermarkets now sell ready-to-drink tea in bottles and cans as well as traditional packets of loose tea or tea bags. Compito tea, which has flavour somewhere between Indian Darjeeling and Chinese Keemun, will soon be available en the shelves of the local stores in Italy.

Eteatrade Launched Internet Auction

Eteatrade is a subsidiary of Plantation and General Investments Plc. Located in London, UK, which launched its first Internet auction recently. "A sizeable proportion of the industry does not need a complex network of representatives in every tea growing region. For them it is far more efficient and effective to log on to www.eteatrade.com from their office and buy tea directly from producers around the world", said Nick Hedges, eteatrade's Marketing Director. He further added that "From producers' perspective eteatrade is a first opportunity to expose their produce directly to a global market place. This will give many producers access to buyers that they have never been able to deal with directly before." Initially eteatrade is auctioning African tea, which accounts for nearly 14 per cent of the world's tea exports. Support from African producers is strong; the companies who have registered their intention to sell their tea through eteatrade account for around two-third of Africa's total tea production. Eteatrade has also received considerable response for their service from producers in China, India, and Sri Lanka. To meet the demand eteatrade will have logistic capabilities in Northern India and Colombo by the end ofthe year.

Sri Lanka Tea Exports (January, 2002)

Total exports inclusive of imports *Ire-exported* for the period January,2002 shows an increase of 1.19 million kgs or 5 *Al* per cent when compared with the same period last year. Bulk exports show a growth of *lA* million kgs or 10.9 per cent. Instant tea exports show a growth of 22.7 per cent. Total export earnings of RS.5.1 billion indicate a growth of 6.7 per cent. compared with the *RsA.8* billion earned in 2001. CIS continued to be the Number One market for Sri Lanka teas. Compared with the same period last year, exports to Syria, Iraq, Iran, Japan, UK, Saudi Arabia and Tunisia increased.

Mombasa Tea Auctions, 2006 : Quality

Dry weather during the first three months of the year adversely effected quality. In the second and third quarters, low temperatures and somewhat mixed weather resulted in improved but variable quality. Thereafter, unseasonably cold temperatures produced some attractive quality. With progressively drier weather and reports of lower crop in North-east India, the market was expected to be more buoyant. The average price for all growths opened the year at US $ 1.79 and by the end of the first quarter was US $ 1.80, dropping to US $ 1.76 at the end of June; the third quarter saw an average of US $ 1.75 and closed the year at US $ 1.78 - disappointing wh~n compared to the 2005 closing average of US $ 1.89. A feature of the year was the increasing dominance of Pakistan Blenders over the Bazaar and Afghan markets. Egypt, the Yemen and other Middle Eastern countries lent consistently good support and were often surprisingly quality conscious. The UK was active but generally selective. The Sudan bought with varying strength. Somalia purchased traditional cheaper Fannings types. There were line orders from South Africa and other markets.

In contrast to the excellent growing conditions of 2005 which created a record crop of 294 million kgs the weather in 2006 was mixed with extended periods of dry weather; low temperatures also inhibited growth. The 2006 crop figure is now estimated to be 248 million kgs approximately 16 per cent below the previous year. During the year, the Kenya Shilling weakened against the US Dollar opening the year at a rate of KShs 60.01 to a dollar and this rate increased to KS hs 62.77 in March with a further rise to KShs 70.57 in June; September averaged KShs 73.33, only strengthening slightly to close the year at

KShs 71.68. Although volumes in auction were lower, there was no corresponding correction in prices and 1999 could be considered only a satisfactory year for the Mombasa Auctions.

Chinese Tea Export Not Flourishing

Though Chinese authorities believe there is great potential for increased exports, large number of small scale factories springing up across the country with poor equipment and low quality control mechanisms have been inhibiting the realization of this potential. The quality of the product from such enterprises affects the reputation of the country's teas on world markets, and makes the market chaotic by the introduction of cutthroat competition. Improper management of tea fields deteriorates the environment and stands in the way ofproqucing quality tea and hence increased exports.

Vietnam Planning to Increase Export

Vietnam, the competitor of China in World Green Tea Market, whose tea output in 1997 dine to 45 million kg~and exports to 31 million kg as planned to export between 120 million kg; to 150 million kg of tea by the year 2010. The country has enlarged national tea area to 100000 hectares.

Sri lanka's National Safety Award: The following Estates managed by Maskeliya Plantations Limited won the Safety Awards in 1999 Forbes & Walker Tea Brokers (Pvt. Ltd), reported.

All Island Merit Award	Medium Scale	Poonagalla Tea Factory
Provincial Winners	Uva Province	Poonagalla Tea Factory
Provincial Winners up:	Central Province	StrathspeyTea Factory
Provincial Merit Award	Central Province	Brunswick Tea Factory

Maskeliya Plantations Limited was also adjudged the First Runner Up in the National Productivity Award in 1998 and is the sole award winner in the National Quality Award contest in 1999. This Company was also selected as the "Top 10" best-managed companies in Sri Lanka this year.

Tea Auctions on the Internet

According to Tea & Coffee Asia, the oldest tea broking firms in London, Thomson Lloyd & Ewart Ltd., hold tea auctions on the Internet. It may be mentioned that tea auctions in London was closed in 1998. Thomson Lloyd & Ewart introduced "Automated Tea Marketing On Line System". The website is www.atlJlostea com. Mr.Robin Harrison, Director of the company said, "it will mirror the traditional tea auction but on an electronic tea platform". In his opinion, the system will massively reduce the costs for a lot of producers.

HACCP Certification to Great Western Estate

Great Western Estate, Sri Lanka, a property of Talawakelle Plantations Limited, managed by Hayles Plantation Services Limited noted for its commitment to quality has been certified as an Estate that conforms to "Hazard Analysis and Critical Control Points System (HACCP) as set out by the Sri Lanka Standards Institution.

O-Cha Festival in Japan

The World O-Cha Festival, 2001 was held at Shizuoka, Japan between October 5 and 8 '2001. The festival was organized to provide the people of Japan and the world with latest information on tea. Tea festival included fairs, exhibition, seminars and international conference. Teas from 12 countries and 13 districts in Japan were displayed, which facilitated the visitors to taste and buy teas. About 31 rare variety of teas had also been exhibited in the Tea Fair. Besides, manufacturing machinery, tea producing machines, mechanical harvesters, sprayers and fertilizer applying equipment, packing machines, etc. were displayed. As the part of festival, around 350 products using tea were exhibited in "Am-Am" O-Cha Plaza. Tea candles, tea soba noodles, cosmetics made with Green Tea ingredients, bath salt, skin cream, T-shirts dyed with tea and bed sheets with antibacterial treatment were exhibited which indicated a broad scope in product diversification using tea.

First World Tea Festival In Russia

The First World Tea Festival which was organized in Moscow continued upto May, 2003. Mr. Vladimir Volkov, the Festival's Director of International Programme said: "We believe that a global event connected with tea and the cultural tradition of various nations will draw worldwide attention to the cultural, historical, health-improving, aesthetic and economic value of tea". A number of tea related events were arranged. Pavilions for main tea producing and consuming countries, namely China, Japan, India, Sri Lanka, Kenya, England, Russia were set up.

Pakistan Trade Delegation In Sri Lanka

Sometime in the first week of October, 2002 a trade delegation led by the then Pakistan's Minister of Commerce, Industries and Production, Mr. Abdul Razak Dawood, visited Sri Lanka to finalise the Free Trade Agreement (FTA) between the two countries. The Pakistani Minister visited the country earlier by bilateral trade discussion when the two countries signed the framework agreement of free trade. Pakistan is the second large trading partner of Sri Lanka in the SAARC region. The Sri Lanka Government expects to increase exports to Pakistan and thereby to reduce its existing trade deficit. The agreement includes the free movement of goods between the two countries through the elimination of tariffs.

Pakistan Preparing for Tea Production

Pakistan is getting prepared to produce tea. It has 500 acres under tea production, and in the; next five years the tea-area is likely to be increased to 1500 acres. North Western Province of the country has been selected for tea cultivation. The Managing Director cum owner of UK based Teacraft., Mr. Nigel Melican, is implementing the current project. Tea craft manufacturers various processing machinery for the Tea industry. It has purchased the rights for selling automated withering machined developed by the Tea Research Association at Tocklai in Assam.

Publicity of Indian Tea in Russia

In a bid to regain the lost market in Russia, the Tea Board of India to publicized Indian! Tea through TV channels and popular dailies of that country. The campaign programme, at a cost of RS.6 crore, started on October 24, 2002. India's export to Russia has sharply declined in the last couple of years due to Russia's leaning on Sri Lanka. This situation has prompted India to launch massive campaign.

15th Session of IGG on Tea

The Food and Agriculture Organisation (FAO) of the United

Nations Organisation (UNO) has informed that the 15th Session of the Inter Governmental Group (IGG) on Tea was held in Sri Lanka from August 19 to 20, 2003.

Trade Fair in Germany

For the third time, Anuga FoodTec brought Food Processing and Packaging Industry at a Trade Fair in Cologne, Germany. The Fair was held from April 8 to 11, 2003 and covered the sectors like (i) Process Technology, (ii) Packaging Technology, (iii) Food Safety and Quality Management, (iv) Enviromental Technology, (v) Bio-engineering, (vi) Informational Technology, (vii) Technological Process Materials & Ingredients and (viii) Services.

Liya Lifted Ban On Indian Tea

At the 8th Session of the Indo-Libyan Joint Commission, Libya lifted the ban on Indian te~. The minutes of the session indicates that NASCa, the buying Agency for Libya is now registering Indian companies which have applied for enlistment as a supplier of various commodities, including tea. According to an official release, both the countries agreed to increase the volume of bilateral trade. An exhaustive list of tradable goods was exchanged to enhance the two-way trade.

Indian Chai Achieves Major Success in UK Market

After stagnating for over a decade, Indian tea has achieved a major breakthrough in the UK market with the introduction of 100 per cent Indian tea product with Indian spices - Chai - by the leading British tea company Twinings. The success is the outcome of a series of campaigns launched by the London office of the Tea Board to popularize Indian Tea. The Twinings 'Chai' package mentions India as the origin of the tea and Nilgiri tea as th core of the blend. The Indian teas were displayed in popular departmental stores like the Harrods, Selfridges, Fortnum and Masons.

India is the largest tea producing country in the world but its share in the global market and particularly in the UK market is not commensurate with its potential. Although India exports 200 million kgs of tea annually, exports to UK stand about 20 million kg with an earnings of about 33 million pounds (Rs.230 crore) per annum. India's exports to the UK have been stagnant for over a decade now. According to market sources, Indian tea had a very dominant share in the UK market till the 1980s. Since then, India lost the market share to African tea primarily due to inconsistent export policy of the country and lack of long-term vision. During 1990-2000 the share of India's exports to the UK declined from 20 per cent to 14 per cent. But in the same period exports to Russia increased form 28 per cent to over 60 per cent. It was at this time the UK companies made good investment in African teas changing the blend to substitute Indian tea with African tea. As a result, the sophisticated tea consumers of the UK got accustomed to Kenyan blend. In this situation, introduction of Indian Chai in the UK market is a grand success .

George Promoted Indian Tea in USA

Indian tea was an unlikely promoter in the country's, the then Defence Minsiter, Mr. (George Fernandes, who impressed upon the US importers of the product as adoritly as he sold his views to America's political bosses. Mr. George Fernandes, who came to New York after his discussion in Washington in January, 2002 had visited and actyd as a compaigner for Indian tea. The Indian Deputy High Commission had arranged a meeting with the US tea importers for Mr. Fernandes, who formally presided over the gathering. But to every one's surprise, he turned out to be a connoisseur of tea.

Emergence of Other Countries as Major Suppliers and Improper Use of Funds for Development of Tea Industry

The emergence of Sri Lanka as a major supplier of tea (with lower cost of production) to the global market in 1965 found Ir.dia's share of world consumption declining from 45 per cent in 1958 to 18 per cent in 2004. In subsequent period, Kenya became a sizeable exporter followed by other East African and Asian countries including China. This situation limited prospects of common tea from India which account for over 60 per cent of country's production. The situation was compounded in 1990s by the uncertainity of the Indian tea's over-dependent Russian market following disintegration of the USSR. What went wrong on the Indian scene? Various reasons are cited and it would be prudent to highlight one of the aspects. A spokesman of the Kolkata-based United Bank of India which has fairly large accounts of tea producers in North-East India indicated that the funds allotted to the borrowers against hypothecation of tea crop were not being properly utilized towards development (not applicable to all) of the respective tea estates. In course of time, the lended sum turned out to be unproductive or became non-performing assets, as known in banking parlance. When the cumulative liabilities of the producers mounted, the banks exerted pressure on the former to sell the properties to clear the dues which ran into crores of rupees .

Sri Lankan Tea Import Permitted

Sometime in February, 2000 India and Sri Lanka agreed to operationalise the free trade pact that provides for removing duty and providing preferential access on a range of items before March, 2000. Among the items tea is also included. India permits import of Sri Lankan tea to the extent of 15 m. kgs per annum with a fixed tariff preference of 50 per cent.

Tata Tea Plans Retail Outlets

Tata Tea opened retail outlets for the promotion of Tetley in the premium category with the expertise of Barista outlets. While iced tea is another product rolled out by Tata Tea variants rolled under Tetley were flavoured tea and ready-to-drink mixes. Tata Tea launched Tetley in India to take on brands such as Taj Mahal Tea, Society Tea and Wagh Bakri. 'There has been tightened advertising activity in anticipation of the launch of Tetley. You are about to witness a very exciting combat in the tea industry. We are launching at a time when the industry is under severe pressure," said Mr. Krishna Kumar, the Vice-Chairman of Tata Tea.

Tea Board Office at London

The Tea Board has been contending for some time that it did a good job in promoting the sale of Indian Tea at the Harrods exhibition in London. But, a programme on tea management sponsored by the London-based Commonwealth Secretariat in 2001 observed that Harrods hardly represented the buying place for the common British. Teas went up for sale at Harrods for any price equivalent of RS.l ,000 a kg and most Indian teas could not qualify for a sale through the Harrods departmental stores. The worst point was that Harrdos fair etc exhausted almost half the total budget of the London office of the Tea Board. Therefore, practically, nothing was left for the office to promote the Indian tea in the UK or the other centers coming under its jurisdiction. That is why, it become difficult to see a good advertisement on Indian tea anywhere in the UK. Nor, was it possible to see the Indian teas figuring prominently in the various fairs around the region. The Tea Board, for instance, was a conspicuous absentee at the world's largest food ingredient exhibition, FI Europe 2001, held in London, even as Sri Lanka promoted its various forms of teas including organic teas. That is why, Indian tea and the London Tea Board were not seen at the right places like the Wimbledon tennis or the L~rds cricket tourney. So, it is a case of Indian Tea Board having a Director of Tea Promotion (DTP) in London and still not seen at the right places to promote the Indian tea. The Government of India, particularly the Commerce Minster, should realize that tying up the hands of the DTP helps none, least of the Indian tea industry.

Director's of Tea Promotion Office, London, located at High Rising "*Indian House*":

The indifference shown by the Government to put the Tea Board Office in London in the right perspective is already costing heavily. For instance, none of the dozen long time residents of London whom Shri P S Sundar, the Special Correspondent asked to guide him to the Tea Board Office, could, by themselves, locate the office. They referred to the Telephone Directory and asked the Indian High Commissioner's Office etc. The truth was that this office is located on one of the floors of the high rising "India House" which houses the office of the High Commissioner. So, all the formalities for entry to the High Commissioner's office are followed leaving an impression that one is entering the department of yet another Indian bureaucracy, not a commodity promotion office. Besides, there is no name Board for the Tea Board Office.

DTP's Office has Contingency Staff: Although the DTP is an IAS officer, he is not adequately staffed. He has only contingency staff paid a low salary with a mandatory technical break in service every three months. Therefore, there is neither loyalty nor continuity in the staff strength. Moreover, the DTP has no place to hold public relations meet. Nor are there good materials to highlight Indian teas or tea packets. Many a time, the guests are not even provided with a cup of tea as a matter of hospitality in the Tea Board Office. After all, the DTP has power to spend only 74 pound and for expense above this, he has to seek specific permission taking almost a month. Therefore, with half the budget going in for the in-store promotion at Harrods, the London office does not spend any money for media publicity, product or logo promotion or the development of market intelligence. It is spending less than one per cent of its total budget on buyer-seller meets and tea events.

UK Market is too Important to India: For all this, the UK market is too important to India to be ignored. For one, it is the world's second largest tea importer with a high per capita consumption of 2.7 kg, the consumption growing at 1 per cent per annum. For another, there has been some increase in the demand for the Indian teas of late, despite the Tea Board office's inability to promote the teas adequately, which should enable the country to find a good berth for some varieties of its teas. Now the UK imports around 150 million kg annually, but India supplies only 20 million kg fetching foreign exchange of around 33 million pound, Kenya is the largest supplier with a share of around 43 per cent and the British look to the Indian teas only when the Kenyan supplies dry up. On the other hand, the UK has a specific market for the PF/PD CTC grades for which India is looking for buyers. Again, while Indian teas are sold for an average price of 1.5 pound a kg, Sri Lankan teas fetch 1.6 pounds and Kenya 1.65 pounds. So, India should know to encash on this price advantage.

UK Imports and Exports after Value Addition: Another sphere for entry is the re-export segment. The UK imports teas, on an average, price of 1.3 pound a kg, but exports them after value addition, at 5 pounds a kg. These tea, branded and attractively packed, are sold to France, Canada, Ireland and the UAB. Presently, people drink tea in the UK thinking it from India. Some 10 brands are popular, but six of them are well known. Tetley and VDB brands account for 25 per cent of the UK market each, Premier 8 per cent, Taylors 5 per cent and Twinning 3 per cent. However, they do not disclose the country of origin for the teas. Thus, there is a definite need to promote the Indian tea highlighting its strengths, but for this, the London office of the Tea Board should be upgraded. It should be adequately staffed, duly empowered to carry a corporate identity and build brand equity for the Indian teas. It should become the hub of information on Indian teas. As of now, it is grossly under-equipped to face the challenge

Generic Promotion within the Country and Outside Well

It is not only the generic promotion within the country, but outside as well that there is a lot of lacuna. As the Food Ingredients Europe 2001 exhibition held in London, for instance, while Sri Lanka displayed its teas, the Indian Tea Board did not show any interest despite it holding a Tea Promotion Office in London. Sri Lanka even displayed its organic teas and started attracting importers from Germany and parts of Europe at the fair. It will do a lot good to the Indian tea to utilize all possible channel like the Food Ingredient Fairs to put up whatever role as deemed fit and possible. On the campaign itself, the impact has been highly negligible. A sporadic full page ad on a particular week day in some select newspapers alone cannot help much. A lot of professional work has to go into this campaign programme so that the consumers are made to drink the Indian tea for its health benefits.

Conclusion

To strengthen the tea industry and face with other competitions there is a need to have a holistic approaches. All sectors of tea i.e. Producers Association manufacturers Association, Tea Board, Research Institutes (11 PM, TRA, UPASI, NTRF etc), Govt. of India may dortail a detailed plan which is based on SMART (Specific, Measureable, Attainable, Reasonable and Time Bound) principles. That may generate a momentum in the growth process. Further, face to face interface is required to sort out the burning issues.

Chapter 13

The Panacea of All Ills

Introduction

The reasons for the widespread popularity of tea are numerous. Some attribute it to custom while others to habit, tradition or belief. In many regions of China where water generally contains harmful bacteria, tea is considered a safe drink. In some parts of the world, tea is the panacea for all ills from common cold to gout and lumbago. In the United Kingdom, some believe that the country's cold climate is the reason for its popularity. But the English weather cannot be the essential reason for its popularity because tea is equally popular in the hot and dry climates of West Asia, Australia and India. According to Mr. C.R.Harler, an expert, tea is consumed chiefly for its stimulation of the nervous and muscul systems which induces a state of consciousness mid-way between gentle excitement and easy repose. It is not drunk on account of its food value for it is merely an auxiliary food as are many other beverages, A cup of tea is said to take away 50 times as much heat as it brings to us. History has made a significant contribution to the popularity of tea. It became as household word in England, thanks to the East India Company. The Dutch drink tea for similar reasons. The Booston Tea Party, which sparked off the American War of Independence, had a significant effect on the consumption of tea in USA. From being a favourite American drink, tea became a hated symbol of oppression. To boycott tea was the mark of the American patriotism and ever since December 16,1773, the night of the Boston Tea Party, the Americans have drunk more coffee than tea. To an Iranian, tea is a status symbol. In an Iranian family, prior to being served to guests, tea is displayed, depending upon the host's prosperity, on a gold, silver or a chin a platter, and then sent back to the kitchen for brewing.

The Japanese are apparently more concerned with the ritual rather than the actual tea itself. The Japanese tea ceremony known as "Chinoyu" was introduced around 700 A.D. from China but it became popular from the early 14th century. Chinoyu is something which is more than a refined form of taking refreshment. Its purpose and essence, according to a Japanese source, is difficult to express in words. It has played an important role in the artistic life of the Japanese people. As an aesthetic pursuit, it involves the appreciation of the room in which it is held, the garden attached to the room, the utensils used in serving tea and the decor of the setting, including the flower arrangement. The development of Japan's architecture, landscape, gardening, ceramics and the floral arts owe a great deal to the tea ceremony. The spirit of Chinoyu, representing the beauty of studied simplicity and harmony with nature, has moulded the basis of these traditional forms of Japanese culture. As a result, it is a rather common practice for young ladies to take lessons in art of the tea ceremony before marriage in order to cultivate the poise and refinement stemiming from Chinoyu etiquette.

Many doctors believe that tea drinking helps in keeping better health.

UK Tea Convention- Health Benefits of Tea

The first UK tea convention was held in 1990. The second UK tea convention was held at Jersey-channel Islands, between 17th and 20th May, 1993. Twenty-eight countries were represent and 275 delegates participated. It has been claimed that tea is the whole-some healthy beverage.

Tea is rich is vitamins and minerals as shown in the following two tables :

Table 13.1 Content of Black Tea B- Vitamin Group

Vitamin	G/100g leaf	g/cup	Percentage daily requirement from cup of tea
Thiamine	135	2.3	0.8
Riboflavin	1266	21.5	5.7
Niacin	75.00	127.5	5.2
Folic Acid	76	1.3	6-13
Pantothenic Acid	1260	21.4	1.46
Biotin	82.6	1.4	3.1

Source - The Assam Review and Tea News, May 1993

Table-13.2 Content of Black Tea Principal Minerals

Mineral	Daily intake from 5-6 cups of tea (mg)	Percentage requirement from 5-6 cups
Potassium	982.0	25
Manganese	1.8	45
Magnesium	17.5	5
Copper	0.17	7
Zinc	2.4	10
Sodium	5.4	1

Source-The Assam Review and Tea News, May 1993

Polyphenols are abundant in tea. Polyphenols in tea have helped in curing cancer. Also, research has shown there is link between higher levels of tea consumption and lower levels of cholesterol. The claim that "Tea is the Wholesome Healthy Beverage" suggested by history, hinted at by analytical evidence, and supported by the fact that over half the world's population drinks the beverage is now being confirmed by a variety of scientific experiments.

Important Massage of the UK Tea Convention Tea as Health

The most important message of the UK Tea Convention was that tea should be promoted as a healthy drink. The convention agreed that the future possibilities for the emerging research evidence on the health benefits of tea consumption were exciting and the timing of the research efforts was appropriate. To summarise :

1. Given the fact that the population is aging and health care budgets are projected to escalate, governments will place increasing priority on the identification and dissemination of behavioural modifications which can reduce the risk of developing chronic degenerative diseases, notably heart disease and cancer.
2. There is increasing evidence that diet can influence the risk of these diseases and this recognition in the formulation of national nutritional recommendations and dietary guidelines can be expected.
3. The consumer is increasingly becoming aware of the association between diet and the development of heart diseases and cancer and there is evidence that consumers are responding to this information.
4. The potential protective effect of tea polyphenols can be presented within the context of a substantiated and credible platform, i.e.. that of antioxidants.
5. Efforts must be taken to disseminate information in a reliable and cautious manner and through appropriate channels, i.e. scientific journals first.
    a) Caution must be exercised not to overextend the interpretation of scientific evidence.
    b) The message should recognise the fact that tea is not the only food which contains antihelix dants; rather should highlight the fact that tea is an appropriate choice within a healthy diet and lifestyle context.

At present, preliminary evidence suggests that tea may have many potential positive health benefits; hopefully future research on the possible protective effects of black tea consumption will continue to be positive. Only time will tell and the outcome of the proposed research must be patiently awaited. In the meantime, an International Research Programme has been funded by the United Kingdom. United States and Canada to look further into the effects of black tea on cancer and cardiovascular diseases.

The United States Tea Association's Attempt To Scientifically Document Tea As Good For Health

The United States Tea Association has for several years been attempting to scientifically document the traditionally held belief that tea is good for health. Health issues have become of more interest in the USA, as they are in other parts of the world, and consumers are becoming increasingly concerned about the effects the foods they eat may have on their health. The Food Marketing Institute in 1989, conducted a study. The findings of the study stated that 99 per cent of consumers surveyed were either "very" or "somewhat a concerned" about the health and nutritional values of the food they bought. The Government, too, has shown more concern in various nutritional areas and the food and Drug Administration has explored new approaches to nutritional labelling that will be more meaningful to consumers addition, significant improvements to consumers' nutritional guidelines and truth in advertising guidelines were made. Such activities obviously have significance for our tea industry in developing and promoting any health benefits of tea.

With these expanding concerns about food and health, the International Agency for Research on Cancer, which evaluated environmental and food chemicals for possible carcinogens and cancer-causing agents, had convened a group of 21 world experts to review all of the published literature on tea, coffee and look for possible carcinogenicity. It also reviewed several of the significant components of these beverages-caffeine, theophylline, theobromine—present in tea and methylglyoxal found in coffee. Tea received a very favourable rating on their scale of 1 to 4. With rating "1" being definite carcinogenic, tea was rated "3" indicating no known data to denote any carcinogenicity. In addition, caffeine, theophylline and theobromine were also rated "3". Another major concern for many Americans is the presence of pesticides in food with the mind, the US Tea Association authorised a screening of pesticide resides in tea. Forty-one samples from ten producing countries were analysed, each in proportion to their share of the US market. The majority of the samples were clear and, overall, showed a lower favourable trend compared to previously reported results. This was especially true of the teas from China which showed DDT residue 95 per cent lower than those of 15 years earlier.

Scientific Advisory Panel on Health Benefit of Tea

In 1987 the United States Tea Association formed a 4-number Scientific Advisory Panel having expertise in nutrition, heart diseases, cancer and pharmacology, to investigate the health benefits of tea and to review all available credible research on tea. The Panel endorsed modest health claims and of their suggestions the USTA published a paper and distributed it to all health professionals stressing the need for proper fluid balance and while recognising water as the quickest and most readily available fluid replacement, endorsing tea as an alternative because of absence of harm in it. The panel also found some indication that tea consumption may have potential ability to lower blood cholesterol and stated that tea may be found to have substantial health benefits if further tests were conducted. Funds were approved for an international tea symposium held in early 1991 under the auspices of the New York Academy of Science with scientists from around the world invited to present papers on the health benefits of tea, with emphasis on cholesterol reduction and cancer prevention. The benefits to the consumer and to the world tea industry of such a symposium was significant.

Establishment United Nations Common Fund

Of greater significance for the tea industry is the creation of a $270 million United National Common Fund for commodities. This Fund, established in 1989, started operating from 1990. At the FAO meeting in Rome in 1989, the Secretariat, enthused by the UK Health Benefits of tea initiative, encouraged the tea industry to apply to the Fund for monies stating that the Health Benefits concept was exactly the type of project to receive a favourable hearing. The United States Tea Association believes that the best way to approach the Common Fund and the FAO is on team basis comprising both producing and importing countries. The United Kingdom Tea Association indicated its support to this approach and in turn received tacit encouragement from the Ministry of Agriculture, Fisheries and Food. Such an approach provided an opportunity for the international tea community, working together, to apply for funds for research on larger-scale and to publicise the result responsibly and credibly. It also appraised the beneficial aspects for our industry throughout the world. Credible and responsible health claims for tea have the potential to increase sales of our product faster than any other vehicle. We ask for the help and encouragement from the tea industry at large in an effort which has an inherent potential to usher in an era of growth for us all.

Healthy Drinks Report-Tea The Most Popular Drink

Our perceptions of what is healthy are not far from the truth, but are not wholly correct. An examination of our actual behaviour reveals that where health is concerned, we are led by guilt reduction rather than any specific health motivation. Dietary guidelines appear to have made some impact, although overall, the there is a tendency towards acceptable "alternatives". In a time of increasing consumer confusion and often inadequate labelling in the drinks area, it is simpler of choose a healthy drink based on what it does not contain. Fluid is a lubricant fuel the body needs like an engine needs oil, and this years long hot summer in Britain highlighted the need to maintain a healthy fluid balance in the body. A survey report reveals that one in four respondents have an insufficient fluid intake. It appears that people are simply not aware just how much fluid should be consumed by the average individual to keep the body healthy.

"You can never drink too many fluids," says Vincent Marks, Professor of Biochemistry at the University of Surrey. This may sound like a sweeping statement, in that certain fluids such as alcohol should never be taken in excess. However, it is generally true that the more one drinks, the better it is for one's health-unless one is already sick from some illness such as kidney or heart disease. On an average, the minimum amount of water one needs each day to function properly is 1.75 litres (approximately 3 pints) and comes from food, drink, and as a by-product of metabolism of food to provide energy within the body. The minimum amount one needs to drink each day is 1 litre (1.75 pints). The body naturally eliminates at least 1.2 litre (2 pints) of water daily and there is no way in which one can prevent this. This is termed an obligatory loss. It is very important that we consume this amount of fluid each day as a minimum. Professor Marks points out, "The amount of total fluid lost daily varies enormously, from the minimum of 1.1 litre to a maximum 2.5 litres."

The amount of fluid needed varies from person to person who are older, overweight, working or living in an air-conditioned environment people who exercise more will need more fluid," he continues. "In general, the more fluid we lose, the more we need to take in." As fluid intake increases, urine volume increases and is more dilute. The more dilute the urine passed the better, as highly concentrated urine pass infrequently can lead to medical problems such as kidney stones and cystitis. As one drinks more, the extra fluid passing through the body helps to wash out waste products.

So the message is clear,one should drink a lot of fluids, particularly after exercising, when one really should think about putting back the water one has lost. Make sure to take in the right kind of fluid-tea is an excellent example as, next to water, it is one of the healthiest drinks around and contains no calories other than those one may add milk or sugar to suit one's own taste. The good news arising from the Healthy Drinks Report is that tea is the most popular drink the world over and by drinking one's favourite drink, one can keep up the fuid intake in one of the healthiest ways.

Tea Minimises Alzheimer's' disease

Xu Chang He, a medical chemist at the Shanghai Institute of Materia Medica, China observed from a research study that tea brewed from the leaves of *Huperzia serrata* could prove an invigorating drink for those affected by Alzheimer's Disease (AD). The symptoms of AD—progressive loss of memory and reasoning power—though resemble the normal process of aging are not quantitatively to the same between early stages of AD and minor event of forget-fullness typical of old age. The genetic organism of the disease have been traced to chromesome 19 recently. Scientists have reported very low levels of acetylcholine an important neurotransmitter involved in memory and learning, in the brain tissues. It is believed that Huperzine-A has the capacity to stand for acetylcholine. And it has been reported that a Chinese team isolated an active ingredient Huperzine-A from tea leaves but the amount of this ingredient in tea leaves is very little, of course.

Tea and Health

Tea has come a long way ever since the father of modern chemistry in India, Sir P.C. Roy, FRS, equated tea drinking with the drinking of poison. No doubt the great scientist was moved in making this statement more out of nationalistic urge as tea once was a symbol of imperial power and repression. Despite Sir P.C. Roy's reservations, tea has warmed its way into the hearts of millions, and it can be said euphemistically that taste of tea has indeed withstood the test of time. Today tea is an integral part of the personal life and social milieu of a large segment of populace the world over, and to cap it all, more and more people are getting intitiated into the charming world of tea drinking. But why this unique phenomenon? No doubt tea is the cheapest drink anywhere in the world, but in ultimate analysis, is it not the cup that cheers that counts the most? Undoubtedly, tea is a stimulant of a very high order, invigorating the body and mind, apart from energizing the drinker. No other beverage works the wonder the way tea does, and with it, if aroma or fragrance component of tea is considered, tea would stand head and shoulder above any other beverage. What is in there tea that permeates as an overriding influence in human system? The answer obviously is the in chemical compounds some 400 of them in the last count— in the leaves. Some of these compounds have been identified their structures enunciated, but it is difficult to partition them as causal chemicals for aroma or stimulants. Possibly interactions between various compounds, rather than their individual functions, are of importance but we really do not know what is happening here.

Medicinal Properties

The intriguing part of the story is that some of these compounds are supposed to have medicinal properties as well. Polyphenols—an interesting group of compounds—are of particular importance in this context in various forms, they and their derivatives have the attributes to cure a wide range of human maladies, from caries to cancer and from diarrhoea to dichotomy of heart. Nothing, of course , could be better than have a cup that cheers and cures as well. But in reality, simple drinking does not ensure effective medication the way standard medicines do. The need, therefore, is to identify and isolate the pharancologically important compounds and test their efficasies clinically against specific diseases, leaving the drinking part alone. In a classical investigation in China, patients suffering from fibrogenesis of heart were claimed to have been cured by feeding them with pigments isolated from green tea. Such studies are, however, few because bulk of the evidence is based on experiments involving laboratory animals and green teas which could retain some of the suspected pharmacological compounds in situ because of non-disruption of cells during processing. Whether under the rigours of rolling black teas could retain the pharnacologically important compounds in the disrupted cells is worth knowing. There is of course the need for well planned clinical investigations using these compounds from black tea, but after pre-testing with laboratory animals. Little at present is documented of the probable and possible medicinal effects of black teas except for their stimulating properties.

An area unexplored is whether the pluckable shoots are the only repositories for the beneficial compounds. What about the maintenance foliage and green branches—do they have or have not these compounds? It would be interesting to know if these compounds get concentrated more in the buas. Also if tea is not plucked, i.e., allowed to grow freely flower and seed, will their leaves retain the pharnacologically active compounds at the same level as the pluckable shoots are supposed to have?

Tea has its complements of bad compounds as well if one were to go by the findings published sometime back in the famous British science journal, *Nature.*

They elaborate on the negative aspects of tea drinking based on data at best subjective and at worst confounded. There have also been subtle hints about possible carcinogenic effects of tea! All these may not withstand the rigrous of scientific scrutifiny, but can resurrect the spirit of Sir P.C. Roy, unless such notions are scientifically dispelled.

An objective, balanced and realistic appraisal of the health benefits of tea drinking, as opposed to evaluation of tea compounds of pharmacological importance, is therefore of primary importance. But in the process it has to be ensured that tea does not turn into a medicinal plant, and a cup of tea into a cup full of medicines.

Physiological and Pharmacological Effects of *Camellia Sinuses*

New York-medical Researchers and health professionals representing a variety of specialities attended a two-day symposium on the health benefits of tea, the first international scientific conference ever held on this subject. Speakers included scientists from the United States, Japan, China, Norway and British Columbia, who described a growing body of research on potential protective effects of tea in the development of cancer and cardiovascular diseases. In addition, the role of tea in fluid balance and renal diseases was addressed. "This is an interesting area that hasn't been looked at previously a clinical and public health nutrition perspective," said George Christakis, M.D., M.P.H., the conference chairman. "When you consider that besides water, tea is that most widely consumed beverage in the world, it becomes clear that the potential public health implications might be enormous."

Among the presentations at the tea symposium were animal experiments by Dr. A.H. Conney of Rutgers University and Dr. Hirota Fujiki of the National Cancer Centre Research Institute, Tokyo, suggesting that green tea might be protective against cancer.

In Dr. Fujiki's studies, epigallocatechingallate (EGCG) (a substance in green tea) inhibited the formation of skin tumours in mice. In these experiments the mice had been exposed to tumour promoters typical of those that humans commonly encounter in everyday life. Dr. Conney and his colleagues found that administration of green tea to mice protected them from skin tumors caused by exposure to ultra violet light. EGCG is one of a class of chemicals called catechin.

John Weisburger, Ph.D., (hc), chairing of the session on carcinogenesis, commented that although much more research was needed, these preliminary animal results were an encouraging sign that yet another common foodstuff may have unsuspected benefits in huma/n health.

Henry Ginsberg, M.D., who chaired of the session on cardiovascular diseasee, reviewed the evidence of association between tea and serum cholesterol levels.

From the epidemiologic data and the few clinical studies available, the evidence is strong that tea drinking is not associated with increased plasma cholesterol levels. There is also suggestive evidence that tea may lower cholesterol levels under certain experimental conditions," he said. Dr. Ginsberg described the existing epidemiological and clinical data as "intriguing." However, he cautioned that any cholesterol lowering effect of tea remained to be proved. Dr. Yukihiko Hara of the Mitsui Noria Company, Japan, discussed experiments in which tea cachines including EGCG, reduced plasma total cholesterol and LDL cholestral in rats. In another set of experiments, catechins were able to lower blood pressure in rats and the life span of stroke-prone animals was extended by supplementing with catechins. Dr. Ginsberg advised caution in interpreting these results because "rate and mice are poor models of atherosclerosis and hyperlipidaemia" and said future research needed to determine the effects of tea in human atherosclerosis.

The conference entitled " Physiological and Pharmacological Effects of *Camellia Siensis* (Tea)," was organised by the American Health Foundation, the Tea Council of the U.S.A. and the Tea Association of the U.S.A. It was organised to raise professional awareness of the potential health benefits of tea and to encourage additional research in this area.

Tea Is A Herbal Drink

Tea is more than just a pleasant beverage. It provides essential minerals, vitamins and possibly it has therapeutic value. Tea aids digestion and the body's fluid balance. It has some action on atherosclerosis. Caffeeine in tea possibly has both good and bad side of it. Russian, Chinese and the Japanese have recognised the therapeutic value of tea. Although many claims are coming to light on the beneficial effects of tea. Further in depth research is required.

The details of the health aspests of tea are presented below:

Plain Type

1. *Anti-inflammatory action* :-Natarajan et al reported that theaflavins and the arubigin from black tea have a pronounced antagonistic action on bradykin which are secreted in vivo during certain inflammatory responses. The same authors have also reported an antispasmodic action against prostaglandins. The efficiency of tea extract was found to decrease as the oxidised polyphenol content increased at the expense of flavonoids. In this regard Indian teas had less of effect than the green teas. In view of this the Russians have modified their processing technology to increase the flavonoid content of some of their teas .
2. *Some recent work on the health effect of tea* : Given below are some of the recent findings of the Chinese, Japanese and American research workers on the beneficial effects of tea.
3. *Antimutagenic and carcinogenic effects of tea* : Green tea polyphenols are strong oxidants. The crude extracts of both green and black teas inhibited MNNG (N-methy N-nitrosoguanidine) induced mutagenecity in *E. coli, in vitro*. Green tea polyphenols exhibited tumor genic activity of induced skin cancers by DBNA (dimethylbena) (a) anthracene: TPA, according to the research workers at the Chinese Academy of Medical Sciences, Beijing, China.

   A bio-antimutagen isolated from Japanese tea reduced high mutations due to altered DNA-polymase-III in a mutator strain of *Bascillus subtitles*. Chemical studies showed that the factor according to Kada *et al* was epigallocatechingallate. Antimutagenic and anti-promoting effect of tea extracts was investigated both stages of initiation and promotion of carcinogenesis in vitro by Nakamura et al at the University of Shizuoka, Japan. Crude extracts of tea and some of its ingredients inhibited the MNNG-induced mutagenecity at doses of 1 mg per plate.
4. *Lung neoplasia*: Wu Ruirong and others of the Department of Biochemis try, Fuzhow, China have reported that lung neoplasia induced by urehane is reduced in animals treated with some

types of tea like oolong tea. Histological lung neoplasia comes under adenocarcinoma.

5. *Anti-tumor activity:* The death rate from stomach cancer in both males and females in Shizuoka prefecture is markedly lower than in the average Japanese people. People here drink lot of green tea. Standard Mortality Ratio (SMR) revealed statistically significant correlation as assessed by poison distribution with the tea drinking habit. Laboratory studies also revealed inhibitory effect of green tea extracts on mouse sarcoma 180. This is particularly so with green polyphenols which could be due to (i) inhibition of the ultimate carcinogen formation, (ii) modulation of the metabolism of the initiating agent, (iii) direct interaction of the electrophillic ultimate careinogenic metabolite, (iv) scavenging and free radicals, (v) inhibition of ornithine decarboxylase activity and (vi) inhibition in the covalent binding of carcinogen to DNA.
6. *Blocking of endogenous nitrosamine*: Some of the varieties of tea containing higher quantities of Vitamin C, according to the research workers, were found to block synthesis of endogenous nitro-samines which are considered carcinogenic. Polyphenols, especially catechins in tea, also show blocking activity. Results of experiments on human volunteers showed that some of the teas could effectively block the synthesis of endogenous nitrosamines of humans.
7. *Inhibition of heptocarcino genesis induced by aflatoxins:* Work done in China has shown that green tea, possesses reasonable inhibitory activity on the AFBI carcinogenesis when tested for GT (r-glutamyltranspeptidase) positive heptocelluarl foci.
8. *Tea catechins and cardiovascular conditions:* Work has been reported at a recent seminar organised in China on the effects of tea catechins on atherosclerosis and the results indicate that the tea flavonoids act as anti coagulants and inhibit rabbit platelet aggregation induced by ADP. Rabbits fed with tea flavonoids showed normal liver in spite of their being given high doses of cholesterol. The total lipid decreased and the concentration of lipoprotein also decreased. Slides of the plaque revealed disappearance of normal endothelial cells and hyperplasia of

fibrous tissues. Control groups exhibited only slight hyperplasia of fibrous tissue. Work done in China has also shown that there is clinical evidence of reduction of serum cholesterol triglyceride in animals treated with tea liquor. Tea flavonoids possessed anti-coagulation activity and inhibited platelet aggregation. Tea pigments in clinical tests were found to have notable effect in reducing fibrinogen in cardiovascualr diseases in experimental animals.

9. *Tea and hypertension*: In Japan, work done with a particular type of anaerobically treated tea called gabarone tea was shown to be good on the blood pressure of spontaneously hypertensive rats. This atributed to gamma aminobutyric acid (GABA). The hypotensive effects of tea disappeared when be animals returned to fresh water intake. Green tea catechins (EGCG) epigallocatechingallate was found to have profound effect on lipid metabolism, according to the work at Shizuoka University. Tea catechins also lowered cholesterol. There is also evidence that there is reduction in the triglyceride levels. There is an indication that successive administration of tea could situate the degradation of triglyceride in the adipose tissue, thereby reducing the weight. Recent work in Japan indicates that dimeric compounds, particularly theaflavins produced oxidatively in the manufacture of black tea inhibited angiotensin 1 covorting enzyme.
10. *Tea pigments*: work in the Chinese Hangzhou Medical University has shown that tea pigments have action on atherosclerosis and promoted fibrinolysis in rabbits. There is also indication that these decreased platelet aggregation and reduced proliferation of smooth muscle cells of iorta in culture. No side effects were noticed in human subjects treated with 250 mg of tea pigments daily for two months, administered orally.
11. *Selenium content of tea:* There are reports that selenium content, when found high in tea, had many special qualities. There have been correlations particularly with tea having high selenium content and less incidence of cancer through interpolative studies in Japan.
12. *Prevention of caries:* Work done both in China and Japan has

shown that toothpaste containing 2 per cent of tea infusion that was specially prepared from low grade tea in high fluorine areas and weas added with the natural pigment for the improvement of colour, prevented caries. Work done on children and in wistar rats has shown that tea toothpaste as good as monofluorophosphate 0.7 per cent toothpaste and it is very likely that the tea polyphenols suppressed the proliferation of carries producing bacteria. Experiments indicate that the content of tea polyphenols in 2 per cent tea infusion containing toothpaste is higher than the minimum bacteria suppressing concentration.

To sum up tea is more than just a pleasant beverage. It provides essential minerals, vitamins and possibly it has therapeutic value. Tea aids digestion and the body's fluid balance. It has some action on ather sclerosis. Caffeine in tea possibly has both good and bad side of it. Russian, Chinese and the Japanese have recognised the therapeutic value of tea. Although many claims are coming to light on the beneficial effects of tea further in depth work is required.

Green Tea's Health Benefits

Writing in the World Coffee & Tea (June 1991) Mr. J. G. Wells stated that the Chinese have been saying for centuries that green tea is good for health and since they consume much of the green tea in the world—almost 20 percent of global production—they have put their belief into practice. Now there is growing scientific evidence to suggest green tea is a protective agent against a surprisingly long list of ailments. Further, preliminary experimental work has verified that green tea has emerged as a practical and effective weapon against a number of chronic ailments. Various studies indicated that green tea contains substances that have the effect of lowering blood pressure and cholesterol, stabilise blood sugar, kill decay-causing bacteria, block the action of many carcinogens and even inhibit the growth of cancerous tumors.

If the preliminary research findings can be verified, marketing campaigns for green tea would be made a great deal easier, and an emphasis on the health properties of tea could give a big boost to tea consumption around the world.

Many of the possible health benefits from tea have been identified as a result of studies conducted in laboratory animals and cell cultures. Most of the research has been focused on the individual constituents of tea. In a number of research studies using laboratory animals, polyphenls, the prime biologicially active ingredients of tea, have been shown to help inhibit the activation of some cancer-causing chemicals, thus preventing these agents from transforming normal cells into cancer cells.

Dr. Fung Lung Chung of the American Health Foundation said that micing given green tea or one of the polyphenols derived from it in their supplies of drinking water developed fewer lung tumors after being exposed to a cancer-causing nitrosamine from tobacco smoke. Researchers working with laboralory animals also reported beneficial effects of green tea extracts in protecting arteries against the damage caused by high-fat diets, in inhibiting the proliferation of precancerous cells and in preventing skin cancer. Dr. Junshi Chen of the Chinese Academy of Preventive Medicine in Beijing showed in studies on rats exposed to a different nitrosamine that two Chinese speciality teas—Fujian Oolong and Jasmine—inhibited the development of esophageal tumors. Dr. Yukihiko, a food scientist with Mitsu. Norin Coin Fujida City, Japan, said 25 years of research with laboratory animals had served to persuade him that tea is a health-promoting and life-prolonging beverage. It is also interesting to observe that the Japanese like the Chineses, are large consumers of tea and have low death rates from cancers of all types.

Cancer-Preventing Substance in Tea

Research findings in Japan indicate that drinking of green tea reduces the risk of colon cancer. Further studies carried in UK and USA hint that black tea also possesses the protective qualities.

Scientists in Britain have found the existence of a substance in tea leaves which is likely to reduce the spread of the disease by blocking the cancer-causing agents in the blood stream.

Research study on mice by Professor Allan Conney, Director, Cancer Research Laboratory at Rutgers University, New Jersey, showed that skin cancer could be markedly reduced with tea. Dr. John Weisburger's study establishes that the properties of tea block the spread of cancer linked to diet. He has conducted a series of studies which reveal that the risk to rats of contracting cancer of the breast, colon and pancreas from carcinogens commonly found in cooked meat and fish is significantly reduced by regular doses of tea.

Tea Trade Heath Research Association (TTHRA) Scientific Knowledge About Human Benefits of Tea

Most Tea Association members are familiar with the Tea Trade Health Research Association (TTHRA). The Association was created to manage and administer a joint research effort between the Tea Council of the USA, the Tea Council of Canada, and the UK Tea Packer Association to further scientific knowledge about the human heath benefits of tea. This project research effort is part of an international project funded by the Common Fund of Commodities under the auspices of the FAO and various producer countries. Set up as a charitable organisation in the UK in November 1993, the TTHRA has raised funds and managed the research project. The focus is specifically directed to the black tea and its role in preventing/ inhibiting the formation of cardiovascular diseases and certain forms of cancer. The TTHRA is guided by a stearing committee made up of technical countries. The committee last met to discuss interim results on January 23 & 24, 1997 at the offices of the Tea Council of Canada. To date, eight research grants have been issued with funds remaining to sponsor three additional studies. Most of the research is still in progress, with at least three of the projects showing positive signs; two of the studies dealing with cancer in animals and one of the studies dealing with animal cardiovascular disease (Chung, Yang & Chait).

Dr. Chung of the American Health Foundation, is studying the effect of tea on lung and liver carcinogenesis. He measured 8-OH-dG in DNA exposed to tea in the diet and animals not given tea. DNA damage is a bio-marker which is frequently a forenunner of cancer. The liver levels of 8-OH-dG in animals fed the 2 per cent tea extract (with or without exposure to the carcinogen were significantly lower. A similar trend was seen in DNA taken from lung tissue but the effect was not statistically significant. DNA is harder to extract from lung issue and the data is more variable. However these results are suggestive of a protective effect of tea. While the data were generated from too few animals to warrant separate publication, they were included along with longer chronic study.

Dr. C.S. Yang of Rutgers conducted a study entitled "Effect of Black Tea and Green Tea on Spontaneous Tumorigenesis in A/J mice" Dr Yang is investigating spontaneous cansers. This means that instead of exposing his animals to treatment like a chemical injection that causes a specific tumor, he has a strain of mice genetically selected to be predisposed to so called natural cancer of the type seen in humans in real life. While the study completed a histopathological analysis, mice fed 2 percent black tea solution significantly in hibited all parameters investigated, including tumor incidence, multiplicity and size. More analysis determined the effect of the lower bady weight before the results were assessed.

Dr. Chait of the University of Washington in Seattle studied the effect of tea fed to mice relative to the incidence of cardiovascnlar disease. In the first set of experiments, using a dietary manipulation to produce CVD, tea did not show any effect. However, in a second set of experiments, using mice which are genetically susceptible to, tea appears to have a modest inhibitory effect against the oxidation of LDL. In addition to the studies funded by the TTHRA, many of the independent studies were made by scientists around the world. Nearly every week Tea Council hears of a new study tonting various health benefits attributed to tea consumption.

Study conducted in the University of Australia revealed that laboratory mice fed black tea suffered 54 per cent fewer concerns than mice fed water on even green tea when they were exposed to damaging ultraviolet rays. The study was undertaken by the Commonwealth Scientific and Industrial Research Organisation (CSIRO). They conducted a human social in early 1997. The Tea Council in January 1998 released a video news release (VNR) for Hot Tea Month. The VNR was structured in such a way to benefit from the news about tea health benefit while positioning hot (and iced) tea as a pleasant beverage. A transcript of the VNR follows for reading pleasure. Two scientists Dr. Jeffrey Blumberg of Tufts University Boston and Dr. Carol, Green-wood University of Toranto were predominantly featured in the VNR. To date, the preliminary andiance figure is well over 7 million viewers which is expected to climb even further the next couple of weeks. This equates to cost of less than $ 00.35 per impression or $3.50 per thousand viewers. As the Tea Council has stated before, the making of tea as a healthy beverage poses tremendous challenges to the global tea industry.

To move aggressively in this directions risk attracting the attention of regulatory authorities and/or communicating to wrong message to consumers. Given the patential for error, the fast policy for industry is to focus their marketing efforts on the sensory plesasures of consuming tea and the leave the dissemination of patential health benefits to the medical and scientific communities. Given the abundance of emerging scientific data identifying a broad spectrum of health benefits associated with tea consumption, the progress or future growth is indeed healthy.

The General Trend of Tea Among the Beverages

Currently, of the ten competitive sorts of products, the health-giving sort, i.e. product possessing health-giving properties, stands foremost. In broad sense, tea belongs to the category of food. There are proper in the present world who are obese due to excessive nutrition, typified by west europe, and others who lack nutrition are underfed. The latter accounts for about few million people and the former represents small percentage (about 8 percent) of total world population. The food structure and features have gradually undergone changes since 1950's. From requiring highest wheat calorie to giving consideration to nutrition, the emphasis of healthfulness is the feature of a-days food structure.

Mankind is always hoping to enjoy a better life and improvement in food system is one of the important aspect. The present food and its requirements can be grouped into the following ten heads :

* "Four features"- diversification, convenient, earthful and practical
* "Three lows"-low fat, low cholesterol and low sugar
* "Two highs"- high protein and high fibre
* "One less"- without pollution

Tea has the advantage to give full play over the other beverages

New Nutritional Theory and Efficaey of Tea

Recently the then membrane hypothesis advanced by the cardiologis and other on findings supplemented and substandard food digestion mechanisms, have been establishing a new theory in nutrition.

Highlighting Health Benefits Necessary for Tea Market

Consumption of tea is lesser than it ought to be in U.S.A. as well as in the EEC countries, excluding the U.K. Even in the U.K., the world's largest importer, consumption of tea is dwindling, the present figure is a staggering 30,000 tonnes. Against this backdrop, the tea producing countries will put an additional tonnage of 8,50,000 at 2000 A.D. provided there does not occur any natural crisis. This situation is suggestive enough as to how supply is outstripping demand at the time when in the beverage market and soft drinks are posing serious threat to tea. The international tea community has, in fact, done little so far to check this situation. Of course, it sounds nice to create demand to absorb the supply. But in the event of promoting individual brand the experience of tea packers in the developed markets is bitter due to cut throat competition among themselves.

Obviously, in this situation the necessity is to develop a common understanding to serve both the individual packer and tea industry in totality.

Tea is generally a third world crop, inheriting a variety of ecofriendly features. The crop is renewable and providing ideal soil cover. The necessity of fertiliser and pesticides in limited. The end product has not much cherishables but some minerals. Still 13 per cent of the UK population favour it an in ideal.

Residual Pesticide In Tea

Existence of pesticide in tea had been apprehended by many consumers. It was reported from different countries too. There have been various studies in India on the subject and some in Sri Lanka also. An interesting note has recently been published in the Observer. Sri Lanka produces the cleanest among teas in the world in terms of pesticide residue levels, an international scientist has affirmed. Dr. R.D. Collier the then Chairman of these European Tea Technical Committee told an international forum in Colombo that the level of pesticide residue in Sri Lankan teas was of no consequence being insignificant when compared with other tea producing countries. Addressing the Seventh International Standards Organisation (ISO) Technical Committee meeting, Dr. Collier assured the Sri Lanka delegation of the satisfaction of the Pesticide Regulatory Authorities in Europe with the continuing high standards of Sri Lanka teas. He was responding to questions during a discussion on Pesticide Reside in Tea, attended by representatives of the major tea consuming countries of USA, UK and Germany and representatives for producer countries India, Kenya and host Sri Lanka.

Quoting Dr. Collier's remarks, the Secretary General of the Planters' Association of Ceylon Mr. S. K. Seneviratne said credit should be given to scientists of the Tea Research Institute (TRI) whose work has given Sri Lanka's tea the image of being one of the cleanest in the world. Dr. Wester Modder, Director of the TRI and the leader of the Sri Lanka delegation, explained that the low levels of pesticide residue in Sri Lanka teas were largely due to the effort of the Tea Research Institute of Sri Lanka (TRI) and the effective management of pests in their tea lands.

This management has a multi pronged approach. Essentially it includes cultural measures, some pesticide usage, resistant clones and biological control methods. However, each one of these elements has its own limitation, making it necessary to bring these elements into an integrated pest management (IPM)" strategy. Pesticide use is resorted to only when large pest outbreaks occur.

The natural control agents of pests include parasites, predators and pathogens. The ecology and inter-relations of most of these have been studied, and measures to preserve the natural balance have been identified and adopted Dr. Modder explained.

Residue Limit of Pesticides : German Regulations

Being the largest supplier of tea to Germany, tea-exporters in India have to comply with the current German legislation stipulating maximum residue limits of pesticides on tea as indicated below:

Table-13.3 Residue Limit of Pesticides

Pesticide	MRL (mg/kg tea)
1. HCH (except Lindane)	0.2
2. Lindane	0.5
3. Hexachlorobenzene (HCB)	0.1
4. Dieldrin	0.1
5. Endosulfan	30.0
6. Chlordane	0.05
7. Endrin	0.1

Source : The Assam Review and Tea News, January 1994 and August 1997

8. DDT	1.0
9. Heptachlor	0.1
10. Methoxychlor	10.0
11. Quintozone	0.3
12. Dicofol	2.0
13. Tetredifon	0.01
14. Ethion	2.0
15. Quinalphos	0.2

Source : The Assam Review and Tea News, August 1997

Residue Limite Or Pesticides : Japanese Regulations

Recently the Food Sanitation Law has been revised by the Japanese Ministry of Welfare, stipulating the maximum residue limits of certain chemicals in tea as shown:

Table 13.4 Residue Limits of Pesticides

Pesticide	MRL (mg/kg tea)
1. Ethiofencarb	30.0
2. Glyphosate	0.5
3. Clofentezine	20.0
4. Chlorpyrifos	3.0
5. Fenbutatinoxide	10.0
6. Dichlorfluanid	5.0
7. Cyhalothrin	15.0
8. Diflubenzuron	20.0
9. Daminozide	0.5
10. Cypermethrin	20.0

11. Deltamethrin	10.0
12. Parathion-methyl	0.2
13. Trichlofon	0.5
14. Flucythrinate	20.0
15. Permethrin	20.0

* **Source** : Japan Tea Association

EEC's Regulations Allowing Pesticide Residue Limits in Tea

On June 29, 1993, the European Economic Council (EEC) issued a directive to the member countries which include the maximum residue limits (MRL) of different pesticides in tea and, were of immediate relevance to those exporting tea to member countries.

The directive further adds that the member countries shall bring into force not later than 31.12.93 the laws, regulations, etc. to comply with this Directive.

Survey of Pesticide Residues In Tea

USA and member states of the Council of European Communities are revising their regulations on pesticide registration and stood safety. In USA the Maximum Residue Limits (MRL) or tolerance levels of pesticides in food are governed by the Federal Food. Drugs and Cosmetic Act while in the EC countries a new directive, 93148/EEC-1993, will be applied for this purpose. The Codex Ammentanus Commission of FAO and WHO has also committee on pesticide residues which stipulates the MRL of pesticides on food items. Unfortunately, several countries do not routinely accept the MRLs proposed by Codex.

Among the various pesticides noted in the EEC last Ethion and Dicofol deserve special mention in view of their extensive use for mite control

A few basket surveys for determining the residues of these two acaricides in South Indian teas were conducted in 1993 and 1994, respectively. The results of the surveys are reproduced below.

Table 13.5 Residues of Dicofol in Black Tea (1993)*

Residue Level (ppm)	% Samples
Not Detectable	25.00
> 0.01 and < 0.05	12.50
> 0.05 and < 0.50	37.50
> 0.50 and < 1.00	25.00

Source : Nilgirs The Assam Review and Tea News, January (1995)

Table 13.6 Residues of Dicofol in Black Tea (1994)*

Residue Level (ppm)	% Samples
Not Detectable	17.39
> 0.01 and < 0.10	17.39
> 0.10 and < 0.50	56.52
> 0.50 and < 1.00	8.70

*Estates in Kerala and Tamilnadu

Source: The Assam Review and Tea News, April (1996)

Table 13.7 Residues of Ethion in Black Tea (1994)*

Residue Level (ppm)	% Samples
Not Detectable	13.64
0.01 - 0.20	72.72
0.21 - 0.33	13.64

*Estates in Kerala and Tamil Nadu

Source : The Assam Review and Tea News, April (1995)

Table 13.8 Residues of Ethion in Black Tea (1995)*

Residue Level (ppm)	% Samples
Not Detectable	21.43
< 0.01	21.43
> 0.01 and < 0.1	17.83
> 0.1 and < 0.5	28.57
> 0.5 and <1.0	3.57
> 1.0 and < 2.0	0.00
> 2.00	7.14

* Nilgiris

Source : The Assam Review and Tea News, April (1995)

Caffeine in Tea

Caffeine is the most widely used stimulant drug in the world though few people consider their morning cup of tea or coffee to be a drug. As a matter of fact one of the perceived benefit of tea is the feeling of "well being" it creates.

Caffeine can be credited with stimulating the heart and respiratory system increasing an individual's producrtivity and efficiency. But after consuming too much caffeine, an individual may feel, jitterly irritable and anxious. In addition high levels of caffein can cause insomnia or an irregular heartbreak.

Caffeine levels in a tea are affected by the type of tea bush how it is grown and processed and the length of time the tea is brewed. But general black teas have the most caffeine. Black teas tend to range from 30-60 milligrams of caffeine per cup with an average of roughly 40 milligrams. The more intense black teas for example certain Assam teas tend to have higher caffeine levels. Oolong teas usually have the next highest caffeine content at 12-55 milligrams per cup. Green teas typically have the lowest caffeine content at between 8 and 36 milligrams per cup. Herbal teas are virtually caffeine-free for they do not contain actual tea leaf.

Conclusion

While coffee was entangled in the a dispute, coca emerges as an excellent high energy food (beverage) very tasty and much enjoyed, but shunned by people who nowadays fear becoming obese, and believed to be the source of some child diseases. According to a report published by the University of Californais (Berkeley) Convalescent Bulletin, two ounces of chocolate contain the equivalent of four teaspoonfuls sugar, indicating that chocolate is fattening. Tea, on the other hand, has weight reducing and anti-sunscreen properties, is a time-honoured health-giving beverage, in which respect it excels coffee and cocoa.

Due to the changes in current food structure, the three-high (high-fat, high cholesterol, high sugar) components have become the food source of human obesity. Obesity not only causes one to lose figure, but is even considered a dreadful condition second to cancer. Alimentary therapy directed against obesity is based on the principle of creating "deficit spending" in heat calorie of the human body, called "negative heat calorie balance". Thus it is recommended that people drink less coffee, take less alcohol and eat less chocolate (cocoa product). In contrast, tea is considered a highly valued weight-reducing item, and is even listed as one of the six foods that possess anti-carcinogenic properties.

The evaluation of coffee in relation to benefit for the body is the major cause of the great change in the consumption of coffee and tea. Despite the fact that besides coffee, tea, cocoa and even some other beverages contain a certain amount of caffeine, yet in comparison to coffee the caffeine content of tea is very low. According to the paper "The Coffee Controversy" by Ronald Troya and Gerald Mark (Compilation on American Life Problems, 1984), experiments have shown that 5 ounces of coffee contain about 100-150 mg caffeine, and British workers believe that the caffeine content of tea is only half that of coffee. In addition, tea has many other pharmacological properties, and a this make people think even more that "tea is a genuine health giving beverage".

Chapter 14

Tea – India and World

Area under tea — India and world

The first recorded mention of tea in India was in 1780 when a few bushes from cantor are said to have been planted in Calcutta. Subsequently, Major Robern Bruc discovered indigenous tea plants growing wild in some parts of Assam in 1834 and then experiments were made in various regions of India. The Britishers took up the pioneering work of tea cultivation and their efforts put India to the premier position which it occupies today in the world of tea. The number of tea producing countries in the world has been increasing since 1958 and at present there are 40 countries that have taken to plantation. Among the principal producing countries of the world, India occupies the first place in terms of area. The number of countries cultivating tea in the world is given in Table 21 of the Appendix which depicts the fact that India's area under tea presents a picture of stagnation. World area under tea registered a significant increase during the period 1958 to 2004. While world tea area increased by 189 percent, India's rose by 34 per cent. India's tea area as percentage to total tea area declined to 18.78 per cent in 2004 from 34.5 percent in 1958. India's total area under tea in 1958 was 327,000 hectare which increased to about 521,000 hectare in 2004. The comparative picture is given in Table 14.1 on the following page:

Table 14.1 India's share in world Tea Area during 1958 to 2004

Area under Tea (ha)			
Year	**World**	**India**	**India's share to world**
1958	949	327	34.5
1968	1065	353	33.2
1978	1725	369	21.4
1988	2475	414	16.7
1991	2488	421	17.2
1994	2494	426	17.0
1995	2443	427	17.5
1996	2443	431	17.6
1997	2432	434	17.8
1998	2450	438	17.8
1999	2452	440	17.9
2000	2550	480	18.82
2001	2638	510	19.33
2002	2646	516	19.50
2003	2713	520	19.16
2004	2774	521	18.78

Source : (i) Tea Plantation in India between 1958 and 1992 - Structural changes, 1996 (ii) Darjeeling Tea- The Golden Brew, 2007 by Dr. G.D. Banerjee.

Production of Tea— India and world

Industrial in world production started declining over the years. It was 35.8 per cent in 1958 and 27.4% in 2004. Production of tea in different producing countries is given the Table 22 of the Appendix. Table shows India's share in world production during 1958-2004

Table 14.2 India's share in world production during 1958 to 2005

Year	World	India	India's share to world production
1958	911	326	35.8
1968	1038	402	38.7
1978	1762	564	32.1

1988	2472	700	28.3
1991	2585	742	28.7
1994	2573	752	29.2
1995	2584	756	29.3
1996	2702	780	28.9
1997	2790	810	29.1
1998	2921	870	29.7
1999	2950	860	29.8
2000	3000	850	30.0
2001	3035	854	28.23
2002	3036	838	27.61
2003	3174	878	27.75
2004	3306	892	27.9

Soruce : (i) Tea industry 'A Road Map Ahead', 2007, (ii) Tea plantation industry in India between 1958 and 1992 – structural changes and (iii) Darjeeling Tea-The Golden Brew by Dr. G.D. Banerjee.

It is evident from the Table that world production increased to 330 million kgs in 2004 from 911 million kgs in 1958 displaying a rise of 262.90 percent while India's production enhanced by 173.62 percent from 326 million kgs to 892 million kgs during the period under reference.

Export of Tea—India and world

India is the largest exporter of tea in world. However, Sri Lanka has been closely following India's foot steps. India's share in the world exports expressed in terms of percentage has indeed declined between the period 1958 and 2004 but there is marginal decline in absolute quantum of exports. In spite of many ups and downs of Indian tea, it has remained, on an average, at a level of 200 million kgs. The main reason for fall of India's share for the last fifty years is that a large quantum of tea has been retained in the domestic market. The picture of tea exports – of Indian world is depiceted in 14.3.

Table 14.3 India's share in world Tea Export

(in million kgs)

Year	World	India	Share of India's Export to world
1958	565	230	40.5
1968	624	208	33.3
1978	812	205	25.3
1988	1036	200	19.3
1991	1148	202	17.6
1994	1033	151	14.6
1995	1083	168	15.5
1996	1115	162	14.5
1997	1179	203	17.2
1998	1254	206	16.2
1999	1308	190	14.5
2000	1367	198	14.8
2001	1391	183	13.2
2002	1441	201	14.0
2003	1401	173	12.3
2004	1540	197	12.8

Source : (i) Global Tea Trade-Dimensions and Dynamics, (2007) (ii) Tea plantation in India between 1858 and 1992 structural changes (1996), (iii) Export potentials of Indian Tea, (iv) Tea Industry A Road Map Ahead (2007) by Dr. G.D. Banerjee

It is interesting to note that world tea exports increased sharply over the years. In 1958 it was 565 million kgs which enhanced to 1540 million kgs in 2004. In other world tea exports sparked by 173 per cent while India as share in world tea export was 40.5 per cent in 1958 and 12.8 per cent in 2004.

World Production and Exports

Global production of tea in 2003 registered in increase (3174 million kgs) as against 2002 (3055 million kgs). Global exports however, declined to 1401 million kgs in 2003 compared to the level achieved in 2002 (1441 million kgs). The fall in global export was due to substantial decline of exports of tea from India, Indonesia, China, Vietnam Tanzania, Malawi etc. During the year 2003, production of tea in world improved by 119 million kgs. Indonesia (8 million kgs), Bangladesh (4 million kgs), China (23 million kgs), Turkey (7 million kgs), Vietnam (5 million kgs), Turkey (13 million kgs). Details of World production and exports by major tea producing countries are given in table below:

Table 14.4 World production and Exports by country

(in million kgs)

	Production				Export			
Country	1996	1999	2002	2003	1996	1999	2002	2003
India	780	805	838	878	162	190	201	174
Sri Lanka	259	284	313	303	234	264	286	291
Indonesia	144	165	162	170	102	85	100	88
Bangladesh	53	47	54	58	26	15	14	12
China	593	676	745	768	170	200	252	260
Kenya	257	249	287	294	244	242	272	269
Tanzania	20	23	28	29	19	21	23	20
Malawi	38	38	39	42	37	40	39	42
Turkey	-	171	142	155	-	4	5	7
Argentina	43	50	58	60	41	52	57	58
Others	495	337	391	417	81	104	192	180
Total	2682	2845	3055	3174	1116	1217	1441	1401

Source – Darjeeling Tea Industry – The Golden Brew, Dr. G.D. Banerjee, 2007

Others include Taiwan, Japan, USSR/CIS, Iran, Uganda, Mozambique, Zaire, Mauritius, Rwanda, Brundi, Cameroon, Brazil, Peru, Ecuador, Zimbabwe, Myanmar, Thailand, Malaysia, South Africa, Australia and Ethopia.

Data further revealed that world production in 2003 increased by 492 million kgs over 1996. Similarly world exports improved by 285 million kgs during 1996 to 2003. In other world production enhanced by 18.25 per cent and world exports by 25.53 per cent. Export of Tea in quantity and value terms from different producing countries are outlined in Tables 24 and 25 of the Appendix. It is also evident from the Tables 26 and 27 of the Appendix that Indian share in world production and exports over the years have been declining while share of Sri Lanka and Kenya have been improving. This shows that India must adopt such policy that may enhance her shares in respects of production and exports.

World Imports

World tea imports for consumption registered an increase of 234 million kgs as compared to 1996. Imports of tea in CIS countries including Russian Federation hiked by 71 million kgs, followed by Asia (west Asia including Afganistan, 54 million kgs, South East Asia (including Pakistan and Japan) 48 million kgs, North Africa 7 million kgs, other Africa 43 million kgs. Decline in tea imports were noticed in United Kingdom (23 million kgs), Ocennia (5 million kgs) etc. The position in respect of tea imports for consumption is illustrated below:

Table 14.5 Region wise imports for consumption on 1996 to 2004

Region/Year	1996	1997	1998	1999	2002	2003	Percentage increase/decrease of 2003 over 1996
1. United Kingdom	148	151	146	137	137	125	(-)15.54
2. Other West Europe	81	77	76	79	74	82	(+)1.23
3. CIS countries including Russian Federation	158	188	179	182	223	229	(+)44.93
4. Other East Europe	35	33	34	30	39	39	(+)11.42
America							
North America	104	99	115	113	112	115	(+)10.58
South America	16	14	17	16	20	21	(+)31.25
Asia							
Asia (west Asia including Afganistan)	182	180	201	163	277	254	(+) 39.56
South East Asia (including Pakistan and Japan)	188	167	223	228	229	236	(+)25.53
Africa							
North Africa	137	155	160	151	163	144	(+)5.11
Other Africa	45	50	57	63	80	88	(+)95.55
Oceania	23	21	22	19	19	18	(-)21.79
Total	1117	1135	1230	1181	1373	135	(+)20.95

World Tea Prices

The annual average prices of tea in respect of all auction centres of the world registered an increase during 1999 to 2004 except Amritsar and Jankarte auction. Avearage quantum of tea sold and price realised in Kolkata auction centre increased by 34125 thousand kgs and Rs. 21.58 per kg respectively during 1996 to 2004 followed by Siliguri auction (11923 thousand kgs and Rs. 16.40 per kg), Comibatore (3343 thousand kgs and Rs. 5.20 per kg). In case of Guwahati auction centre average quantity decline by 20334 thousand kgs lent average price fetched enhanced by Rs. 1825 per kg. Similarly in coonoors average quantum reduced by 12715 thousand kgs lent price realisaion rose by Rs 5 per kg. Taking both teas in North India and South India into account, quantity and price realised increased over this year. Teas in Colombo, Chillenganj, Mumbasa and Limbe auction centres increased in quanity terms as also price relationship per kg. Detalis are brought out in Table 14.6.

Tea Prices

Average price per kg of tea in Indian auction centers in 2003 and 2004 registered on fall compared to 1998 and 1999 resulting in hardship to the Indian Tea plantation UPASI has been taking up the issue at various foras but the remedial measures announced by the Government have only been peripheral. These included increasing the basic import duty on tea from 15 per cent to 35 per cent, lowering of the state sales tax from 8 per cent to 4 percent and Central Sales Tax (C.S.T.) from 4 percent to 2 percent by Tamil Nadu and Kerala governments in respect to teas sold through auctions, exemption from excise duty for co-operative and bought leaf factories, announcement by the Tea Board of a subsidy to small growers etc.

From a long-term perspective it has been felt that a campaign for generic promotion of tea in the domestic market should be launched. Another aspect that has been engaging the attention of the members is the need to improve upon the quality profile and the image of the south Indian tea.

Table 14.6 : Prices of Tea at Differnet Auction Centres

Auction centers	1996		1997		1998		1999		2003		2004		Absolue increase or decrease in 2004 over 1996		Precentage increase (+) or decrese (-) in 2004 over 1996	
	Qty.	Price	Qty.	Price	Qty.	Price	Qty.	Price	Qty.	Price	Qty.	Price	Qty.	Price	Qty.	Price
1	2	3	4	5	6	7	8	9	10	11	12	13	14	15	16	17
Kolkata	85194	58.76	83316	79.88	82381	87.83	89172	88.60	133874	68.71	119319	80.34	(+)34125	(+)21.58	(+)40.05	(+)36.72
Gawhati	147429	50.13	148670	67.76	140226	78.76	145072	80.53	138664	59.01	127095	68.78	(-) 20334	(+)18.25	(-)3.79	(+)37.22
Siliguri	80066	47.73	67001	65.47	72356	74.66	86793	72.56	87090	54.58	91989	64.13	(+)11923	(+)16.40	(+)14.89	(+)34.57
Amritsar	681	29.54	744	41.89	718	51.96	556	46.66	190	28.62	149	26.04	(-)532	(-)3.50	(-)78.13	(-)11.84
North India	313,370	51.82	305731	70.69	295681	80.22	321593	80.56	359818	61.33	338552	71.59	(+)25182	(+)8.04	(+)19.77	(+)38.15
Cochin	57698	44.42	63523	61.67	58586	73.31	59573	62.06	50633	45.78	54599	52.30	(-)3099	(+)7.88	(-)5.37	(+)17.79
Conoor	56994	38.40	73298	57.13	70847	65.06	79285	53.34	40586	34.55	44279	43.40	(-)12715	(+)5.00	(-)22.30	(+)13.02
Coimbatore	15057	41.30	16474	60.13	17246	68.74	20262	57.26	22331	38.30	18400	46.50	(+)3343	(+)5.20	(+)22.02	(+)12.59
South India	129746	41.42	153295	59.31	146679	68.78	159120	57.10	113550	40.29	117278	47.01	(-)12198	(+)5.59	(-)9.40	(+13.49)
All India	443116	48.77	459026	66.89	442360	76.43	480713	72.79	473368	56.28	455830	64.55	(+)12714	(+)15.77	(+)2.86	(+32.34)
Colombo	229979	104.04	254966	119.36	256033	134.25	260448	114.96	273230	148.32	269870	180.18	(+)39896	(+)76.14	(+)17.35	(+)73.18
Chillagong	48653	46.35	43666	71.93	44897	69.96	39873	58.85	47790	67.77	52930	63.72	(+)4277	(+)17.37	(+)8.79	(37.48)
Jakarta	22423	114.41	29826	164.64	35144	170.25	24167	105.27	33770	95.49	32310	102.22	(+)9887	(-)12.19	(+)44.03	(-)10.65
Mombasa	189800	142.00	166617	200.00	243566	189.00	210785	178.00	285840	154.00	298090	155.00	(+)108290	(+)13.00	(+)57.05	(+)9.15
Limbe	14433	78.96	17208	124.79	18029	119.21	12972	93.74	15900	93.39	17220	100.27	(+)2787	(+)21.31	(+)19.31	(+)26.98
London	17368	113.47	11208	135.06	-	-	-	-	-	-	-	-	-	-	-	-

Source : (i) Global Tea Trade-Dimensions and Dynamics, (2007) (ii) Tea plantation in India between 1858 and 1992 structural changes (1996), (iii) Export potentials of Indian Tea, (iv) Tea Industry A Road Map Ahead (2007) by Dr. G.D. Banerjee

Remedial Measures

With a view to mitigating the hardship to the tea producers, arising from the crash in prices, UPASI represented to the Government on certain remedial measures that included:

- Excise duty on tea be abolished; if this cannot be done in total, it be withdrawn or suspended in respect of South India. Since the duty had already been abolished for the Bought Leaf and Co-operative Factories and, further, since full refund of excise duty is being granted on exports, the revenue implication for the latter option will not be much.
- Basic import duty on tea be enhanced from 15 per cent to at least 35 per cent. (This has already been acceded to.) We have now sought further hike, even 150 per cent, which is still permissible under WTO Agreement.
- Import from Sri Lanka at concessional import duty be suspended, till prices improve in South India.
- Government of India should initiate measure to revive tea export to Russia. As a special case, Indian Government could consider repaying an additional Rs. 200 to Rs 300 croer to Russian debt during the current financial year with an explicit stipulation that this will be exclusively used by them for import of tea from India. Further, Russia should be requested to have the same rate of import duty at 5 per cent both for bulk tea as also packet tea in respect of tea imports under Rupee Debt-Repayment Route.
- Under Section 5 of the Provision of Food Adulteration Act, no tea can be imported into India which does not conform of PFA standard for tea. This provision should be strictly implemented in respect of teas imported with for re-exports or for domestic consumption in order to ensure that substandard teas do not land on our shores.
- Presently, lower quality from teas countries are being imported, blended with a small proportion of India tea and is an-exported with a certificate of origin that the consignment is Indian tea. This practice should be stopped. Certificate of origin should not issued for blends which do not have 100 per cent Indian tea

terming it as India tea. At best, such certificates should indicate the blend percentage on the label. The organisations issuing such certificates of origin should also check up if the export contract was being effectively executed in accordance with the terms of the contract.

- Any tea imported by paying foreign exchange should be allowed to be re-exported only if payment for such re-export for teas is also in foreign exchange. This will stop the practice of importers in India importing tea by paying foreign exchange from countries like Sri Lanka, Indonesia, Kenya etc and re-exporting it to Russia under rupee payment mechanism.

Export Measures Promotion

A number of export promotion measures were undertaken. These included the following:

- UPASI, jointly with the tea Board and the tea Trade Associations of Cochin, Coonoor and Coimbator, organised an International Tea Convention in Cochin sometimes in September 1999. About 450 delegates including 40 from overseas, participated in the convention which turned out to be a fruitful get-together of the various segments connected with the tea industry and trade.
- The Consultative Committee of plantation associations, of which UPASI is a constituent, organised another International Millennium Tea Convention in Delhi during March 2000. About 700 delegates including 20 from overseas countries, participated in it.
- Mr. M. H. Ashraff, UPASI Vice-president joined a delegation led by Tea Board Chairman to Russia and Ukrain in July 1999. He joined yet another delegation that visited Turkey in May 2000. President, Chairman an UPASI Tea Committee and a few other leading members joined another delegation to U.A.E., Jordan and Syria in June 2000.

Excise Duty

The Co-operative and Bought Leaf Factories purchasing green leaf from small growers holding 10 hect or less land under tea cultivation, subject to certain conditions, were exempted from payment of excise duty w.e.f. 10th December 1999. One of the conditions in respect of Bought Leaf Factories was that not less than two-thirds of their total green leaf shall be purchased from small growers.

Cess

The cess of 30 paise per kg is to be paid on all teas produced under Tea Act. However, in certain cases Central Excise authorities had been demanding cess at two stages at the time of bulk tea manufactured and again at the time of consumer packaging. This was taken up with the Commerce Ministry which, vide Standing Order dated 11 November 1999, made it clear that cess under Tea Act is payable only once.

Sales Tax

Arising from the crisis faced by the tea industry and in order to give a fillip to sales through auctions, the Tamil Nadu Government reduced the state sales tax on tea from 8 percent to 4 percent for the period from 2nd June 2000 to 1st December 2000 in respect of teas purchased through Coonoor and Coimbatore auctions. Further, inter-state sales tax for the same period was reduced from 4 percent to 2 percent in respect of inter-state sales of teas purchased at the above auction centres with or without 'C' Form. The Kerala Government also reduced C.S.T. for sales through Cochin auction to 2 percent for the period 9-6-2000 to 30-11-2000 and the State S.T. from 8 per cent to 4 percent for the period 27-6-2000 to 1-12-2000.

Price Subsidy

The Tea Board announced a scheme of subsidy to be given to the small tea growers owning upto 10-12 hectare as and when the fortnightly average auction price of a particular factory happened to be bless than Rs 55 per kg; the maximum subsidy for green leaf will be Rs 1.25 per kg. The scheme was effective from 1 May 2000 and the Board has decided to operate it through tea factories. The small growers intending to benefit from the scheme have to register themselves with the Tea Board along with appropriate proof of tea cultivation.

Export to Russia: The RBI decided to allow export of goods on consignment basis to the Russian Federation against repayment of state credits. Initially this facility has been made available to export houses/trading houses/star trading houses and superstar trading houses with good track record for export of tea. Exporters desirous of availing this facility have to apply for permission to the RBI.

Quality Assurance: The Tea Board introduced a scheme on quality assurance in respect of export of tea. The scheme stipulates an optional provision for quality assurance for export of tea from India. Details of the procedure to be followed have been circulated to the exporters.

UPASI Tea Research Foundation: The Foundation was registered as a trust in March 2000. The Commerce Ministry a approved on outlay of Rs 44.39 lakh for the Foundation for the financial year 1999-2000 and asked the Tea Board to release the funds.

International Tea Convention

The twelfth session of the inter-governmental group (IGG) on tea under aegis of FAO was held at Bali in Indonesia from 2-4 July 1997. Prion to that the First International Tea Business Conference (ITBC) organised by the Indonesian Tea Association was held from 30 June to 1 July 1998. Both the sessions were attended by delegates from a number of countries. The then Chairman of Tea Board attended both the sessions. During the meeting of the IGG, the following items were reviewed :-

1. The overall aspects of economic and trade issues in connection with :
   - i) Tea market situation and short term outlook.
   - ii) Identification and development of markets.
   - iii) Price deteriorating export earnings and food scenario of small growers.

iv) Policy consideration to strengthen economic prosperity.

2. Inter-governmental action on :-
   i) Progress Report on tea consumption and Human Health Project.
   ii) Production and market proprovement measures.
   iii) Statement of priorities of the group for the common fund for the commodities.
3. Outcome of the report of the International Tea Business Conference.

FAO meet

The 13th session of the inter-governmental group of tea of the Food and Agricultural Organisation was held in Ottava, Canada, during 22-29 September 1999. Mr. M.H. Ashraff, President, United Planters' of Southern India (UPASI) attended the session as a delegate.

The meet reviewed short and medium term market prospects, market development strategies, tea consumption, human health projects, quality control etc.

Indian Tea Scene

Production: Indian tea production during 2003 stood at 878.13 million kgs as against 848.47 million kg in 2002. This showed an increase of 39.66 million kg when compared with previous year. The rise in Indian tea crop was attributed towords improvement in production of tea in both North Indian and South Indian crops 16.53 million kgs and 23.12 million kgs respectively over 2002.

Marketing

a) Indian Auction : The overall percentage of sale through Indian auction in relation to total production during 2003 was 54.41 per cent The percentage sale of tea through North India auctions in relation to total North Indian production during 2003 stood at 54.59 percent, whereas the tea sold through South Indian auctions in relations to South Indian production was 51.36 percent.

b) London auction: The sale at London auction was totally closed down by the London Tea Trade with effect from 30th June, 1998.

c) Ex-garden sale: Ex-garden sale within the country during 2003 was worked out to 40.62 percent as against 40.78 percent in 2002. The overall picture of primary marketing of Indian teas by different channels is given in the Table below :-

Table 14.7 : Primary Marketing of Indian Tea

Year	Qty. Sold through Auction			Exgarden Export under forword contact	Ex garden private sale
	India	London	Total		
2001	464 (54.31)	-	464 (54.31)	39 (4.57)	351 (41.12)
2002	457 (54.45)	-	457 (54.45)	40 (4.77)	341 (40.78)
2003	478 (54.41)	-	478 (54.41)	43 (4.97)	357 (4.62)

Prices

At the close of the year 2003 the annual average prices of tea at All India auctions stood at 56.03 as against Rs. 55.96 of 2002, which shows a marginal increase of Rs. 0.07 per kg i.e. 0.13 per cent over the year 2002. During the year 2003, the average prices of tea in South Indian auctions registered a decline of 4.08 per cent at the close of the year and reached to the level of Rs. 39.93 per kg as against Rs. 41.63 per kg of 2002. Also the average prices of tea at North Indian auctions registered a decline of 2.15 per cent and reached to the level of Rs. 61.31 per kg as against Rs. 62.66 per kg of 2002 because of decline in prices at all major north Indian auction centers during 2003 over 2002.

Exports

The export of tea from India during the complete calendar year 2003 stood at a level of 173.68 m kg in quantum and Rs. 1590.21 crores in export earnings as against 201.0 million kgs and Rs. 1753.39 cr in 2002 and thereby showing a decline of 27.32 million kgs and Rs

163.18 crore. The unit export price during 2003 stood at Rs 91.56 per kg as compared to Rs 87.23 per kg in 2002. During the financial year 2003-04 the export of tea from India reached a level of 183.09 million kgs and Rs. 1636.99 crores in value realisation as against 184.39 million kgs and 1664.92 crores in value realisation achieved. This indicates in the coresponding period of 2002-03. a decline of 1.32 million kgs and Rs. 27.93 crores during 2003-04.

The decline in export of tea from India during 2003-04 was mainly attributed to the set back in export of Iraq, Russia Federation Poland Germany and Ireland etc. Total export of tea including instant tea from India during the last five years are given below:

Table 14.8 : Exports of Tea from India during 1999 to 2004.

Calender year	Quantity	Value	Unit volume	Financial year	Quantity	Value	Unit value
1999	191.72	1965.87	102.54	1999-00	192.44	1932.66	100.43
2000	206.82	1898.61	91.80	2000-01	203.55	1889.79	92.84
2001	182.58	1682.11	92.13	2001-02	190.00	1695.79	99.25
2002	201.00	1753.39	87.23	2002-03	184.39	1664.92	90.29
2003	173.68	1590.21	91.56	2003-04	183.07	1636.99	89.42

Source : Tea plantation Industry – A Road Map Ahead by Dr. G.D. Banerjee

Direction of Exports

Druing 2003, the export of tea from India to both CIS and Non-CIS countries registered a decline of 4.03 million kgs and 23.50 million kgs respectively. Under CIS countries the export to Russian Federation (5.29 million kgs) and Ukraine (1.08 million kgs) exhibited a set back, where as Kazakhustan and Belarus have shown an improvement during 2003 over 2002. Under non-CIS countries, the exports of tea from India to Iraq declined substaintially to the level of 30.80 million kgs which was the main reason for the fall in export during 2003 over 2002. Decline in export to Poland, UK, UAE was noticed by more than 1.0 million kgs each. Significant improvement in export has been achieved in countries such as Australia (3.34 million kgs), Pakistan (2.06 million kgs), Afganistan (2.80 million kgs), USA (1.33 million kgs), Canada (0.26 million kgs), Saudi Arab (0.49 million kgs) etc during 2003 over 2004.

Product diversification

Efforts were made to increase export of tea from India in bulk, value teas, organic and flavoured teas. During 2003-04 export of value-added teas touched the level of 42.37 million kgs in quantum and Rs. 599.68 crores as against 39.84 million kgs in quantum and Rs. 563.41 crores achieved during 2002-2003. A marginal increase in quantum and value earnings was noticed during 2003-2004 to the extent of 2.53 million kgs and Rs. 36.27 crores respectively over 2002-2003. The information on tea exports from India in the aforesaid forms can be seen from the following tables :

(A) Exports of Bulk Tea from India

Year	Quantity (m.kgs)	Value (Rs. Cr.)	Unit Price (Rs/Kg)
1999-2000	124.01	1137.23	91.70
2000-2001	129.54	1048.60	80.95
2001-2002	142.15	1040.74	73.21
2002-2003	144.55	1101.51	76.20
2003-2004	140.70	1037.31	73.72

(B) Exports of packet Tea from India

Year	Quantity (m.kgs)	Value (Rs. Cr.)	Unit Price (Rs/Kg)
1999-2000	63.52	674.33	106.16
2000-2001	69.31	719.56	103.81
2001-2002	42.72	521.14	121.99
2002-2003	33.61	408.43	121.54
2003-2004	34.01	405.80	119.31

(C) Exports of Tea Tea Bags from India

Year	Quantity (m.kgs)	Value (Rs. Cr.)	Unit Price (Rs/Kg)
1999-2000	2.31	55.72	241.21
2000-2001	1.92	38.52	200.63
2001-2002	2.54	59.71	234.89
2002-2003	3.18	66.85	210.37
2003-2004	4.90	94.31	192.46

(D) Exports of Instant Tea from India

Year	Quantity (m.kgs)	Value (Rs. Cr.)	Unit Price (Rs/Kg)
1999-2000	2.60	65.38	251.46
2000-2001	2.78	83.10	298.92
2001-2002	2.59	74.20	286.04
2002-2003	3.05	88.13	288.66
2003-2004	3.46	99.57	287.71

Internal consumption

Major share of the Indian tea production is consumed within this country. However, there is a perception that the rate of growth of tea consumption in India has declined from the earlier levels. In order to increse the domestic demand for tea, the tea industry along with tea Board has started a generic promation campaign propagating the health aspects of tea. The internal consumption of tea has been estimated at 714 million kgs in 2003 as against 693 million kgs in 2002 showing an increase of 21 million kgs over the preceeding year.

Taxes & Duties

Cess at the rate of 30 paise per kg levied on tea in India with effect from 1st April 1997, except Darjeeling tea where it was levied at a concessional rate of 12 paise per kg.

Excise Duty

(a) Rs 1 per kg on teas falling under heading 09.02 has been established with effect from 01.03.2003. However, an overall execise duty of Rs 1 per kg has been introduced for development purposes with effect from 01.03.2003.

(b) 16 per cent advolerem on instant tea falling under heading 21.01.02.

Export Duty

There is no export duty on tea exported from India at present.

Import Duty

Basic duty fo 100 per cent plus 10 per cent sur charge on basic import duty plus special additional duty of 4 per cent of basic duty and surcharge (w.e.f. 1st March 2002). Concessionary rate of 7.5 per cent basic duty plus other normal surcharges apply to import from Sri Lanka under Indo-Sri Lanka free trade aggrement attracts upto a volume of 15 million kgs per calender year under EXIM policy, the import of tea continued to be allowed without payment of import duty for the purpose of re-exports by the export oriented unit (EOU), Export processing zone (EPZ) and special economic zone (SEZ) units and also under Duty Exemption Scheme.

Chapter 15
International Tea Promotion

Part-I

Promotion - The Tools

Marketing or Products

Promotion is one of the essential tools for the marketing of any product along with the other three essential p's of marketing, namely product improvement pricing and packaging. Even for a primary commodity like tea, as distinguished form a product, promotion is important in sustaining the long-term demand. Tea has in the past experienced long spells of low prices when supply was said to be in excess of demand. Promotion tends to take a back seat when prices are ruling at high levels but one would forget the role of promotion only at one's peril. In this chapter an attempt has been made to underline the importance of international tea promotion and trace is history.

Promotional Campaigns As early As 1894

India is the undisputed leader among the tea producing and exporting countries. Efforts to promote Indian tea abroad were started as early as 1894, when tea industry started promotional campaigns in US, Germany, Italy, etc. Voluntary contributions were asked for by the Indian Tea Association from among its members for the purpose of tea propaganda in other countries. For about 75 years now statutory basis has been provided for the promotion of Indian tea. In 1903, Indian tea cess committee was formed under the Indian Tea Cess Act and this laid the formulation for systematic propaganda for Indian tea which has been carried on by the successor organisations namely, the Indian Tea Market Expansion Board (ITMEB) which came into being in 1936 and the Central Tea Board which was constituted in 1949. Since 1954, the Tea Board has been continuing the efforts at promoting tea as a beverage as well as promoting Indian tea. Of late, these two types of promotion have been supplemented by assistance in the promotion of tea packets, tea bags, etc. marked under Indian brand names.

Organised Internal Efforts form Promotion of Tea As Beverage

Organised Internal efforts to promote tea as a beverage did not start until prolong depression in tea prices brought the tea producing countries together and made them realise that joint action was necessary for their survival. After the conclusion of International Tea Agreement between the representatives of the principal producing countries of that period namely India, Ceylon, Indonesia and others which was later on joined by the East African tea producing countries, the ITMEB was formed in 1935 with the objective of creating an environment, in principle, of joint generic promotion for tea by the principal tea producing countries of the world. This was the first attempt made in the history of tea economy in the World. Extensive tea promotion campaigns were carried out in the main tea consuming countries at that time-namely the U.K., the USA, Canada, Australia West Germany, Sweden, Belgium, the Netherlands and Egypt. After the Second World War, campaigns were also started in New Zealand, Iraq various parts of Africa, Ireland and Denmark. The campaigns by the ITMEB succeeded in achieving noticeable improvement in which campaigns were undertaken, although the extent of improvement naturally varied from country to county. After less then 20 years of good work, difference of opinion developed among the participating countries and this body ceased to have International backing. This was a big set back in the generic promotion of tea as a beverage.

Absence of International Body

In the absence of an international body like ITMEB, other institutional arrangements had to be made for the promotion of tea as a beverage. Under these arrangements, the concentrated interests namely the tea producing and exporting countries on the one hand and the tea trade in the importing countries on the other, came together with the common purpose of enlarging the market for tea in arrangements called the Tea Councils brought into being in eight different countries. These were the USA (1950), Ireland Canada and West Germany (1954), Australia (1963). France & the U.K. (9165) and New Zealand (1966). These tea councils have been doing very useful work for tea as a beverage and in the better dissemination of knowledge about it. It, however follows form this type of arrangements that the gains out of the additional tea consumption are shared by all the producing countries, exporters and the tea trade although the actual buying of tea from different countries depends on the commercial decisions by the various importers. Since the dissolution of the ITMEB, these Tea Councils have been the only institution for the generic tea exporting countries and the tea trade in importing countries. The promotion methods followed by the Tea Councils vary from country to country. So does the level of expenditure. But is clear that the promotional activities of the Tea Councils have led to a fairly sustained improvements in tea consumption in the countries concerned.

Scheme of Generic Promotion

It has been the task of the generic promotion to protect the beverage tea from the onslaught of other competing beverages-especially in the context of fast changing economic pattern and consumers habit depending on his income. For example, over the years, tea has been promoted as a drink which is, the cheapest next to water. By overemphasising this aspect the good qualities of tea as a beverage has not received due notice As a result in many countries, the younger generation started considering cold drinks and coffee as the 'in drinks'. It is only now that qualities of tea as a beverage are beginning to be appreciated.

It has sometime been thought that for a big tea producing countries like India, there is no point in undertaking or participating in the schemes of generic promotion of tea as a beverage. India would do well to undertake what is called 'uninational promotion' and see that its own tea is promoted separately. This point of view is only partially correct. There is no doubt that the aim of generic promotion as well as uninational promotion is the same-namely share of Indian tea in the world market-should go up. There is, therefore, no basic conflict between generic promotion on the one hand and uninational promotion on the one hand and uninational promotion on the other hand while generic promotion is necessary in order to enhance the size of the market, uninational must come close on its heels so as to take a bigger share of the increased market. But the question arise about the form which uninational promotion should take. This form has to be decided keeping in view the realities of the world marketing of tea. It would be well to recognise the fact that at present the actual marketing of tea to the consumers is in the hands of foreign companies which buy teas not only from one tea producing country but from a number of such companies. These marketing companies find it more convenient to mix and blend the teas of various origins and then sell them to the consumer under their own brand names. As a result they spend large amounts of money to promote the names of their own brands. In this context it becomes irrelevant for them to promote the name or names of the countries from which their teas comes, as only the brand name is of the primary significance to these companies. Until Indian companies become strong enough to undertake world marketing of tea under for Indian tea would remain largely a public relations venture seeking to promote Indian tea in a 'generic' way interalia by maintaining constant contacts with the tea traders of the countries concerned, by spreading greater understanding of Indian tea among the consumers and by removing any snags which might develop in the export of tea.

Generic promotional Programmes

To come back to international promotion, at present the various tea councils function independently of each other. Moreover, all the tea exporting countries are not participating in the various tea councils. As a result, generic promotional programmes had in many cases to be undertaken on a rather ad hoc and peicemeal manner without any co-ordination with similar programmers being undertaken with other tea councils. There is no overall objective review of the work that has been done and an assessment of what requires to be done in various markets both actual and potential.

In several meetings of the inter-governmental group on tea which was constituted under the auspices of F.A.O. in 1970, the importance of 'Generic Promotion' and the need for its coordination and intensification has been fully recognised by all the tea exporting countries especially in the as late as 1974. This trend, however, afterwards but it did not continue. Thus at the initiative of India and Sri Lanka, the inter-governmental group on tea adopted a multidimensional approach and recognised that regulation of exports was not necessarily the only means to solve the problem of long-term decline in the prices of tea in the World. It was equally necessary to stimulate demand by intensive promotion of tea as a beverage. An international symposium on Tea Market Expansion was held in London in December 1974 under the joint auspices of International Trade Centre of UNCTADGATT and the Common wealth secretariat. This symposium discussed all aspects of tea promotion and evaluated the experience of Tea Councils and made a review of the selected areas with the greatest potential for tea consumption. This symposium came to the conclusion that the existing promotional activities through Tea Councils which were confined to individual markets were not enough for ensuring a sustained increase in tea consumption all over the World. The symposium also strongly recommended the setting up of a central body for deciding the promotional strategy, identifying prospective markets for undertaking promotion and for monitoring the implementation of promotional programmes in tea markets.

Follow-up action on these recommendations has been taken by International Trade Centre and after Intensive consultations with the various interests concerned. A conference was held in Geneva sometime in 1980's to draft an agreement for setting up an International Tea Promotion Association. This conference which was presided over by Shri S.G. Bose Mullick, the then Commerce Secreatary in the Government of India, was successful in agrreing to the text of an agreement. Already Government of nine countries Malwai, Burundi, Rwanda and Mauritius, who account for one-third of world exports, have notified their acceptance of the text of the agreement. Moreover, Kenya, Bangladesh and others have also joined the Association.

International Tea Promotion Association A Mile-Stone

The setting up of this Association is a mile-stone in the history of generic promotion of tea in the World. After about a quarter of a century, International cooperation for organising generic promotion has been revived. The new Association has provided for larger membership than the erstwhile ITMEB. What is more significant is the involvement of various tea exporting countries whose tea cultivation is based on the efforts of a large number of small growers and who looks to stability of earnings from this source. India has been a film champion of generic promotion of tea along with Sri Lanka. She has been supporting such efforts in many countries of the World for so many decades. As the biggest rea exporting country of the World, India looks forward for a sustained increase in tea consumption all over the World resulting in better returns to all involved in tea industry specially the humble workers in far flung areas where tea is grown and the small grower contributed his little mile in effort of tea growing. Generic promotion will only help in indirect expansion of scope for Indian tea in various markets of the World. India is spending huge amounts in promotional activities. This amounts also involve financial support to various Tea Councils in the task of genetic promotion and promotional interest of Indian tea abroad.

The Tea Board (India) has its office in various countries of the World to intensify their efforts to take advantage of the favourable climate created for tea as a beverage so as to increase the share of Indian tea in the global set up.

Part - II

Roles of Food and Agriculture Organisation (FAO), United Nations Conference on Trade and Development (UNCTAO), General Agreement on Tarriffs and Trade (GATT) and International Tea Promotion Association (ITPA)

A stable market depends on a equilibrium between supply an ddemand at a price which is remunerative to producers and aeceptable to consumers. This is an essential condition for accelerating the growth of any industry and particularly for an agro-industry like Tea. For an export commodity a stable international market is also essential for earning steady foreign exchange from export of the commodity in question.

Prior to the 1950s the price of tea did not cause much concern. However, since the 1950s world tea economy has been experiences a state of disequilibrium as a result of (i) the slow rate of growth of tea consumption and (ii) the emergence of other producitng countries who were more dependent on export markets. The rate of increase in world comsumption of tea tended to slow down froman average of 4.1 per cent per year during 1950-55 to 2.8 per cent per year in the following five years. In importing countries it was developing only at a rate of 2 per cent per year. This has resulted in an imbalance in the supply of tea and the demand for the same. Tea prices showed a gradula erosion in the world market since 1954. This had been a matter of concern for the tea exporting countries and since 1964 onwards discussions have been going on under the auspicus of the Food and Agriculture Organisation. As a result of such discussions, a permanent machinery for consultation was established under the FAO and certain informal regulatory schemes for tea are already in operation.

The 37th session of the CCP (Committee and Commodity Problems) fo the FAO held on 1964 noted the slow erosion of tea prices and decided that in consultation with the principal countries concerned, the FAO., Director General, should convene an ad-hoc meeting of Governments interested in the production and consumption of tea to report of what action might be taken.

The first Ad-hoc Meeting on tea was held in Sri Lanka on May 1st 1965. The meeting agreed that, while the outlook for the world tea economy did not justify the establishment of a permeanent international machinery in the shape of a tea study group, thesituation and outlook should be kept under review, and recommended that another ad-hoc meeting be held after eighteen months to review developments in the tea industry and trade and a conference on tea statistics shold be held by the exporters as there was considerable scope for improvement in istatistics of production and consumption mentioned by FAO. Following these recommendations a meeting on tea statistics was held in Rome in 1966. The meeting considered the question of the reporting year to be adopted for tea statistics. The meeting also made certain recommndations regarding working out of representative price series by collection of data on retail prices and their dissemination among member Governments.

The second ad-hoc consultation on tea was held at London from the 20th to 28 February, 1967. This meeting considered the outlook for tea in the light of the continuing decline in the unit value of tea exports. It was recognised in this meeding that the pressure of supplies wa the major factors depressing the unit value. Production continued to expand and the implementation of the development plans in most producing countries especially in Africa signalled an increase in the rate of expansion of tea prodction in the coming years. In view of the incresing weight of plain varieties of tea coming to the market and helping to depressthe price of tea as a whole, the possibility of forbidding the export of tea below certain standards was suggested but it was recognised that this would imply evolving international standards of tea.

An informal group on promotion met during the consultation. It was emphasized that price increase could adversely affect consumption potential in developing countries. However, in developed countries increase in consumption would rather depend on promotion and quality. The meeting emphasized that consultations should continue and that the situation and outlook should be kept under review.

The third ad-hoc consultation met in Kampala (Uganda) in Janurary 1969. The meeting concluded that any feasible scale of effort devoted to promotin was unlikely to expand consumption so as to prevent the downward trend in tea prices. The producing countries felt that urgent action was required on their part while importing countries emphasized that they wre anxious to co-operate in securing stable prices remunerative to producers and acceptable to consumers. A group of exporters was proposed to facilitate the development of an action programme. It was agreed at a continuing body was required to examine the problems of tea and to evolve proposls for international action. This proposal was approved by the committee on Commodity Problems in its Forty Forth Session held in September - October, 1969 and the '*Consultative Committee on Tea'* was thus established which has been subsequently renamed as 'Intergovernment Group on Tea (Intergovernmental Group of Tea) cover a continous review continuation of studies on market structures and the promotion of tea consumption, the improvement of tea statistics, the proparation Governemtn. For this last purpose, an ad-hoc working party was held in Rome in May, 1969 which discussed issues regarding international regulations of exports. As no satisfactory result was achieved, the party decided to meet again at Mauritius.

A subsequent meeting of the group of exporting countries was held at Mauritius in July 1969. In this meeting a scheme was agreed upon for removing from the export market in 1970, some 45,000 tonnes of balck tea that would otherwise have been available for export. A proposal was also submitted on the distribution among exporting countries of export quota of 598800 tonnes of tea. The first session of the Consultative Committee on Tea (held in Rome in December

1969) approved this interim arrangement. The exproter's group was established as a standing group (subsequently called the sub-group of exportes). The terms of reference of thestanding exporters group were framed so as "to provide a regular forum in which the tea exporting countries can discuss matters of common interest and formulate proposals and recommndations for consideration by the "Consultative Committee". The conultative Committee agreed to establish also a working group on long term measures with the following terms of reference :-

(i) To take into account after detailed study, all availabel information on production, quality the market structure foteas as well as consumption trends in making its recommendations concerning the need and justification for long term action;

(ii) To consider long-term international co-operationto achieve prices that are equitable to the consumer, remunerative to producers and capable of ensuring satisfactory levels of export earnings for exporting countries vis-a-vis their Governments for consideration;

In the preparation of such schemes, consideration should be given to the interests and problems of all producing, exporting and consuming countries, with due weightage to the need for protection of the interests of smaller tea producing countries, particularly those in which opportunities for other cash crops are very limited and in which tea is involved in crop diversification programme.

The members of the working group consisted of the exporting countries of Argentina, Sri Lanka, Congo, India, Indonesia, Kenya, Malawi, Mauritius and Uganda and the importing countries of U.K., USA., Canada, Netherlands, Poland, Australia and Japan.

In Search of Long Term Agreement

The Mauritius Agreement was not a signed and scaled treaty similar to the similar to the International Agreements of Coffee and Sugar - but gentlemen's understanding of only one year's duration, and its enforecement and inplementation depended on goodwill and the honour by the participants. Yet, weak as it was, it proved significant in many ways viz, (i) it demostrated that even moderate co-operation among exporters can achieve price stability, (ii) it revealed a positive attitude of the importing countries. They took the view that the Accord was a first constructive effort and could help to prevent excessive pressure of supplies.

The working group on long-term measures for tea met in Rome in April, 1970. While, in principlem a quota type agreement appeared to be most suitable for tea, the exporting countries felt that they shold reconcile differences among themselved with regard to distribution of quotas and that the best way to achieve this would be to appoint an '*honest broker*' whose task would be to carry out confidential talks with all the exporters and to bring forth compromised proposals. Subsequently, tow confiliators, one from FAO and the other from UNCTAD were appointed. They requested the exproting countries to submit a report as soon as possible, on domestic consumption and export availabilities of tea.

The second meeting of the Consultative Committee on tea was held in New Delhi during 30th December 1970. Before this, the standing Exporters Group held two meetings, one in September 1970 and the other during 26th to 28th November 1970. In these two meetings of the standing Group of Exporters, the quota adjustments for Kenya and Malawi were agreed upon keeping the total unchanged. In the second session of the Consultative Committee and exporting countries it was emphasized that any interim arrangement for 1970 should be in the framework of negotiations for a long term agreement. It was also decided that the quota for 1971 should remain the same as hat for the year 1970. A standing group on promotion was set up (This was subsequently renamed 'The Sub-group on Promotion'). At the Third Session of the Standing Exproter's Group held in Rome in April 1971, there was disagreement between the producing countries whether prioirty for discussion would be given to the principles of a long term agreement or to the quota arrangement for 1971. A compromised solution was reached through the conciliators by extending the quota period by 3 months upto 31st March, 1972 leaving the quota for the extended 15 months period to be decided in the next meeting.

The Fourth Session of the standing Exporter's Group was held in Rome in September 1971. It was decided in this meeting that a global export quota of 727.6 thousand metric tonnes may be fixed for the 15 months period from 1st January, 1971 to 31st March, 1972. Individual quotas were also fixed. The meeting also discussed in interim report of a conciliators on the principles of a long term international agreement for tea. It was agreed that the Secretariat should circulate a paper setting out views expressed which would be considered by Governments. The consiliators were also requested to continue their work and to report to the next session.

The Fifth Session of the Sub-Group of Exporters and the interim Govt. Group on Tea (which is the new names for the Standing Exporters' Group) wa held in Rome from 18 to 22 September, 1972. It was attended by 48 delegates of 15 countries, including Bangladesh as an observer, accounting for 92 percent of world exports of black tea. The meeting wa preceded by a report of the Conciliators which came to the conclusion that no real progress could be made until exporting countries had reched a common view about the outlook for the world tea market and prospects for production, exports and import requirements. They had, therefore, propsoed that a meeting of the Sub-Group of Exporters should be convened at which the outlook for the world tea market over the coming ten years should bethe main item on the Agenda. For the first time it was possible to arrive at an understanding that pending finalization of an international agreement, quotas should be fixed on a rolling three-year basis. It was agreed that for the countries participating in the Session, the global quota for the year 1st April 1972 to 31st March, 1973, should be 6,19,000 metric tonnes and for the year 1973-74 the global quota for the year 1974-75 was fixed at 6,70,000 tonnes. The estimates of exports by individual countries for 1972-73 and 1973-74 were also proposed.

The sixth session of the Sub-Group of Exporters was held in July 1973 in which the export arrangements for 1972-73 were reviewed and the quotas for 1973-74 and 1974-75 were revised to 6,57,000 tonnes and 6,81,000 tonnes respectively. However, although there was increase in prices of tea in the London auctions in 1970 (45.7 new pence a kg) the average price of all types of tea in London declined to 43.3 new pence a kg. in 1971 and further to 42.2 new pence. Besides, wages costs of insecticide, fertilisers, the cost of transportation and shipping have risen greatly in recent years. In view of this the sub-group decided to examine the possibilities of a multi-dimensional approach in interantional co-operation to solve the persistent problem of lower prices. Studies on various techniques for improving prices were requested from FAO and UNCTAD. Further, it was agreed that promotion was an essential part of a comprehensive approach to the solution of the tea industry's problem. It was also agreed that an international symposium on promotion and market expansion should be organised as early as posible. It was decided that a global study to evaluate the cost-benefit impact on promotion should also be undertaken. The International Trade Centre of GATT/ UNCTAD was to explore ways to finacne these projects. In the meantime, the common wealth Secretariat, London has agreed to finance the symposium which will be jointly organised by the Commonwealth Secretariat and the I.T.C. - UNCTAD/GATT in co-operation with Food and Agricultural Organisation.

A. Breakthrough

The seventh session of the sub-group of Exporters held at Rome on the 10th June, 1974 and the special session of the Inter Government Group on Tea held on 17th to 19th June, 1974 marked a turning pon in the efforts of the tea exporting countries for stabilising prices of tea. This session reviewed the developments in the World Tea situation in the context of the declining trend of "real" prices of tea, on the one hand and steady escalation of costs as a result of increase in cost of petroleum products which affected ocean freight, cost of manufacture, transport etc. on the other. The Sub group observed that although the average price durng the period from January to May, 1974 was higher than that of the same period of 1973 by about 32 percent, producers had not generally been benefitted by increse in cost of all inputs. It was also apprehended that shortage and high cost of fertilisers as well as various other inputs would adversely affect production during 1974. In view of these, the Sub-Group decided to reduce the overall export quota for 1974-75 from 681 million kgs. to 658 million kgs. - A reduction by 23 million kgs. Such a reduction wa achieved for the first time since the begninning of the "Quota system" and it is bound to have a long term effect on the fixation of future "Quotas". The global quota for 1975-76 was also reduced and fixed at 682 million kgs. - about the same quota originally fixed at 682 million kgs - on provisional basis. A global quota of 693 million kgs. was fixed for the year 1976-77. Time alone will tell wheather this will also not have to be reduced.

A Multi-Dimensional Approach

The Sub-Group was unanimously of the view that immediate steps to increse the "real" prices of tea were necessary for the survival of the industry. An agreement was reached for examining in depth the following elements of a multi-dimensional international agreement for tea:

(a) A minimum export price arrangement should be made below which exports should not be allowed,

(b) Co-ordination and regulation of marketing to avoid building up of stocks in importing countries which would have depressing effect on prices.

(c) Intensification of and co-operation in global promotion including new markets,

(d) Rationnalization of marketing so as to achieve the most favourable prices with special references to the feasibility of extending auctions in producing countries,

(e) Provision of an independent market intelligence service for tea exporting countries designed to provide uptodate and regular information and marketing development and future outlook for various types of tea.

The Sub-Group requested the Director General of F.A.O to set-up and convence a meeting of a working group to examine the above proposals and to report their findings to the Sub-Group as early as possible. The recommendations of the Sub-Group on tea as well.

Maximum Return for Promotional Expenditure

The Sub-Group also discussed about the study on cost-benefit impact on promotion to be undertaken jointly by the International Trade Centres of United Nations Conferrence on Trade and Development/ General Agreement on Tariffs and Trade (UNCTAD)/(GATT) and the Commonwealth Secretariat. Discussion were also held regarding a symposium on export promotion. The object of this symposium was to pool the experience of different countries in the field of promotion so as to chalk out a programme for generic promotion of tea in various important markets including new markets. It was agreed that in selecting markets for promotion, preference should be given to those having the largest potential so that there may be maximum possible return for the promotional expenditure incurred.

The meeting of the working party of the Sub-Group of Exporter's of the Inter-Governmental Group on Tea was held at Rome from 2nd to 8th April, 1975 which recommended the following:

(i) that the technical difficulties in determining the minimum export price for all countries in an equitable manner, and the difficulties in their adoption should be removed.

(ii) that non-adoption of the export quota type of scheme in view of the lack of effectiveness of the informal quota arrangements for the previous few years should be enforced.

(iii) that the International Trade Centre and Commonwealth Secretariat should be invited to submit report on the joint missioni, in the next session, of the Sub-group of exporters for considering the establishment of Internatinal Tea Promotion Council (ITPC).

(iv) that a study on marketing and distribution system for tea should be conducted and made available to the Sub-Group of exporters for consideration and

(v) that the Director General of Food and Agriculture Organisation should be invited to explore the possibilities of improving the availability, timeliness and of statistical data relating to tea to the Sub-Group of exporters and Inter-Governmental Group on Tea for consideration of the establishment of a Marketing Intelligence Service for tea exporting countries. However, the Director General of FAO suggested to the member Governments of the Sub-Group to submit the report on the respective market situation in the next session.

The Eighth Session of the Sub-Group of exporters of the Inter-Governmental Group on Tea was held in Rome on 20-23 Apri, 1976. It was suggested in the Session that a draft of economic provision of long term agreement on tea between exporting and importing countries will be examined in a subsequent meeting of the Inter-Governmental Group. The meeting was subsequently conducted in London in February, 1977. As a result an International Programme for tea was accepted by the Group which established an ad-hoc working party including 14 countries to consider in depth the techniques and measures required for the achievement of objectives of the programmes. The big powered Indian Deligation suggested the various elements of the Action programme for Tea which was got approved by the Sub-Group of exporter and later on by the Inter-Governmental Group on Tea. The first meeting of the Sub-Group on statistics was set up following the recommendations of the Inter-Governmental Group, the meetig of which was held in India in April 1976 and also in London in February 1977 which recommended various measures relating to improvements in Tea Statistics so as to ensure more scientific study on various aspets of the World Tea situation.

In May 1976, the UNCTAD met in Nairobi to discuss the integrated programme of commodities and adopted resolution No. 93(iv) indicating the main objectives of the integrated programme for commodities which broadly explained the Action Programme for Tea. Another point of discussion was the proposal for creation of international buffer stock of few commodities of strategic importance in the developing exporting countries (including tea which is susceptible to price fluctuations).

In September 1976, a meeting was held in Geneva under the auspices of UNCTAD/GATT and the tea producing countries approved the constitution of International Tea Promotion Association (ITPA). The Association started functioning since January 1980 with headquarters at Totterdam. The question of introduction of Export Regulations Scheme and revival of International Tea Agreement (ITA) for the propose had been under active consideration of FAO/UNCTAD since 1965. The producing countries had in a meeting held in November 1976 finally agreed to the introduction of a Export Regulation Scheme combined with buffer-stock-holding agreement. The matter was discussed further in the UNCTAD meeting held in December 1976.

Further, in order to make a common understanding between the leading tea producing countries in respect of export quotas and buffer stock, a tea delegation visited the various African countries in the first week of May 1980 and Sri Lanka in the middle of 1980. Another round of discussions among the tea producing countries took place in the first week of May 1980 at Jakarta (Indonesia) so as to give a formal shape to the export quota and buffer stock arrangements. In September/October 1980 another meeting was held at Geneva to discuss further about introduction of export quotas for all the tea producing countries. This was followed by November 1980. Subsequently in May 1981, a meeting of the tea producing countries was convened by UNCTAD at Geneva.

The meeting of the producing countries convened by UNCTAD at Geneva in the last week of May 1981 also ended without any agreement. The impasse arose only because of Kenya's insistence of adopting a Seven Year time-lag for working out export quota as a basis for the agreement. In June 1981, there was an informal discussion at Geneva between the representatives of the Government of India, Sri Lanka and UNCTAD Secretaries for finding out a way out of the impasse. The UNCTAD Secretaries after holding similar informal discussion with the representative of Govt. of Kenya suggested a compromised formula which proposed a three-tier system under which different countries were allocated varying lag periods for working out the export quota. The lag period in respect of India and Sri Lanka under the revised formula was to be four years and six years respectively and five years for other countries. At the initiative and request from the Govt. of Kenya a meeting of the representatives of India, Sri Lanka and Kenya was held in Nairobi in September 1981. The representatives of the Kenyan Government expressed their willingness to consider the revised formula as a basis for working out export quotas. They also agreed to give up the instance of seven year lag period. The meeting in Kenya thus proved to be a major break-through so that for the first time in three years the tea producing and exporting countries of world reached an accord regarding the basis for working out the extra quota.

In a meeting of the tea producing countries held at New Delhi from 8 to 12 February 1982 under the auspices of UNCTAD it was agreed, in principle, that export quota was, necessary for achieving the price objective. In that meeting a draft element of the proposed international tea agreement was also approved. In the meeting of the tea exporting and importing countries held in Geneva in May 1982 the various aspects of international tea agreement were discussed. The talks ere, however, inconclusive. The UNCTAD was making efforts to bring India, Sri Lanka and Kenya under a common understanding in respect of sharing of export quotas.

Subsequently, the Ninth, Tenth and Eleventh Sessions of the Sub-Group of Exporters of the Inter-Governmental Group on Tea was held during the period 1983 to 1987. Lastly, the Twelfth Session of the sub-Group of Exporters of the Inter-Governmental Group on Tea was held in Rome from 22-25th February 1988. It was agreed in the meeting that production expansion should take place in the sector but the quality standard should not deviate significantly from ISO standard 3720.

Apart from the various measures discussed above, the impediments in the path of the tea imports in developed countries viz., tariff/ nontariff barriers etc. were also examined by the Inter-Governmental Group on Tea and remedial measures suggested. The importing countries were requested to remove those barriers as early as possible. The reaction of the importing countries was apparently quite encouraging.

International Tea Convention

The eighth International Tea Conventional of the Inter-Governmental Group on Tea under the aegies of FAO was held in Rome during October 1990. It was attended by the delegates of a large number of countries. The Indian delegation was led by the Chairman, Tea Board. Short-term and longterm outlook for tea, taking into consideration the global supply and demand position, were discussed at length.

Part III

Inter-Governmental Group on Tea (IGG) : (FAO)

The Inter-Governmental Group on Tea held its twelfth session from 2nd to 4th July 1997 at Bali, Indonesia. It was attended by the member countries including India. The Chairman and Vice Chairman of the Board attended the meeting. Following issues were discussed at the above session.

1. Economic and trade issues which included :
   a) Market situation and short-term outlook.
   b) Identification and development of markets.
   c) Price deterioration, export earnings and food security of small tea growers.
   d) Policy consideration for strengthening economic viability.

2. Inter governmental action included :
   a) Progress report on tea consumption and human health project.
   b) Production and market improvement measures.
   c) Statement of priorities of the group of the common fund for commodities.

In regard to Inter-governmental action, the Technical Advisory Committee (TAC) presented its report to the group covering the research activities on health aspects on consumption of black tea as of December 1996. Subsequently, the Project Executing Agency (PEA) presented a progress report updating information on findings of health related research upto the second year of the project. Evidence indicated that black tea consumption could protect against lung cancer developments. Tea drinking was most likely to protect against breast cancer.

On the promotional phase of the project, the group received a report from the PEA relating to the work which had been completed and extensively researched to develop a communication package to convey a general health message for black tea globally. Due to stands taken by different countries a compromise formula was arrived at by having an international logo (Rising Sun in a Tea Cup) as well as a message (Tea; Discover the Goodness).

The IGG considered property rights governing the communication in package developed on its behalf by the PEA. It was decided that the ownership of the communication package symbol, strapline and trademark would be registered in the name of Food and Agriculture Organisation (FAO).

FAO in co-operation with the PEA and its Steering Committee would prepare a proposal as to the usage of the communication package following completion of the test markets and the overall project.

South Asian Association for Regional Co-operation (SAARC)

An Indian tea delegation visited Pakistan in July 1997. Reciprocating this visit, an 8-member tea delegation from the Pakistan Tea Association led by its the then Chairman, Mr. M M Ispahani, visited India for the first time after Independence between16th and 25th November, 1997. During the visits of these two delegations some contracts were signed to export tea from India to Pakistan. The delegation had an introductory round of discussions in Tea Board and with the tea trade as well as Indian exporters in Kolkata. The delegation represented around 70 per cent of the tea trade in Pakistan. During their visit a proposal had been mooted for setting up an auction centre in Karachi or Dubai. It was decided that M/s J Thomas & Co Pvt Ltd would prepare a feasibility report on this proposal.

It was noted that in the second round of trade negotiations under the SAARC Preferential Trade Agreement (SAPTA), a National Schedule of Concessions granted by Pakistan to India had been listed where tea had not found place. The matter was taken up with SAARC Chamber of Commerce. The Association thereafter represented to the Union Commerce Ministry that a tariff concession to tea imported from India could substantially address the high cost of imports which continued to constrain the Pakistan tea trade. The Association also submitted that tea should be brought under the umbrella of concessional tariff when the third round of SAARC Trade agreement (SAPTA) negotiations commence under the SAARC. Ministry's response, however, was not available by the end of this reporting period.

Nivedan teas

Following sharp increase in tea prices during the period from 1995 to 1997 there was considerable pressure from the Government to offer tea at a concessional price. The subject was discussed at a meeting of the CCPA held on 28th November 1997 following which a Nivedan Co-ordination Committee was constituted by the Chairman, CCPA under the convenorship of Mr D L Thapar of Assam Co Ltd and with representatives of all constituent associations and members of the ITA Export, Promotion & Marketing sub-committee as members. The committee worked out the modalities of the offer. Producers offered teas in designed polypacks of two sizes, 250 gms and 100 gms, at a price of Rs. 88 per kg. All tea producing companies were thoroughly advised on the modalities. They were also advised to put out advertisements in local papers and/or banners to in form the public on the retail outlets. The position was reviewed at several committee meetings held on different dates. The committee decided to place teas in retail outlets in some selected towns/cities all over India by 31st January 1998. The committee closely monitored the offers made by members of all CCPA constituents. The subject was also discussed with senior Government officials at New Delhi. By the end of this reporting period, it was noted that while about 6.5 lakh kgs were already despatched out of total agreed quantity of 1.3 million kgs, ITA members had nearly fulfilled their obligations. Being approached by the Union Commerce Ministry, the Association advised certain major tea producers to offer a total 13000 kg of tea (packed in 100 gm polypouches) to National Co-operative Consumer Federation of India Ltd. (NCCF) which producers obliged.

Generic promotion of Indian tea

The Indian Tea Association and UPASI jointly commissioned ORG-MARG in July 1995 to conduct a study on tea consumption patterns in India towards examining the feasibility of generic promotion of tea in India as a measure to stimulate per capita tea consumption. Total cost of this study (Rs.20.04 lakhs) was borne by these two Associations. A working group was constituted to guide the Secretariat in this project.

ORG-MARG submitted the study report in August 1996. The Working Group as well as the General Committee of ITA and UPASI deliberated on the report. On the recommendation of the General

Committee a Task Force was, thereafter, constituted which interacted with six advertising agencies who placed their proposals for generic promotion campaign in certain selected states on the basis of each state's potential. It was decided that instead of launching the campaign all over India, initial campaign could cover on two states, one in North India and one in South India, primarily because of cost involvement. Finally M/s Hindustan Thompson Associate (HTA) was selected which presented the following two options :

Option I	:	To cover West Bengal and Karnataka Total cost: Rs 2.82 Cr.
Option II	:	To cover North India belt and Karnataka Total cost : Rs 6.15 Cr.

HTA presented its final proposal in June 1997 to the ITA General Committee which was in favour of Option I. The matter was thereafter placed at a CCPA meeting held on 28th November 1997 where the constituents' participation was sought keeping in view that the entire tea industry could benefit from the exercise. Response received from constituent associations, however, was not favourable. Finally the ITA General Committee decided that while efforts should continue to pursuade UPASI on participation in the promotion campaign, ITA members should be prepared to go with the launching alone even if UPASI declined to participate. At the end of the year it was noted that UPASI did not confirm its participation.

Later the Association approached the Tea Packeter Association of India (TPAI) which expressed its willingness to participate and contribute to the project. At an informal meeting between the chairmen of Hindustan Lever Ltd and association, the former generously agreed to financially contribute in the promotion campaign. A considerable time was spent to decide on the theme and story of the campaign. At a meeting the General Committee suggested that a tightly knit Steering Committee comprising marketing personnel with adequate exposure to A&P from the member companies as well as TPAI and HLL could be constituted for taking up the exercise to its logical conclusion. Thereafter, a Steering Committee was formed under the convenorshipc of Mr P Siganporia, Tata Tea Ltd in January 1998.

Cess under the Tea Act

The Central Government, Ministry of Commerce, vide their notification dated 27th March 1997 revised the rate of cess on tea from the existing 8 paise to 12 paise per kilogram in respect of Darjeeling Hill areas and from 15 paise to 30 paise per kilogram for all other areas. The Association at once represented to the Union Commerce Ministry against this move. Although the Commerce Ministry had conveyed that the additional revenue would go towards increased development outlays, the industry felt that part of the increase should go towards meeting R&D and HRD activities and that the industry should, in the circumstances, desist from separately contributing to its research institutions such as TRA, UPASI, TRI, DTRC and IIPM. The matter was raised by ITA Chairman at a meeting with Commerce Ministry at New Delhi where it was pointed that the annual budgetary allocations of the Tea Board should reflect total funding of R&D and HRD activities both in the North and the South. While the matter was slated for discussion at the Central Advisory Committee meeting, it was decided that the CCPA should seek a separate meeting with the Union Commerce Ministry to exclusively review its research and the funding of research institutions. The Association also represented to the Tea Board that the increase in cess for non-traditional areas should not be more than what was notified for the two sub-divisions of Darjeeling, and the Board was requested to take up the matter with the Commerce Ministry. No further development was recorded on the subject during this reporting period.

Tea Marketing control order

Following the rising tea prices and lower offerings of teas in the Indian auctions against the background of higher production in India, Tea Board requested the CCPA to ensure strict compliance with the provisions of the Tea Marketing (Control) Order 1984 regarding sale of tea. Although the CCPA responded to the Tea Board by stating that regulatory measures such as TMCO are obsolete and should be dispensed with in the present era of liberalisation, CCPA/ITA advised their members on several occasions to comply with the provisions of TMCO pertaining to the sale of tea through auctions.

Tea Board complained that a large number of tea companies were not furnishing the annual information regarding production and marketing for the year 1996. The Board pointed that non-submission of such information would constitute violation of Clause 5 of the TIMCO. CCPA/ITA had advised members accordingly.

Tea Board vide letter No. 11(1)/DTD/1997/3527 dated 32.1.98 informed CCPA that they had decided that fulfilment of the provisions of the TMCO would be henceforth treated as one of the pre-requisites for financial assistance under the on-going development schemes of the tea board. Members were advised vide ITA Circular No.16 dated 5.2.98.

Export of Packet Tea Bags and Instant Tea

The Union Commerce Ministry reportedly reviewed the policy in connection with the tea import through EOU/EPZ units and decided to relax certain conditions in regard to DTA sales by EOU/EPZ units engaged in manufacture of packet tea, tea bags and instant tea for a period of 6 months w.e.f. 1.1.98. The ministry, in this connection, issued a Circular No. 8/1/91-EPZ dated 2.2.98 (reproduced in Appendix No. 11). The Association vigorously protested against this dilution. (The ministry, however, did not extend the relaxation after 31.6.98).

The Russian Federation increased basis of customs duty imposition on packet tea import into Russia w.e.f. 1.6.97. The duty, which was 10 per cent of CIF value subject to a minimum of 0.1 ECU per kg, was revised to 20 per cent of CIF value subject to a minimum of 0.4 ECU per kg. This disproportionate rise in minimum Duty Clause was discriminatory against Indian packet tea exports a major part of which averages between $1.70 to $2 per kg (CIF). Apprehending that this discrimination puts India among others at a disadvantage vis-a-vis packet teas imported from the West which comes in at higher CIF values, the Association urged the Commerce Minister to take up the matter appropriately with his counterpart in Russian Federation towards rationalising the position.

London auction

During the period under review the Association was informed by one of its member companies (M/s Assam Tea Co Ltd) that their application to the customs authorities seeking customs approval for notional price for the London auction was kept pending for quite some time. The Association took up the matter with the customs authorities that export of tea on consignment basis be ultimately sold through the London auctions as it formed a significant part of Indian tea exports, and as tea prefixed contracted value could not be indicated on consignment of such teas, it was the long-standing practice for consignment exporters to indicate a notional price which had been accepted by the customs authorities for many years. The Association, therefore, requested the customs authorities to expedite approval of Assam Company's application. The customs authorities complied with the Association request and accorded necessary approval to the Assam Company in this regard.

Guwahati Tea Auction Centre

During the year under review GTAC witnessed higher level of the withdrawl of teas from the auction which was causing a lot of concern to the trade. With a view to resolve the matter, a meeting of the Sales Sub-Committee of the GTAC was convened on 12th June 1997. It was decided in this meeting that as per the Ahuja Committee recommendations, the last day for withdrawal of teas by sellers at the GTAC would be Thursday of the week preceding the week prior to the sale in question and broker would put "Withdrawal Notices" on the Notice Board of the GTAC on the same day during office hours with effect from Sale No.28 onwards.

In another development, the Association's Export Promotion & Marketing Sub-Committee in a meeting reviewed the overall tea market situation where it was felt that the throughput at the Guwahati Auction Centre might require some scrutiny. As a case in point it was highlighted that after Sale 40 which closed on the same date as last year, the quantity of unsold teas amounted to 39,000 packages as compared to 2,29,000 packages last year. The Association, therefore, felt that without compromising the overall volumes routed through the Guwahati Auction there might be a case for appropriately staggering subsequent offerings to ensure that enough teas were retained to cover the lean period till March 1998. It would be pertinent to mention that the centre had dropped some sales in March 1997. Summing up the above points the Association requested the GTAC to examine these aspects and adopt appropriate measures.

Siliguri Tea Auction Centre

During the period under review a crisis was developed at the Siliguri Tea Auction Centre arising out of the resignation of buyers from the Governing Body of the STAC following a hard stand taken by the STAC to deal with the buyers who had failed prompt in respect of Sale No.6. Later with the assistance of the Minister and the District Magistrate, Darjeeling the impasse at STAC was resolved and buyers were granted extension of a day prompt.

It was noted during the year that two Auction Buyer's Associations at Siliguri had appealed for a concession on the existing sampling qualification norms for the year 1998-99 on the purchase on 1997-98 and that it was represented that if the existing qualification norms for free trade sample were applied, about 30% of buyers at Siliguri would not qualify for samples. At the meeting of the Governing Body of STAC, Seller members had indicated that the matter would have to be considered at the CCPA level. The matter was thereafter discussed threadbare in the CCPA (West Bengal Interest) meeting held on 17th February 1998.

In this meeting the seller's position was summed up as follows :

- There should be no concession/relaxation on the prevailing sampling qualification norms at any auction centre.
- Buyers at Siliguri should agree, in principle, to the introduction of the 3 years' aggregate purchase norm.
- Minimum percentage qualification (0.2%) for small buyers should be increased in order to make the auction system attractive and competitive.

Auction matters

In the Annual Report for 1996-97 it was stated interalia that the CCPA had written to the Tea Board for introduction of the consecutive 3-year aggregated purchasing norms as qualification for entitlement of free trade sample.

During this year the Tea Board, vide their letter No.13(23)/ML/98/482 dated 8.5.98, favourably considered the CCPA's proposal and issued instruction to all auction centres in North India to abide by the 3 year's aggregated purchase norms to qualify for free trade sample as follows:

Sampling Year 1998-1999 : Purchase Year 1997-98.

Sampling Year 1999-2000 : Purchase Year 1998-99.

Sampling Year 2000-2001: Purchase Years 1998-99 and 1999-2000.

Sampling Year 2001-2002 : Purchase Years 1998-99, 1999-2000 and 2000-2001.

For sampling year 2002-2003 and onwards, aggregate purchases in the previous three consecutive purchase years would form the basis for eligibility to free trade samples. With effect from sampling year 2001-2002 a buyer would not be eligible to free trade samples if his purchases in any relevant purchase year falls below 25% of the minimum qualifying quantity. The text of the Tea Board's above mentioned letter is reproduced in Appendix No. 12. The Association advised members accordingly vide Circular letter No. 1216 dated 19.5.98.

In another development, a message dated 24.12.97 was received from Tea Board regarding the rate of bidding for CTC teas in case of price per kg goes beyond Rs. 100/- with immediate effect. The Board decided to relax the provisions of the Auction Rules pertaining to bidding and the incremental bids in case of CTC teas until further orders. The Board directed that for CTC teas in all auction centres in India, if the price per kg went beyond Rs. 100/- per kg, the incremental bid would now be only Rupee one. This would be applicable to CTC leaf and all dust teas, all other conditions would remain unchanged.

Tea Board vide letter dated 1.1.98 advised all auction centres that no withdrawals of CTC lots, including Leaf, Brokens. Fannings and Dust grades, will be allowed exception unavoidable and exception circumstances until further orders. Tea Board later rescinded this directive vide letter No. 13(23)/ML/98 dated 30th July 1998.

Marking ink

The Indian Tea Association had from time to time advised members to remain vigilant against complaints in respect of marking ink used on tea chests. The Association, during this reporting period, had received a letter from a reputed Merchant Exporter conveying their concern over the lack of corrective steps to address this problem and highlighting the fact that powdered ink continued to be used to mark tea chests. Following this the Association suggested to the members that following precautionary remedial measures should be taken at the tea estate level viz:

Patenting of CTC manufacturing process including vacuum packaging

A patent application had been filed by M/s George Williamson & Co Ltd, a British Company, for method and apparatus for preparing processed tea leaf which essentially pertain to CTC manufacture and subsequent vacuum packaging of tea. Several companies, however, filed objection petitions with the Patent Office in Chennai contesting the application on the ground that the claims made were nothing novel as the manufacturing process and vacuum packing methods had been in use in the industry for many years. It was, however, clarified that the application by M/s George Williamson & Co, UK was not attempting to patent the existing CTC manufacturing process, instead this was intended to patenting a combination of the manufacturing process and vacuum packing of bulk tea.

Conclusion

The problem of falling prices in the world Market is a matter of serious concern for all the tea producing countries. It is sincerely hoped that combined thrust of various measures indicated in the foregoing paragraphs will enable them, in not too distant future, to achieve a sustained increase in "real prices" of tea which will neutralise the effect of all round escalation of costs and will at the same time enable the exporting countries to prevent the erosion of their foreign exchange earnings from export of tea due to decline in prices, on the one hand and depreciation of the purchasing power of almost all the international currencies due to world wide inflation on the other.

Chapter 16

India International Millennium Tea Convention - Recommendations

The India International Millennium Tea concention was organised in Taj Palace Hotel, New Delhi from 22-24 March 2000 with the objectives of (i) upgrading the value perception of tea, especially in the light of emerging research findings on health benefits, (ii) considering tea as the drink of the new millennium and crating awareness on the entire range fo possibilities of India tea. The convention was attended by the degegated who were involved in tea production, trade and research etc., from National and International organisations etc. with a view to attain the objectives, the entire convention concentrated on the following areas:

1. To review the Tea Industry Scenario.
2. To establish health eredentials of tea
3. To review the emerging marketing concepts that could also draw on health aspects of tea and hellp reposition it as a beverage of the new millennium.

The Details of recommendatins are highlighted below:

- Mr. R.S. Jhawar, Chairman, CCPA, in his welcome address highlighted the following aspects:
- The" Tea Industry", employing over 1.1 million workers directly, the largest in any industry, looking after more than 4 million dependents of these employees, and supporting more than 50,000 small tea growers, along with its associated and ancillary activities in distribution, retailing, warehousing, tea shops, etc., is directly and indirectly supporting almost 2% of the population of the country.

- This for an industry which has a turn over of only RS.6000 crores (US $ 1.5 billion).
- Of the working population directly employed by the Tea Industry, 50% are women.
- In the world where ecological degradation is reaching alarming proportions and the management of the environment is now a primary concern of the policy makers around the world, the Tea Industry provides a non-polluting atmosphere through miles and miles of lush green plantations.
- With 31 % of the total Tea produced in the world, India continues to mair:tain its leadership in the international market.
- Since the country's Independence, the production of Tea has increased from 251 million Kgs. to about 850 million Kgs, an increase of 250%. Additional land availability during this period was only 40%.
- This was possible due to investments by the industry in Research & Development and development of Human Resources.
- The Tea Research Association, Tea Research Institute of Coonoor, Darj eeling Tea Research Centre and the latest, the Indian Institute of Plantation of Management, are the finest institutions established in this direction.
- It is basically on these pillars that the industry has been able to retain its global leadership over the last 150 years.
- Tea is also a healthy drink. Polyphenol content of Tea has superior anti-oxidant properties which helps in preventing and controlling several chronic diseases, including cancer and cardiovascular. Tea also plays a vary positive role in contributing to dental care, beauty care and in improving longevity. Antioxidant properties in two cups of tea are supposed to be equal to 3 or 4 glasses of orange juice or 20 glasses of apple juice.
- It is this new role of tea which is going to be of extreme value to the world community, particularly as medical is progressively becoming more and more expenSIve.
- Unlike alcohol or colas, or even coffee, we do not have any

negative health effects in Tea. The image of tea is not only one of a stimulant but also that of health promotion. If 3.5 billion cups of tea consumed daily across the world could convey this message, Tea could playa very significant role in transforming human values.

- Tea is set to be the" Wonder Beverage of the New Millennium"
- India's per capita daily consumption is less than a cup. Globally, daily consumption per capita is just about half a cup, and there lies a vast potential.
- There is a need to work together towards a generic campaign to strengthen the brand equity of tea.
- " Drink Tea and Stay Healthy" is our motto.

Addressing the convention, Sri Murasoli Maran, the then Minister of Commerce & Industries, Government of India, observed that:

- The tea industry in India is now more than 160 years old and, though as an export item it has ceased to be an important commodity for India, it still holds a considerable potential of the economic development of the country.
- It is one of the most organised industries employing more than a million people and generating a revenue of about Rs.6,000 crore.
- Tea occupies the pride of place in the plantation sector in India, as it is the common man's beverage popular all over the country.
- Tea is an important agricultural product traded all over the world. It plays a key role in the economy of more than 30 developing and least developed countries (LDCs), as it is grown mostly in Asia, Africa and some South American countries.
- Around 1260 million kgs. of tea was exported in the year 1998, giving invaluable foreign exchange to the exporting countries.
- During the last one and a half decades, the tea industry has witnessed an increase in production worldwide, exceeding the increase in demand during that period.
- The disproportionate increase in demand and supply has left a surplus of about 150 million kgs. of tea by the end of 2110.

- The period has also seen increasing uncertainties in market conditions, giving rise to increased price volatility in tea markets.
- There is an emergent need to arrest the wild price fluctuations, as they may discourage long term investments in tea.
- The trading of 85% of the total world tea production through auctions, which are spot markets, is the peculiarity of the tea industry.
- One method to achieve stability in tea prices may be to develop forward and future markets.
- Risk management tools, which have been used by traders and producers very effectively to deal with price uncertainties in important commodity markets like Coffee, Cocoa and Sugar, perhaps need to be evolved keeping in view the specific situation in tea trade. May be it is not easy but it may be worthwhile examining the alternative.
- Traditionally tea faces stiff competition from coffee. Of late, however, a much stiffer challenge has come from carbonated drinks.
- This is one of the important reasons for a rather not so encouraging demand-supply projections of tea over the next decade.
- It is worth noting that consumption is projected to increase only in the countries where tea has firmly established itself.
- As per Food and Agriculture Organisation's projections, world black tea consumption will increase between 2000 and 2005, at an annual growth rate of 2.8%. Developing countries would account for the largest part of the increase with a growth rate estimated at 3 % per annum during the period, whereas the developed countries, including the countries in transition, are likely to register a moderate annual growth of 2.2%.
- The tea industry must go in systematically for generic promotion of tea.
- The entire tea fraternity should look above the brand loyalties and cooperate in generic promotion.

- If there were to be serious mismatch between demand and production, the brand image alone cannot help the producer much.
- Discovery of the anti-oxidants viz., flavonoids, in both black and green teas, help neutralise 'free radicals' produced in the body as part of the normal functioning and thereby decreasing incidence of heart attack or stroke caused by blocked arteries.
- Discovery of anti-carcenogenic properties and the re-discovery of extra-ordinary revival and relaxing properties of tea, are bound to give added advantage to generic promotion programmes.
- There is an urgent need to harmonise the standards for MRL (Minimum Residue Limits) in Tea.
- It will be proper that all the tea exporting and importing countries follow the technical standards set by the "Coded Alimentarious Commission", under the aegis of the WTO (World Trade Organisation)

Session (i) The World Tea Scenario - Mr.Kaison Chang, Secretary, IGG, FAO

- Tea is grown widely in countries of Asia, Africa and the Near East.
- It has widespread implications for the earnings and food security of farm communities, particularly small holders in these countries.
- Historically, tea has competed effectively in an increasingly crowded beverage market, but indications are that it has lost ground, particularly in the early to mid-nineties.
- Demand has become sluggish and even declined in some of its traditional markets.
- Consequently, prices have fallen in real terms as the imbalance between production and consumption has grown.
- The production to consumption ratio needs to be rationalised in order to attain remunerative prices and hence ensure the viability of the global tea economy.

Current Tea Situation:

- World tea production in the last decade has grown at an yearly rate of 1.81 per cent until 2004 and consumption has kept pace at a slightly higher growth rate of 2.05 per cent per year.
- However, global consumption has consistently been significantly less than production.
- Global production is dominated by India.
- The second largest producer is China with its highest output also recorded in 1998, when its production reached 665 000 tonnes.
- Kenya follows as a distant third at 294 200 tonnes and Sri Lanka at 280 100. Argentina and Bangladesh follow as fifth, sixth and seventh respectively.
- Preliminary estimates available to F AO indicate that world tea production in 1999 declined down from a record 1998 output of nearly 3 million tonnes to 2.7 million -t:onnes.
- Smaller crops are harvested in all major producing countries, except in China and Sri Lanka. as unfavourable weather affected in Bangladesh, India, Indonesia, and Kenya.

Exports:

- World Tea Exports have grown by almost 2 per cent over the last decade.
- Sri Lanka is the largest exporter, followed by Kenya, China and India.
- In the year 1998, global exports expanded by more than 7 per cent, compared to 1997, to reach 1.27 million tonnes.

Imports:

- World imports grew yearly at 1.2 per cent over the last decade. The United Kingdom was the largest importer until 1997, when the CIS surpassed its imports. Pakistan is the third largest importing country followed by the United States, Egypt, and Japan.

- In 1998, world tea imports rose by 2.4 per cent compared to volumes in 1997, with most growth occurring in developing countries, mainly Pakistan, where demand expanded by 28 per cent.
- Significant growth was also experienced in the United States, as imports expanded by 19 per cent in 1998, potentially attributable to the impact of consumer promotion of health benefits of tea consumption in that country.
- However, the expansion was not sufficient to offset declines in other developed countries, such as the 4 per cent decline in the EC and 5 per cent in the Russian Federation.
- A marked trend in recent years has been the shift in demand towards the import of Quality teas, not only in mature markets such as United Kingdom and Russian Federation, but also in the rest of Europe and North America.

Prices:

- The price of black tea generally declined in all auction markets in the first of half of 1999, due to forecast of larger crops in major producing countries and weaker demand in the Russian Federation.
- However, prices recovered as revised production estimates indicated lower harvests.
- The F AO composite price trend of tea (a weighted average price oftea traded in the major auction markets of Kenya, India, and Sri Lanka) indicated as sustained price decline in the first half of 1999, from an average of US 166 cents to US 161 cents per Kg. However, in the third quarter prices recovered by 11 per cent to US 178 cents per Kg. Prices further improved in the fourth quarter and averaged US 183 cents per Kg, up 3 per cent from the previous quarter.

Developments in Enhancing Demand:

- Previous efforts at improving prices were production oriented, and focused on decreasing the cost of promotion and increasing yields.

- *A programme to create an Increased Demand/or Tea Through Research on the Human Health Benefits of Black Tea Consumption and Generic promotion, concluded at the end of 1999.*
- The project was significant in that it was the first "intergovernmental" coordinated effort at the world level, at generically promoting tea in market place.
- The objectives of the project were to provide scientific data on health benefits of black tea consumption, and to demonstrate the cost effectiveness of a health based generic campaign. It was implemented by the United Kingdom Tea Council and supervised by the FAO Intergovernmental Group (IGG) on Tea.
- Generally, the scientific and test market results were favourable. However, the scientific research results still have to be peer-reviewed and published, while the test marketing results will have to be quantitatively analysed to evaluate the impact of the generic promotion campaigns carried out, in various countries, on consumption.
- *One of the most tangible and immediate benefits that have emerged from the project has been the creation of the international Tea Mark.*

Medium Term Developments:

Production:

- World Black Tea production is projected to reach 3.1 million tonnes by 2005, an annual average growth rate of 3 percent from the 1993-95 base period.
- Production in India is estimated at 1.15 million tonnes in 2005.
- **Production expansion programmes initiated by major exporting countries have contributed to previous increases in output of black tea in recent years, and the impact of these programmes, particularly as bushes reach optimum production age, may continue.** Consumption:
- World Black Tea consumption is projected to increase by 3 per cent per annum to 3.0 million tonnes by 2005, with developing

countries accounting for the largest part of the prospective increase. Consumption in these countries would reach 2.15 million tonnes by 2005, an annual growth rate of more than 3 per cent.

- Black tea consumption in India is projected to reach 820 000 tonnes by 2005.
- The reduction of import tariff and declining prices could have a more pronounced effect on consumption in countries like Pakistan, the Islamic Republic of Iran and Egypt.
- In developed countries, including countries in transition, black tea consumption would increase more moderately to 850 000 tonnes in 2005.

Imports:

- Import requirements at 2005 are projected at 1.55 million tonnes, an average annual increase of 3.6 per cent from the base period average.
- Import requirements by developing countries would increase more rapidly to reach 850,000 tonnes.
- In volume terms, the major importers would be the CIS (mainly Russian Federation), Pakistan, the United Kingdom, Egypt and the United States. Together these countries would account for 51 per cent of the total import requirements.

Exports:

- Export availabilities are projected to reach 1.6 million tonnes in 2005, an "average annual increase of 3.8 per cent from the actual exports during the base period.
- China, India, Indonesia, Sri Lanka and Kenya are expected to account for 78 per cent of the total projected export availabilities.
- The balance would largely be sourced from Bangladesh, Malawi, Tanzania, Turkey and Zimbabwe, where export availabilities are expected to increase significantly over the medium term.

Conclusion:

Given the prospect of downward pressure on prices, the commodity policy for tea for the next decade should largely concentrate on the exploration of possible new market-oriented approaches.

Session (ii) :The Tea Situation In India : by Deepak Atal - M.D., Rossel Industries.

Tea Production:

- It is time for the Indian tea industry to take stock of itself in this kaleidoscope of change for no industry can remain an island in the waves of transformation that are hitting the global market place.
- In the tleld of production, India holds a dominant position, as a global leader.
- The Indian Tea Industry has recorded enviable growth intlwpost independence period barring a few setbacks in some years. The year 2005 saw an all time record 889 million kgs.
- Growth in productivity during the above period was 1.5%.
- Taking 1951 as the cut off year, India produced 42% of the world's production of 683 million kg. In 1997. world production rose to 2,667 million kg. and the Indian share was around 30%. By 1998. India accounted for approximately 29% of the world production.
- India's percentage share against global production has been dropping. This is a result of quantum jump in the production of other tea growing countries as well as new entrants. The fact that India remains the largest producer of tea is an achievement in itself, as the growth in planted area is a mere 0.5%.
- This is a tltting tribute to the dedication and commitment of the planting community, backed by in-house R&D, and the systematic and continuous upgradation and modernisation of operations in the sphere of both tleld and factory.
- There is no room for complacency. Two stark realities face the industry. One is the reality of the global market place. Consumption trends indicate that the growth of markets is particularly in the underdeveloped and developing parts of the world with limited purchasing power and therefore, demand is

governed by the value for money options.

- The second factor is that the economics of scale can only be achieved by sustained increase in production to balance cost, quality and market share in order to achieve and maintain a competitive advantage.
- This predetermines a greater thrust into the areas of tea technology than ever before. Keeping in view the constraints of land, biotechnology to overcome present yield barriers, need to be explored with greater urgency.
- The global warming and the changes in weather pattern underscore the need to increase the momentum for genetic engineering to achieve production of plants with increased resistance to drought, frost, water logging, apart from inter flush and seasonal dormancy. To keep pace with the increasing requirement of hygiene in manufacturing standards, the application of "Hazard Analysis Critical Control Point", generally referred to as HACCP (Haccup) will need greater thrust.
- What is required is an acknowledgement for the need and renewed dedication to research and development.
- India as a signatory to the W.T.O. would have to dismantle its import restrictions by the year 2002.
- To be in shape to compete globally, one of the areas that needs to be given greater priority would be research and development in derivatives of tea.

Exports:

- In the area of exports, the Indian tea industry has been to some extent a victim of circumstance. Unlike other major producing countries, India has seen a significant increase in domestic consumption and as a consequence, out prices itself in the international markets for the bulk of its tea.
- In 1951, India held 45% of the world's total exports. By 1998, the figure declined to around 17% in spite of maintaining a level of 190-200 million kg.
- The disintegration of the USSR, the financial constraints in Iran

and Iraq, the growing domestic market erratic policies of the Indian government in the earlier years, all impacted negatively on India's market share.

- Yet, tea exports are vital to the Indian economy and the health of the industry.
- Traditional trading routes and export of bulk tea alone will not suffice for India's export efforts. Strengthening of supply chain management, linking up with major distribution networks, opting for alliances and partnerships with international marketeers would need a greater thrust.
- In the developed world, the traditional fashion of tea consumption is on a down swing. Yet markets are growing for canned tea, organic tea and derivatives of tea.
- Apart from servicing the traditional buyers ofIndian tea such as UK, Germany and Japan, India will need to look beyond- to the USA and Canada, for example, where tea consumption though small, is on the rise, and where the current presence of Indian tea is limited.
- Russia and CIS continue to be critical to Indian export efforts. It is estimated that total imports into the CIS from India are in the region of 68-70%.
- Quite clearly, India's compulsion today is to diversify her export market.
- The Indian Tea Industry must look to develop and strengthen its national brand equity, catering to Western and Oriental tastes that are prevalent in this region. The "Nargis" brand is a step in that direction.
- It is incumbent on the Indian tea industry to work towards regional brand building and to assure the world markets that quality and volumes are available.
- The "India Tea Logo" together with the logos of Darjeeling, Assam and Nilgiris need to be promoted and endorsed by the Government of India with support from industry.

The domestic market:

- The domestic market is the bedrock of the Indian Tea Industry.

- According to a recent survey undertaken by ORG, India's total consumption of tea in 1999 was estimated at 638 million kg. and per capita consumption at 0.66 kg.
- This has been further broken down to the packet market share at an estimated 264 million Kgs. against loose tea consumption of 374 million Kgs.
- Taken as a composite whole, the emerging trend of tea consumption in India is a marked shift to quality and this is reflected in the price differential between quality and common categories of tea.
- This is a natural corollary to the growing sophistication of the consumer and whilst demand in the next decade may be in the region of 730 million Kgs.
- The changing consumer profile has led to increasing competition from aerated beverages f and other soft drinks. This underscores the need for a cohesive the consumer friendly campaign of generic promotion of tea not only to highlight the health benefits of tea, but to, change the positioning of tea as a beverage with particularly the below 35-year olds, be in the urban or rural markets.
- In a nutshell, the Indian tea industry is confronted with:
- Increased competition
- A need to search for and develop new markets
- To strengthen the competitive edge of quality and costs
- To boost demand on the platform of a healthy, youthful beverage.
- To maintain a steady increase in production so as to adequately serve international demand. Indian has huge potential as is seen by a surge in tea plantations by small gowers in various areas.

Session (iii) : The Kenyan Tea Situation - Mr. N.G.Waireri - East African Tea Trade Asso'ciation.

- Kenyan tea industry is an young, the oldest tea bush is only 70 years old,
- Growth in production is 7-10 per cent annually,

- Even on small holdings the average yield is 2000 kg / hectare, while those holdings on a commercial scale have yields of 4000 kg / ha.
- The climate in the country allows harvest of tea all year round.
- Kenya consume only 4 per cent of tea it grows. So exportable surplus is greater.
- Tea is Kenya's number one forex earner.
- Most of the tea is grown by family holdings rather than large plantations.
- Pakistan is one of the largest importers.

Session (iv) : The Sri Lankan Tea Situation: Mr.C.Ratwatte, Chairman, Sri Lanka Tea Board.

- The total extent of tea land in Sri Lanka today is around 1,87,000 hectares.
- According to the latest land survey, the high grown varieties now cover an extent of 51 ,500 hectares; mid-grown 56,000 ha.; and the low grown 79,711 ha.
- Tea production in 1999 — 283,760 metric tonnes. Tea exported during 1999 — 269,261 metric tonnes.
- The per hectare yield is around 1,500kg. The yield of high-grown tea is 1450kg, mid grown is 900 kg and low-grown is 1,800 kg per hectare.
- Tea small grower sector is steadily expanding.
- Future of the tea industry to a great extent will depend on the performance of the small tea cultivator that form the core of the private sector.
- Out of the total holdings (188,867 ha), 56% is under public management and 44% under the management of the small holder.
- In small holder sector 82,916 hectares are cultivated by 206,652 tea growers, as against 106,047 hectares in the public sector with 404 management units.
- The status of cultivation of both sectors seems well balanced.
- With a balanced growth in tea production, the tea export sector has performed well to absorb all the excess.

- The value added exports are well maintained, but had shown a decline in the recent past. The Middle East and West Asian sectors are the main buyers.

Session (v): The Tea Scene in Indonesia - Mr.R.Badruddin, Chairman, Tea Association of Indonesia.

- Tea plantations in Indonesia, covering about 140,000 ha, belong to mostly variety Assamica, with an annual production of about 160,000 metric tonnes, consisting of about 120,000 MT of black tea and 40,000 MT of Green tea.
- Being a tropical country, Indonesia has two seasons, rainy and dry weather, and therefore production is carried out all year round.
- The main producing area is West Java province, contributing about 70 per cent of the national production, balance are produced in North, West and South Sumatra provinces and some are in East and Central Java provinces.
- West Java mountain area is emiched with sufficient rainfall is one of the reasons why tea grows very well in this province.
- The Tea area and production in Indonesia are given below:

Indonesia: Tea Area & Production - 2005

Particulars	Area (Ha)	Production (MT)
Smallholders	62027	33,824
Private	44675	38,407
State-owned	55298	93,796
Total	16200	166027

Source : Tea statistics Tea Board

- Policy: The Indonesian Government po icy conveyed through the Dept. of Agriculture made it clear that there are three duties to be adhered by the tea plantation companies; know as "Tri Dharma Perkenunan" are:
- To emphasise the plantations activity on export, thus to earn foreign exchange
- To create employment
- To conserve environment.

- Consumption: The per capita consumption per year is about 250 grams.
- The most popular tea is Jasmine Tea, which originates from Green Tea mixed with Jasmine flower to give specific fragrance and taste. This tea is also the raw material for the first tea-drink introduced in bottle as Ready to Drink Tea, which now is a life style.
- In the past 10 years, there were 3 droughts which have affected the production of tea in Indionesia, during 1991, 1994 and 1997.
- 80 per cent of the tea produced in Indonesia is black and the remaining is green. 90% of the black tea is Olihodox and only 10 per cent CTC.
- 80 per cent of the tea produced is exported and 20 per cent is left for domestic consumption.

Session (vi) : The Tea Scenario in Bangladesh - By M.A.Rahman, Director Operations, Duncan Brothers (Bangladesh) Ltd.

- Bangladesh tea industry comprises of 158 tea estates.
- Developed and owned almost entirely by the private sector over past 100 years.
- Grown mainly in the marginal undeveloped lands of the two districts of Sylhet and Chittagong. Total allocation of plantation area is 112,291 hectares.
- Total area under actual tea cultivation is 49,155 ha.
- Produces mainly CTC Black Tea and also some green tea.
- 80% of the yearly crop is produced between the period May to October.
- Current national average productivity is 1168 kg.! ha. However, the average of well managed estates ranges from 1700 to 2500 kg. / ha.
- Average annual production for the last five years is 52 million kgs, with production in 1998 being 55.6 million kg.
- Contributes about 0.81 % of country's GDP.

- Total work force depending on the industry is about 400,000 people, which is 3.3% of the total employment of the country.

Session (viii) : Indian Exports to CIS market: by Mr. M.H. Ashraff, President, UPASI

- India is better placed than most other countries as a consistent supplier of tea, in view of the large volumes, different types and varieties.
- India has CTCs, Olihodox, Green Tea, and Instant Tea. It has Darjeelings, Dooars, Assams, Cachars, Nilgiris, High Ranges, Wynaads and so on.
- Many factories have dual manufacturing facilities and the manufacture can be attuned to market demand at any given point of time.
- The Russian Federation, representing the preponderant Republic of the former USSR, is by far, India's single most important economic partner in the Region.
- Russia occupies a prominent place on the global tea map.
- It is the third largest consumer of tea in the world, only after India and China.
- More significantly, it is the largest importer of tea in the globe.
- Currently, the per capita consumption of tea in Russia is nearly 1 Kg.
- In fact, the erstwhile USSR was itself a major tea producer and at the output level of 152 million Kg. in 1985, it was the fourth largest producer in the world, after India, China and Sri Lanka.
- Records show that over 80,000 hectare were under tea cultivation.
- But the disintegration of the unified USSR has resulted in a sea change in the entire scenario.
- The local production in the region has reportedly come down to a mere 10 million Kg. or so by now.
- Russia has been for decades, and continues to be so even now, the largest single tea import market for India.

- The total tea export from India to USSR in 1951 was at the level of 200 million Kg.
- In 1960 the export to Russia was 10 million Kg.
- India exported as much as 98 million Kgs. to Russia and the CIS, with Russia alone accounting for 88 million Kgs.
- Russia imports tea from India through three main routes - normal dollar payment, escrow account, and the debt-repayment mechanism, under which India is repaying about RS.3000 crores a year.
- Another significant feature of the Indo-Russian tea trade is that a sizable chunk ofIndian Tea exports used to be in the form of consumer packs. This has enabled establishment of Indian brands in that country and create consumer preferences and brand loyalty.
- However, Russia introduced a differential import duty of 20 per cent on packet teas against 5 per cent for bulk teas apparently to encourage domestic packing industry.
- Admittedly, this has affected Indian Packet Tea exports to that country.
- Unfortunately, it has also resulted in a very marginal quality tea entering the Russian market thus having a negative impact on the image ofIndian teas.
- Indian strategy should be towards improving the quality profile and image of Indian Tea .

Session (ix) : Tea Market in Russia - by Mr. V.A.Paulius, MD, Nikitin Ltd.

- Tea, Beer and Vodka are three important beverages. Modern beverages and Beer are replacing Tea in Russia
- Market for Tea is presently "Price driven" rather than" Quality driven" Indian Tea samples contain Vietnamese and Chinese teas
- Establishment of a j oint quality control mechanism is needed. Advertisements on TV and news media on Indian Tea is necessary.

Session 9 : Tea Market in Russia - by Mr. Avanesov

- China replaced India in exports of tea to Russia.
- Market changed to low quality to doubtful quality teas.
- Russian standards of tea should go up to arrest low quality imports.

Session x : Trends of Development of Tea Markets in Russia & CIS - by Mr.Vladimir Kabloukov, Orimi Trade Ltd.

- Preferences towards cheaper product (Tea) will stay important. Promotion of locally branded teas.
- Cost reduction as a part of marketing strategy. Increment of tea consumption in Russia. Increment of consumption of better quality tea.

Session (xi): Human Resource Development in Tea - by Dr.Subhash Sharma, Director, Indian Institute of Plantation Management

- Three eras of plantation industry - Romantic era: Scientific / Technical era; and Liberalisation / Knowledge era.
- The framework of total resources management - Land use management; Man management; Money Management; Knowledge management.
- Expanding circle of knowledge management concerns ofIndian Tea Industry — Estate Management: Eco- friendliness; E-commerce ; futures; Intellectual Property Rights; Bio-diversity; WTO
- Typology of workers: Knowledge workers; Acknowledged workers; Unacknowledged workers.
- Creation of a Strategic Institution for HRD : Indian Institute of Plantation Management

Session (xii) : E-commerce in Tea - by Anjan Majumdar, Executive Director, Price Waterhouse Coopers.

- New sales & marketing take place within four phases of a company's e-business evolution -Channel enhancement; Value Chain Integration; Industry transformation; and Convergence.

Session (xiii) : Tea and Disease Prevention - The relevant mechanisms: by John H.Weisburger, Ainerican Health Foundation, USA

- The beverage tea has been drunk by human beings for over 4000 years.
- By tradition, it has been thought that tea not only serves for health maintenance, but would lower the extent of diseases such as influenza, if it were consumed in the early stages of the disease and through out.
- However, detailed research on the possible health benefits on tea is fairly new and has contributed much valuable information.
- Tea has antibacterial and anti-viral attributes, probably involved in the control of infectious diseases.
- Of greater current importance is the fact that tea drinking decreases the risk of a number of chronic diseases of world wide importance.
- These are coronary heart disease, and cancers of lung, pancreas, breast, colon, and prostate, prevalent in the western world.
- They include hypertension and stroke and cancers of the stomach and oesophagus, present in many parts of Asia, with emphasis in China and Japan.
- Tea contains some caffeine, about 50 mg. per cup, in contrast to 125 mg. in a cup of coffee. The caffeine adds to the beneficial effects of the tea polyphenols.
- The black or green tea polyphenols are powerful antioxidants. The risk of coronary heart disease (CHD) involves the oxidation of a blood protein, actually made in the liver, LDL-Cholestrol. The antioxidant properties of the tea polyphenols prevents this oxidation and thus account for the lower risk of heart disease in regular tea drinkers.
- Regular intake of 7-10 cups of tea per day is actually better. Tea under these conditions potentiates the wholesome action of vegetables and fruits.
- The antioxidant properties of tea lessens the risk of many types of cancer is decreased. Milk about 2% added to black tea, does not affect the beneficial, health promoting effect of tea.

- Regular tea drinkers have a lower risk of heart disease, stroke, many types of cancer and even may be beneficial in controlling several types of cancer and even may be beneficial in controlling several types of infectious diseases.

Session (xiv): Tea and Cancer Prevention; by Chang S Yang, Professor of Pharmacy, Rutgers State University, New Jersey, USA.

- Tea drinking is associated with many other life style characteristics which influence the onset of cancer.
- Modification of tea manufacturing technology and tea drinking habits may be needed to gain the full benefits of consumption of black tea.

Session (xv): Health Promoting Functions of Tea Polyphenols: by Yukihiko Hara, Director, Food Research Laboratories, Mitsui Norin Co. Ltd.

- Today. tea is widely cultivated all over the world in both tropical and subtropical regions (annual production totalling 2.5 million tons) and has even become the second most popular drink after water.
- Since ancient times tea has traditionally known to be effective in keeping the body and soul in good condition.
- In modern times, as chemical research on tea ingredients has progressed, many studies have been conducted, linking the various traditionally acclaimed effects of tea drinking to the components oftea. e.g. caffeine or vitamin C.
- Most recently tea polyphenols, the major components of the soluble constituents of tea. were fractionated and purified.
- Tea polyphenols were proved to be multifunctionally effective in preventing putrefaction of rancidity of foods. infection of alimentary or respiratory diseases, occurrence of cardio-vascular diseases or development of malignant tumors.
- The separation methods of tea polyphenols from either green tea or black tea bas been discussed.

Session (xvi) : It is your Cup of Tea - How to reduce the risk of Cancer: by Dr.M.Siddiqi, Director, Chittarajan National Cancer Insititute, Calcutta, India.

- The use of Green Tea dates back to 7th Century China, where it was recommended for its medicinal properties.
- It is now known that tea (*Camellia sinensis*) leaves contains several hundred chemical compounds including flavonoids, vitamins, polysaccharides, amino acids and many essential micro-nutrients and anti-oxidants which have a positive influence on human health. Chemoprevention or dietary intervention has emerged as a promising strategy toreduce the risk of human cancer.
- Tea has the potential of emerging as an ideal agent for dietary intervention against human cancer. The presentation reviewed the available information on the role of tea as a cancer chemopreventive beverage and discussed results from epidemiological studies on reduced risk of cancer in susceptible human population.

Session (xvii) : Tea in Prevention of Cancer, Heart Diseases, Stroke and Arthritis: by Hasan Mukhtar, Professor and Research Director, Department of Dermatology, Case Western Reserve University.

- Tea is an inexpensive, and next to water, the most widely consumed beverage in the world.
- Tea is derived from the plant *Camellia sinensis*, an evergreen shrub of the theaceae family.
- The tea plant originated in Southeast Asia and is presently cultivated in over 30 countries around the world.
- Of the total tea produced and consumed in the world, 78% is black tea, 20% is green tea and less that 2% is Oolong tea.
- Black tea is mainly consumed in western countries and some Asian countries, including India.
- Green tea is consumed mainly in China, Japan India and a few countries in North Africa and Middle East.

- Oolong tea production and consumption is confined to south-eastern china and Taiwan.
- The water extract of the dry tea leaves, as is consumed by humans, contains compounds including a mixture of polyphenols,
- It is no wonder that tea which is rich in antioxidants possesses numerous health promoting effects,
- Recent studies have shown that green as well as black tea may prevent Prostate Cancer.
- Tea consumption may lead to the prevention of heart disease. Tea has been shown to strengthen blood vessels and to decrease the cholesterol level in the blood stream.
- Some studies have shown that tea consumption may reduce the risk of stroke.
- The polyphenolic fraction prepared from both green and black teas have been shown to prevent inflammation caused by chemicals and ultraviolet radiation.
- **Now, since the health promoting benefits of tea drinking are becoming apparent, TEA should be declared as the** *Drink of the Millennium.*

Session (xviii) : Consumer connectivity - International Experience: by Ken Pringle, Chief Executive, Tetley Group.

- The opportunity for tea -
- Demand set to rise due to population growth and considering tea as a health drink
- Demand quality will improve - by branding and added value products
- Supply growth will be limited.
- Prices will rise - long term

Session (xix): Marketing among the youth segment: by Vikram Kaushik, Executive President, Marketing, Colgate-Palmolive India.

- Youth are the consuming class
- Almost 6 out of 10 Indians are youth

Age (Years)	%	Cumulative %
< 15	38.1	38.1
16-24	18.4	56.5
25-44	26.3	82.8
45-59	9.9	92.7
60	7.3	100

- The youth angle - perceptions: Impulsive, Rebellious, Western oriented, AmoraL Adventurous / irresponsible.
- Youth today are modern but traditional (opinion statements) : Open minded, fashionable, and traditional but conservative.
- Newer parental approach driving today's youth
- Implication for the marketeers:
- The demographic logic dictates products for the youth
- Positioning and adveliising strategies must take cognisance of these values
- A new-Indian language is emerging
- What is local today will be global tomorrow and vice-versa.

Session (xx): Tea for Two Thousand: by Chris Bell, Regional Director, Central Asia & Middle East (Lipton Brands), J.Walter Thompson, UK.

- Tea is the largest beverage by volume
- There is significant opportunity to upgrade tea.
- There is a need for improving the advertising technique to make tea fresh and relevant for a new generation of drinkers.

GLOBAL OPPORTUNITIES

Session (xxi) : The North American Tea Market: by Danielle J.O'Rourke, President, Tea council of Canada.

- Opportunities for Indian Tea in Canada:
- Upward trend especially blends benefits North Indian Teas: Darjeeling, Assam, Estate teas.
- Southern Indian teas well suited to Canadian mainstream blends
- Green tea offers potential if similar taste profile to Japanese and Chinese origins.

- Momentum established with tea essences and extracts should continue with strength of iced tea
- Quality attracts premium price - assurance sought by consumers via Tea Councilor other third party.

Session (xxii) : The Evaluation of Tea in the US : by Joe Simrany, President, Tea Association of the USA.

- Historically, tea has not done so well in the United States.
- Although it is the most popular beverage in the world, it falls into 5th or 6th place in the United States following Soft Drinks. Beer, Coffee, Milk, Bottled Water, and Juice.
- American consumption of tea : Black tea (92%); Green Tea (7%) ; Oolong tea (1 %)
- Over 80% of the tea that is consumed is consumed over ice.
- Iced Tea, Tea Bag, Instant Tea and Iced Tea mix, are discovered in USA
- Besides the above USA has also contributed Ready to Drink (RTD) tea.
- USA has contributed" The Focus on Tea and Health".
- What is the next trend:
- Organic Tea
- Pesticide free tea
- Estate Teas
- Tea pairings
- Nutraceutical Teas
- Tea Supplements
- Tea Creams
- Tea Therapy
- Tea Ceremonies
- Tea Novelties
- Genetically Engineered Teas.
- India is well positioned as consuming countries begin to demand higher quality teas from both a standpoint of their sensual qualities as well as the composition of their chemical components.

- India also leads the way in organic farming and traditionally has produced some of the finest teas with very low reliance on pesticides.
- India's biggest challenge in future will not concern having the types of tea available to satisfY the world market but with the quantities available to satisfy that demand.
- As the domestic market for tea grows in India, as it absolutely will, the amount of tea available for the export market will become a significant concern.

Marketing in India

Session (xxiii) : Branded Tea - growth opportunities: Mr.Harish Bhat, GM, Marketing, Tata Tea.

- Tapping the potential for branded tea is necessary.
- Branded tea occupies 38% of the market share.
- Loose tea conversion to branded tea - is a big growth area.
- Tea bags - convenience is the key.

Session (xxiv): Consumer promotions - Thus far and no further: by Prosenjit Nag, Sr.Vice President, Duncan Industries.

- Market Research findings indicate that:
- Brand loyalty in packet tea is declining at a frightening pace
- Only 15% consumers are brand loyal
- Consumer promotions are here to stay
- Specially for Packet tea as products
- Key lies in Brand Building.

Session (xxv) : Growth of Local Brands: by RMukherjee, General Manager, Eveready Industries:

- The presentation attempts to paint a picture of the current status in terms of market share and geographical spread, understand the success factors from the consumer and trade point of view, some thoughts on what could be competitive response and finally the implications on the Industry.

Region	Urban	Rural	All
North	29	51	39
East	13	23	18
West	17	48	33
South	3	7	5
All India	**18**	**39**	**28**

- The Percentage of Total Packet Tea Market in India is given below:

A recipe for competitiveness:

- Building the brand experience Product innovation
- Deeper and deeper into rural Management of price differentials

Session (xxvi) : Innovations in Tea: by Mr.V.S.Sitaram, Marketing Controller, Hindustan Lever ~(Limited.

- Soft drink consumption - increased from 28% (1992) to 38% (1998)
- Liptons cold brew tea brews within 5 minutes in cold water, against 39 minutes it takes normally.

Session (xxvii) : Changing Consumer Concerns - MS.Sundanda Brahma, Senior Vice-president, Quantum Market Research.

- Change can take place at many levels and impact on other levels. Process of change is not hierarchical, but dialectical
- Congruence at all levels suggests cultural synchronicity and incongruence at any level suggests change
- Types of social change, Indian consumer and change, Significant social trends, Masculinisation of the Feminine Prototype, The Cyber Revolution, etc. were discussed.
- Under implications for the tea Industry the following observations were made:
- Creation of new paradigms in tea consumption - Health, Revitalisation, Spiritual well being.
- Integration of tea as a beverage into mainstream youth preferences.

- Product innovations to complement the woman of the millennium - Convenience, Choice, Pathways to upgrade lifestyles.
- Establishment of tea as a global bench mark of taste style, finesse.
- Tea marketing promotions, using the internet - focus on direct marketing, address a wider, varied audience.
- Strategic review, among marketers, to enhance e-commerce capabilities.
- Internet based tea retailing.

Session (xxviii): Rural Market opportunities - by Ms.Sukanya Pal, General Manager, ORG-MARG.

- Discussed rural market patterns and opportunities for tea.

Address by Chief Guest - Mr. Omar Abdullah, the then Minister of State for Commerce,

Government of India.

- Tea, the ubiquitous beverage, represents one of India's finest agro-assets and an industry that has already spanned over 160 years.
- Because of special flavour and taste, tea has become a beverage liked by one and all.
- The percentage of people drinking tea daily provides a tangible and interesting marker on the relative strengths of the main constituents of the overall beverage market.
- India is the largest consumer as well as producer of tea in the world.
- The consumption of tea has grown world over despite severe competition from the soft drinks, coffee, and other similar industries.
- The majority share of world production came from India with a contribution of 870 million kgs. in 1998, which is 30%.
- While the performance of India during 1998, in terms of trade was commendable, it could not sustain its performance during

1999 of reasons beyond the control of the industry.

- The exports of tea in 1999 came down to 190 million kgs as compared to 210 million kgs in the year 1998.
- The set back in expOlis must be overcome and industry should work in consultation with the trade partners to improve performance in the coming years.
- India has to her credit the world's finest teas with a wide range of varieties and grades. Although, India can now supply a wide range of varieties and grades of teas, her teas however, continue to rely on commodity level trading.
- There is quite clearly the need for Indian tea producers to now squarely address the more intricate and strategic issues of value added marketing.
- Tea producers have started establishing their brands in a strong bid to enhance and stabilize their earmngs.
- The key to success in the Tea Business is the establishment of Brands.
- Branded packet tea constitutes some 40% of the total Indian tea consumption.
- The Government is strongly committed to supporting the plantation sector which over its long history has not only sustained a huge employment base but also remained one of the most consistent foreign exchange earners.

Action Points

- In Kenya, Sri Lanka, Indonesia Small Growers have contributed for increasing the Tea production. The" Small Grower Sector" can play an important role for increasing the production in India too.
- Separate scheme is formulated by Regional offices ofNABARD to encourage tea growing by Small Tea Growers. Keeping in view the need for increasing the tea production, further necessary steps may be taken up to encourage tea growing by Small Tea Growers.
- There is a need to improve the Quality of Tea. Replacement /

Updating the machinery, besides other factors, will add to quality improvement of tea. Thrust in this direction may be given and needed credit support may be extended to the tea industry.

- Demand for "Organic Tea" is on the increase in the international markets. Proposals for Organic tea production (on the approved scientific norms) need to be considered. A paper on Organic Tea Production on scientific lines may be prepared in consultation with Tea Board and Tea Research Association.

Appendix

Table 1 : Number of Tea Estates - North India

Districts/State	1951 (+)	1961	1971	1990	1995	2000	2001	2007
Darrang		98	94	93	116	829	829	829
Goalpara		10	10	13	13	249	249	249
Kamrup		15	14	15	13	54	54	54
Lakhimpur		229	233	15	20	326	326	326
Dibruqarh		@	@	280	385	21388	22392	23890
Nowgong		22	23	24	34	213	213	213
Sibsagar (a)		254	262	264	471	15735	16375	17932
Cachar		116	114	121	115	206	206	206
North Cachar		-	-	9	9	8	8	8
Karbi Anglong		-	-	14	20	143	143	143
Total Assam	**785**	**744**	**750**	**848**	**1196**	**39151**	**40795**	**43850**
Darjeeling		99	97	102	83	85	85	85
Dooars		155	151	163	168	545	548	548
Terai (b)		47	48	82	92	910	921	921
Total West Bengal	**296**	**301**	**296**	**347**	**343**	**1540**	**1554**	**1554**
Tripura	55	55	53	58	57	292	292	292
Bihar	9	3	3	1	17	244	244	244
Uttar Pradesh	45	33	30	8	11	11	11	11
Himachal Pradesh	1115	1385	1385	1660	3679	3679	3679	3679
Manipur		-	-	2	5	39	39	39
Sikkim		-	-	1	1	74	74	74
Arunachal Pradesh		-	-	6	21	50	50	50
Nagaland		-	-	1	8	94	94	1
Orissa		-	-	1	2	1	1	1
Meghalaya		-		-	-	15	15	15
Mizoram		-	-	-	-	12	12	12
North India Total	**2305**	**2521**	**2517**	**2933**	**5340**	**45202**	**46860**	**49822**

(a) Including Karbi Anlong & North Cachar upto 1989, (b) Including West Dinajpur, (c) Including Coock Behar, + Break up by district are not available

@ Figures prior to 1981 included with Lakhimpur, * Provisional

Source - Darjeeling Tea - The Golden Brew, Dr. G.D. Banerjee and Srijeet Banerji, 2007

Table 2 : Number of Tea Estates South India

Districts/State	1951	1961	1971	1990	1995	2000	2001	2007
Kanyakumari		6	7	7	7	7	7	7
Tirunelveli		3	3	4	4	4	4	4
Madurai		4	4	6	6	6	6	6
Coimbatore		34	31	40	45	52	52	52
Nilgiris		4942	6405	6760	25749	60549	62145	65855
Total Tamil Nadu	**2772**	**4989**	**6450**	**6817**	**25811**	**60618**	**62214**	**65924**
Cannanore		8	11	-	-	-	-	-
Palghat		5	5	32	33	33	33	33
Kozhikode		22	19	-	-	-	-	-
Malapuram (d)		-	1	1	1	1	1	1
Trichur		1	1	1	1	1	1	1
Trivandrum		6	6	6	6	6	6	6
Quilon		28	110	104	104	104	104	104
Ernakulam		4	16	2	2	2	2	2
Kottayam		1902	2863	3705	953	954	954	1005
Idukki (e)		-	-	204	4978	4967	4967	5085
Wynaad (+)		-	-	34	53	85	85	85
Total Kerala	**1125**	**1976**	**3032**	**4089**	**6133**	**6153**	**6153**	**6322**
Chikmagalur		11	14	14	29	29	29	29
Coorq		1	1	6	7	7	7	7
Hassan		1	1	1	1	1	1	1
Total Karnataka	**12**	13	16	21	37	37	37	37
Total South India	**3909**	**6978**	**9498**	**10927**	**31979**	**66808**	**68404**	**72283**
Total All India	**6214**	**9499**	**12015**	**13860**	**37319**	**112010**	**115264**	**122105**

(d) New District formed since 1969 out of Kozhikode District., (e) New District formed since 1972 out of Kottayam & Ernakulam District., + Break up by districts is not available

* Provisional

Note : Since 1998 figures are inclusive of Small Growers operating in different tea producing District/States

Source : Darjeeling Tea - The Golden Brew by Dr. G.D. Banerjeeand Srijeet Banerji 2007.

Table 3 : Area under Tea in India North India

Districts/ State	1951 (+)	1961	1971	1990	1995	2000	2001	2007
Darrang	25320	26509	30897	39989	40284	41037	41233	43233
Goalpara	1467	1603	2098	3141	3176	3460	3454	3454
Kamrup	1881	2074	2713	3557	3013	3442	3436	3436
Lakhimpur	46926	50243	57297	4212	4494	4815	4727	4727
Dibrugarh	@	@	@	68207	68998	93076	94080	96880
Nowgonq	5064	5577	6372	7780	7723	7994	8001	8501
Sibsagar (a)	44571	46433	51930	63348	62810	74807	75864	77854
Cachar	30445	29928	31018	35075	29969	32008	32272	33875
North Cachar	-	-	-	3696	4263	4004	4047	4050
Karbi Anqlong	-	-	-	1358	1550	1869	1869	1870
Total Assam	**155674**	**162367**	**182325**	**230363**	**226280**	**266512**	**268983**	**277880**
Darjeeling	16569	18605	18245	20065	18932	17228	17318	17518
Dooars	54609	54756	59485	67760	69175	69703	70017	70417
Terai (b)	8402	9344	10769	13345	13083	20548	21467	21554
Total West Bengal	**79580**	**82705**	**88499**	**101170**	**101190**	**107497**	**108802**	**109492**
Tripura	4773	5055	5444	5778	5952	6623	6700	6700
Bihar	1644	534	460	22	76	1350	1445	1445
Uttar Pradesh	2605	2084	1818	876	1068	1068	1068	1068
Himachal Pradesh	4317	4183	4183	2063	2312	2325	2325	2325
Manipur	-	-	-	140	347	907	950	950
Sikkim	-	-	-	171	172	296	300	300
Arunachal Pradesh	-	-	-	195	1361	2176	2250	2250
Nagaland	-	-	-	13	256	1214	1270	1270
Orissa	-	-	-	213	219	214	214	214
Meghalaya	-	-	-	-	-	351	370	370
Mizoram	-	-	-	-	-	391	400	400
North India Total	**248593**	**256928**	**282729**	**341004**	**339233**	**390906**	**395077**	**404664**

(a) Including Karbi Anglong & North Cachar upto 1989, (b) Including West Dinajpur, (c) Including Coock Behar, + Break up by district are not available,

@ Figurs to 1981 included with Lakhimpur, * Provisional

Source : Darjeeling Tea - The Golden Brew by Dr. G.D. Banerjee and Srijeet Banerji 2007.

Table 4: Area under Tea in India - South India

Districts/State	1951	1961	1971	1990	1995	2000	2001	2007
Kanvakumari		451	484	434	434	434	434	434
Tirunelveli		449	509	800	800	800	800	800
Madurai		734	944	945	946	973	973	973
Coimbatore		10249	10058	10187	11241	11764	11784	12584
Nilgiris		20840	22651	26237	35537	60427	61634	62634
Total Tamil Nadu	**33375**	**32723**	**34646**	**38603**	**48958**	**74398**	**75625**	**77425**
Cannanore		1448	1505	-	-	-	-	-
Palghat		574	635	681	829	850	850	850
Kozhikode		4014	3874	-	-		-	-
Malapuram (d)		-	174	174	174	174	174	174
Trichur		401	459	466	496		530	530
Trivandrum		1082	1057	1023	965	965	965	965
Quilon		3006	2673	1362	1348	1348	1348	1395
Ernakulam		161	147	2	2	2	2	2
Kottayam		29098	26747	2019	776	840	840	850
Idukki (e)		-	-	23584	26710	26748	26748	28303
Wynaad (+)		-	-	5375	5475	5483	5483	5683
Total Kerala	**33203**	**39784**	**37271**	**34686**	**36775**	**36940**	**36940**	**37987**
Chikmagalur		1168	1222	1320	1414	1428	1434	1434
Coorg		178	205	261	290	299	299	300
Hassan		448	443	395	395	395	395	395
Total Karnataka	**1669**	**1794**	**1870**	**1976**	**2099**	**2122**	**2128**	**2130**
Total South India	**68247**	**74301**	**73787**	**75265**	**87832**	**113460**	**114693**	**117542**
Total All India	**316840**	**331229**	**356516**	**41269**	**427065**	**504366**	**509770**	**522206**

(d) New district forme dsince 1969 out of Kozhikode District., (e) New District formed since 1972 out of Kottayam & Ernakulam District.

\+ Break up by district are not available, * Provisional

Note : Since 1998 figures are inclusive of Small Growers operating in different tea producing District/States.

Source : Darjeeling Tea - The Golden Brew by Dr. G.D. Banerjee and Srijeet Banerji, 2007.

Table 5: Production of Tea - North India

Districts/State	1951(+)	1961	1971	1990	1995	2000	2001	2007
Darranq	26909	31194	41283	79632	80538	77030	78224	78224
Goalpara	1616	1717	2428	5027	5779	6297	6223	6313
Kamrup	1157	1668	2557	4702	4766	4302	4585	4385
Lakhimpur	5996	73339	91949	8257	8678	9068	9113	9000
Dibrugarh	*	*	*	140047	143931	163426	166504	163504
Nowgong	3691	5643	7423	11690	13846	11788	11793	11800
Sibsaqar (a)	41174	48569	55289	92331	98186	119978	119626	116621
Cachar	19827	20181	22736	40174	40180	49206	50296	45296
North Cachar	-	-	-	4873	5115	6179	5643	5643
Karbi Anglonq	-	-	-	1048	1598	1945	1929	1920
Total Assam	150370	182311	223665	388181	402617	449219	453936	43614
Darjeelinq	7838	10107	10293	14499	11298	9281	9742	9241
Dooars	63944	66898	80840	114124	121420	128964	130739	126915
Terai (b)	6376	9253	12954	21130	24804	43291	46395	43395
Total West Bengal	**78158**	**86258**	**104087**	**149753**	**157522**	**181536**	**186876**	**179551**
Tripura	1873	2689	2960	5205	5679	6431	6506	6400
Bihar	1098	55	41	76	130	538	543	500
Uttar Pradesh	901	804	690	534	341	264	327	300
Himachal Pradesh	1125	1188	888	1180	1359	1247	1022	940
Manipur	-	-	-	18	102	96	101	100
Sikkim	-	-	-	90	83	105	110	105
Arunachal Pradesh	-	-	-	38	707	993	1047	937
Naqaland	-	-	-	-	74	43	45	41
Orissa	-	-	-	31	17	105	105	100
Meghalaya	-	-	-	-	-	140	148	140
Mizoram	-	-	-	-	-	39	41	41
North India Total	233525	273305	332331	545106	568631	640756	650807	625296

(a) Including Karbi Anglong & North Cachar upto 1989, (b) Including West Dinajpur, (c) Including Cooch Behar, + Break up by district are not available

* *Provisional*

Source : Darjeeling Tea - The Golden Brew by Dr. G.D. Banerjee and Srijeet Banerji, 2007.

Table 6: Production of Tea - South India

(in million and kg.)

Districts/State	1951	1961	1971	1990	1995	2000	2001	2007
Kanvakumari		267	247	182	120	137	117	117
Tirunelveli		444	858	2262	2447	990	1779	1643
Madurai		1062	1738	3397	2906	2660	3152	2960
Coimbatore		13913	18434	28210	28168	32831	31261	29854
Nilgiris		24082	36254	76525	84274	95194	96092	92636
Total Tamil Nadu	25225	39768	57531	110576	117915	131812	132401	127210
Cannanore		1175	1441	-	-	-	-	-
Palghat		720	975	1697	1999	2267	1898	1698
Kozhikode		4827	6140	-	-	-	-	-
Malapuram (d)		-	138	97	NA	NA	NA	NA
Trichur		669	674	1503	1553	1896	1668	1668
Trivandrum		1058	940	744	433	399	124	124
Quilon		1878	1648	423	438	364	364	364
Ernakulam		46	67	-	-	-	-	-
Kottavam		29172	30706	324	140	308	245	245
Idukki (e)		-	-	46697	49473	51406	46439	46093
Wvnaad (+)		-	-	9180	10742	12307	14413	12113
Total Kerala	25775	39545	42729	60665	64778	68947	65151	62597
Chikmagalur		1157	2022	2701	2993	3521	3606	3388
Coorg		192	273	497	606	687	797	796
Hassan		430	582	793	1093	1199	1161	1161
Total Karnataka	874	1779	2877	3991	4692	5407	5564	5345
Total South India	51874	81092	103137	175232	187385	206166	203116	195154
Total All India	285399	354397	435468	720338	756016	846922	853923	820451

(d) New District formed since 1969 out of Kozhikode District., (e) New District formed since 1972 out of Kottayam & Ernakulam District., + Break up by district are not available

* Provisional

Note: Since 1998 figures are inclusive of Small Growers operating in different tea producing District/States

Source : Darjeeling Tea - The Golden Brew by Dr. G.D. Banerjee and Srijeet Banerji, 2007.

Appendix

Table 7: Average Yield of Tea - North India

(kg. in ha.)

DistrictslState	1951 (+)	1961	1971	1990	1995	2000	2001	2007
Darrang	1063	1177	1336	1991	1999	1877	1897	$
Goalpara	1102	1071	1157	1600	1820	1820	1802	$
Kamrup	615	804	942	1322	1582	1250	1334	$
Lakhimpur	1193	1460	1605	1960	1931	1883	1928	$
Dibrugarh	-	-	-	2059	2086	1756	1770	$
Nowgong	729	1012	1165	1503	1793	1475	1474	$
Sibsagar (a)	924	1046	1065	1458	1563	1604	1577	$
Cachar	651	674	733	1145	1341	1537	1559	$
North Cachar	-	-	-	1318	1200	1543	1394	$
Karbi Anglong	-	-	-	772	1031	1041	1032	$
Total Assam	966	1123	1227	1685	1779	1686	1688	1569
Darieeling	473	543	564	723	597	539	563	$
Dooars	1171	1222	1359	1684	1755	1850	1867	$
Terai (b)	759	990	1203	1583	1896	2107	2161	$
Total West Bengal	982	1043	1176	1480	1557	1689	1718	1640
Tripura	392	532	54489	901	954	971	971	$
Bihar	668	103	380	3455	1711	399	376	$
Uttar Pradesh	346	386	212	610	319	247	306	$
Himachal	261	284		572	588	536	440	$
Manipur	-	-	-	129	294	106	106	$
Sikkim	-	-	-	526	483	355	367	$
Arunachal Pradesh	-	-	-	195	519	456	465	$
Nagaland	-	-	-	0	289	35	35	$
Orissa	-	-	-	146	78	491	491	$
Meghalaya	-	-	-	-	-	399	400	$
Mizoram	-	-	-	-	-	100	103	$
North India Total	939	1064	1175	1599	1676	1639	1647	1545

(a) Including Karbi Anglong & North Cachar upto 1989, (b) Including West Dinajpur, (c) Including Cooch Behar, + Break up by district are not available, @ Figures prior to 1981 included with Lakhimpur

* Provisional

$ Detailed break-up Not Available

Source : Darjeeling Tea - The Golden Brew by Dr. G.D. Banerjee and Srijeet Banerji, 2007.

Table 8 : Average Yield of Tea - South India

(kg. in ha.)

Districts/State	1951	1961	1971	1990	1995	2000	2001	2007
Kanyakumari		592	510	419	276	316	270	$
Tirunelveli		989	1686	2828	3059	1238	2224	$
Madurai		1447	1841	3595	3072	2734	3239	$
Coimbatore		1357	1833	2769	2506	2791	2653	$
Nilgiris		1156	1601	2917	2371	1575	1559	$
Total Tamil Nadu	**756**	**1215**	**1661**	**2864**	**2408**	**1772**	**1751**	$
Cannanore		811	957	-	-	-	-	$
Palghat		1254	1535	2492	2411	2667	2233	$
Kozhikode		1203	1585	-	-	-	-	$
Malapuram (d)		-	793	557	-	-	-	$
Trichur		1668	1468	3225	3131	3577	3147	$
Trivandrum		978	889	727	449	413	128	$
Quilon		625	617	311	325	270	270	$
Ernakulam		286	456	-	-	-	-	$
Kottayam		1003	1148	160	180	367	292	$
Idukki (e)		-	-	1980	1852	1922	1736	$
Wvnaad (+)		-	-	1708	1962	2245	2629	$
Total Kerala	**776**	**994**	**1146**	**1749**	**1761**	**1866**	**1764**	$
Chikmagalur		991	1655	2046	2117	2466	2515	$
Coorg		1079	1332	1904	2090	2298	2666	$
Hassan		960	1314	2008	2767	3035	2939	$
Total Karnataka	**524**	**992**	**1539**	**2020**	**2235**	**2548**	**2615**	$
Total South India	**760**	**1091**	**1398**	**2328**	**2133**	**1817**	**1771**	**1660**
Total All India	**901**	**1070**	**1221**	**1730**	**17770**	**1679**	**1675**	**1571**

(d) New District formed since 1969 *out of Kozhikode District.,* (e) *New District formed since* 1972 *out of Kottayam & Emakulam District., + Break up by district are not available*

* Provisional

Note: Since 1998 *figures are inclusive* of *Small Growers operating in different tea producing District/States*

$ Detailed break-up Not Available

Source : Darjeeling Tea - The Golden Brew by Dr. G.D. Banerjee and Srijeet Banerji, 2007.

Appendix

Table -9

Area Production and Yield Rate of Indian Tea during 1918 to 2007

Year	Area in hectares	Production in thousand kg.	Avg. yield in kg./ hectare	Year	Area in hectares	Producti on in thousand kg.	Avg. yield in kg./hectare
(1)	(2)	(3)	(4)	(1)	(2)	(3)	(4)
1918	274,592	172,578	629	1958	325,357	325,225	1,000
1919	279,948	171,031	611	1959	326,924	325,955	988
1920	284,922	165,645	549	1960	330,738	321,077	971
1921	286,924	124,405	434	1961	331,229	354,396	1,070
1922	286,597	141,359	493	1962	332,524	345,735	1,043
1923	287,816	170,260	592	1963	334,036	346,413	1,037
1924	289,232	170,215	588	1964	337,874	372,485	1,102
1925	294,474	164,886	559	1965	341,762	366,374	1,072
1926	299,232	178,233	595	1966	345,256	375,983	1,089
1927	305,939	177,320	579	1967	342,653	384,759	1,107
1928	313,994	183,322	584	1968	351,065	402,489	1,146
1929	318,892	196,336	615	1969	353,359	393,588	1,114
1930	325,177	177,393	546	1970	354,133	418,517	1,182
1931	326,512	178,755	547	1971	356,516	435,468	1,221
1932	237,574	196,711	601	1972	358,675	455,996	1,271
1933	331,000	174,033	526	1973	360,108	471,952	1,311
1934	334,406	188.099	541	1974	361,663	489,475	1,353
1935	336,572	178,912	331	1975	363,303	478,137	1,341
1936	337,553	179,252	531	1976	364,275	511,817	1,405
1937	337,630	195,160	578	1977	366,276	556,267	1,519
1938	337,414	204,963	608	1978	369,184	563,846	1,527
1939	336,901	205,296	610	1979	372,980	543,776	1,458
1940	337,034	210,415	624	1980	381,086	569,172	1,494
1941	339,832	226,844	688	1981	383,629	560,562	1,422
1942	310,081	233,502	752	1982	394,170	560,427	1,461
1943	309,919	237,834	768	1983	369,066	581,484	1,468
1944	308,518	213,856	693	1984	398,453	639,894	1,606
1945	308,922	229,038	741	1985	398,966	656,162	1,645
1946	309,256	246,068	796	1986	407,647	620,803	1,523
1947	309, 986	254,801	822	1987	411,335	665,251	1,617
1948	310,798	262,092	843	1988	414.347	700,014	1.689
1949	312,398	236,753	850	1989	414,953	688,105	1,658
1950	315,656	278,212	881	1990	416,269	720,338	1,731
1951	316,870	285,399	901	1991	420,470	754,192	1,754
1952	317,916	278,671	877	1992	420,289	732,322	1,742
1953	318,642	278,777	875	1993	418,363	760,826	1,819
1954	319,418	295,519	925	1994	425,966	752,895	1,768
1955	320,238	307,704	961	1995	427,065	756,016	1,770
1956	320,588	308,719	963	1996	431,204	780,140	1,809
1957	323,285	310,802	961	1997	434,294	810,031	1,865

				1998	474024	874108	1844
				1999	490200	852935	1684
				2000	504366	846922	1679
				2001	509806	853923	1675
				2002	515832	838474	1625
				2003	519598	878129	1690
				2004	524403	892965	1713
				2005	527942	888654	1683
				2006	528124	888985	1699
				2007	528234	89100	1720

Note : (a) Figures prior to 1947 relate to combined figures of India and present Bangladesh. (b) From 1980 onwards area as on 31st December.

Source – *Darjeeling Tea – The Golden Brew by Dr. G.D. Banerjee* and Srijeet Banerji, 2007.

Table 10. Size wise Distribution of Tea Estate during 1957

South India					North India			
Size group (mha)	**No. of tea estate**	**Area (ha)**	**Prod. (Th kgs)**	**Yield**	**No. of tea estate**	**Area (ha)**	**Prod. (Th kgs)**	**Yield**
Up to 10	3918 (85.58)	8101 (4.58)	4663 (3.64)	675	58 (4.67)	291 (0.04)	104 (0.02)	367
Above 150 to 300	375 (8.22)	13,714 (7.76)	2874 (2.24)	210	241 (20.10)	17713 (2.92)	7897 (1.44)	446
Above 300 to 500	73 (1.60)	16,438 (8.30)	10088 (7.88)	613	186 (15.51)	41806 (6.90)	26,998 (4.77)	821
Above 500	59 (1.29)	23,476 (13.28)	16777 (13.11)	715	190 (15.84)	75,218 (12.59)	56496 (10.38)	751
	139 (3.04)	1,15,000 (65.08)	935 (73.13)	813	526 (43.88)	4,69,115 (77.55)	454478 (83.39)	968
Total	4562 (100.00)	1,76,730 (100.00)	127929 (100.00)	723	1,199 (100.00)	605142 (100.00)	544973 (100.00)	901

Table 11. Size wise Distribution of Tea Estate by Area, Production and yield during 1971

	South India				North India			
Size group (mha)	**Number of tea estate**	**Area (ha)**	**Prod. (Th kgs)**	**Yield**	**Number of tea estate**	**Area (ha)**	**Prod. (Th kgs)**	**Yield**
Up to 5	8802 (93,78)	7298 (17.90)	19512 (33.26)	2673	24 (2.12)	65 (0.02)	79 (0.02)	1215
Above 5 to 50	446 (4.75)	5684 (13.94)	2242 (3.82)	394	144 (12.72)	3984 (1.42)	7920 (0.81)	484
Above 50 to 100	47 (0.50)	3605 (8.60)	2942 (5.02)	893	132 (11.66)	9805 (3.52)	8140 (2.58)	830
Above 100 to 200	60 (0.03)	8985 (21.93)	11599 (19.78)	1264	253 (22.36)	36201 (13.00)	32,738 (10.35)	904
Above 200 to 400	31 (0.33)	15326 (37.58)	22335 (38.12)	1459	342 (30.22)	98512 (35.37)	108337 (34.25)	1100
Above 400	–	–	–	–	237 (20.93)	129,996 (46.67)	185,118 (52.19)	1270
Total	9386 (100.00)	40778 (100.00)	58656 (100.00)	438	1132 (100.00)	278,543 (100.00)	316,370	1138

Source : Tea plantation industry between 1850 and 1992 - Structural change by Dr. GD Banerjee, 1996.

Table 12. Distribution of Tea Estate by Area Production and Yield in 1982

	South India				North India			
Size group (mha)	**Number of tea estate**	**Area (ha)**	**Prod. (Th kgs)**	**Yield**	**Number of tea estate**	**Area (ha)**	**Prod. (Th kgs)**	**Yield**
Up to 8.09	10273 (95.6)	9,347 (12.5)	3000 (2.71)	321	49 (4.25)	172 (0.05)	39 (0.01)	227
Above 8.09 to 50	238 (2.22)	4,321 (5.79)	2,722 (2.48)	630	148 (12.84)	3,694 (1.27)	4,444 (1.10)	1.203
Above 50 to 100	42 (0.39)	3,106 (4.16)	2,584 (2.34)	832	143 (12.41)	9,611 (3.3)	10,491 (2.45)	1092
Above 100 to 200	64 (0.59)	9,644 (12.93)	14,937 (13.50)	1,548	256 (23.11)	36,555 (12.50)	41,986 (98.3)	11,48
Above 200 to 400	101 (0.94)	29,173 (39.3)	53,276 (48.16)	1,827	358 (31.09)	140390 (48.3)	229974 (53.87)	1,638
Above 400	37 (0.34)	18,989 (25.51)	34,085 (30.83)	1,796	181 (16.32)	99,847 (34.58)	1,39,930 (32.80)	1,401
Total	10,719 (100.00)	74,580 (100.00)	4,10604 (100.00)	1483	1152 (100.00)	2,90,269 (100.00)	4,26,846 (100.00)	1,470

Source : Tea Plantation Industry in India between 1850 and 1992 - Structural changes by GD Banerjee, 1996.

Table 13. Distribution of Tea Estate by Area, Production and Yield during 1990

	South India				North India			
Size group (mha)	**Number of tea estate**	**Area (ha)**	**Prod. (Th kgs)**	**Yield**	**Number of tea estate**	**Area (ha)**	**Prod. (Th kgs)**	**Yield**
Up to 8.09	10,488 (96.05)	10,676 (14.15)	–	NA	29 (2.75)	117 (0.03)	235 (0.05)	2,009
Above 8.09 to 50	188 (1.75)	3,454 (4.58)	2436 (1.87)	706	83 (7.86)	2,490 (0.79)	3,229 (0.63)	1,300
Above 50 to 100	43 (0.39)	3,11 (4.12)	2,744 (2.11)	882	131 (12.41)	9,794 (3.12)	13,489 (2.60)	1,377
Above 100 to 200	57 (0.52)	8570 (11.36)	13,978 (10.75)	1,631	221 (20.92)	32,468 (10.34)	40688 (7.86)	1,253
Above 200 to 400	108 (0.98)	31,377 (41.59)	67,258 (51.70)	2,143	288 (27.27)	84,081 (26.78)	1,31,858 (25.41)	1,564
Above 400	35 (0.33)	18255 (24.20)	43,683 (33.57)	2,392	304 (28.79)	185051 (58.94)	3,28,633 (63.45)	1,776
Total	10919 (100.00)	75,443 (100.00)	1,30,100 (100.00)	1,724	1056 (100.00)	3,14,011 (100.00)	5,17,869 (100.00)	1,649

Table 14. Distribution of Tea Estate by Area, Production and Yield 1999

	South India				North India			
Size group (mha)	**Number of tea estate**	**Area (ha)**	**Prod. (Th kgs)**	**Yield**	**Number of tea estate**	**Area (ha)**	**Prod. (Th kgs)**	**Yield**
Up to 10.12	61403 (99.25)	45648 (42.24)	698.88 (34.48)	1530	35890 (97.45)	58,083 (15.20)	1,07,161 (17.19)	1844
Above 10.12 to 50	174 (0.28)	5084 (4.70)	4245 (2.09)	835	170 (0.46)	6037 (1.58)	4472 (0.72)	741
Above 50 to 100	68 (0.10)	6277 (5.80)	3110 (1.53)	500	92 (0.25)	10,241 (2.68)	13650 (2.19)	1333
Above 100 to 200	175 (0.08)	7299 (6.75)	15677 (7.74)	2147	170 (0.45)	31,145 (8.15)	42460 (6.82)	1636
Above 200 to 400	136 (0.20)	28746 (26.60)	60244 (29.72)	2095	221 (0.60)	81,240 (21.26)	118641 (19.03)	1460
Above 400	57 (0.09)	20100 (18.60)	49512 (24.43)	2463	291 (0.79)	1,95,384 (51.13)	336875 (54.05)	1724
Total	62013 (100.00)	108070 (100.00)	202676 (100.00)	1875	36836 (100.00)	382130 (100.00)	623259 (100.00)	1631

Table 15. Distribution of Tea Estates in Area, Production and Yield during 2005

	South India				North India			
Size group (mha)	**Number of tea estate**	**Area (ha)**	**Prod. (Th kgs)**	**Yield**	**Number of tea estate**	**Area (ha)**	**Prod. (Th kgs)**	**Yield**
Up to 10.12	67998 (99.41)	78788 (42.34)	89799 (38.93)	1840	59368 (97.92)	61999 (15.26)	11216 (16.94)	1809
Above 10.12 to 50	156 (0.22)	3246 (2.82)	4347 (1.84)	1339	233 (0.39)	5858 (1.53)	4988 (0.75)	851
Above 50 to 100	47 (0.07)	3399 (2.95)	3114 (1.35)	916	146 (0.24)	10979 (2.71)	14356 (2.17)	1307
Above 100 to 200	53 (0.08)	7938 (6.87)	16306 (7.06)	2054	234 (0.39)	32976 (8.13)	48160 (7.27)	1460
Above 200 to 400	104 (0.15)	30534 (26.50)	67295 (29.17)	2203	302 (0.49)	86370 (21.27)	125641 (18.98)	1456
Above 400	40 (0.07)	21308 (18.50)	49920 (21.65)	2342	346 (0.57)	208008 (51.10)	356878 (53.89)	1715
Total	68398 (100.00)	115213 (100.00)	230781 (100.00)	2003	60629 (100.00)	406190 (100.00)	662184 (100.00)	1630

Source : Tea Plantation Industry in India between 1850 and 1992 - Structural Changes, 1996

Dr. G.D. Bangerjee and Global Tea Trade - Dimensions and Dynamics, 2007 by Dr. G.D. Banerjee and Srijeet Banerji.

Table -16

Quantity and Value of Tea Exports from India (Excluding Instant Tea) during 1954-55 yo 2005-06

(Quantity in th. kg. Value in th. Rs.)

Year	Financial Year				Calendar Year		
	Quantity	Value	Unit Price Rs./Kg.	Year	Quantity	Value	Unit Price Rs./Kg
(1)	(2)	(3)	(4)	(5)	(6)	(7)	(8)
1954-55	208,462	14,82,316	7.11	1954	203,195	13,07,523	6.43
1955-56	183,769	10,96,448	5.97	1955	166,708	11,36,132	6.82
1956-57	233,088	14,51,344	6.23	1956	237,484	14,28,249	6.10
1957-58	191,755	14,36,435	5.93	1957	200,786	12,33,859	6.15
1958-59	217,322	12,96,953	5.97	1958	229,503	13,65,859	5.95
1959-60	215,459	12,90,846	5.99	1959	213,680	12,60,135	5.90
1960-61	196,437	12,22,549	6.22	1960	193,063	11,99,883	6.21
1961-62	205,329	12,21,680	5.95	1961	206,292	12,42,513	6.02
1962-63	220,800	12,96,000	5,87	1962	211,826	12,35,339	5.83
1963-64	209,328	12,31,885	5.88	1963	223,542	13,23,710	5.92
1964-65	212,325	12,46,657	5.87	1964	210,523	12,49,012	5.91
1965-66	197,385	11,48,374	5.82	1965	199,365	11,49,747	5.77
1966-67	190,383	15,62,189	8.21	1966	179,205	15,65,921	8.74
1967-68	203,333	18,01,974	8.86	1967	213,676	18,90,384	8.85
1968-69	200,824	15,65,092	7.79	1968	208.440	16,64,825	7.99
1969-70	174,112	12,45,029	7.15	1969	168,709	12,05,317	7.14
1970-71	199,139	18,42,470	7.44	1970	202,016	14,87,533	7.36
1971-72	214,317	16,09,204	7.51	1971	202,052	15,36,678	7.61
1972-73	193,228	14,72,935	7.62	1972	198,195	15,11,439	7.00
1973-74	190,268	14,48,490	7.61	1973	188,192	14,27,072	7.58
1974-75	225,057	12,35,355	9.93	1974	210,583	19,27,972	9.16
1975-76	211,409	23,82,948	11.27	1975	218,128	24,46,592	11.22
1976-77	242,418	29,54,777	12.19	1976	233,611	27,31,364	11.09
1977-78	221,522	56,37,117	25.45	1977	229,637	54,16,157	23.59
1978-79	177,327	35,91,193	20.25	1978	176,051	36,28,916	20.61
1979-80	208,448	37,68,961	18.08	1979	199.639	36,18,401	18.12
1980-81	231,736	43,52,730	18.78	1980	224,026	42,90,277	19.15
1981-82	224,200	40,68,252	18.15	1981	241,246	43,42,541	18.00
1982-83	194,090	36,94,482	19.03	1982	189,933	35,55,525	18.72
1983-84	202,312	55,75,549	27.56	1983	208,476	51,68,145	24.79
1984-85	217,401	77,13,889	35.48	1984	217.040	74,04,551	34.12
1985-86	214,234	64,79,796	30.25	1985	214,021	69,52,966	32.49
1986-87	196,232	57,94,783	29.53	1986	203,149	58,08,510	28.59
1987-88	201,830	62,77,688	31.10	1987	201,891	63,92,465	31.66
1988-89	204,075	63,52,799	31.13	1988	200,956	61,26,397	30.49

1989-90	210,615	90,47,231	42.96	1989	211,622	84,00,923	39.70
1990-91	198,240	106,20,939	153.58	1990	209,085	110,41,507	52.81
1991-92	215,166	119,64,625	55.61	1991	201,720	112,03,136	55.54
1992-93	178,950	103,16,425	57.65	1992	173,358	97,17,402	56.05
1993-94	153,427	103,98,935	67.78	1993	173,726	113,25,271	65.19
1994-95	150,836	96,35,458	63.88	1994	149,317	96,52,334	64.64
1995-96	166,239	12,184,898	73.29	1995	167,143	119,08,077	71.24
1996-97	167,172	12,568,167	75.18	1996	160,004	120,70,978	75.44
1997-98	208,773	19,453,207	93.18	1997	200,713	172,18,472	85.79
1998-99	203431	212,88,720	104.65	1998	207,640	223,83,087	107.80
1999-2000	189837	186,72,822	98.38	1999	189,092	190,24,369	100.60
2000-01	200770	180,66,853	89.99	2000	204,353	182,70,324	89.41
2001-02	187407	162,15,897	86.53	2001	179,859	160,22,060	89.80
2002-03	181341	157,67,963	86.95	2002	198,087	166,97,757	84.30
2003-04	183070	1636990	89.42	2003	183640	1673520	91.93
2004-05	185830	1688440	90.86	2004	193,540	1783471	92.15
2005-06	191450	1770913	92.50	2005	201000	1753390	87.23

Source – *Tea Industry - A Road Map Ahead, 2007 by Dr. G.D. Banerjee and Srijeet Banerji.*

Table 17 : Exports of Value Added Items of Tea from India during 1973-74 to 2006-07

Year	Quantity in Thousand Kgs				Value in Thousand Rs				Unit Value (Rs/Kg)			
	Packet Tea	Tea Bags	Instant Tea	Total	Packet Tea	Tea Bags	Instant Tea	Total	Packet Tea	Tea Bags	Instant Tea	Total
1	2	3	4	5	6	7	8	9	10	11	12	13
1973-74	4744	144	295	5183	50206	3571	9217	62994	10.58	24.80	31.24	12.15
1974-75	6095	108	255	6458	83851	2752	8563	95166	13.76	25.48	33.58	14.74
1975-76	10787	157	478	11422	172457	5914	19162	197533	15.99	37.67	40.09	17.29
1976-77	12612	285	584	13481	193635	10560	25066	229261	15.35	37.05	42.92	17.01
1977-78	25187	390	598	26175	519834	18522	31533	569889	20.64	47.49	52.73	21.77
1978-79	38599	238	685	39523	787384	10570	35500	833454	20.40	44.41	51.75	21.09
1979-80	30024	493	656	31173	580703	20275	30509	631487	19.34	41.13	46.51	20.26
1980-81	32322	754	761	33837	699835	32591	36608	769034	21.65	43.22	48.11	22.73
1981-82	20493	777	832	22102	468216	33531	41712	543459	22.85	43.15	50.13	24.59
1982-83	10101	618	799	11518	263232	23172	43185	329589	26.06	37.50	54.05	28.62
1983-84	17368	514	1049	18931	521288	24259	66874	612421	30.01	47.20	63.75	32.35
1984-85	21841	631	1138	23610	930552	36551	95538	1062641	43.61	57.93	83.95	45.01
1985-86	25690	590	938	27218	994063	37839	80428	1112330	38.69	64.13	85.74	40.87
1986-87	16847	467	1134	18448	595727	31845	94896	722468	35.36	68.19	83.68	39.16
1987-88	21142	498	861	22501	785994	32424	66611	885029	37.18	65.11	77.36	39.33
1988-89	25541	626	733	26900	879841	44409	65909	990159	34.45	70.94	89.92	36.81
1989-90	75817	546	1147	77510	3548148	46875	100986	3696009	46.80	85.85	88.04	47.68
1990-91	71514	490	925	72929	3904642	43715	90068	4042425	54.66	89.21	97.37	55.43
1991-92	78321	483	1283	72929	452097	71408	158039	4750364	57.72	147.84	123.18	59.32
1992-93	65245	520	1740	67505	4040263	72536	270592	4383391	61.92	139.49	155.51	64.93
1993-94	64917	1007	1121	67045	4685722	101456	221463	5008641	72.18	100.75	197.56	74.71
1994-95	52042	1008	1320	54370	3577669	144180	228667	3950516	68.75	143.04	173.23	72.66
1995-96	83965	861	1230	86056	6162394	125811	260940	6549145	73.39	146.12	212.15	76.10
1996-97	81016	1716	1868	84600	5714458	252479	446403	6413340	70.53	147.13	238.97	75.81
1997-98	78115	2169	2483	82767	7490434	449957	578336	8518727	95.89	207.45	232.92	102.92
1998-99	82013	2415	2428	86856	8904328	498180	629703	10032211	108.57	206.29	259.35	115.50
1999-00	63518	2305	2602	68425	6743290	557207	653770	7954267	106.16	241.74	251.26	116.25
2000-01	69315	1917	2783	74015	7195601	385232	831013	8411846	103.81	200.96	298.60	113.65
2000-02	42719	2542	2594	47855	5211372	597103	741979	6550454	121.99	234.89	286.04	136.88
2002-03	33606	3178	3053	39837	4084322	668547	881282	5634151	121.54	210.37	288.66	141.43
2006-07	34013	4900	3461	42374	4057973	943075	995752	5996800	119.31	192.46	287.71	141.52

Table 18 : Country wise Region Wise Exports of Total Tea from India (Financial Year)

Name of the Countries	Quantity in Thousand Kgs			Value in Thousand Rupees			Unit Price in Rs/Kg		
	2001-02	**2002-03**	**2005-06**	**2001-02**	**2002-03**	**2005-06**	**2001-02**	**2003-04**	**2005-06**
West Europe									
(a) E.E.C.									
United Kingdom	16856	19574	20752	1515649	1778000	1771154	89.92	90.83	85.35
Ireland	2988	2439	2553	392372	374499	373872	131.32	153.55	146.44
Denmark	92	66	63	13961	10097	10518	151.72	152.98	166.95
Netherlands	3463	2599	3390	423068	352251	391363	122.17	135.53	115.45
Germany	4406	4805	5128	725005	905344	1073166	164.55	188.42	209.28
Belgium	51	2	1	9912	609	1406	194.35	304.50	1406.00
Italy	102	88	151	31263	29218	46379	306.50	332.02	307.15
France	95	158	166	26999	48909	48279	284.20	309.55	290.84
Spain	29	17	17	2508	2411	2075	86.48	141.82	122.06
Portugal	1	5	10	111	466	1607	111.00	93.20	160.70
Reunion	-	1	4	-	94	790	-	-	55.40
Greece	10	-	20	839	-	1108	83.90	-	5540
Sub – Total (a)	**28093**	**29754**	**32255**	**3141687**	**3501898**	**3721717**	**111.83**	**117.70**	**115.38**
(b) Other West Europe									
Austria	1	19	1	416	3337	211	416.00	175.63	211.00
Finland	360	8	61	39055	1392	4164	108.49	174.00	68.26
Norway	1	1	-	573	302	-	573.00	302.00	-
Sweden	102	7	4	6285	1344	1320	61.62	192.00	330.00
Switzerland	31	98	99	12337	35997	39274	397.97	367.32	396.74
Sub – Total (b)	**495**	**133**	**165**	**58666**	**42372**	**44969**	**118.52**	**318.59**	**272.54**
Sub – Total (I)	**28588**	**29887**	**32420**	**3200353**	**3544270**	**3766686**	**111.95**	**118.59**	**116.18**

Contd.

Table 18 : Country Wise Region wise Exports of Total Tea from India (Financial Year)

Name of the Countries	Quantity in Thousand Kgs			Value in Thousand Rupees			Unit Price in Rs/Kg		
	2001-02	2002-03	2005-06	2001-02	2002-03	2005-06	2001-02	2002-03	2005-06
II East Europe :									
Russian Federation	61875	46411	42762	4209617	3027431	2740974	68.03	65.23	64.10
Ukraine	3054	2361	1487	286701	180092	102922	93.88	76.28	69.21
Latvia	160	28	15	11781	2399	857	73.63	85.68	57.13
Kazakhstan	12478	12854	13069	1290017	1296378	1209555	103.38	100.85	92.55
Turkmenistan	34	17	-	2189	1410	-	64.38	82.94	-
Estonia	26	25	5	2705	3099	811	104.04	123.96	162.20
Lithuania	12	6	-	1095	466	-	91.25	77.67	-
Uzbekistan	182	130	2	12270	10431	63	67.42	80.24	31.50
Kyrgyzstan	333	118	112	20928	5865	5727	62.85	49.70	51.13
Georgia	5	14	-	1602	1784	-	320.40	127.43	-
Moldavia	6	6	-	1410	838	-	235.00	139.67	-
Azerbaijan	-	-	18	-	-	2135	-	-	118.61
Tajikistan	-	-	19	-	-	961	-	-	50.58
Belarus	43	81	65	3421	7843	5045	79.56	96.83	77.62
Armenia	4	-	-	598	-	-	149.50	-	-
Total CIS	**78212**	**62051**	**57554**	**5844334**	**4538036**	**4069050**	**74.72**	**73.13**	**70.70**
Czechoslovakia	181	265	317	13190	15786	17009	72.87	59.57	53.66
Poland	8669	6401	5714	525949	339452	330087	60.67	53.03	57.77
Hungary	102	104	103	4493	4300	4937	44.05	41.35	47.93
Romania	-	17	-	-	1104	-	-	64-94	-
Yugoslavia	17	16	-	1068	1111	-	62.82	69.44	-
Kosovo and Metohija	18	35	32	1115	2305	2514	61.94	65.86	78.56
Sub – Total II	**87199**	**68889**	**63720**	**6390149**	**4902094**	**4423597**	**73.28**	**71.16**	**69.42**

Contd.

Table 18 : Country wise Region Wise Exports of Total Tea from India (Financial Year)

Name of the Countries	Quantity in Thousand Kgs			Value in Thousand Rupees			Unit Price in Rs/Kg		
	2001-02	**2002-03**	**2005-06**	**2001-02**	**2002-03**	**2005-06**	**2001-02**	**2002-03**	**2005-06**
III Amercia									
(a) North America & West Indies									
U.S.A.	6074	7635	8449	910502	1081913	1107603	149.90	141.70	131.09
Canada	861	1091	1689	83706	109344	163076	97.22	100.22	96.55
Sub – Total (a)	**6935**	**8726**	**10138**	**994208**	**1191257**	**1270679**	**143.36**	**136.52**	**125.34**
(b) Latin America									
Mexico	-	-	1	-	-	1297	-	-	1297.00
Suriname	-	-	6	-	-	917	-	-	152.83
Brazil	4	-	0	1783	-	12	445.75	-	199.07
Trinidad & Tobago	-	7	0	-	2137	6	-	305.29	539.82
Venezuela	-	2	-	-	1428	-	-	714.00	-
Chile	88	48	24	6747	2612	1251	76.67	54.42	52.13
Sub – Total (b)	**94**	**57**	**31**	**8975**	**6177**	**3483**	**95.48**	**108.37**	**112.35**
Sub – Total (III)	**7029**	**8783**	**10169**	**1003183**	**1197434**	**1274162**	**14.72**	**136.34**	**125.30**
IV West Asia & (a) North Africa									
A. R. E.	370	336	232	22638	17004	9440	61.18	50.61	40.69
Sudan	420	115	153	21109	12157	7228	50.26	105.71	47.24
Tunisia	1140	635	727	70783	35557	31321	62.09	56.00	43.08
Sub – Total (a)	**1930**	**1086**	**1112**	**114530**	**64718**	**47989**	**59.24**	**59.59**	**43.16**
(b) West Asia									
Iran	1437	1349	1634	152074	106543	102281	105.83	78.98	62.60
U. A. E.	25793	24728	25701	3154568	2914517	2808438	122.30	117.86	109.27
Qatar	107	247	178	14439	33302	26812	134.94	134.83	150.63
Kuwait	253	332	350	35567	45978	40980	140.58	138.49	117.09
Saudi Arab	671	579	994	56767	60433	87572	84.60	104.37	88.10

Contd.

Table 18 : Country wise Region Wise Exports of Total Tea from India (Financial Year)

Name of the Countries	Quantity in Thousand Kgs			Value in Thousand Rupees			Unit Price in Rs/Kg		
	2001-02	**2002-03**	**2005-06**	**2001-02**	**2002-03**	**2005-06**	**2001-02**	**2002-03**	**2005-06**
Bahrain	111	178	154	16995	27329	23872	153.10	153.53	155.01
Muscat	358	265	368	40126	31519	46737	112.08	118.94	127.00
Jordan	146	139	189	13089	15044	20485	89.65	108.23	108.39
Yemen	704	416	213	35873	17695	9075	50.96	42.54	42.61
Turkey	910	864	75	118705	123938	9254	130.45	143.45	123.39
Syria	-	103	84	-	7454	5003	-	72.37	59.56
Israel	14	75	15	761	5794	1756	54.36	77.25	117.07
Sub – Total (b)	**55828**	**62741**	**44225**	**5239267**	**5613689**	**4056359**	**93.85**	**89.47**	**91.72**
Sub – Total IV	**57758**	**63827**	**45337**	**5353797**	**5678407**	**4104348**	**92.69**	**88.97**	**90.53**
V Asia Other Than West									
Afghanistan	437	652	4414	35813	44185	215335	81.95	67.77	48.78
Bangladesh	-	29	31	-	1833	3291	-	63.21	106.16
Hong Kong	6	69	498	2080	10174	82806	346.67	147.45	166.28
Japan	2040	2272	3520	438016	455398	746543	214.71	200.44	212.09
Malaysia	30	120	240	1966	7405	16750	65.53	61.71	69.79
Singapore	430	541	1435	43111	46393	101591	100.26	85.75	70.80
Nepal	120	139	272	12965	9712	22310	108.04	69.87	82.02
Philippine	100	178	208	26250	42958	52720	262.50	241.34	253.46
Pakistan	2614	3535	6541	130483	204615	289515	49.92	57.88	44.26
Taiwan	95	389	527	12605	34995	41400	132.68	89.96	78.56
Korea	7	7	17	4050	2374	5170	578.57	339.14	304.12
Sri Lanka	1117	1331	2226	98924	122324	164587	88.56	91.90	73.94
China	90	83	98	9511	8969	18942	105.68	108.06	193.29
Indonesia	409	1323	124	35026	73451	8519	85.64	55.52	68.70
Thailand	32	26	55	4857	5598	14183	151.78	215.31	257.87

Contd.

Table 18 : Country wise Region Wise Exports of Total Tea from India (Financial Year)

Name of the Countries	Quantity in Thousand Kgs			Value in Thousand Rupees			Unit Price in Rs/Kg		
	2001-02	**2002-03**	**2003-04**	**2001-02**	**2002-03**	**2003-04**	**2001-02**	**2003-04**	**2003-04**
Vietnam	-	39	71	-	1813	21117	-	46.49	297.42
Bhutan	-	-	4	-	-	279	-	-	69.75
Mauritius	-	0	0	-	0	46	-	158.00	632.81
Maldives	1	3	21	89	323	1309	89.00	107.67	62.33
Seychelles	0	-	-	31	-	-	285.10	-	-
Sub – Total (V)	**7528**	**10736**	**20302**	**855777**	**1072520**	**1806413**	**113.68**	**99.90**	**88.98**
VI Africa Other than North									
Djibouti	3	0	-	1009	0	-	336.33	145.50	-
Nigeria	1	-	1	220	-	136	220.00	-	136.00
Macau	-	0	-	-	22	-	-	183	-
Niger	-	13	-	-	541	-	-	41.62	-
South Africa	141	4	5	14778	1050	1364	104.81	262.50	272.80
Kenya	777	582	6479	38203	22607	273861	49.17	38.84	42.27
Ethiopia	13	-	9	4000	-	2393	307.69	-	265.89
Cameroon	-	-	40	-	-	2311	-	-	57.78
Congo	5	3	-	184	808	-	36.80	269.33	-
Benin	-	-	0	-	-	70	-	-	164.62
Algeria	-	174	53	-	11154	3919	-	64.10	73.94
Angola	-	0	-	-	6	-	-	190.50	-
Sub – Total VI.	**941**	**776**	**6587**	**58472**	**36188**	**284054**	**62.14**	**46.63**	**43.12**
VII Australia and Oceania									
Australia	953	1412	4491	93487	211984	706919	98.10	150.13	157.41
New Zealand	5	84	48	2640	6348	3727	528.00	75.57	77.65
Sub – Total VII.	**958**	**1496**	**4539**	**96127**	**218332**	**710646**	**100.34**	**145.94**	**156.56**
GRAND TOTOAL	**190001**	**184394**	**183074**	**16957858**	**1664924 5**	**16369906**	**89.25**	**90.29**	**89.42**

Source - Global Tea Trade - Dimensions and Dynamics 2007, by Dr. GD Banerjee and Srijeet Banerjee.

Contd.

Table 19 : Price Differentials of Value Added Teas in India during 1966-67 to 2006-07

(fob Rs./kg)

Year	Packet tea	Tea bag	Bulk tea	Instant Tea	Percentage of value addition in packet tea/ tea by instant tea		
1966-67	9.88	--	8.21	–	20.34	--	–
1971-72	9.48	20.39	7.51	–	26.24	172	–
1973-74	10.58	24.80	7.61	31.24	27.90	225	311
1974-75	13.76	25.48	9.93	33.58	38.56	157	238
1975-76	15.99	37.67	11.27	40.09	41.88	234	256
1976-77	15.36	37.05	12.19	42.72	26.01	204	252
1977-78	20.64	47.49	25.45	52.73	18.90	86	107
1978-79	20.40	44.41	20.25	51.75	0.70	35	155
1979-80	19.34	41.13	18.08	46.51	6.70	77	157
1980-81	21.65	43.22	18.75	48.11	15.28	130	157
1981-82	22.85	43.15	18.15	50.13	25.90	138	176
1982-83	26.06	37.50	19.03	54.05	36.94	97	184
1983-84	30.01	47.20	27.56	63.75	8.88	71	131
1984-85	42.61	57.93	35.48	83.95	20.10	63	137
1985-86	38.69	64.13	30.25	85.74	27.70	112	183
1986-87	35.36	68.19	29.53	83.68	19.70	131	183
1987-88	37.18	65.11	31.10	77.36	19.50	109	149
1988-89	34.45	70.94	31.13	89.92	10.60	128	188
1989-90	46.80	85.85	42.97	88.04	8.90	100	105
1990-91	54.64	89.21	53.58	97.37	3.50	69	81
1991-92	57.72	147.84	55.61	123.12	3.80	62	121
1992-93	61.92	139.49	57.65	155.51	7.41	142	169
1993-94	72.18	100.75	67.78	197.56	6.50	33	191
1994-95	68.75	143.05	63.88	173.23	7.62	121	171
1995-96	73.39	146.15	73.30	212.15	0.12	99	150
1996-97	70.53	147.13	75.18	238.97	-6.18	97	148
1997-98	97.89	207.45	93.18	232.92	5.05	123	150
1998-99	108.57	206.29	104.64	259.35	3.76	97	148
1999-00	106.16	241.74	98.36	251.26	7.90	145	155
2000-01	103.81	200.96	80.96	298.60	28.23	148	269
2001-02	121.99	234.89	73.21	286.04	66.63	221	291
2002-03	121.54	210.37	76.20	288.66	59.50	176	279
2003-04	119.31	192.46	73.72	287.71	61.84	161	290
2006-07	114.23	195.53	76.69	286.50	48.90	155	274

Source : The Plantation Industry, 2007. A Road Map Ahead by Dr GD Baneerjee and Srijeet Banerji

Table 20 : District Wise Estimated Average Daily Number of Labour Employed in Tea Plantation in India during 1992 to 2007

(a) North India

States	District	1992	1993	1994	1998	1999	2000	2001	2002	2003	2007
Assam	Darrang	106655	103268	102945	113208	113611	114629	116220	117841	118730	117785
	Goalpara	9161	10128	10900	9138	9439	9508	9573	9707	9980	9976
	Kamrup	8025	6582	6193	8826	8863	8918	8957	9083	9406	9451
	Dibrugarh	179659	179005	193105	191792	196787	197145	200544	203373	202212	202725
	Lakhimpur	13754	13142	13255	13809	13862	14056	14127	14335	14160	13850
	Nowgong	18452	18201	20962	18719	18737	18910	18958	19228	19260	19125
	Sibsagar	154079	155430	141478	151439	153782	156825	160050	162296	160073	159136
	Cachar	59030	58511	59501	4322	67191	67708	67826	68783	69902	69793
	Karbi Anglong	2839	2835	3342	10286	4396	4512	4506	4570	4898	4905
	N. Cachar	9021	8026	8120	67175	10275	10320	10302	10447	10701	10772
	Total	**560675**	**555128**	**559801**	**588714**	**596943**	**602531**	**611063**	**619663**	**619322**	**617518**
West Bengal	Darjeeling	45638	46586	58814	50289	50964	51515	51938	52671	52547	53363
	Terai (a)	36646	35997	39113	36119	38264	38420	38874	39426	40165	39897
	Dooars (b)	160598	160693	160521	161176	161784	163524	164757	167085	167624	169412
	Total	**242882**	**243276**	**258448**	**247584**	**251012**	**253459**	**255569**	**259182**	**260336**	**262672**
Others	Tripura	10794	13291	11979	12186	12041	12105	12028	12198	11560	11518
	Bihar	58	41	39	42	40	50	108	110	117	117
	Uttaranchal	473	414	381	370	375	387	390	396	320	313
	Himachal Pradesh	982	1019	1021	1029	1030	1033	1035	1050	1001	998
	Sikkim	330	364	365	366	392	392	392	398	413	420
	Arunachal Pradesh	1504	1734	1738	1786	2076	2086	1564	1585	1570	1577
	Manipur	293	447	447	479	504	504	492	499	725	691
	Orissa	444	441	441	281	275	279	254	257	476	455
	Nagaland	32	110	110	199	228	228	231	234	135	135
	Meghalaya	-	-	-	216	239	239	209	212	225	231
	Mizoram	-	-	-	89	105	107	115	116	72	72
	Total	**14910**	**17861**	**16521**	**17043**	**17305**	**17410**	**16818**	**17055**	**16614**	**16527**
North India Total		**818467**	**816265**	**834770**	**853341**	**865260**	**873400**	**883450**	**895900**	**895900**	**896717**

(b) South India

States	District	1992	1993	1994	1998	1999	2000	2001	2002	2003	2007
Tamil Nadu	Coimbatore	25549	25466	27502	24919	25135	25281	25407	26171	28746	29969
	Kanyakumari	144	146	120	131	142	167	174	179	202	206
	Madurai	2242	2154	2242	2951	2907	3078	3117	3211	3286	3412
	Nilgiris	67919	68670	82466	84841	215106	225440	237136	244276	233975	230235
	Tirunelveli	1784	1743	1775	1802	1789	1814	1831	1886	2142	2205
	Total	**97638**	**98179**	**114105**	**114644**	**245379**	**255780**	**267665**	**275723**	**268351**	**2666027**
Karnataka	Coorg	630	599	612	625	618	647	656	676	810	829
	Chickmagalur	2745	2901	2881	2511	2503	2531	2552	2629	2879	2975
	Hassan	702	615	581	546	559	611	629	648	714	704
	Total	**4077**	**4115**	**4074**	**3682**	**3680**	**3789**	**3837**	**3953**	**4403**	**4508**
Kerala	Kottayam	1056	1080	1081	1061	1109	1109	1109	1142	1325	1357
	Idukki (c)	49893	50863	54025	55696	56133	58399	58457	60218	65749	68086
	Palghat	1673	1654	1937	1924	1945	1958	1952	2011	2381	2464
	Quilon	1331	1420	1385	531	540	546	552	569	674	693
	Trichur	2066	1710	1435	1533	1530	1539	1550	1597	1903	1973
	Trivandrum	1230	1233	1359	832	827	829	829	854	967	1010
	Wynaad	14273	14500	14523	12157	12412	12706	12749	13133	14185	14775
	Total	**71522**	**72460**	**75745**	**73734**	**74496**	**77086**	**77198**	**79524**	**87184**	**90358**
South India Total		**173237**	**174754**	**193924**	**192060**	**323555**	**336655**	**348700**	**359200**	**359938**	**360893**
All India Total		**991704**	**991019**	**1028694**	**1045401**	**1188815**	**1210055**	**1232150**	**1255100**	**1256210**	**1257610**

Source : Tea Plantation Industry-A Road Map Ahead by Dr. G.D. Banerjee.

(a) Including West Dinajpur (b) Including Cooch Behar

(c) Including Ernakulam

Table -21
Area Under Tea in Different Countries during 1987 to 2004

(Area in hectares)

Name of the Country	1987	1988	1989	1990	1991	1992	1993	1994	1995	1996	1997	2001	2002	2003	2007
(1)	(2)	(3)	(4)	(5)	(6)	(7)	(8)	(9)	(10)	(11)	(12)	(13)	(14)	(15)	(16)
India	411335	414347	414953	416269	420500	420289	418331	425966	427065	431245	433759	509806	515832	519598	521403
Bangladesh	46588	47378	47439	47650	47677	47781	47888	47847	48036	47889	48587	49313	49500	50000	504001
Sri Lanka	221498	221683	222110	221758	221619	221836	221834	187310	187310	157310	194000	188971	187971	188199	188720
Indonesia	121322	125245	129375	134934	137055	138736	129231	128503	142202	154185	152847	150938	150723	143620	142782
Taiwan	24571	25595	23914	14315	23863	22117	23087	21218	21552	21221	21567	18938	18329	18500	18600
China	1044522	1056528	1065866	1061864	1060530	1084200	1170800	1134600	1115300	1103000	1076200	1140700	1134200	1207300	1262312
Japan	59900	59600	59000	58500	57600	56700	55700	54500	53700	52700	51800	50100	49700	50000	5000
Malaysia	2565	2669	2666	2513	3056	3039	3005	3000	3099	3053	3100	3100	3100	3300	3500
Turkey	80698	86288	89525	90575	88639	89345	89330	76971	76609	76743	76800	76653	76600	76639	77000
Vietnam	59200	59100	58300	59900	60000	61000	62000	63000	64000	64000	65000	82000	85000	87000	90000
Burnundi	5399	6165	6840	8537	7866	8363	8750	9065	7820	7950	7950	8709	8625	8800	8900
Cameroon	1238	1404	1486	1486	1486	1512	1531	1547	1512	1547	1563	1500	1500	1550	1600
Kenya	85420	86802	87473	97020	100629	101845	104864	110222	112556	117437	117350	131581	139976	131419	131418
Malawi	18786	18831	18507	18204	18300	18587	18705	18801	18963	18986	18966	18761	18800	18694	18663
Mauritius	3661	3386	3071	2905	2869	3133	3151	3028	2077	1109	767	659	680	681	674
Rwanda	11447	11729	11929	12286	12395	12566	12566	12566	12566	12566	12566	12825	12862	12862	12849
South Africa	6273	6534	6721	6326	6721	6164	6164	6130	6307	6327	6657	7335	6597	6435	6401
Tanzania	18875	18875	18875	18875	19415	19415	19415	19881	20153	20564	20600	21371	21317	21984	22287
Uganda	20905	20905	20905	20905	20500	20500	20500	20500	20500	20500	20531	20870	21170	21570	21720

Name of the Country	1987	1988	1989	1990	1991	1992	1993	1994	1995	1996	1997	2001	2002	2003	2007
(1)	(2)	(3)	(4)	(5)	(6)	(7)	(8)	(9)	(10)	(11)	(12)	(13)	(14)	(15)	(16)
Zaire	11800	1000	9906	9860	9500	9000	9000	9000	9000	9000	9000	6000	6200	6200	6250
Zimbabwe	5440	5564	6102	6337	6352	6421	6455	6445	6707	6858	6900	6800	6850	6850	6800
U.S.S.R./ CIS	3200	2830	2730	1650	1800	1600	1600	1600	2600	4300	4500	40600	40500	41300	41800
Argentina	NA	40700	41276	41276	41406	41406	41406	40000	40000	39000	39000	36000	36000	36000	36300
Brazil	NA	5000	5000	5500	5200	6000	6000	6000	6000	6000	6000	5000	5000	5000	5200
Peru	NA	4000`	400	4000	3000	2000	2000	2000	2000	2000	2000	2700	2700	2800	2800
Papua & New Guinea	3950	3880	3850	3906	400	4000	4000	4000	4000	4000	4000	3800	3700	3700	3700
Iran	32026	32026	32000	32000	32000	32000	32000	33000	34000	34000	35000	34664	34500	34500	34000
Myanmar	-	-	58150	58662	57683	59	59	61	64	67	71	75	80	85	90
Ecuador	-	-	6574	NA	NA	890	930	920	910	930	910	950	950	950	960
Ethiopia	-	-	NA	NA	NA	NA	2100	2150	2210	2050	2305	2350	2400	2400	2400
Grand Total	2293503	2355854	2438457	2972917	2448165	2493982	2572564	2494038	2443034	2380490	2432510	2638169	2646461	2713136	2774797

Source : Export Potential of Indian Tea, 2007, by Dr. GD Banerjee and Srijeet Banerji

Table 22

Production Of Tea In Different Producing Countries During 1987 to 2007

(in thousand kgs)

Name of the Countries	1987	1988	1989	1990	1991	1992	1993	1994	1995	1996	1997	1998	2001	2002	2003	2007
(1)	(2)	(3)	(4)	(5)	(6)	(7)	(8)	(9)	(10)	(11)	(12)	(13)	(14)	(15)	(16)	(17)
India	665251	700014	688105	720338	754192	732322	760826	752895	756016	780227	810613	870405	83923	838474	878129	892965
Sri Lanka	214602	228190	207951	234074	241552	178870	233276	243563	246424	258969	277428	280656	296301	310604	303254	308089
Indonesia	127894	133764	146790	160481	152898	144834	136587	128289	143675	166256	153619	166121	166868	1621194	169819	164817
Bangladesh	40611	43581	39076	45894	45030	48935	50507	51655	47673	53406	53495	55700	56820	53624	58298	55627
China	508000	545400	534900	540100	541600	559827	599941	588468	588423	593386	613366	625000	701699	745374	768140	835231
Taiwan	25578	23557	22130	22299	21378	20685	20412	21886	20892	23322	24154	22641	19837	20345	21000	21000
Japan	96301	89801	90501	89903	87903	92103	92103	86303	84804	88709	91211	82609	90371	83677	91930	100262
Malaysia	4725	4929	5678	5621	6984	6499	5886	6091	6403	6141	6200	6300	5431	5060	4040	4500
Vietnam	29000	29700	30200	32200	33000	34000	35000	38000	40000	40000	42000	42000	80000	88000	93000	95000
Papua & New Guinea	6300	6400	6100	6200	5500	5950	6000	6500	6500	7000	6500	6000	6100	6200	6400	6500
U.S.S.R./ CIS	120000	1170000	127000	131000	116000	55000	30000	18000	10000	8000	16000	18000	15000	14300	14500	15650
Iran (a)	45605	55595	46000	44000	45000	48000	50000	53000	55000	58000	60000	60000	59000	49500	58051	55000
Turkey	141029	166442	141582	126768	135304	156269	127715	134350	104680	114540	139523	115000	142900	142000	155000	165000
Kenya	155808	164030	180600	197008	203589	188072	211168	209422	244552	257162	220722	294165	294631	287102	293670	324609
Uganda	3600	3512	4620	6704	8950	9129	12289	13461	12692	17418	21075	26422	33255	33831	36475	35706
Tanzania	14515	14629	16977	18414	19321	18365	23249	23764	23705	19768	22475	24333	24745	27511	29482	30688
Malawi	31908	40157	39476	39059	40530	28136	39497	35140	34526	38312	43930	40360	36770	39185	41693	50090
Mozambique	3000	1500	1800	2000	2000	15000	2000	2000	1500	1600	1600	1600	3000	3000	3200	3100
Zaire	4300	3100	3100	3000	3000	3000	3000	3000	2500	2500	2500	2500	2600	2700	2800	3000

Name of the Countries	1987	1988	1989	1990	1991	1992	1993	1994	1995	1996	1997	1998	2001	2002	2003	2007
(1)	(2)	(3)	(4)	(5)	(6)	(7)	(8)	(9)	(10)	(11)	(12)	(13)	(14)	(15)	(16)	(17)
Maunitius	7147	6854	5500	5751	5918	5844	5930	5089	3784	2496	1787	1488	1612	1382	1436	1482
Rawanda	11677	12286	12971	12854	13546	13643	9500	6000	4500	9000	13228	12000	17809	14948	15484	14191
Burundi	4383	3784	3862	4040	5320	5921	5523	6864	6994	5728	4189	6669	9011	6605	7308	7500
Cameroom	2882	2452	2407	2941	3351	3417	3903	3568	3873	3581	4189	4000	4200	4200	4300	6300
Argentina	35000	35000	40000	43000	43700	44000	46000	42000	32000	43000	55000	50000	59000	58000	60000	63000
Brazil	10000	10000	11000	9500	9500	9000	10000	10000	10000	9000	8000	8000	4417	4561	4800	4900
Peru	3000	3000	3000	3500	35000	3000	3000	2700	2500	2500	2500	2400	2600	2700	2700	2750
Equador	2000	2000	2000	1500	2036	1574	1489	1768	1836	2000	2000	1900	1600	1700	1800	1850
Zimbabwe	15081	16612	17948	17092	15613	7797	14091	13437	15659	16822	17098	17845	22382	22544	21973	18734
Myanmar	-	48	49	36	47	50	53	54	53	54	55	56	65	70	75	80
Ethiopia**	-	-	-	1500	1500	1500	1550	4600	4500	4500	4500	4550	4600	4700	4800	4700
Other Countries	12210	12728	13452	13006	12872	10262	11594	13045	11611	10204	12000	12095	113514	19768	119021	131906
Grand Total	2341408	2524880	2494505	2583822	2635487	2508754	2613436	2573158	2584422	2702047	2790402	2921759	3035273	3055041	3174061	3305965

Source : Export potential of Indian Tea, 2007, by Dr GD Banerjee and Srijeet Banerji.

Table 23

Average Yield Of Tea Per Hectare in Principal Producing Countries During 1961 to 2007

(Kg. per hectare)

Year	India	Sri Lanka	Bangladesh	Indonesia	Kenya	Japan	U.S.S.R	Turkey	Argentina	Papua & New Guinea	Tanzania	Mauritius	Brazil
(1)	(2)	(3)	(4)	(5)	(6)	(7)	(8)	(9)	(10)	(11)	(12)	(13)	(14)
1961	1070	869	821	552	712	1614	850	1050	758	940	745	1120	1250
1971	1221	901	292	726	828	1724	909	1138	802	945	805	1250	1300
1977	1519	862	895	927	1262	1714	1386	1482	503	985	855	1345	1305
1978	1527	819	894	1056	1292	1746	1437	1631	645	995	860	1360	1345
1979	1458	846	826	853	1334	1614	1494	1902	784	1025	870	1390	1360
1980	1494	782	911	887	1178	1677	1647	1782	499	1035	891	1450	1400
1981	1461	858	928	958	1152	1670	1746	798	724	1065	920	1475	1405
1982	1422	776	916	834	1184	1615	1776	1055	889	1078	925	1505	1420
1983	1468	743	966	1036	1469	1648	1829	1565	896	1105	930	1545	1430
1984	1606	918	843	1137	1393	1521	1872	1767	985	1150	935	1595	1442
1985	1645	929	932	1156	1755	1576	1848	2048	679	1160	934	1605	1450
1986	1523	954	805	1043	1846	1597	1801	1723	966	1165	930	1625	1458
1987	1617	969	872	1039	1824	1608	1845	1743	NA	1195	925	1645	1465
1988	1689	1029	920	1068	1890	1507	1745	1775	860	1235	930	1680	1475
1989	1658	936	824	1093	2065	1534	1645	1519	969	1285	940	1700	1480
1990	1780	1056	963	1076	2031	1537	1542	1448	1042	1370	945	1745	1490

Year	India	Sri Lanka	Bangladesh	Indonesia	Kenya	Japan	U.S.S.R	Turkey	Argentina	Papua & New Guinea	Tanzania	Mauritius	Brazil
(1)	(2)	(3)	(4)	(5)	(6)	(7)	(8)	(9)	(10)	(11)	(12)	(13)	(14)
1991	1794	1090	946	974	2039	1526	1501	1563	1055	1425	950	1795	1498
1992	1742	806	1024	1044	1847	1624	1437	1749	1063	1488	946	1865	1500
1993	1819	909	1055	1057	2014	1654	1875	1430	1111	1500	1197	1882	1667
1994	1768	1300	1079	998	1900	1584	1125	1745	1050	1625	1195	1681	1333
1995	1770	1368	992	1010	2172	1579	1045	1366	800	1602	1100	1600	1245
1996	1809	1401	1115	1078	2190	1683	745	1493	1103	1625	1125	1541	1200
1997*	1869	1447	1146	1087	2507	1595	565	1497	1282	1640	1130	1600	1170
2001	1675	1568	1152	1106	2239	1804	369	1864	1639	1605	1158	1929	885
2002	1625	1652	1083	1076	2051	1684	353	1854	1611	1676	1291	2031	912
2003	1690	1611	1166	1182	2235	1839	351	2022	1667	1730	1341	2109	960
2007	1712	1633	1104	1154	2470	2005	374	2143	1736	1757	1377	2199	942

Source : Tea Statistics, Various Issues, Tea Board, India, Kolkata

Table 24

Exports Of Tea From Production Countries During 1987 to 2007

(in thousand kgs)

Name of the Country	1987	1988	1989	1990	1991	1992	1993	1994	1995	1996	1997	1998*	2001	2002	2003	2007
(1)	(2)	(3)	(4)	(5)	(6)	(7)	(8)	(9)	(10)	(11)	(12)	(13)	(14)	(15)	(16)	(17)
India	202753	201747	212662	210024	202918	174962	175318	150691	167996	161696	202995	205659	182588	201002	173685	197668
Sri Lanka	200774	219710	203763	215251	210823	177801	209942	224235	235036	233573	257273	265305	287503	285985	290561	290604
Indonesia	90422	92667	114709	110964	110218	121243	123926	84916	79227	101532	66843	70000	99721	100185	88175	98572
Bangladesh	21606	21687	23426	26970	25381	27160	31914	23640	25428	26146	25155	22215	12925	13653	12173	13435
China	174274	198289	204584	195471	184872	1755200	201435	179679	166573	169670	202464	217152	249678	252273	259980	280193
Taiwan	7375	7631	6745	5835	5317	5296	5142	4373	3172	3475	2918	2482	2451	2592	2713	2388
Japan	1107	1260	671	322	289	290	328	345	492	495	580	752	760	806	845	923
Malaysia	400	350	300	300	300	286	272	378	293	492	600	600	400	440	640	690
Vietnam	13000	14849	15016	13681	10002	12967	1800	2000	22000	24000	26650	29450	68217	74812	59000	70000
Papua & New Guinea	5491	5834	4539	5375	3743	5648	6441	6300	5800	6300	5000	5000	6100	5500	5600	6500
Iran	1300	1500	1600	1500	1500	1000	1700	1038	1600	1700	2500	1600	4000	8457	7014	800
Turkey	177	234	24943	27654	2314	5048	39611	5200	2301	4011	19103	4500	4809	5160	7042	5904
Kenya	134779	138201	163188	169588	175557	166518	188290	183147	237498	244226	198375	263023	258118	272459	269268	333802
Uganda	2079	3078	3134	4760	7050	7817	10251	10971	10682	14982	18260	23355	30427	31073	34069	29686
Tanzania	11441	10034	12015	14908	17494	17835	19387	18570	20511	18443	19006	22218	22060	22563	20416	24170
Malawi	33404	36989	39891	41024	37054	35363	35270	38672	32648	36661	49223	41000	38261	39386	42015	46599
Mozambique	2100	800	1000	750	1339	600	300	500	400	450	500	500	700	750	800	900
Zaire	1784	2200	2764	2000	2027	1500	2353	1501	2000	2000	2000	2000	2000	2100	2200	2200
Mauritius	6595	5436	4638	4414	4502	5461	4398	4036	2894	1381	436	194	41	39	41	42
Rwanda	7096	8574	10830	10225	11013	13034	7000	5000	3000	4000	5000	5000	11000	11200	11500	13000
Burnmdi	4265	3659	3696	3802	48004	5651	5760	6009	7079	4408	5457	5784	8709	6510	6926	7000
Argentina	33647	34258	43335	45966	36029	36529	43549	43230	41113	41307	56409	59021	56645	57107	58191	66374

Brazil	8073	9686	9000	7500	7347	8211	8335	8377	7252	3891	3404	3208	4082	3979	4209	3593
Peru	100	100	200	200	196	248	388	205	72	50	200	200	100	100	100	100
Ethiopia	400	400	400	300	1444	1458	1200	1500	1074	1198	1195	1200	1000	1100	1200	1200
Zimbabwe	11819	12700	12768	11507	11304	6089	8065	9688	9156	11570	11205	10800	17154	17634	17056	14912
Other Countries	400	400	4319	445	3346	3279	6780	4476	4958	5708	5770	5250	5852	5960	4001	4762
Grand Total	973437	1036793	1125036	1134734	1078183	1016820	1153655	1032677	1082555	1114865	1179371	1254518	1391651	1440840	1400796	1540001

Source : Export potential of Indian Tea, 2007, by Dr. GD Banerjee and Srijeet Banerji

Table 25

Value of Exports of Tea from Major Producing countries During 1987 to 2007

(Figures in Thousand U.S. Dollars)

Name of the Country	1987	1988	1989	1990	1991	1992	1993	1994	1995	1996	2001	2002	2003	2007
(1)	(2)	(3)	(4)	(5)	(6)	(7)	(8)	(9)	(10)	(11)	(12)	(13)	(14)	(15)
India	493170	440209	517745	492619	374927	372164	315273	372534	351896	488745	356485	360787	34194	406290
Bangladesh	29166	40206	38800	28061	32434	42627	29000	32071	32284	40449	16037	16237	15736	15984
Sri Lanka	358676	385671	376182	426257	328307	390964	408035	462593	582871	679696	654674	639636	653368	700564
Indonesia	118737	125308	162734	143130	140823	155698	96181	87719	112343	88838	99854	103426	95818	116018
Japan	2637	3311	2833	3652	3883	4981	5494	7766	7464	8144	9961	11766	13765	16748
Turkey	469	439	38225	3089	6200	45807	5529	5506	5024	4521	4078	4400	5389	6854
Kenya	198369	208782	264277	277469	294818	321903	325889	365707	378509	383508	450705	431712	451167	548750
Malawi	27613	31042	38222	35792	30565	34530	29907	27127	25410	31907	35476	34697	37635	47212
Maurtius	6887	6534	5891	5267	6118	5821	4623	2926	1565	610	216	223	231	348
Zimbabwe	10755	13945	13596	12571	7355	9999	11322	10992	12955	24293	6571	6842	6924	7045
Rwanda	12791	15028	19771	21125	23913	22521	23151	23561	23851	24100	24150	24350	24480	24480
Tanzania	15279	13280	16679	22072	21432	23992	19807	20082	18794	29088	27967	27493	24663	30059
Uganda	2495	2657	2507	6934	7762	11232	11765	8698	17300	32811	33165	34802	34069	46200
Argentina	16621	23491	32349	27661	28515	38225	36850	31582	31572	44491	40462	39471	33205	39181
Taiwan	28377	NA	24057	19323	17011	20772	21937	18702	21253	NA	15277	16043	17921	16758
Papu & New Guinea	6105	7377	7005	4393	6728	7341	7124	7245	7285	7100	7000	7200	7000	7000

Source : I.T.C. Bulletin, London

Table-26

Share of Major Countries in Total World Production During 1987 to 2007

(in percentage)

Name of the Countries	1987	1988	1989	1990	1991	1992	1993	1994	1995	1996	1997	1998	2001	2002	2003	2007
(1)	(2)	(3)	(4)	(5)	(6)	(7)	(8)	(9)	(10)	(11)	(12)	(13)	(14)	(15)	(16)	(17)
India	28.41	28.27	28.21	28.05	28.95	29.53	29.28	29.43	29.44	28.85	29.04	29.79	28.15	22.45	27.67	27.01
Sri Lanka	9.17	9.22	8.53	9.11	9.27	7.21	8.98	9.52	9.60	9.58	9.94	9.61	9.76	10.17	9.55	9.32
Indonesia	5.46	5.40	5.80	5.65	5.12	5.88	5.48	5.07	5.66	6.15	5.51	5.69	5.50	5.31	5.35	4.99
Bangladesh	1.73	1.76	1.60	1.79	1.74	1.97	1.94	2.03	1.86	1.97	1.92	1.91	1.87	1.76	1.84	1.68
China	21.70	22.03	21.93	21.03	20.79	22.58	23.09	23.10	22.92	21.94	21.98	21.39	23.12	24.40	24.20	25.26
Taiwan	1.09	0.95	0.91	0.87	0.82	0.83	0.79	0.86	0.81	0.86	0.87	0.77	0.65	0.67	0.66	0.64
Japan	4.11	3.63	3.71	3.50	3.37	3.71	3.54	3.39	3.30	3.28	3.27	2.83	2.98	2.74	2.90	3.03
U.S.S.R. / CIS	5.13	4.73	5.21	5.10	4.45	2.22	1.15	0.17	0.39	0.30	0.57	0.62	0.49	0.47	0.46	0.46
Iran (a)	1.95	2.25	1.89	1.71	1.73	1.81	1.73	1.77	1.28	2.14	2.15	2.05	1.94	1.62	1.83	1.66
Turkey	6.02	6.72	5.80	4.94	5.19	6.30	4.91	5.27	4.08	4.24	5.00	3.94	4.71	4.65	4.88	4.99
Kenya	6.65	6.62	7.40	7.67	7.82	7.58	8.13	8.22	9.52	9.51	7.91	10.07	9.71	9.40	9.25	9.82
Uganda	0.15	0.15	0.19	0.26	0.34	0.38	0.47	0.12	0.49	0.64	0.76	0.90	1.10	1.11	1.15	1.08
Tanzania	0.62	0.59	0.70	0.72	0.74	0.74	0.89	0.93	0.92	0.73	0.81	0.83	0.82	0.90	0.93	0.93
Malawi	1.36	1.62	1.62	1.52	1.56	1.13	1.52	1.38	1.34	1.42	1.57	1.38	1.21	1.28	1.31	1.52
Zimbabwe	0.64	0.67	0.74	0.67	0.60	0.31	0.54	0.53	0.61	0.62	0.61	0.61	0.74	0.74	0.69	0.59
Mozambique	0.13	0.06	0.07	0.08	0.08	0.06	0.08	0.08	0.06	0.06	0.06	0.05	0.10	0.10	0.10	0.09
Zaire	0.18	0.13	0.13	0.12	0.12	0.12	0.12	0.12	0.10	0.09	0.09	0.09	0.09	0.09	0.09	0.09
Mauritios	0.30	0.23	0.23	0.22	0.23	0.24	0.23	0.20	0.15	0.09	0.06	0.05	0.02	0.05	0.05	0.04

contd.

Argentina	1.49	1.41	1.64	1.67	1.68	1.77	1.77	1.65	1.25	1.59	1.97	1.71	1.94	1.90	1.89	1.91
Myanmar	-	-	-	1.42	1.41	1.49	1.46	1.47	1.44	2.00	1.97	1.92	0.00	0.00	0.00	0.00
Equador	0.01	0.02	0.02	0.02	0.03	0.05	0.05	0.03	0.04	0.05	0.05	0.05	0.06	0.06	0.07	0.08
Ethiopia	-	-	-	0.06	0.06	0.06	0.06	0.06	0.06	0.06	0.05	0.05	0.04	0.05	0.05	0.05
Other Countries	3.71	3.51	3.69	3.55	3.64	3.77	3.54	3.97	4.44	3.60	3.62	3.47	3.49	3.51	3.52	3.53
Grand Total	100.0	100.0	100.00	100.00	100.00	100.00	100.00	100.00	100.00	100.00	100.00	100.00	100.00	100.00	100.00	100.00

Table -27. Share of Major Countries in World Tea Exports During 1987 to 2007

Name of the Country	1987	1988	1989	1990	1991	1992	1993	1994	1995	1996	1997	1998*	2001	2002	2003	2007
(1)	(2)	(3)	(4)	(5)	(6)	(7)	(8)	(9)	(10)	(11)	(12)	(13)	(14)	(15)	(16)	(17)
India	20.83	19.45	18.89	18.50	18.81	17.20	15.20	14.61	15.51	14.51	17.21	16.39	13.12	13.95	12.40	12.84
Sri Lanka	20.63	21.18	18.10	18.96	19.54	17.47	18.21	21.75	21.69	20.96	21.81	21.15	20.66	19.85	20.74	18.87
Indonesia	9.29	8.93	10.19	9.77	10.22	11.91	10.75	8.24	7.31	9.11	5.67	5.58	7.17	6.95	6.29	6.40
Bangladesh	2.22	2.52	2.08	2.38	2.35	2.67	2.77	2.30	2.35	2.35	2.13	1.77	0.93	0.95	0.87	0.87
China	17.90	19.11	18.17	17.22	17.14	17.25	17.47	17.43	15.37	15.23	17.17	17.31	17.94	17.51	18.56	18.19
Taiwan	0.76	0.74	0.60	0.51	0.49	0.52	0.45	0.43	0.29	0.31	0.25	0.20	0.18	0.18	0.19	0.16
Japan	0.11	0.12	0.06	0.03	0.03	0.03	0.03	0.03	0.05	0.04	0.05	0.06	0.05	0.06	0.06	0.06
Papua & New Guinea	0.56	0.56	0.48	0.47	0.35	1.27	1.40	0.33	0.58	0.57	0.42	0.40	0.44	0.38	0.40	0.42
Iran	0.13	0.14	0.14	0.13	0.14	0.10	0.13	0.15	0.15	0.15	0.21	0.13	0.29	0.59	0.50	0.52
Turkey	0.02	0.02	2.22	2.24	0.21	0.51	3.43	0.51	0.21	0.36	1.62	0.36	0.35	0.36	0.50	0.38
Kenya	13.85	13.33	14.50	14.94	16.27	16.36	16.34	17.86	21.92	21.92	16.82	20.97	18.55	18.91	19.22	21.68
Uganda	0.21	0.30	0.28	0.42	0.65	0.77	0.89	1.07	0.99	1.34	1.55	1.86	2.19	2.16	2.43	1.93
Tanzania	1.17	0.97	1.07	1.31	1.63	1.75	1.68	1.81	1.89	1.66	1.61	1.77	1.59	1.57	1.46	1.57
Malawi	3.43	3.56	3.54	3.61	3.43	3.48	3.06	3.76	3.01	3.29	4.17	3.27	2.75	2.73	3.00	3.03
Mozambique	0.22	0.08	0.09	0.07	0.12	0.06	0.03	0.05	0.04	0.04	0.04	0.04	0.05	0.	0.06	0.06
Zaire	0.18	0.21	0.25	0.18	0.19	0.15	0.13	0.20	0.18	0.18	0.17	0.16	0.14	0.15	0.16	0.14
Mauritius	0.68	0.52	0.41	0.39	0.42	0.54	0.38	0.39	0.27	0.12	0.04	0.02	0.00	0.00	0.00	0.00
Argentina	3.46	3.30	3.85	4.05	3.34	3.59	3.78	4.19	3.79	3.71	4.78	4.71	4.07	3.96	4.15	4.31
Brazil	0.83	0.93	0.80	0.66	0.68	0.81	0.72	0.82	0.69	0.35	0.29	0.26	0.29	0.28	0.30	0.23
Zimbabwe	1.21	1.2	1.13	1.01	1.05	1.60	0.70	0.83	0.85	1.04	0.95	0.86	1.23	1.22	1.22	0.97
Other Countries	2.31	2.81	3.15	2.95	2.94	3.00	2.45	3.24	2.86	2.76	3.00	2.73	2.80	2.86	2.94	2.96
Grand Total	**100.00**	**100.00**	**100.00**	**100.00**	**100.00**	**100.00**	**100.00**	**100.00**	**100.00**	**100.00**	**100.00**	**100.00**	**100.00**	**100.00**	**100.00**	**100.00**

Source - Global Tea Trade - Dimensions and Dynamics, 2007 by Dr. GD Banerjee and Srijeet Banerji

Annexure 1

Rates of Daily Wages for Tea Plantation Labour in North India

Area	Daily Wages 1.11.97 to 31.10.98		Daily Wages 1.11.98 to 31.10.99	
	Adult	Non Adult	Adult	Non Adult
(1)	(2)	(3)	(4)	(5)
1 ASSAM				
Zone - A :				
Dibrugarh, Tinsukia, Jorhat, Sibsagar and Golaghat districts	31.60	15.82	34.10	17.07
Zone - B :				
Sonitpur, Lakhimpur and Dhemaji districts	31.53	15.78	34.03	17.03
Zone -C :				
Darrang district	31.50	15.77	34.00	17.02
Zone - D :				
Nogaon, Morigaon, Nalbari, Barpeta, Kamrup Bongaigaon, Kokajhar, Dhubri & Goalpara district	31.43	15.77	33.93	17.02
Zone - D :				
Karvianglong dist. excluding tea plantations situated within the radius of 16 kms from Dimapur	31.43	15.74	33.93	16.99
Zone - E:	1.8.98 to 31.7.99		1.8.99 to 31.7.2000	
Cachar, Karvianglong, Hailakandi, N.C. Hills Districts and tea plantations situated within a radius of 16 kms from Dimapur in Karvianglong dist.	26.85	13.50	29.35	14.75
2. WEST BENGAL				
Dooars				
For tea plantations of 500 acres and above	29.90	19.90	31.80	21.15
For tea plantations below 500 acres	25.37	16.98	27.87	18.23
Terai	29.30	19.90	31.80	21.15
Darjeeling	29.30	19.90	31.80	21.15

Annexure 1 cont.

3. TRIPURA (from 1.12.97)	20.63	10.31	NA	NA
4. **HIMACHAL PRADESH** (From 1.3.96)	36.00	NA	NA	NA
5. **SIKKIM** (from 1.4.95)	40.00	-	NA	-
6. **UTTAR PRADESH**	42.84	-	NA	-

Plucking incentive Rates (paise per kg) in West Bengal w.e.f. 12.7.94

Dooars 32 paise

Terai 32 paise

This terms of settlement for West Bengal is valid upto 31.3.98

Source : *Tea Board, India, Kolkata; Various Issues*

Annexure 2

Rates of Daily Wages for Tea Plantation Labour in South India

KERALA

	Worker	Basic (Rs.)	D. A. (Rs.)	Total (Rs.)
(1)	(2)	(3)	(4)	(5)
From 1.4.98 to 30.6.99	Adults Adolescent	28.25 21.19	30.66 24.27	58.91 45.46
From 1.10.99 to 31.12.99	Adults Adolescent	28.25 21.19	35.94 28.45	64.19 49.64

Note : (A) Dearness Allowance : The basic wages mentioned for the workers are equated to 400 points of the Consumer Price Index Numbers published for the Ernakulam centre (Base 1970 = 100). The workers shall be eligible to D.A. for the increase in the average Consumers Price Index Numbers of the Ernakulam centre for the previous three months above 400 points. The rate of D. A. will be as follows.

Adults — 6.00 paise per point per day/paise

Adolescent —4.75 per point per day/paise

The adjustment of D.A. shall be made on 1st January, 1st April, 1st July and 1st October of every year on the basis of average consumer Price Index Number published for the previous three months beginning from 1st October, 1st January, 1st April 1st July, respectively.

(B) Incentive scheme :

i) A gtime rate worker: Rs. 17.05 per day.

ii) Minimum price rate for output.

1) Rs. 1.13 per kg. upto 10 kg of leaf plucked during a day in the months of January, February and August.

2) 81 paise per kg. upto 14 kg of leaf plucked during a day in the months of the year.

3) 37 paise per kg. for the first 10 kgs over and above the standard output and 41 paise per kg for the next 10 kgs and 47 paise per kg thereafter.

The terms of the settlement are to be effective from 1.4.95 and shall be valid upto 31.3.1999, and negotiations for a fresh settlement are on.

KARNATAKA

	Worker (Rs.)	Basic (Rs.)	D. A. (Rs.)	Total (Rs.)
(1)	(2)	(3)	(4)	(5)
From 1.4.98 to 30.6.99	Adults	40.00	5.62	45.62
	Adolescent	32.00	5.62	37.62
From 1.4.99 to 31.3.2000	Adults	52.00	4.25	56.25
	Adolescent	45.00	4.25	49.25

Note : (A) Dearness Allowance : The calculation of the variable D. A. will be once in a year. The D.A. shall be calculated every year on the 1st April on the basis of the average of the indices of proceeded 12 months i.e. January to December. The Employees shall be paid cost of living allowance at the rate of 0.2 paise per point per day over and above 976 points of price increase in the C.P.I. for industrial workers on the basis of state average of 1960 = 100 base.

(B) Incentive scheme :

Pluckers are paid a guaranteed wage equal to their daily time rate of wage irrespective of crop collected upto a base standard output. For a crop gathered by the plucker over and above the base output an incentive rate is paid. The prevailing rates are as follows.

District	Base Output	Crop gathered above base and upto 18 kgs.	Crop gathered above 18 kgs.
Chickmagalur	12 kg	12 p. / Kg	13 p. / Kg
Hassan	12 Kg	12 p. / Kg	13 p. / Kg
Coorg	12 kg	11.5 p. / Kg	12.5 p. / Kg

This terms of settlement is valid until 30.9.1993. The new settlement valid thereafter is not available.

(C) The Government of Karnataka notified Rs. 42.72 as the minimum wages per day for tea plantation workers w.e.f. 1.4.97. There is an industry-wide wage settlement under which the basic pay is

Rs. 31.00 and D.A. is Rs. 11.05. Since the total adds up to less than the minimum wage of Rs. 42.72, the industry is paying a wage of Rs. 42.72.

Field Workers : TAMIL NADU (Figures in Rs. and P.)

	Workers	Basic (Rs.)	D. A. (Rs.)	IR (Rs.)	Total (Rs.)
(1)	(2)	(3)	(4)	(5)	(6)
Estates Above 100 Acres					
From 1.10.99 to 31.12.99	Adults	30.27	26.11	6.25	62.63
	Adolescent	21.19	18.28	4.38	43.85
From 1.4.96 to 30.6.96	Adults	30.27	16.10		46.37
	Adolescent	21.19	11.27		32.46
From 1.4.97 to 30.6.97	Adults	30.27	19.90		50.17
	Adolescent	21.19	13.93		35.12
From 1.4.98 to 30.6.98	Adults	30.27	22.94		53.21
	Adolescent	21.19	16.06		37.25
Estates Below 100 Acres					
From 1.10.99 to 31.12.99	Adults	30.27	26.11	6.10	62.68
	Adolescent	21.05	18.28	4.27	43.60
From 1.4.96 to 30.6.96	Adults	30.07	14.13		46.20
	Adolescent	21.05	9.91		30.96
From 1.4.97 to 30.6.97	Adults	30.07	14.13		44.20
	Adolescent	21.05	9.91		30.96

Note :

a) The above rates of wages are linked to 1051 points, i.e. average Consumer Price Index for the year 1991 for Chennai centre (with base 1960 = 100) and for every rise of one point over and above 1051 points the employee working in tea plantation shall be paid D.A. at the following rates :

Adult worker — 2 paise per point per day.

Adolescent worker — 1.4 paise per point per day.

b) The D.A. shall be revised on the 1st January, 1st April, 1st July and 1st October of every year based on the average Consumer Price Index of Madras centre (with base 1960=100) for the second previous quarter from 1st July, 1st October, 1st January and 1st April, respectively.

c) The wage settlement expired on 31.12.98 and negotiations are in progress. Meanwhile, an interim relief was granted.

Source : *Tea Board, India, Kolkata, Various issues*

Annexure 3

Rates for Daily Wages for Tea Plantation Labour

(A) North India

Area	Wage Rates in Rs.		W.e.f	As per Agreement Dated
	Adult	Non-Adult		
Assam Valley	48.50	29.70	01.09.2002 to 31.12.2003	16.03.2000
Cachar	46.25	23.21	01.06.2004 to 31.05.2005	18.07.2001
Dooars	45.90	28.62	01.04.2002 to 31.03.2003	03.02.2001
Terai	45.90	28.62	01.04.2002 to 31.03.2003	03.02.2001
Darjeeling	45.90	28.62	01.04.2002 to 31.03.2003	03.02.2001
North Dinajpur	45.90	28.50	01.04.2002 to 31.03.2003	03.02.2001

Note : (A) Dearness Allowance :

The basic wages mentioned for the workers are equated to 400 of the Consumer Price Index Numbers published for the Ernakulam Centre (Base 1970 = 100). The workes shall be eligible to D.A for the increase in the average Consumers Prices Index Numbers of the Ernakulam Centre for the previous three months above 400 points. The rate of D.A will be as follows :

Adults 6.00 Paise per point per day

Adolescent 4.75 Paise per point day

The adjustment of D.A shall be made on 1st January, 1st July and 1st October of every year on the baiss of average consumers Price Index Number published of the previous three months beginning from 1st October, 1st January and 1st April and 1st July respectively.

(B) Incentive Scheme :

(i) A guaranted time rate worker Rs. 17.05 per day

(ii) Minimum Price rate for output

(1) Rs. 1.13 per kg. upto 10 kgs. If leaf plucked during a day in the months of January, February and August

(2) 81 paise per kg. upto 14 kgs. of leaf plucked during a day in the months of the year.

(3) 37 paise per kg for the first 10 kgs over and above the standard output and 41 paise per kg for the next 10 kgs and 47 paise per kg thereafter.

(B) South India

Area	**Worker**	**Basic (Rs)**	**D.A. (Rs)**	**Total (Rs)**	**w.e.f**
Kerala	Adults	34.72	43.32	78.04	01.04.2005
	Adolescent	26.04	43.32	69.36	
Karnataka	Adults	(The DA upto 2703 points have been merged with basic wages)		71.00	01.04.2005
	Adolescent			63.90	
Tamil Nadu a) Nilgiris	Rs. 72/- (Plus Attendance Bonus of Rs. 2/-)				01.10.2004
b) Nilgiri - Waynad	Rs. 73/- (Plus Attendance Bonus of Rs. 1/-)				
c) Anamallais	Consolidated pay of Rs. 72/- per day and there is not time limit prescribed. The wage matter is pending before the special Industrial Tribundal, Chennai.				01.01.2002

Note :

(A) Dearness Allowance :

The Calculation of the variable D.A. will be once in a year. The D.A. shall be calculated every year on the 1st April on the basis of the average of the indices preceding 12 months i.e. January to December. The Employees shall be paid cost of living allowance @ 0.2 paise per point per day over and above 976 point of price/increase in the C.P.I. for industrial workers on the basis of the state average in the services of 1960 = 100 base.

(B) Incentive Scheme :

Pluckers are paid a guaranteed wage equal to their daily time rate of water irrespective of crop collected upto a base standard output. For extra crop gathered by the plucker over and above the base output an incentive rate is paid. The prevailing rates are as follows:

District	Base Output	Crop gathered above base and upto 18 kgs	Crop gathered above 18 kgs
Chickmagalur	12 Kgs	12 P./Kg	13 P./Kg
Hassan	12 Kgs	12 P./Kg	13 P./Kg
Coorg	12 Kgs	11.5 P./Kg	12.5 P./Kg

The term of settlement is valid until 30.9.1993. The new settlement vaiid thereafter is not available.

(C) The Government of Karnataka notified Rs. 42.72 as the minimum wages per day for tea plantation workers w.e.f. 01.04.1997. There is an industry wise wage settlement under which the basic pay is Rs. 31.00 and D.A. is Rs. 11.05. Since the total adds upto less than the minimum wage of Rs. 42.72. The industry is paying a wage of Rs. 42.72.

Annexure 4

Labour wage settlement between January and March 2000 in South Indian Tea Plantations

Kerala : In Kerala, a three-year wage settlement was signed in the Plantations Labour Committee on 6th March 2000, revising the wages with retrospective effect from 1st April 1999. The salient features of the settlement were:

* The basic wage rates were increased by Rs. 6.47, Rs. 6.17 and Rs. 6.00 in tea/cardamom, coffee and rubber plantations, respectively. Accordingly, the revised basic wages in the different crops from 1st April, 1999 were as follows :

Tea/Cardamom	:	Rs. 34.72
Coffee	:	Rs. 34.42
Rubber	:	Rs. 39.29
Cardamom other than mixed	:	Rs. 34.12

* No change was effected in the D.A. scheme.
* Job differential for factory workers and all other categories receiving job differentials were increased by 25 p. and fixed at a uniform level of Rs 2.00.
* While there is no change in the standard output in tea, the incentive rates for output above standard were raised by 3 p./kg. in every slab.
* Supervisors and selected special categories were given an increase on Rs 225 and other special categories were given an increase of Rs. 205 before fitment in the revised scales.

The movement of wages for the four quarters commencing from 1st April, 1999 was of the following order :

Adult Daily Wage (Basic + D.A.)

PERIOD	Tea Cardamom (mixed) Rs.	Coffee Rs.	Cardamom other than mixed Rs.	Rubber Rs.
April/June 1999	68.80	68.50	68.20	73.37
July/Sept. 1999	69.64	69.34	69.04	74.21
Oct./Dec. 1999	70.66	70.36	70.06	75.23
Jan./March 2000	71.38	71.08	70.78	75.95

b) Tamil Nadu

i) Tea/Coffee :

In Tamil Nadu, the wages in tea/coffee plantations were revised through a bipartite settlement signed on 12/13th January 2000, with retrospective effect from 1st January 1999. The main features of the settlement were :

* The total wage from 1st January 1999 was fixed at Rs 69.
* The relative average index for January/March quarter 1999, being 2047 points, D.A. was payable for 1047 points (2047 - 1000 points) at 2.6 p. per point, which worked out to Rs. 27.22. Deducting D.A. of Rs 27.22 from the total wage of Rs 69 the revised basic wage of Rs 41.78 was arrived at.

The movement of wages from 1-1-1999 to 31-3-2000 was as follows :

PERIOD	Adult Daily Wage (Basic + D.A.)
January/March 1999	Rs. 69.00
April/June 1999	Rs. 71.42
July/September 1999	Rs.70.71
October/December 1999	Rs. 70.07
January/March 2000	Rs. 71.32

Subsequently, by another bipartite settlement dated 2nd May 2000, the wages of supervisors, non-staff and skilled categories were also revised with retrospective effect from 1-1-1999.

ii) Kanyakumari:

In rubber plantations in Kanyakumari, consequent to the expiry of the last wage settlement on 31-12-1997, a tripartite settlement revising the wages with retrospective effect from 1-1-1998 was arrived at on 15-12-1999. The main features of the settlement were :

* The settlement covered two distinct periods, i.e. from 1-1-1998 to 31-12-1999 and from 1-1-2000 to 31-12-2001.
* The pre-revised basic wage of Rs. 41.15 was increased by adding Rs. 8.05 and merging D.A. on 80 point at 15 p. per point; thus arriving at a total basic wage of Rs. 61.20 for the period 1-1-1998 to 31-12-1999. From 1-1-2000, D.A. for another 70 points amounting to Rs. 10.50 was further added to the basic pay, bringing the basic wage to Rs 71.70 from that date.
* No change in the D.A. rate of 15 paise/point.
* A service weightage was introduced for the first time with three service slabs of 10 to 20 years, 21 to 30 years and above 30 years at the rates of 20 p. to 30 p. and 40 p. per day respectively.
* The rainy day allowance was raised from Rs. 20 per day to Rs. 25 per day up to 31-12-1999 and Rs. 30 per day thereafter.
* The incentive rate for latex was increased from Rs. 1.90/kg. to Rs. 2.60/kg. up to 31-12-1999 and to Rs. 2.80/kg thereafter and for scrap from 70 p./kg to Rs 80/kg and 90/kg respectively.

The movement of wages from 1-4-1999 was as follows :

PERIOD	Adult Daily Wage (Basic + D.A.)
April/July 1999	Rs. 79.80
August/November	Rs. 79.50
December 1999/March 2000	Rs. 80.85

c) Karnataka: Consequent to the adjustment of VDA under the settlement dated 11th February 1999, the wages payable in coffee/tea/rubber and mixed estates from 1-4-2000 was as follows:

	Adult Wage
Basic Rs.	52.00
VDA	6.80
	58.80

During the year, revision of wages of non-staff categories, which was pending for quite some time, was also settled through a bipartite settlement dated 10th June 1999, with retrospective effect from 1st April, 1998, valid until 31 March, 2002. The settlement granted a fitment increase of Rs. 325, besides a service weightage of Rs. 10 per year of service.

Source : *United Planters Association of South India (UPASI) Year Book and Annual Report, 2000*

Annexure 5.

Guidelines on wage issues by Labour Liason Committe in Kerala, Karnataka and Tamil Nadu

The developments on the issue of wages in the three States were deliberated and guidelines were issued at various meetings of the Labour Liaison Committee.

Legislations

a) Employees' Provident Fund Scheme, (EPF) 1952

Paras 68-B and 68-BB of the EPF Scheme were amended so as to make the withdrawal provisions for construction of house, purchase of site, etc. liberal. By amending Para 68-B, the requirement to produce documentary evidence to the effect that the house/site is free from encumbrances was done away with and in its place a mere declaration was to be made to the members to the effect that the house/site was free from encumbrances and the same was under the title of the member and/or the spouse. By the amendment to Para 68-BB, the withdrawal from the Fund for repayment of housing loan was extended to loans availed from Housing Board, nationalised banks and public financial institutions, besides loans from State Governments, registered co-operative society, etc. Further, the withdrawal for this purpose could be availed by a member even in respect of a loan taken in the name of his/her spouse.

b) Employees' Pension Scheme, 1995

Para 16 of the above Scheme was amended to increase the minimum widow pension from Rs. 250 p.m. to Rs.450 p.m., the minimum children pension from Rs. 115 to Rs. 150 p.m. and the minimum orphan pension from Rs. 170 to Rs. 250 p.m.

Members were advised of the above amendments.

Second National Commission on Labour

By a notification dated 15th October 1999, issued by the Ministry of Labour, Government of India, the Central Government has constituted the Second National Labour Commission. The Commission consisted of Mr. Ravindra Varma as Chairman, one full time member, seven part time members and a member Secretary. Mr. Arvind R. Doshi, president, Employers' Federation of India is a part-time member of the Commission.

The terms of reference of the Commission are :

a) to suggest rationalisation of existing laws relating to labour in the organised sector;

b) to suggest an 'umbrella' legislation for ensuring a minimum level of protection to the workers in the unorganised sector.

As per newspaper reports, the Commission has constituted six Study Groups to be operational shortly. The six Study Groups would deal with legal (labour laws), social security, globalisation, unorganised sector, skill development and women workers.

The Commission has also issued a very elaborate questionnaire for eliciting information covering its terms of reference.

Suitable submissions from the plantation industry's perspectives would be made to the Commission at the appropriate time, in liaison with the Central Organisations of Employers.

Source - UPASI Year Book and Annual Report

Annexure 6

Present Taxes and Duties on Tea in India

Central Levy:

1.	Tea Cess	(a)	30 paise per Kg on tea produced except in Darjeeling Plantation Deistrict.
		(b)	12 paise per Kg on tea produce in Darjeeling
2.	Excise Duty	(a)	Re. 1 per Kg on teas falling under heading 09.02 has been abolished w.e.f. 01.03.2003. However, an additional excise developmental purposes w.e.f. 01.03.2003
		(b)	16% ad valorem on Instant Tea falling under heading 2101.20
3.	Export Duty		- NIL -
4.	Import Duty	(a)	100% ad valorem on teas falling under heading 09.02
		(b)	30% on Instant tea falling under heading 2101.20
		(c)	7.5% on teas imported under Indo-Sri Lanka FTA
		(d)	NIL-when imported for re-export under Duty Exemption Scheme and / or by EOU/ EPZ/ SEZ units
5.	Corporate Tax		35% plus 2.5% Surcharge
6.	Education Cess on all duties & taxes		2% of the levy amount.
7.	Service Tax		10% on taxable services.

State Levy

Assam :

1.	Agricultural Income Tax (levied on 60% of the total income)		Upto income of Rs. 1,00,000 ----- 30% Above Rs. 1,00,000 ----- 35% w.e.f. 01.04.2004 For teas routed through ICD Amingaon an admissible deduction @ 50 paise per Kg.
2.	Green Leaf Cess payable under Assam Taxation on Specified Land (Amendment) Act, 1994	(a)	Upto 14 hectares : Nil.
		(b)	20 paise per kg. of green leaf produced by producers having an area above 4 hectares but within 40 hectares.
		(c)	32 paise per Kg on Green Leaf produced by producers having an area above 40 hectares in Brahmaputra Valley.
		(d)	29 paise per Kg on Green Leaf produced by producers having an area above 40 hectares in Cachar/ Barak Valley.
3.	Land Revenue under Assam Land Revenue Reassessment Amendment Act		@ Rs. 12 per Bigha for Tea estates in Brahmaputra Valley @ Rs. 9 per Bigha for Tea Estates in Barak Valley Plus Local Tax on Land Revenue @ 25% and surcharge on Land Revenue @ 30%.

4.	Assam Sales Tax	(a)	1% on sales through Guwahati Tea Auction Centre (including Private Sales through GTAC). Orthodox teas purchased for export exempted.
		(b)	8% on sales outside Auction but within Assam.
		(c)	4% on ex-gardem inter state sales. 1% on inter-state sales through Guwahati Tea Auctions Centre.
5.	Entry Tax under Assam Entry Tax Act, 2001 on several inputs (both Revenue and Capital Items) used by the Tea Industry	(b)	8%

West Bengal :

1.	Agricultural Income Tax (levied on 60% of the total income)		30% (W.E.F.01.04 2003)
2.	Green Leaf Cess payable under WB Rural Employment & Production Act WB Primary Education Act.		8 paise per Kg of Green Leaf. 4 paise per Kg of Green Leaf.
3.	Land Revenue		@ Rs. 30/- per acre under West Bengal Land Reforms Amendment Act, 1955 plus --- Road Cess - @ 6% of land rent --- PWD Cess - @25% of land rent -- Rural Employment Surcharge- @ 15% of land rent.
4.	Salami (payable on transfer of properties other than by way of inheritance at the time of renewal)		Rs. 15000 per hectare.
5.	Sales Tax		
	Tea sold in Kolkata or Siliguri Auctions	(i)	Tea sold to registered dealer for exports............NIL
		(ii)	Tea sold to a registered dealer for re-sale In original form.......1%
		(iii)	Tea sold to an unregistered dealer..........8%
	Tea sold other than in Kolkata or or Siliguri Acutions	(i)	Tea sold to registered dealer for exports..........NIL
		(ii)	Tea sold to a registered dealer for re-sale In original form........1%
		(iii)	Tea sold to an unregistered dealer.........8%
	Inter-State Sale	(i)	Tea purchased in Kolkata or Siliguri Auctions In course of inter-state trade.........2% CST.
		(ii)	Tea sold ex-garden in the course of inter-state trade......4% CST.
6.	Agricultural Produce Marketing Fees		@ 1% under West Bengal Agricultural Produce Marketing Act 1972.

Tamil Nadu :

1.	Agricultural Income Tax (levied on 60% of the total income)		Exempted. (Tamil Nadu Government has passed a Bill in the Assembly to repeat the Tamil Nadu Agricultural Income Tax Act, 1955 w.e.f. 1.4.2004)
2.	Land Tax (Land assessment). Including Local Cess & Local Cess Surcharge payable to Panchayats.		Rs. 51.87 per hectare.
3.	Factory Licence fees		Ranging from Rs.6400 to Rs. 54,000.
4.	Dangerous and Offensive Trade licence fees for all factory, machinery, Pumpsets, gensets etc and other service installations.		
5.	House Tax or Property Tax levied by Panchayats/Town Panchayats based on capital quinquenial revision & Library cess		
6.	State Sales Tax	(a)	Tea sold through Auctions.........8% Tea sold through Tea Serve (Auction) 4%
		(b)	Teas sold other than Auctions...........8%
		(c)	Resale i.e. for second and subsequent sale On dealers above Rs. 10 lakhs.........1%
		(d)	Infrastructure Surcharge 5% on Sales Tax
	Inter-State Sale		Tea sold in Auction for inter-state sale.......4% Tea sold through Tea Serve (Auction) 2%
7.	Pollution control consent fee under Water and Air Pollution Acts,		Ranging from Rs. 5,000 to Rs. 25,000 per factory.

Kerala :

1.	Agricultural Income Tax (levied on 60% of the total income)	(i)	Upto Rs. 25,000 ....45%
		(ii)	Above Rs. 25,000 to Rs,1 Lakh 50%
		(iii)	Above Rs. 1 Lakh to Rs.3 Lakhs 55%
		(iv)	Above Rs. 3 Lakhs to RS.10 Lakhs 60%
Agricultural Tax had been exempted for holding of 50 acres and below during the years 2000-01 to 2003-04.			
2.	Plantation Tax (Under the Kerala Plantation Tax Act, 1960)		Plantation Tax on Tea has been exempted for the financial years 2003-04 and 2004-05.
3.	Land Tax (under the Kerala Land tax Act, 1961)	(i)	Panchayat Tax --- Rs. 50 per ha. per annum
		(ii)	Township or Municipal Area --- Rs. 100 per ha. per annum.
		(iii)	Corporation Area --- - Rs. 200 per ha. per annum.
4.	Sales Tax		Tea sold through Auctions 8%
			Teas sold other than Auctions 8%
			Addl. Sales Tax ---------------- 15%
	Inter-State Sale		Tea sold in Auction for inter-state sale. 4%

Karnataka :

1.	Agricultural Income Tax (levied on 60% of the total income)	(i)	Upto Rs.1 lakh 30%
		(ii)	Above Rs.1 lakh to Rs.5 lakh .... Rs.30,000 plus 40% of the amount by which the total income exceeds Rs.1 lakh.
		(iii)	Above Rs.5 lakh ...... Rs.1,90,000 plus 50% of the amount by which the total income exceeds Rs.5 lakh.
2.	Turnover Tax	(a)	Above Rs.5lakhs but less than Rs.5 Crores....2%
		(b)	Above Rs.5 Crores but below Rs.10 Crores...2%
		(c)	Above Rs.10 Crores.........3%
3.	Infrastructure Development Tax		5% on Tax payable
4.	State Sales Tax	(i)	Unbranded 8%-12%
		(ii)	Branded 12%
		(iii)	Central Sales Tax 4%
		(iv)	For Registered Dealer, Sale of unbranded tea grown by him in the State is 9%

Taxes levied in other producing States, non-tea producing States/Union Territories

State	Central Sales Tax	State Sales Tax	Other Taxes
Andhra Pradesh	4%	10%	CST without form 'C' 10%
Bihar	N.A.	10%	Additional tax 1%, CST without form 'C' 10%
Delhi	2%	5.5%	--
Goa, Daman, Diu	N.A.	4% (w.e.f. 30.5.95)	--
Gujarat	4%	8%	12% packages below 20 kgs, 8% for packages above 20 kgs + Surcharge 10%, Octroi 1%
Hariyana	4%	8%	CST without form 'C' 10%
Himachal Pradesh	4%	7%	--
Madhya Pradesh	N.A.	8%	On loose tea and 10% on tea in Packets.
Maharastra	4%	8%	Surcharge 10%
Meghalaya	4%	7%	Surcharge 1%
Mizoram	NIL	Nil	--
Nagaland	4%	6%	--
Orissa	4%	12%	Entry tax 1%, CST without form 'C' 12%
Pondichery	3%	3%	--
Punjab	2%	4%	--
Rajasthan	4%	4%	--
Tripura	4%	8%	--
Uttar Pradesh	4%	6%	Single point and additional tax 2%
Sikkim	4%	8%	

Annexure - 7

Duties and Taxes on Tea in different Producing Countries

(Other than India)

Bangladesh :

(1)	Export Duty	Nil
(2)	Cess	1% Ad Valorem Auction Price
(3)	VAT	15% of Auction price of tea for internal consumption only.

Sri Lanka :

(1)	Export Duty	Nil
(2)	Ad Valorem Sales Tax	Nil
(3)	Cess	(w.e.f. 2 April 1997)
	Medical Aid (not payable on Instant Tea)	0.35 cents per kg
	Tea Board Cess	250.00 cents per kg
	Total	250.35 cents per kg
(4)	Import Duty	25% (w.e.f. 15.02.2000) subject to approval by the Tea Board, Imports for re-exports are exempted from duty.

Indonesia :

(1)	Export Duty	Nil
(2)	Export Tax	Nil
(3)	Import Duty	5%
(4)	Surcharge	Nil
(5)	VAT	10% (on Black Tea only)

(6) Sales Tax Nil

(7) Tea Promotion Charge (On Exports) Rupiah 2.50 per kg.

Kenya :

(1) Export Duty Nil

(2) Manufacturing Cess K Shs. 46 per 100 kgs. of Made Tea.

(3) VAT 18% on local sales only w.e.f. 15.6.00

(4) Local Govt. Agricultural Produce Cess 1% of Gross Income to the Farmer

(5) Presumptive Income Tax 2% of Gross Income to the Farmer (re-introduced w.e.f. 1 January 2002)

(6) Import Duty

0902.10, 20, 30 & 40 15% per kg.

Instant Tea 15% per kg.

Made 15% per kg.

Imports from Countries within COMESA group are free of duty.

Uganda :

(1) Export Duty Nil

(2) Production Cess Temporarily suspended

(3) Import Duty (Payable after 3 months i.e. Tea

Import License required Imported & r-exported exempt)

Tea 1 Shilling per pound

Extracts etc. 50% Ad Valorem

17% on internal sales only

(4) VAT

Tanzania :

(1)	Export Duty	Nil
(2)	Cess	2.5% on FOB Export proceeds Value
(3)	Sales Tax	Nil

Malawi :

(1)	Export Duty	Nil
(2)	Surtax	10% on domestic Sales
(3)	Cess (In Malawi Kwacha) w.e.f.01.4.02	@ US $ 0.0135 per kg of Made Tea
	Out of which paid	
	To Tea Research Foundation	US $ 0.010
	Retained by Tea Association of Malawi	US$ 0.0035
(4)	Import Duty	
	Green Tea (not fermented) in packing not exceeding 3 kgs	10% (Surtax 10%)
	Other Green Tea	10% (Surtax 10%)
	Black Tea (fermented & partly 50%	(Surtax 10%)
	fermented) not exceeding 3 kgs	45% Preferential rate, Surtax 10%
	Other Black Tea	50% (Surtax 10%)
		45% Preferential rate, Surtax 10%

Russian Federation :

(1) Import Duty

Tea in packages not exceeding 3 kgs. 20% on CIF Value

(but, not less than 0.4 Euro per kg)

Availability of certificate of Origin reduces the tariff to 15% on CIF value as per invoice (but not less than 0.3 Euro/Kg inclusive of packaging).

Tea Bags not exceeding 3 kgs. 20% on CIF Value

(but, not less than 0.8 Euro per kg)

Availability of certificate of Origin reduces the tariff to 15% on CIF value as per invoice (but not less than 0.6 Euro/Kg inclusive of packaging).

Bulk Tea 5%

Availability of certificate of Origin reduces the tariff to 3.75% of the product cost as per invoice on CIF value.

Additional Duties & Taxes

VAT	18%
Budgetary Fees as per invoice on CIF	0.15% of the product cost
Special Tax & Sales Tax	Nil

Mozambique :

(1) Export Duty	Nil
(2) Import Duty	Esc. 36 per kg net

Mauritius :

(1) Export Duty	Nil
(2) Import Duty	

(a) Preferential	20% Ad Valorem Value
(b) Fiscal Duty	20 Mauritian Cts./kg of Tea imported
(c) Import Permit:-	
Black Tea	Mauritian Rs. 5,000
Green Tea	Mauritian Rs. 1,000

Taiwan :

(1) Export Duty	Nil
(2) Import Duty	
Green & Black Leaf	20%
Oolong Leaf	25%
Tea Dust	20%
(3) Import Licenses	Not required

Japan :

(1) Export Duty Nil

(2) Import Duty	Developing Countries	Less Developing Countries	Others Countries
Black Tea in Bulk	2.5%	Nil	3.0%
Black Tea in Packets	12.0%	NIl	12.0%
Instant Tea	8.0%	Nil	10.0%
Green Tea	17.0%	17.0%	17.0%

Argentina :

(1) Export Duty 1.5% with effect from 07.04.2003

(2) Import Duty

0902.10 & 30	28%
0902.20 & 40	11.5%
21.01	28%
Additional Duties & Taxes	
Statistical Fee	0.5% (Only for Imports)
VAT	21% (All imported & locally consumed goods)
Tax Reimbursements	Nil (with effect from 01.02.2003); 5.0% on FOB Value of Exports prior to that

Annexure 8

List of Discussions in the Annual General Meeting (AGM) of Bharatiya Cha Parishad

Attempt has been made to highlight the various opinions / views and made by the representatives of the different associations and chief guests invited for attending its annual general meetings held from time to time. The proceedings have been compiled. Gists which are of prime importance have been dealt with. Some of the burning issues relating to the industry have been out lined below.

(i) Shri K.S. Rao, the then Additional Chief Secretary of the Assam Government, in the annual general meeting of Bharatiya Cha Parishad held in 22 May, 1992 said that there were suitable areas available in Mizoram, Nagaland, Arunachal Pradesh and Sikkim for plantation. He also mentioned that "temi" variety of tea grown in Sikkim was very popular in Germany. It was good as any of the Darjeeling varieties. He further, added that industry must strive hard to prove that Indian varieties of tea were the "champagne of teas".

(ii) Sri A.K. Goswami, the then Deputy Director, Tea Board, North Eastern zonal office, Guwahati Assam, asserted that during the last 20 years Assam, on an average, exhibited a growth rate of production at the rate of 2.7 per annum. The North-East zonal Office of the Tea Board had introduced various financial schemes like (i) Replantation and consolidation subsidy scheme for Barak valley and Tripura; (ii) Loan for extension planting under plantation finance scheme; (iii) Supply of machinery and irrigation equipment under the Board's high purchase scheme (iv) Special input interest subsidy scheme for small tea growers in certain districts of Assam. Shri Goswami said that the overall strategy to expand tea cultivation in this region included (a) bringing new areas in non-traditional area and (b) uprooting and replanting the old and uneconomic areas with improved planting materials to boost up the productivity level as well as extension planting in the grant areas of the existing tea estates wherever possible. To encourage tea cultivation by small growers, Tea Board set up a tea advisory committee in Assam Agricultural University, Jorhart to render all financial assistance including training facilities for the small tea growers in this region. Necessary funds have been provided by the Tea Board to Assam Agricultural University.

(iii) Shri Vijay Mehera, the then Chairman, Assam branch of Indian Tea Association, signaled the positive growth of tea production. But the law and order situation, specially in the north bank of the river Brahmaputra, caused anxiety. Security and safety of the worker in the plantations and personnel working in the industry assumed paramount importance. The exorbitant and arbitrary levies have created burden on the industry.

(iv) Shri D.M. Dadich, the then Chairman, Assam branch of Tea Association of India stressed the issues relating to high rate of agricultural income tax and failure to provide power by Assam State Electricity Board.

(v) Shri V.K. Goenka, the then Chairman, Tea Research Association (TRA) mentioned that tea research was initiated in the city of Calcutta (Kolkata) first time in the world and the laboratory was established at the Indian museum. The headquarters of the Indian Tea Association, which also established its scientific department to carry out its R & D is also at Kolkata. From the beginning made in 1891 here, through the establishment of the historical Tocklai Experimental Station at Jorhat in 1911 and other outstations, the TRA has grown as the largest organisation for tea research in the world. The association had organised an international conference on tea science in January 1990 and 1993 at Kolkata. Four more international scientific symposia were organised at the USA, Japan, China and Srilanka. Out of these ones at USA, Japan and Sri lanka were on health aspect. The themes of the symposies in 1991 and 1993 were the cultural practices and agro-techniques together with bio-chemistry of tea and their relation to pharmacology of the human system.

(vi) The Food and Agricultural Organisation (FAO) of the United Nations has already laid emphasis on the health aspect of drinking black tea and association undertook R & D work with some of the prestigious hi-reach areas. Efforts were made to develop more and more planting materials giving higher yield and better quality through conventional breeding. Endeavours were also intensified in the area of biotechnology to develop plants which drew nutrients more efficiently.

Annexure 9

Proceedings of the 112th of Annual General Meeting of Indian Tea Association

In the 112th Annual General Meeting of India Tea Association (ITA) held on 19 March 1994 in Kolkata, Shri H.P. Barooah, the out-going Chairman of ITA expressed great concern over the following issues :-

(i) Although tea production has been increasing over the last few years, exports could not reach 200 million kgs, (ii) Despite the fact that tea convention (1994) offered keen insight into the consumption pattern and preferences in the markets, focus on the quality and price factors is required for competitiveness in different markets. Some tea companies have adopted fresh approaches by way of joint ventures and strategic alliances to take advantage of the opportunities that lie in the international trading arena; (iii) The growing concern of some of the importing countries regarding Minimum Residual Levels (MRL) of pesticides made the industry to take up a campaign at grassroot level to teach and train the workers and the management regarding use of certain pesticides. (iv) The benefit of 33 AB (lock-in period of deposit has been done away with) has not been extended to tea estates manufacturing their leaf in other factories, but selling on their own account. Nothing has been done about 80 HHC, as a result of which the tea industry, which grows, manufactures and exports tea, gets benefits only to the extent of 40 percent of its profits, whereas a merchant-exporter who just buys and exports the teas gets 100 percent benefit of 80 HHC; (v) With the policy of free market economy, GATT has come with the spectre of import of tea in to the country. A small section has supported the idea, a much bigger section has opposed it (vi) Today cost of production is high (Rs. 50 per kg), productivity per worker is about the lowest (730 kg per man year), land productivity is low (1200 kg/ha) etc. If one has to give a level field to our global competition stay in business, one has to be an efficient producer. The productivity of worker and land must improve substantially. (vii) For ecological reasons a certain universally accepted ratio of forest land to other lands must be maintained as such association demands that degraded forest can be given to the industry for growing tea not only in the national interest but also in the ecological interest. And it is in this matter that association wants our newly farmed partnership with the bond to extend its wings and give effective support to the industry by allotting India-a big portion of land which can be degraded. (viii) Taxation must be further rationalised in the true sprit. The West Bengal Government may emulate Assam in taxation and incentives to industrialisation and Assam emulate West Bengal in allotment of further land.

Addressing the 112th A.G.M. of Indian Tea Association held on 14 March, 1994 at Kolkata, Shri Pranab Mukherjee, the then Commerce Minister said "India has to build up an image of sustainable exporter. Domestic consumption should not put pressure on exports from the country. If this necessitates imports will be made. But for tea the country will not allow import. Government's policy for the moment permits imports only for blending purposes for export oriented units on conditions of value additions of a minimum of 40 per cent. Such units are not allowed to sell in domestic market." He pointed out that the industry should take advantage of various research projects undertaken by Tea Board to increase yield per hectare. Dispelling fears of adverse impact of the GATT on agriculture he said, there is no question of diluting incentives for tea industry because threshold limit under GATT is very large. Under GATT, developing countries would gain access to the markets in the developed world where agro-product market was skewed. We have been able to ilinch this because of serious disputes between the developed countries.

Annexure 10

The 104th Annual General Meeting of Indian Tea Association

Shri S.K. Bhasin, the then Chairman of Indian Tea Association (ITA) in its 104th Annual General Meeting held on 15 March, 1993 pointed out a very disturbing fact revolving around absenteeism among workers, rising wage bills and increase in cost of inputs causing increased production costs. But this has to be controlled, otherwise it would be difficult to stand in the market in the face of keen competition. He drew attention of the members to the steady decline in tea exports and deterioration in law and order situation.

Shri Vijay Mehra, the then Chairman of Assam branch of Indian Tea Association (ABITA) in its 104th AGM indicated that the biggest bane of the industry is non-availability of adequate land for extension planting, absence of uprooting / replanting incentives, poor infra-structural facilities in the periphery of the tea estate, maintenance of quality in international standard ISO-9000, residual toxicity of chemicals, abolition of child labour, dismal performance of Assam State Electricity Board (ASEB), consciousness of the importance of human resources, escalating price trend of important inputs and suffocating tax structure.

Annexure 11

107th Annual General Meeting of Kolkata Tea Trade Association

While inaugurating the 107th AGM of (Calcutta) Kolkata Tea Traders Association held on 1 January, 1995, Shri Pranab Mukherjee, the then Commerce Minister said, of late, people worldwide have not only become health conscious but also protesting against use of pesticides residue in tea. As a result they have imposed stricter measures for import of tea in their respective countries. Those who have been able to meet their high quality standard are enjoying booming exports but those who could not, have unfortunately lagged behind. He cautioned unless the exporters ensure steady supply of quality product at competitive price, it would be difficult in catch up with the present world trend. In his opinion, one of the major hurdles in tea export in recent times has been ecological and environmental nature as certain advanced countries like Germany were taking serious exception to the use of chemical fertilisers and pesticides on tea plants. The industry should take note of these developments and make appropriate arrangements. The Union Commerce Minister said that ministry provided all necessary assistance to the Tea Board to set up two testing laboratories at Kalkota and Cochin to conduct proper check on tea consignment before tea exports. On the promotional front, the industry has to emphasise on both domestic and international markets as in the changed world scenario. The laboratories have been established recently and the Board has been conducting the proper check on tea consignment before tea export.

Annexure 12

34th Annual General Meeting of Tea Association of India

34th AGM of Tea Association of India held at Kalkota on 6 February, 1995 stressed that TAI in Assam has been implementing welfare measures for local population like (i) construction of additional school buildings and hospitals; (ii) providing donations to cultural and social organisations; educational institutions, bus stands and (iii) adoption of villages for improved water supply and better agricultural practices, (iv) Arising from the growing global conscious on health vis-a-vis food products, unique opportunities exist to estimate tea consumption on the basis of (iv) health benefits like fluid balance in body, zero caloric content, (v) protective effects on heart diseases and stroke, combacting cancer, and (vi) possessing some anti-viral and anti-bacterial effect, (vii) developing domestic market by making better quality teas, better distribution in the rural areas and more affordable packets. There should not be any compulsion for putting 75 per cent bulk teas in auction and it should be left to the choice of producer how to sell his tea in the context of liberalised economy. (viii) There is need for large area of additional land for extension of tea. Bringing the agricultural income tax rate at per with the corporate tax rate to make tea competitive in the international market. Paying attention to develop and strengthen the infrastructure like roods, bridges, telecommunication etc. and improve the productivity of land and labour.

References

Books (Nine Books and One Phd Thesis)

1. *Banerjee G D , Structural Changes in Tea Industry since 1956 unpublished thesis submitted to Jadhavpur University,Kolkata.,* **1982**
2. *Banerjee G D* **(1996)**, *Tea Plantation Industry in India between 1815 and 1992—Structural Changes, Lawyers BookStall, Guwahati, Assam.* Foreword given by **Chief Regional Executive, IAS, Tea Board, Assam, Guwahati**.
3. *Banerjee G.D. Prof S.G . Hundekar of Dharwad Agriculture University, and Prof. P. Das, Andhra University Edited,* **(1997),** *Challenges before Small Scale Industries, Horizontal Publishers, Darbhanga Castle, Allahbad, UttarPradesh, India..* **Foreword given by Sri P. Kotaih, Ex Chairman, NABARD, Mumbai**
4. *Banerjee G. D. and Karmakar K. G, The Tea Industry in India – A Survey,* **September 2005,** *Department of Economic Analysis and Research, NABARD, Mumbai.* **Foreword given by Mrs Ranjana Kumar Ex Chairperson , NABARD, Mumbai**
5. *Banerjee G.D.and Banerjee and Banerji Srijeet, Darjeeling Tea—The Golden Brew,* **2007,** *,International Book Distributing Company, , Lucknow, Uttar Pradesh, India. ..* Foreword given **by Prof. Emeritus, Sri A. K. Gupta Visva Bharati Central University, santiniketan**
6. *Banerjee G.D.and Banerjee Sarda, Sustainable Tea Plantation Management,* **2008,** *International Book Distributing Company, 2008, Lucknow,Uttar Pradesh,* **Foreword given by Basudeb Banerjee, IAS, Chairman, Tea Board, India. (Under printing)**
7. *Banerjee G.D.and Banerjee Sarda, Agriculture and Rural Development Policy Agendas in the New Millennium,* **2008,,** *International Book Distributing Company, , Lucknow,Uttar Pradesh, India.* **Foreword given by Dr. K.G.karmakar, Managing Director, NABARD, Mumbai., (Under printing)**
8. *Banerjee G.D.and Baneri Srijeet , Tea Plantation Industry A Road Map Ahead,* **2008,,** *M/S Abhijeet Publication , New Delhi, India.* **Foreword given by Sri Kisanjeet Basu, Former Executive Director, NABARD; Former Director, Bankers Institute of Rural development (BIRD), and Former Member, Reserve Bank of India Service Board, Mumbai**

9. *Banerjee G.D.and Baneri Srijeet, World Tea Trade—Dimensions and Dynamics,* **2008,,** *M/S Abhijeet Publication , New Delhi, India.* **Foreword given by Sri Dr Shurhozelie, Minister, Planning & Cordination and Urban Development, Government of Nagaland, New Secretariat Complex, Kohima ,**
10. *Banerjee G.D.and Baneri Srijeet , Export Potential of Indian Tea,* **2008,,** *M/S Abhijeet Publication , New Delhi, India.* **Foreword given by Sri H.K Kukuh, IAS, Principal Secretary and Finance Commissioner, Finance Department Government of Nagaland, New Secretariat Complex, Kohima,**

Reports Published

1. Socio-Economic implications of high yielding varieties of food grains in the eastern region of India, UNDP Global Project, Agro economic research Center. Santiniketan, Visva Bharati
2. Efficiency of small farms under different tenurial conditions with special reference to North Bengal, ICAR, New Delhi – 1, Dept of Economics and Politics, Visva Bharati, santiniketan.
3. Techno-Economic Survey of Darjeeling Tea Industry, Tea Board, India, Kolkata, West Bengal.
4. Techno-Economic Survey of Tripura Tea Industry, Tea Board, India, Kolkata, West Bengal.
5. Techno-Economic Survey of Small tea gardens in Kottayam and Idukki (Kerala), Tea Board,
6. Techno-Economic Survey of Small tea gardens in Kangra (H.P.), Tea Board, India, Kolkata, l.
7. Techno-Economic Survey of Nilgiri Tea Industry, Tea Board, India, Kolkata, West Bengal.
8. Techno-Economic Survey of Cachar Tea Industry, Tea Board, India, Kolkata, West Bengal.
9. Evaluation Study Report on Inland Fisheries in Nadia district, West Bengal., NABARD, West Bengal Regional Office, Kolkata, West Bengal
10. Evaluation Study Report on Inland Fisheries in West Tripura, Tripura, Assam Regional Ofice , Guwahati, Assam
11. Evaluation Study Report on Poultry Farming (Broiler) in Medinipur district, West Bengal, NABARD, West Bengal Regional Office, Kolkata, WestBengal

Papers

A. Indian Journal of Agricultural Economics, Indian Society of Agricultural Economics, Krishi Vikas Sadan, First Floor, (Near Dr Antoni Da Silva, , Technical, High School, Veer Savarkar Marg, dadar (West), Mumbai-400028 E. mail-isae@bom7. vsnl.net.in, Webside—www.isacindia.org

1. Changes overtimes in the levels of income of the weaker section of Rural Community (WB), Annual conference Issue June-July 1972.
2. Impact of agro-processing on incomes of primary producers, Annual Conferences, Dec.2003

B. TAI News Letter - Published by Tea Association of India, Indian Exchange Palace, Kolkata -1, (West Bengal)

3. Problems and Prospects of Tarai Tea Industry, Feb. 1983, Vol.16, No.2.
4. Problems and Prospects of Indian Tea Exports, March 1983, Vol.16, No.3.
5. The role of FAO/UNCTAD and ITPA for Development of World Tea, May 1983, Vol.16, No.5.
6. Export prospects of Indian Tea in Tunisia, July 1983, Vol.16, No.7.
7. Tea Plantation of India (North), September-October 1983, Vol.16, Nos. 9 and 10.
8. Structural Development in Tea Industry, November 1983, Vol.16, No.11.
9. Evolution of Tea Industry in India (Part I), December 1983, Vol.16, No.12.
10. Evolution of Tea Industry in India (part II), February 1984, Vol.17, No.2.
11. Ownership of Tea Estates, March 1984, Vol.17, No.3.
12. Japan as a base of Indian Tea, August 1984, Vol.17, No.8
13. Changes in pattern of Management, September 1984, Vol.17, No.9.
14. Area, Production and yield of Tea in different excise zones, December 1984, Vol.17, No.12.
15. Changes in the pattern of ownership, February 1985, Vol.18, No.2.
16. Market Research, Vol.18 No.3, March 1985.
17. The role of Tea in Indian Economy, April 1985, Vol.18, No.4.
18. Export prospects of Indian Tea in Nigeria, June 1985, Vol.18, No.6.

19. Export prospects of Indian Tea in Singapore, November 1985, Vol.18, and No.11.
20. Tea Plantation in South India, October 1986, Vol.19. No.10.
21. Impact of area, production of tea in new planting, yield rates, export and domestic consumption, November 1986, Vol.19 No.11.
22. Efficiency of tea estates, January 1987, Vol.20, No.1.
23. Role of tea plantation in North India, May 1987, Vol.20,No. 5
24. Export prospects of Indian tea in Iran, January 1988, Vol.21. No.1.
25. Structural changes in tea exports in India, February 1988, Vol.21, No.1.
26. Export Possibility of Indian Tea in Arab Republic of Egypt, May 1988, Vol.21, No.5.
27. Export prospects of Indian Tea in Canada, July 1988, Vol.21, No.7.
28. Export prospects of Indian Tea in Poland, September 1988, Vol.21., No.9.
29. Export prospects of Indian Tea in Syria, January 1989, Vol.22., No.1.
30. International Tea Promotion, March 1989, Vol.22, No 3.
31. Export prospects of Indian Tea in Libya and Jordan, May 1989, Vol.22.
32. Tea in South India, July 1989, Vol.22, No.7.
33. Production and Exports of Value added teas in India, October 1989, Vol.22, No.10.
34. Problems and Prospects of Coimbatore Tea Industry, July 1990, Vol.23, No.7.
35. Problems and Prospects of Wynaad Tea Industry, October 1990, Vol.23, No.10.
36. Tea Statistics, Tea Boards of India, various issues
37. Tea Directory, Tea Boards of India, various issues
38. FAO 1995, 1999: Impact of Uruguay round agreement on the world economists position and current situation and short term outlook, paper presented to Inter Government Group on Tea Ottawa September.

C. The Assam Review and Tea News - Published by Assam Review Publishing Company, 27A, Waterloo Street, Kolkata –69,Phone - 033-22482251

39. World markets of tea and its international arrangements, January 1985, Vol.73, No.1.

40. Tea Economy in South India, February 1985, Vol.73, No.2.
41. Export prospects of Tea in Singapore, July 1985, Vol.74, No.7.
42. Structure of Tea Industry, August 1985, Vol.74, No.8
43. The entire thesis, namely, "Structural Changes in Tea Plantation Industry since 1958' was published by the above publisher in 17 instalments, like,
44. October 1985, Vol.73, No.10,
45. November 1985, Vol.73, No.11,
46. December 1985, Vol.73, No.12,
47. January 1986, Vol.74, No.1,
48. February 1986, Vol.74, No.2,
49. March 1986, Vol.74, No.3,
50. April 1986, Vol.74, No 4,
51. May 1986, Vol.74, No.5,
52. June 1986, Vol.74, No.6,
53. July 1986, Vol.74, No.7,
54. August 1986, Vol.74, No.8,
55. September 1986, Vol.74, No.9,
56. October 1986, Vol.74, No10,
57. November 1986, Vol 74. No 11,
58. December 1986, Vol.74, No.12,
59. January 1987, Vol.76, No.1
60. February 1987, Vol.76, No.2
61. Export possibility of Indian Tea in Iraq-1, January 1989, Vol.77, No.1.
62. Export possibility of Indian Tea in Iraq-II, February 1989, Vol.77, No.2.
63. International Tea Promotion, May 1989, Vol.77, No5.
64. Tea in South American Countries, July 1989, vol.77, No.7.
65. Production and Export of Value added Tea in India, August 1989, Vol.77, No.8.
66. Export prospects of Indian Tea in Jordan, October 1989, Vol.77, No.10.
67. Export prospects of Indian Tea in Iran in February1990, Vol. 78No. 1,
68. Export prospects of Indian Tea Libya in June 1990, Vol. 78,No. 6
69. Export prospects of Indian Tea japan in August 1990, Vol. 78 ,No. 8

70. Eexport prospects of Indian Tea in Argentina, March 1991, Vol.79, No.3
71. Export prospects of Indian Tea in South America, November 1991, Vol. 79, No. 11
72. Export prospects of Indian Tea in Poland, September 1992, Vol. 80, No. 9
73. Export prospects of Indian Tea in Australia, June 1993, , Vol. 81, No. 6
74. Export prospects of Indian Tea in Egypt, October 1993, , Vol. 81, No. 10
75. Export prospects of Indian Tea in Germany, November 1993 Vol. 81, No. 11
76. Export prospects of Indian Tea in Netherland, December 1993, Vol. 813, No.12
77. Export prospects of Indian Tea in Srilanka, January 1994, Vol. 82, No.1
78. Export prospects of Indian Tea in Indonesia, February 1994, Vol. 82, No.2
79. Export prospects of Indian Tea in China, March 1994, Vol. 82, No.3
80 Export prospects of Indian Tea in Peru, April 1994, Vol. 82, No.4
81. Export prospects of Indian Tea in Pakistan, May 1994, Vol. 82, No.5
82. Export prospects of Indian Tea in Canada, June 1994, Vol. 82, No.6
83. Export prospects of Indian Tea in Ethopia, September 1994, Vol. 82, No.9
84. Export prospects of Indian Tea in kenya, October 1994, Vol. 82, No.10
85. Export prospects of Indian Tea in Tanzania, November 1994, Vol. 82, No.10
86. Export prospects of Indian Tea in Uganda, December 1994, Vol. 82, No.12
87. Export prospects of Indian Tea in Vietnam, January 1995, Vol. 83, No.1
88. Export prospects of Indian Tea in South Africa, February 1995, Vol. 83, No.2.
89. Export prospects of Indian Tea in Zimbabwe, March 1995, Vol. 83, No.3
90. Export prospects of Indian Tea in Mozambique, April 1995, Vol. 83, No.4

91. History of Darjeeling Tea, December, 1999,Vol. 87. ,No, 12
92. Development Issues of Tea Industry, February, 2000, Vol 88. No 2
93. Development Issues of Tea Industry, March 2000, Vol 88, No 3.
94. Development Issues of Tea Industry, April 2000, Vol 88, No 4.
95. Structural Issues in Tea industry, May, 2000, *Vol 88.No 5*
96. Tea Trade In Japan, Part-1,April 2008, Vol. 97
97. Tea Trade In Japan, Part2, May 2008, Vol 97

D. Chai ki Bat— published by Bharatiya Chai Parishad, 25 Ballyganj, Circular Road, Kolkata-700 019

98. Export prospects of tea in Canada, January 1988, Vol.33, No.1.
99. Export prospects of tea in Saudi Arabia, February 1988, Vol.33, No.2.
100. Export prospects of Indian Tea in Iran, April 1988, Vol.33, No.4.
101. Export prospects of Indian Tea in Poland, May 1988, Vol.33, No.5.
102. Structural Changes in the Tea Exports of India, August 1988, Vol.33, No.8.
103. Export possibility of Indian Tea in Arab Republic of Egypt, January 1989, Vol.34, No.7.
104. Availability of Tea in Internal Market/ maximisation of export earnings, March 1989,
105. Export prospect of tea in Iraq, May 1989, Vol.34, and No.5.
106. Market Research on Tea Consumption, August 1989, Vol.34, No.9.
107. Market Research on Tea Consumption, October 1989, Vol.34, No.10.
108.Green Tea (Part I), March 1992, Vol.37. No.3.
109. Green Tea (Part II), April 1992, Vol37, No.4.

E. The Northeast Times, G.L.Publications, GS Road, Guwahati.

110. Industrialisation sets back to farm income, 21 January 1992.
111. Economics of Green Tea, 28 May 1992.
112. Indian Tea in Syria, 16 June 1992.
113. Indian Tea in Jordan, June 21, 1992.
114. Indian Tea in Libya, July 07, 1992.
115. National Bank's Role for Tea Development, July 12, 1992.
116. The role of National Bank for development of Tea Industry, July 15, 1992.
117. Dry land and Rain fed Farming, November 18, 1992.
118. Potentials of horticulture crops, November 28, 1992.

119. Market potential of Indian Tea in Syria, December 10, 1992.
120. Cashew nut Plantation, December 19, 1992.

F. Financial Express, Mumbai

121. Green Tea - Peep into the past, 07 November 1992.
122. Rain fed and Dry land Farming - A Balanced Agricultural Strategy Vital, 02 January 1993.

G. Eastern Mirror, Dimapur, Nagaland

Economics of Organic Farming – A case for Banana Plantation (Dec, 27, 2005)

123. Dairy Industry in 21st Century, January 4, 2005
124. Problems of Agricultural Marketing in Nagaland, February 26, 2005
125. The Role of SHGs in Poverty Allivation, October 20, 2005
126. The Development of Handicrafts and Handloom in Nagaland, November 16, 2005
127. Economics of Tea cultivation in Kangra, December,18, 2005
128. Himachal Pradesh Tea Industry –A Revival Package, 15 January, 2006
129. Agricultural Economy of Nagaland— Opportunities and Challenges, 20, February, 2006
130. Village Development Board as Financial Institution—Published in three instalments on15, 16 and17 April,2007

H. National Bank News Review, NABARD, Mumbai

131. A fresh insight into the problems of rural development in the North-East Region, February 1992.
132. Brackish Water Fish Culture - A Cast Study, January-March Issue, 1995.
133. Agro-processing Sector—Some Issues, July- September ,2004

I. Financing Agriculture, Agriculture Finance Corporation, Dhanaraj Mahal, Ist Floor,Chatrapati Shivaji Marg, Mumbai-400001, Tel No 2028924,Fax 022-*2028966,E mail (i) afcl@bom vsnl.net.in, (ii) piplapure@afcmails.com*

134. Horticulture Strives Well in Food and Nutritional Security – April-June 2000, Vol. 32, NO-1
135. Agricultural Extension— Assessment of various Models, October-December 2000, Vo.32. NO-2
136. Bio technology for Indian farmers, July -September 2001,Vol.- 33,

NO- 3

137. Water Resources Management –A long Term Planning and Judicious Use of Water and Food Security, October-December 2001, Vol.- 33, NO-4
138. Evaluation Studies of Self Help Groups, April –June 2002, Vol.- 34, No-2
139. Economics of Medicinal Plants, July –September 2003, Vol.- 34, No-3
140. Boosting of Agricultural Exports—Opportunities and Challenges, Janurary-March,2005
141. Dairy Development in the Context of Globalization, January – March 2006
142. Primary Marketing of Indian Tea, Indian Journal of Agricultural Marketing, Annual Conference Issue, December 2000.

J. Man and Development, Centre for Research in Rural and Industrial Development, Sector19-A.Madhya Marg, Chandigarh-160019, E-mai- crridchd@sancharnet.in

143. Agricultural Extension: A Critical analysis of various models, September 2001, Vol. 33. NO 3

K. Indian Journal of Agricultural Marketing, Indian Society of Agricultural Marketing, Nagpur, 57/IV, Seminary Hills, Nagpur-440006, E-Mail—kumar81@im.eth.net,

144. Marketing of Indian Tea —A Review, Sept 2001, Vol- 33, No- 3

***L.* Afro-Asian Journal Of Rural Development, NO-2, State Guest houses Complex, Chanakyapuri,, New Delhi-110021, Phone-(91-11) 4100475, 6877783,61115936, Fax No-(9-11) 4672045,6115937 ,E mail-aardohq@nde.vsnl.net.in**

145 Marketing of Mango Processing under Institutional Finance—A Case Study in Andhra Pradesh, July-December 2001,Vol.-XXXIV, No-2

M. Indian Association of Social Science Institutions (IASSI) Quarterly Journal, Care of Institute of Applied Man Power Research, Indra Prastha Estate, New Delhi, Gram-Samaj Vidya, New Delhi, Tel- 331-5284, 335-6834, E mail-stiassi@ bol. net. in

146. Indian Tea A No Longer A Fashionable S slogan, April- June 2002,Vol.19, No –4
147. Agro-processing – A Link between Agriculture and Industry.Jan-March,2004 (jointly with (K.G.K)

148. Sustainable Tea Plantation Management, Jan-March, 2004 (jointly with S.B)
149. China's Pure Tea – Tea with Miraculous Function, Oct – Dec 2005.
150. Diversification of India Tea - Value Addition. Oct - Dec 2006.

N. Times Agriculture Journal, The Economic Times and NABARD, The Times of India Building, Dr.D. N.Road,Mumbai-400001,E-mailprittik@marwar.com (ii) b2bedit @ timegroup.com

151. All Hands on Deck, September- October Issue, 2002
152. Horticulture Over View - Poised for Golden Revolution – November - December Issue, 2002
153. Financing Horticulture - January-February Issue, 2003
154. A difficult Terrain - July-August Issue, 2003

O. Waste Lands News —Society for Promotion of Waste Lands Development, 14 – A, Vishnu Digamber Marg , New Delhi-110002, e mail- spwd@vsnl.com, Editor Sujata Kausik

155. Water Vision, Jointly with DR K. G. Karmakar and Sarda Banerjee, November, 2004.,

P. Kurukshetra, A journal of Rural Development, Room No-655/661,Nirman Bhavan, A wing, (GateNo.5) Ministry of Rural Development, New Delhi -110011, E mail-kurupage@ yahoo.Co. in. Editor- Anjani Bhushan, Assistant Editor-Kalama

156. Corporate Partnership for Agricultural Development Vol –53, No. 6, April 2005,
157. Eco labelling in Agriculture, January 2006,

Q. Yojana journal of Rural Development, Yojana Bhavan,, Sansad Marg, New Delhi-110001,

158. Tea Industry at the Cross Roads, Independence Special Issue, 15 August, 2005S

R. Agriculture Today – The National Agriculture Magazine, Editor – M J Khan, C-17, III Floor, Lajpat Nagar-I, New Delhi – 110024, E-amil : agricult@del3.vsnl.net.in and editor@agriculturetoday.org

159. Economics of Organic Farming, October 2005 issue, Volume–VIII, No.10

160. Ecolab ling in Agricultural Products December issue, 2005,

S. NAB LAW, Law Department, NABARD, Plot No. 24, Block-G, Bandra Kurla Complex, Bandra East, Mumbai-400051, Chief Editor—U.N.Srivastava, Chief General Manager E Mail-nablaw@vsnl.com, nablaw@gmail.com

161. Agricultural Marketing Infrastructure in NAGALAND—Challenges and Opportunities Vol.23, No.1 April-June, 2007,

T. Technical Digest, Technical Service Department, NABARD, Plot No. 24, Block-G, Bandra Kurla Complex, Bandra East, Mumbai-400051, Ph-022-26530038, E.Mail-nabtsd@bom5vsnl.net, in,

162. Opportunities and Challenges of Indian Dairy, Issue. 9, 2006, tsd @nabard.org

[illegible]

160. Establishing an Agricultural Products [illegible]

6. NABARD Law Department, [illegible] Plot No. [illegible] Block G, Bandra Kurla Complex, Bandra [illegible] Mumbai [illegible]

[illegible]

[illegible]

161. [illegible]

[illegible] Vol.23, No.1 [illegible] 20[illegible]

T [illegible] [illegible]

[illegible] 24 [illegible]

[illegible]

[illegible]

[illegible]

[illegible]

Index

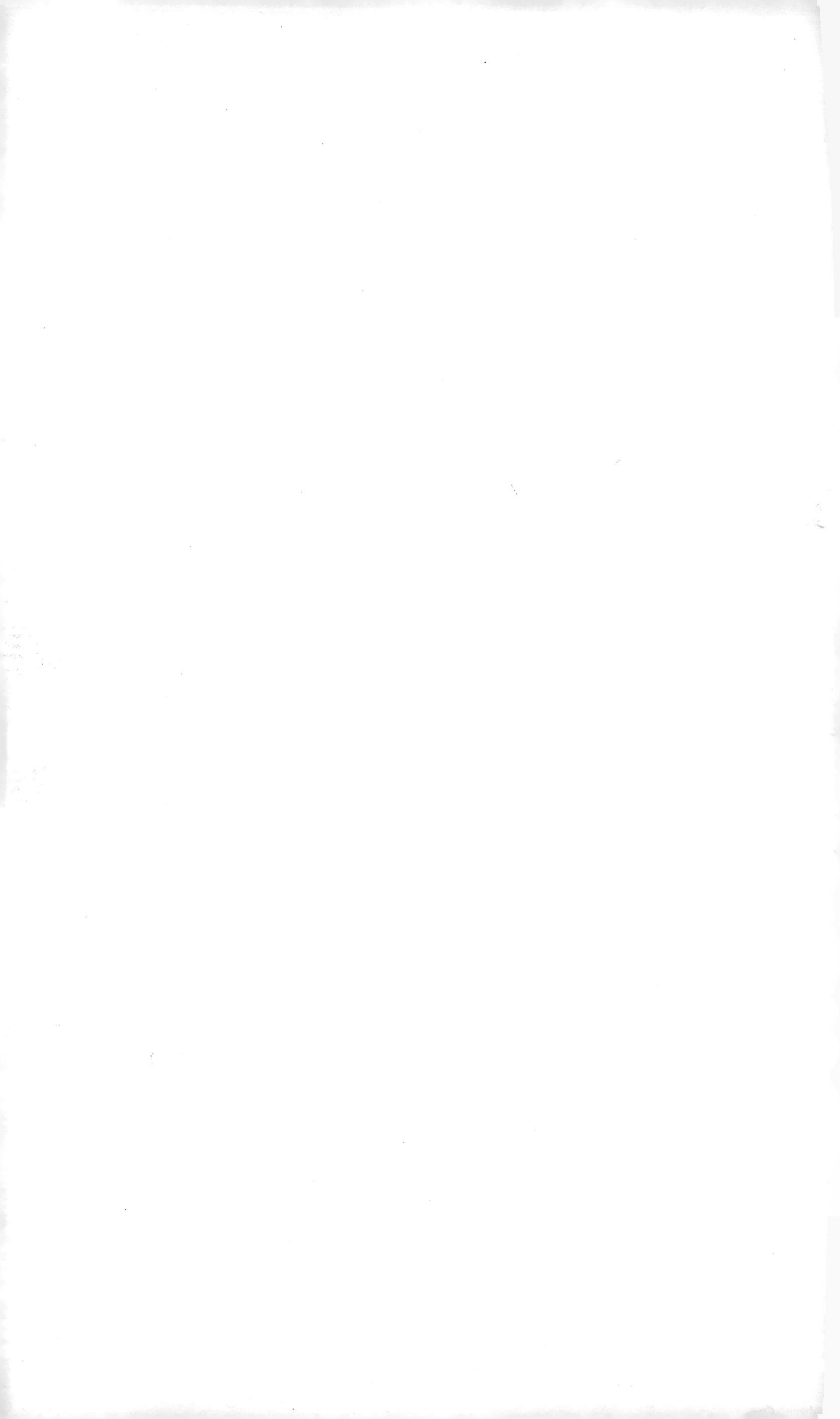